Textbook of Head and Neck Pathology

Margaret S. Brandwein-Weber

Textbook of Head and Neck Pathology

Volume 2: Mouth, Oropharynx, and Larynx

Springer

Margaret S. Brandwein-Weber
Mount Sinai Hospital
New York, NY, USA

ISBN 978-3-030-09403-4 ISBN 978-3-319-76106-0 (eBook)
https://doi.org/10.1007/978-3-319-76106-0

Softcover re-print of the Hardcover 1st edition 2018

Printed on acid-free paper

This Springer imprint is published by the registered company Springer International Publishing AG part of Springer Nature
The registered company address is: Gewerbestrasse 11, 6330 Cham, Switzerland

Dear Shaya, my best life!

Preface

We are the pathologists

Modern-day seers

Our currency consists of precise microscopic measurements and grand intuitive leaps

Lumping and splitting and divining the unseen

Most importantly, we are the anonymous hands, hearts, and minds behind the scenes who give to unknown souls with the greatest of intention, clarity, and impeccability

The universal challenge of writing about diagnostic surgical pathology is the flawed process of distilling experiential learning at the microscopic into words and pictures on a page. Experiencing pathology and reading about pathology are two very different processes that will be forever entwined. One cannot become a pathologist and maintain competency without being grounded in both. Either process alone is incomplete. My goal throughout all these volumes is to strike the right balance of tersely presented information, diagnostic descriptors, pitfalls, histological examples, to companion you as you experience pathology.

Margaret S. Brandwein-Weber
New York, NY, USA

Acknowledgment

Special thanks to Dr. Muhammad S Qazi, MD, for writing the section on gross examination in ► Chap. 3.

Contents

Supplementary Information

Oral Cavity: Anatomy and Histology

M. S. Brandwein-Weber, *Textbook of Head and Neck Pathology*,
https://doi.org/10.1007/978-3-319-76106-0_1

Mucosal lip	Commences at upper and lower vermillion labial borders
	Composed of stratified keratinizing squamous mucosa
Buccal Mucosa	Commences at the angle of mouth. Superior and inferior boundaries are the gingival sulci. Posterior boundary is the pterygomandibular raphe, a fibrous boundary between oral cavity and oropharynx. The buccal space contains adipose tissue, the parotid duct, accessory parotid, when present, and cranial nerves V and VII. The buccal cavity is lined by stratified keratinizing squamous mucosa; submucosal adipose tissue is abundant. The presence of submucosal sebaceous metaplasia (Fordyce spot) can be a useful hint in confirming buccal location
	The Organ of Chievitz (juxtaoral organ) is located in the soft tissue medial to the mandible in the buccotemporal space. It is thought to act as a mechanosensor during swallowing, sucking, chewing and speaking. In adults, the organ of Chievitz is an incidental finding in cancer resections, often adjacent to nerves. In children, it may be discovered as a small cheek mass. It is composed of multilobulated, circumscribed nests of epithelial cells which can appear as either nonkeratinizing squamous epithelium, or columnar glandular cells with clear cytoplasm, or duct-like structures
Alveolar ridge	Stratified keratinizing squamous mucosa, extending from superior and inferior gingival sulci to the maxillary and mandibular alveolar processes. The superior alveolar mucosa ends at the junction of the hard palate. The inferior alveolar mucosa ends at the floor of mouth. The gingival submucosa is comprised of dense fibroconnective tissue, devoid of minor salivary glands
Retromolar trigone	Triangular region posterior to the last mandibular molar is comprised of stratified keratinizing squamous mucosa, and underlying fibroadipose tissue
Floor of mouth	This mucosal crescent extends from lower alveolar ridge to ventral tongue. The posterior boundary is the anterior tonsillar pillars. It is characterized by *nonkeratinizing* stratified squamous mucosa overlying loose submucosa with large ducts leading to minor salivary glands and the sublingual glands. Of note, this region is affected by dysplasia and cancer disproportionately to surface area. This is due to its dependent nature which allows for prolonged exposure to carcinogens dissolved in pooled saliva. As floor of mouth mucosa is normally nonkeratinized, leukoplakia here is especially worrisome
Anterior mobile tongue	This is comprised of the tongue tip, lateral borders, dorsum, and ventral tongue. The line of the circumvallate papillae separates the oral tongue from the pharyngeal tongue base. The lateral and dorsal tongue are lined by stratified keratinizing squamous mucosa; the ventral tongue mucosa is normally nonkeratinizing. The tongue skeletal muscles form densely interlacing horizontal and longitudinal fascicles [1] with interspersed minor salivary glands. The amount of adipose tissue between muscle fascicles increases posteriorly
Extrinsic tongue muscles	The extrinsic muscles have a bony attachment and a tongue insertion. The extrinsic muscles tend to move the position of the whole tongue. The genioglossus arises from the mandible and protrudes the tongue forward. The hyoglossus (also known as tongue root) arises from the hyoid bone and retracts and depresses the tongue. The styloglossus arises from the styloid process of the temporal bone and raises up the lateral tongue during swallowing. The palatoglossus arises from the palatine aponeurosis at the posterior hard palate, and depresses the soft palate, moves the palatoglossal fold to the midline, and raises the back of the tongue during swallowing
Intrinsic tongue muscles	The intrinsic tongue muscles have no bony attachments; they change the shape of the tongue
Hard palate	Semilunar region between the maxillary alveolar ridge to the posterior border of the palatine bone. The lateral hard palate is composed of keratinizing stratified squamous epithelium overlying dense fibroconnective tissue and is devoid of minor salivary glands. Centrally, the hard palate contains mucinous minor salivary glands

1.1

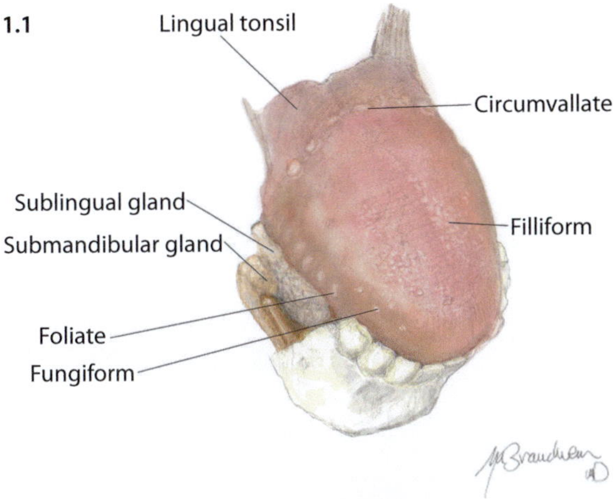

1.2a

1.2b

1.2c

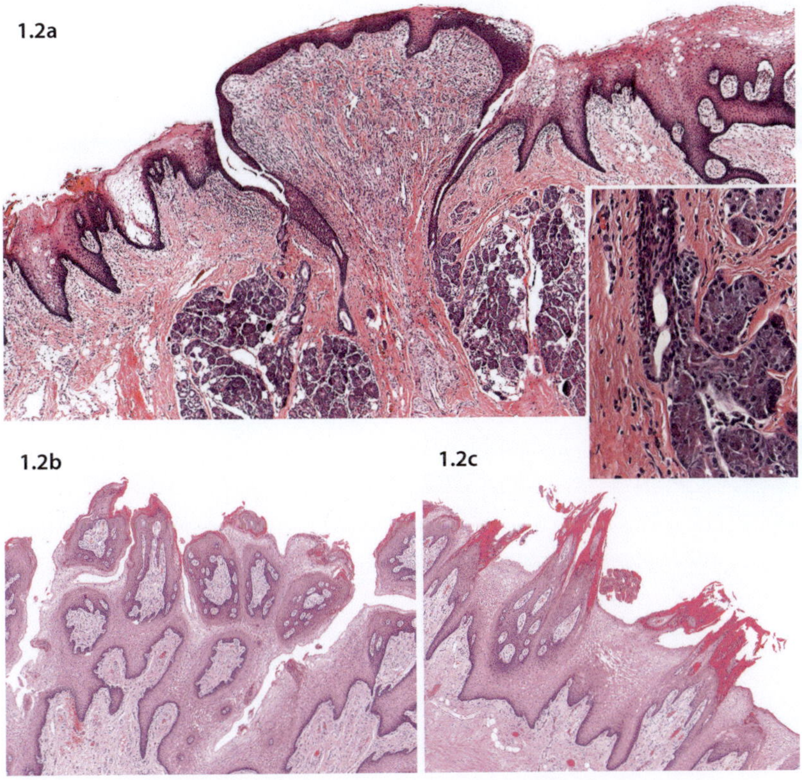

Figs. 1.1 and 1.2 The **circumvallate papillae** form a single V-shaped row which borders between the anterior 2/3 (mobile) tongue and the oropharyngeal tongue base. They represent the largest papillae and are shaped like an inverted triangle surrounded by a depression or "moat" (**1.2a**). Ducts from Von **Ebner's glands** (serous minor salivary glands or gustatory glands) pool secretions into these moats, clearing out food and allowing for new taste stimuli (**1.2 inset**). The **fungiform papillae** are concentrated at the lateral tongue and tip. They are papillary-like (**1.2b**) with a prominent connective tissue core. The **filiform papillae** represent the most common lingual projection. Histologically, they appear as fine, heavily keratinized projections (**1.2c**). The **foliate papillae** represent vertical, nonkeratinized ridges along the posterior lateral tongue, anterior to the circumvallate papillae. The circumvallate, fungiform, and foliate papillae contain **taste buds**, [2] the filiform papillae lack taste buds

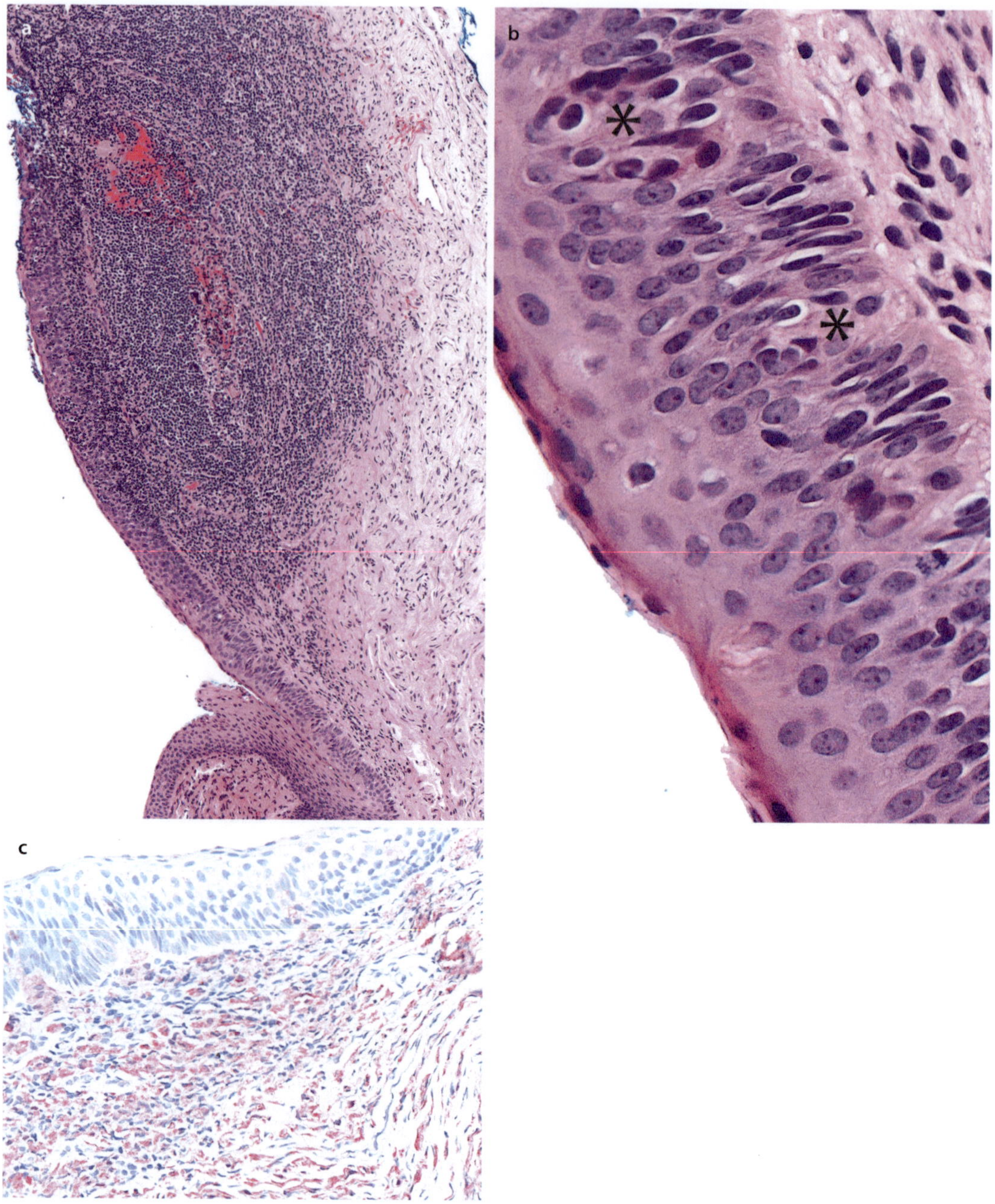

Fig. 1.3 **a** The foliate papillae represent vertical, nonkeratinized ridges along the posterior lateral tongue. Here we also see lingual tonsillar tissue. **b** The actual neuronal "taste buds" appear as flask-shaped collections of innervated specialized epithelial cells (*). **c** S100 stain: Hyperplastic nerves, and collections of ganglion cells may be seen in the region of the foliate papillae, and should not be mistaken for a proliferative neoplasm

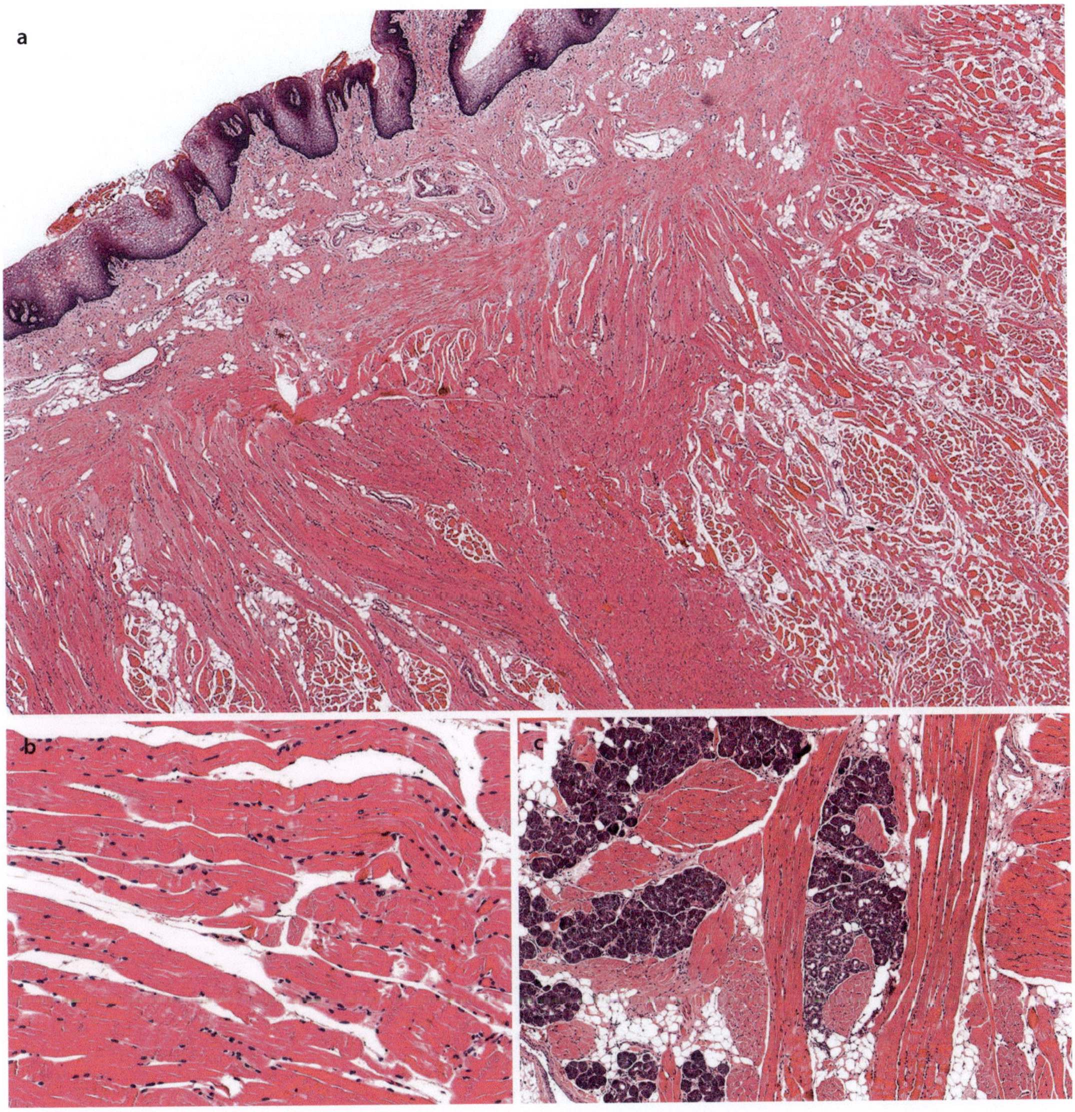

Fig. 1.4 **a**, **b** The tongue muscles form densely interlacing horizontal and longitudinal fascicles. **c** Minor salivary glands are interspersed in the tongue with no apparent subsite predilection

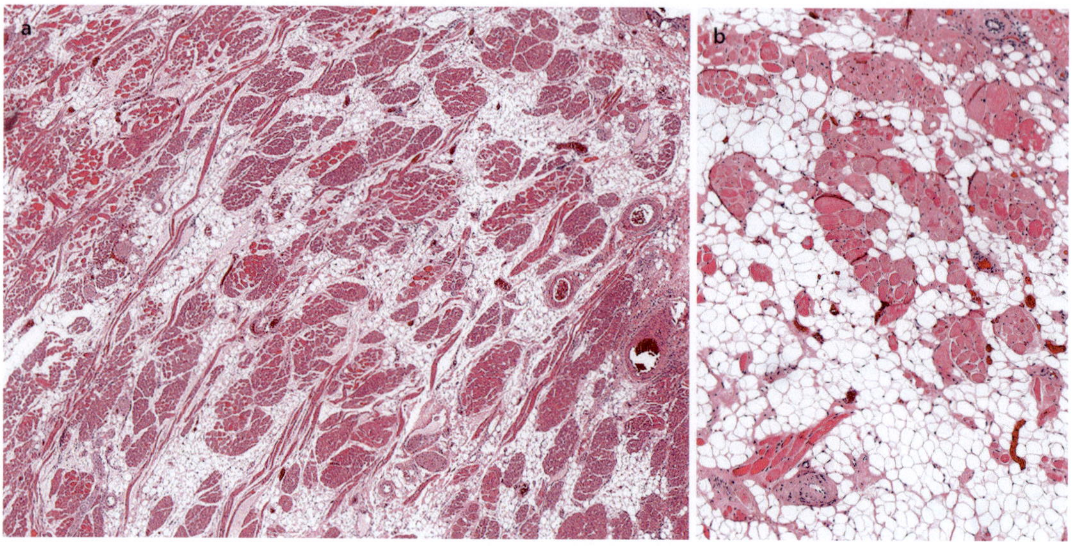

Fig. 1.5 **a, b** Increased adipose tissue is present between muscle fascicles tissue at the posterior tongue

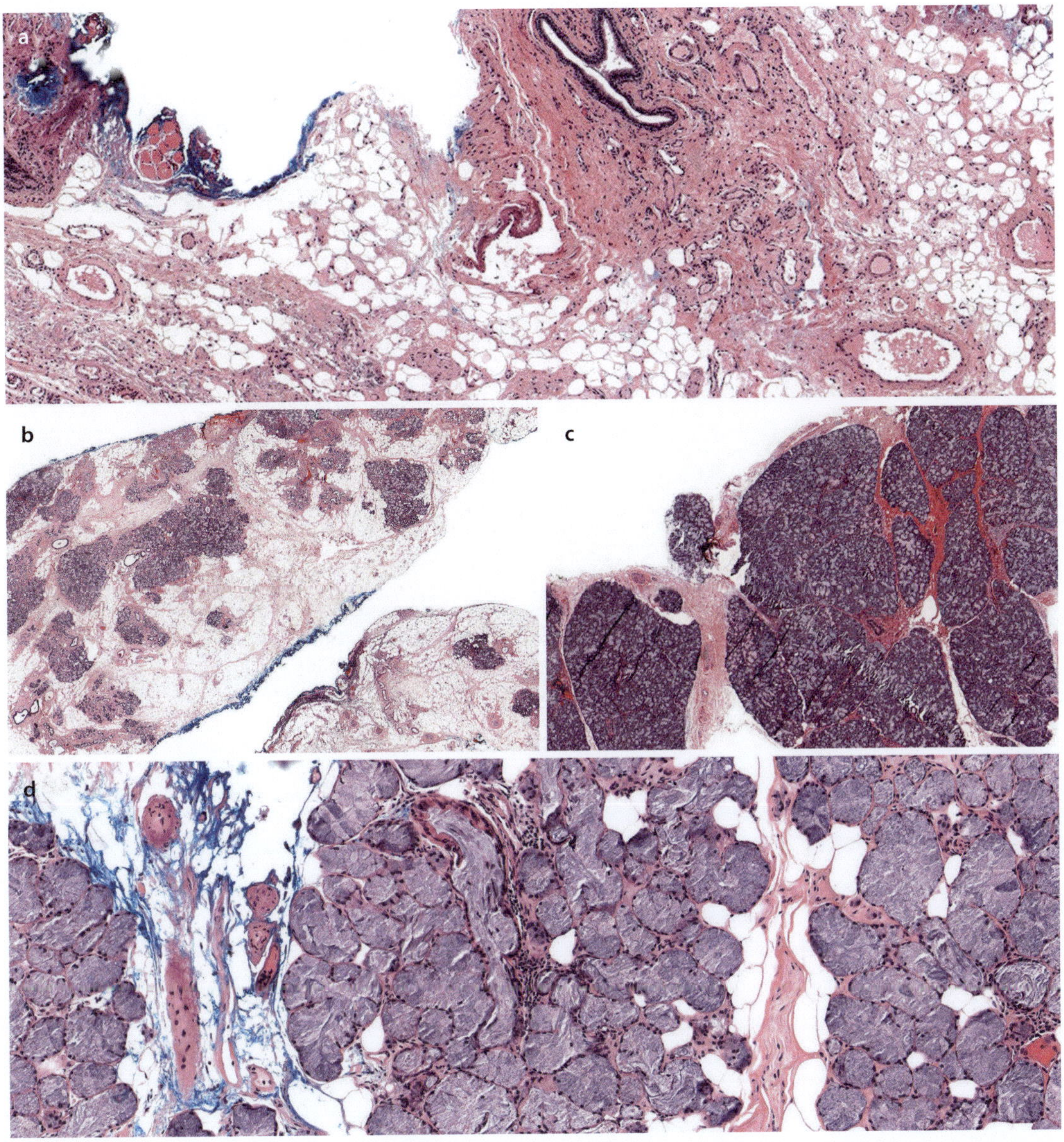

Fig. 1.6 **a** The floor of mouth is characterized by stratified nonkeratinizing squamous mucosa. The submucosal connective tissue contains adipose tissue, some striated muscle bundles, and large salivary ducts **a**. The sublingual glands may be distributed as scattered lobules **b** or as an organized segmented gland **c**. **d** The sublingual gland is usually entirely mucinous

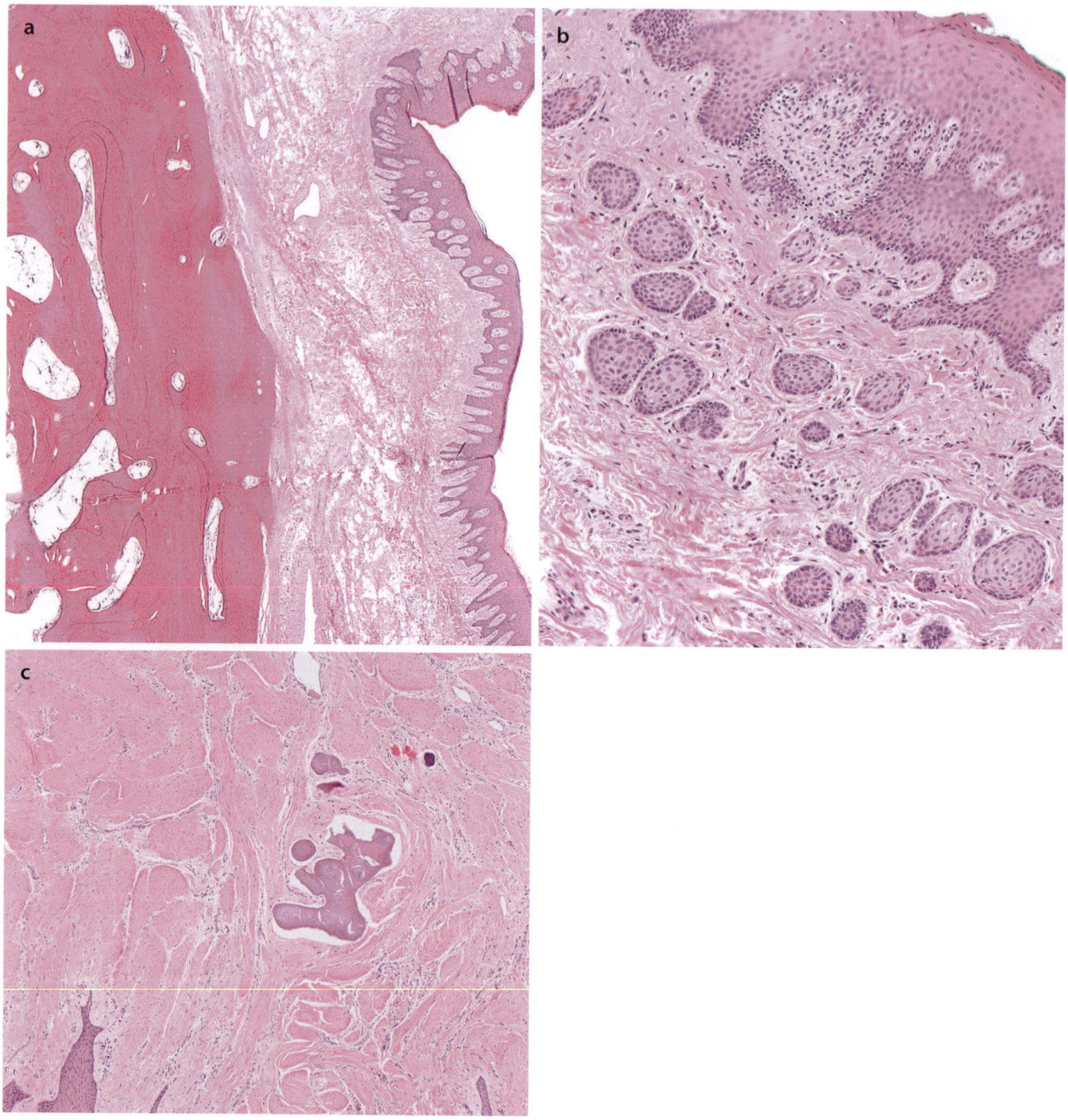

Fig. 1.7 **a** Gingival tissue is characterized by stratified keratinizing squamous epithelium and fibrous submucosal devoid of minor salivary glands. **b** Odontogenic squamoid rests can be abundant. **c** Mineralized odontogenic rests can also be present

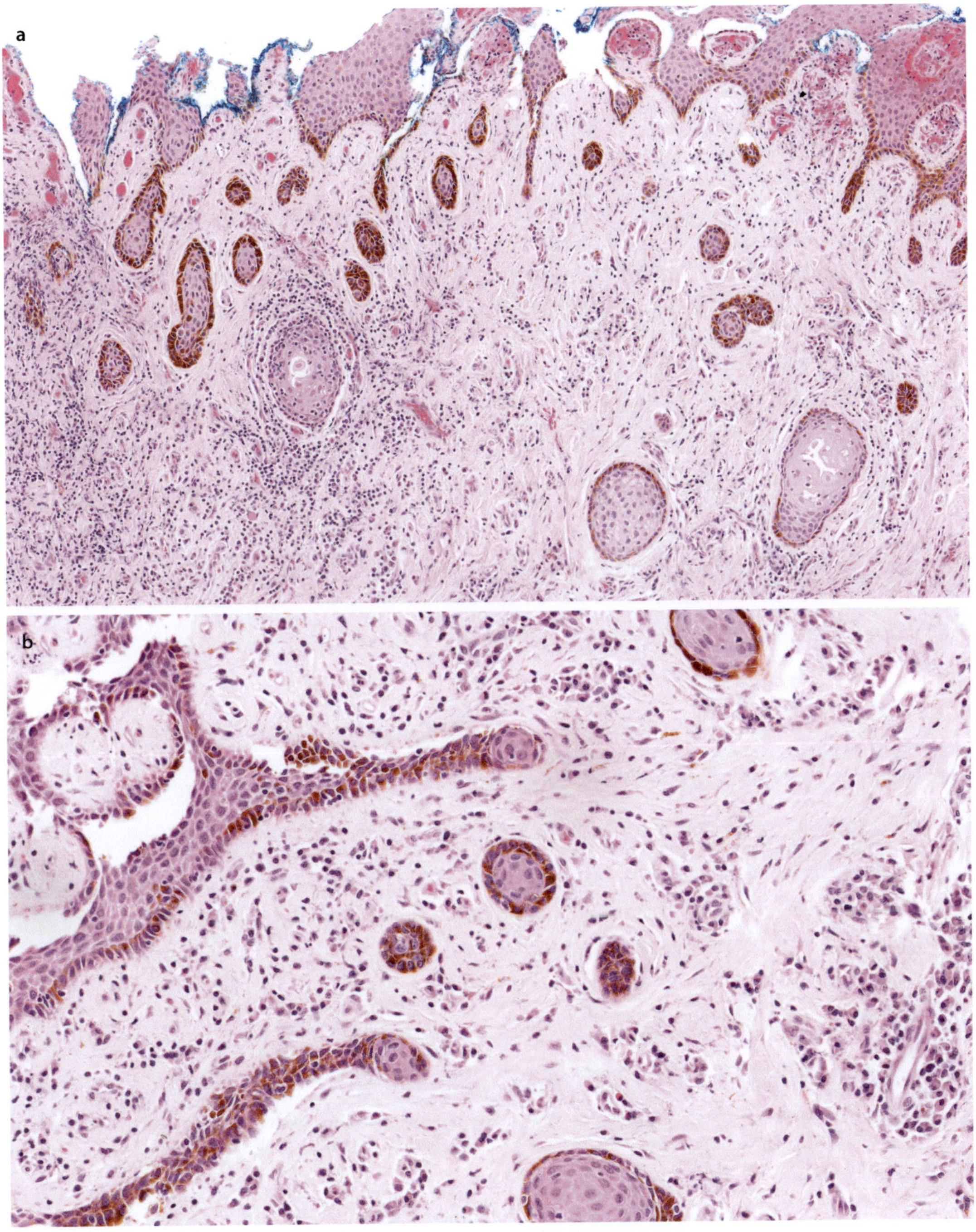

Fig. 1.8 **a, b** Unusual pigmentation of gingival basal reserve cells and odontogenic rests

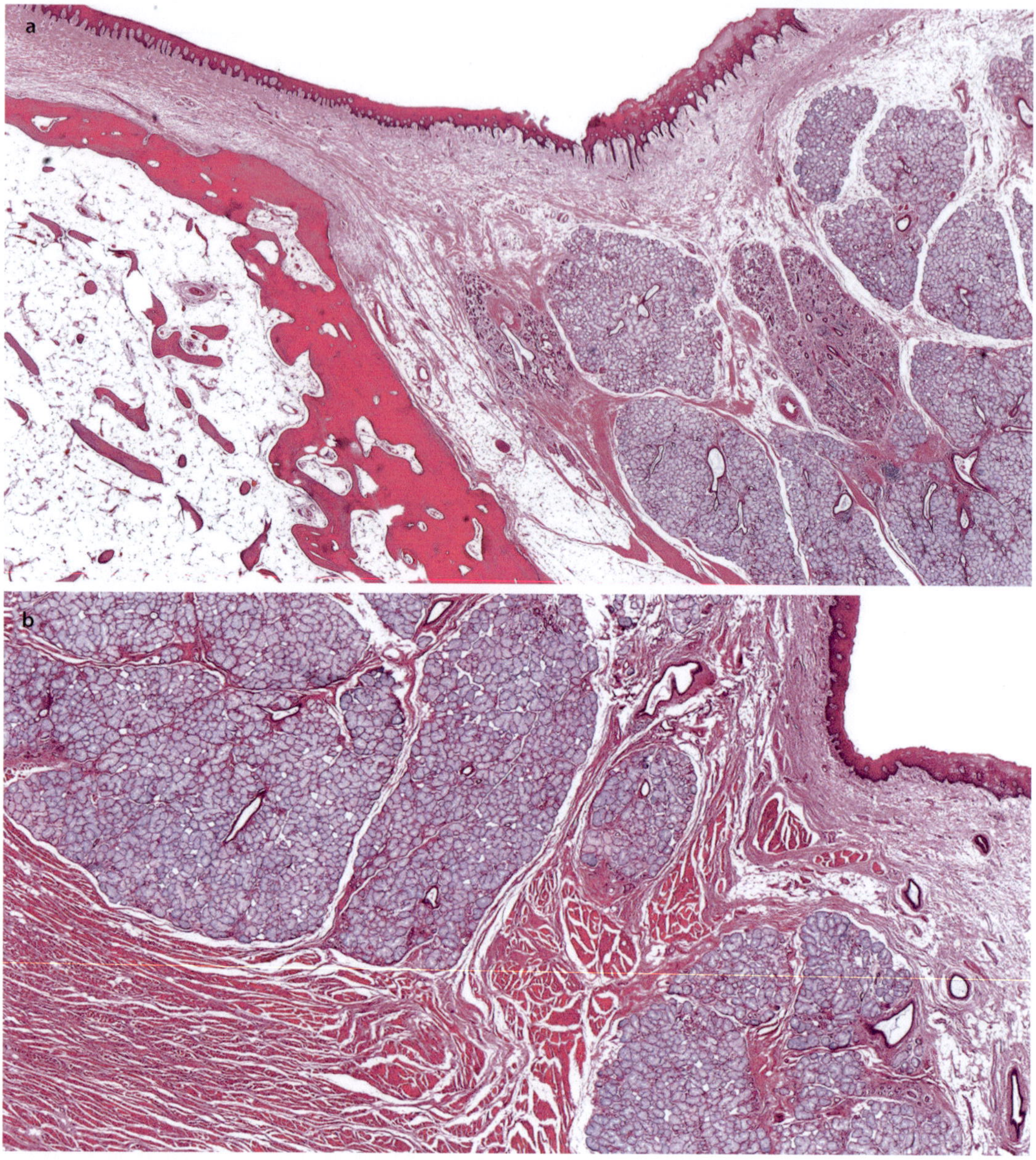

Fig. 1.9 **a** The lateral hard palate resembles the gingiva. Centrally, lobules of mucinous minor salivary glands are present. **b** The soft palate, which is within the oropharynx, is distinguished from the hard palate by the presence of skeletal muscle

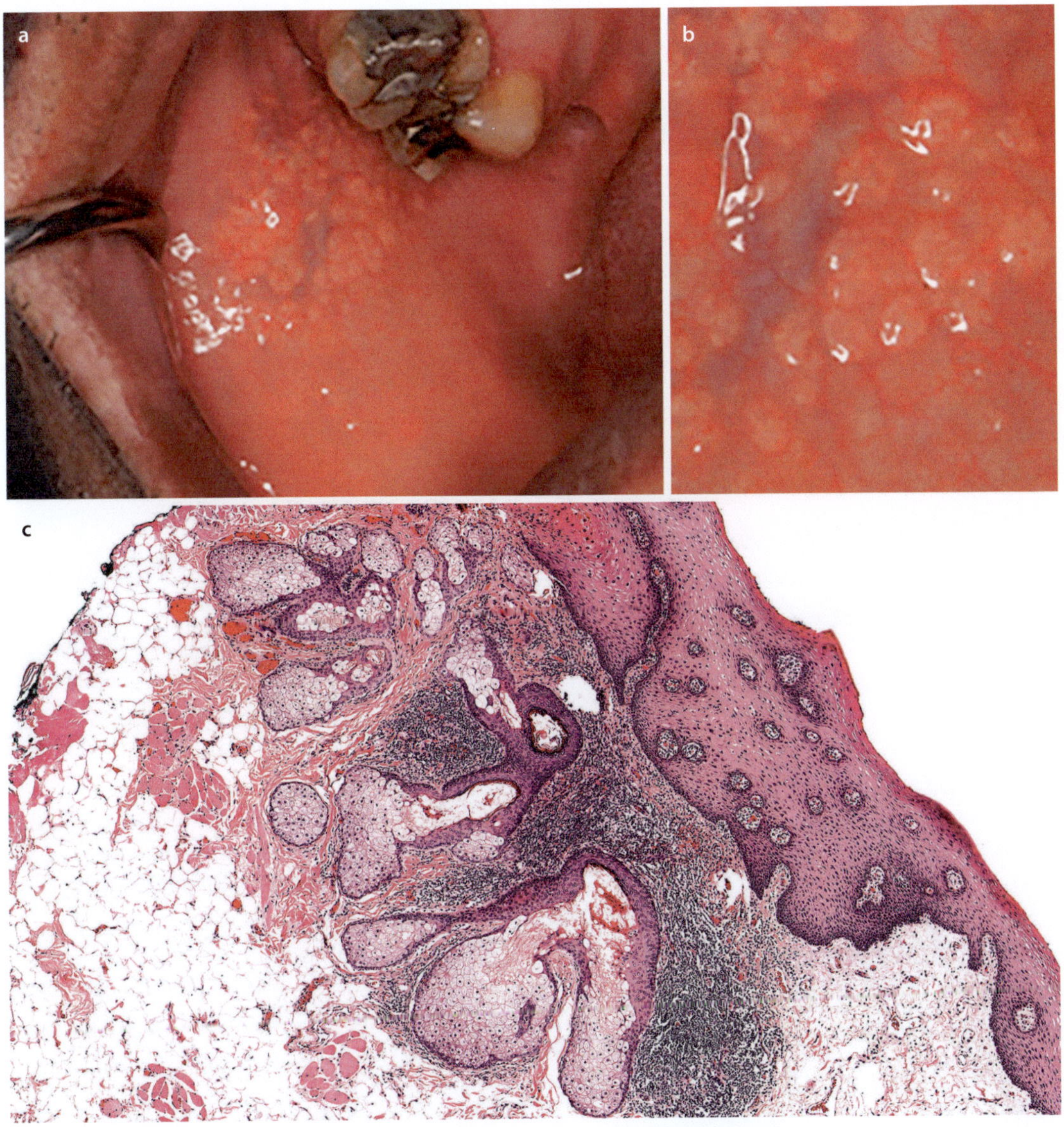

Fig. 1.10 **a, b** Fordyce granules are soft, yellow submucosal nodules occasionally seen in the buccal tissue. **c** Microscopically, they represent ectopic sebaceous glands

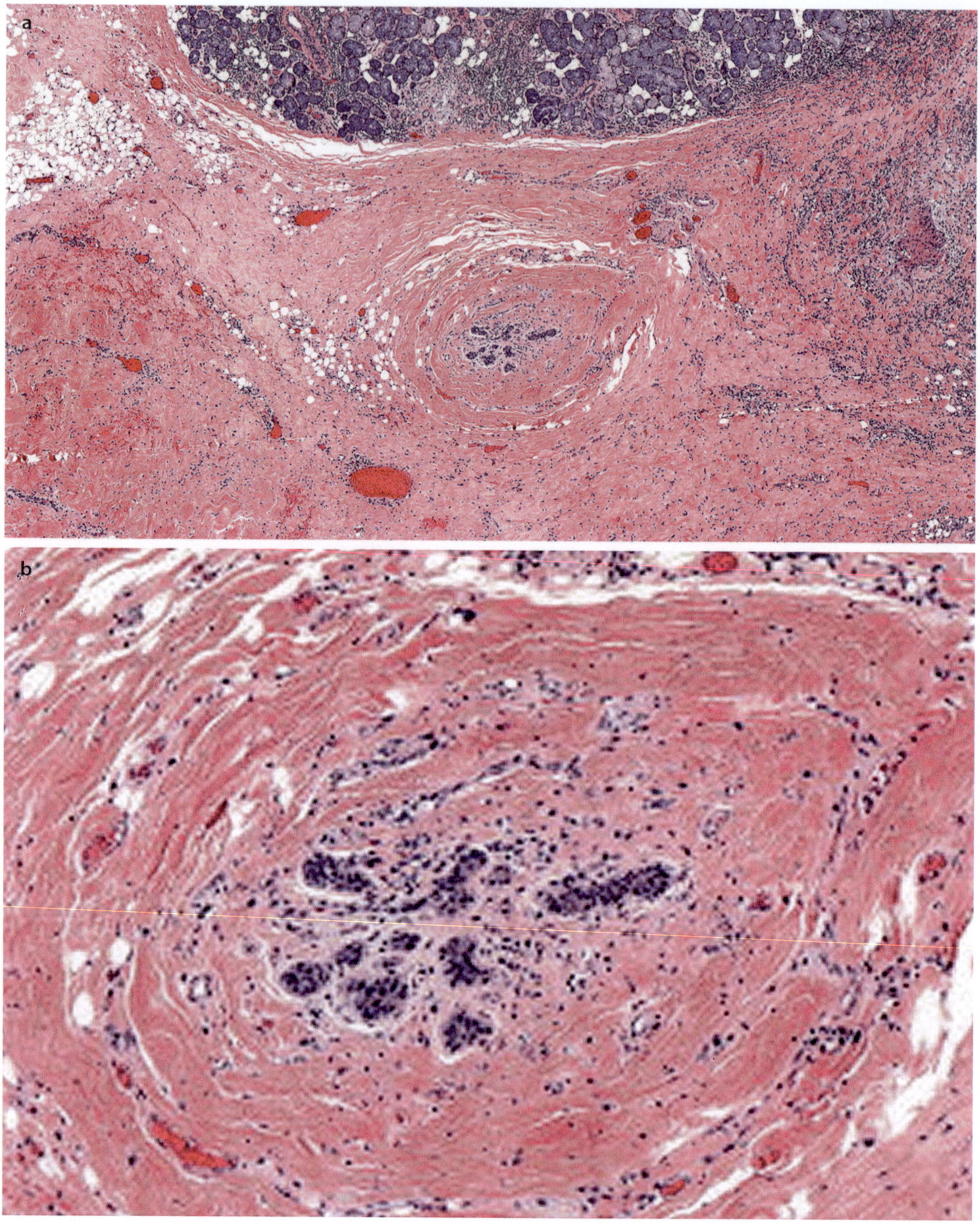

Fig. 1.11 **a**, **b** The organ of Chievitz (juxtaoral organ of Chievitz) Is a distinct anatomic organ situated close to the buccotemporalis fascia [3, 4]. It is composed of multiple epithelial lobules surrounded by a network of nerve fibers. Here we see small nests of these epithelial cells arranged in a lobular pattern

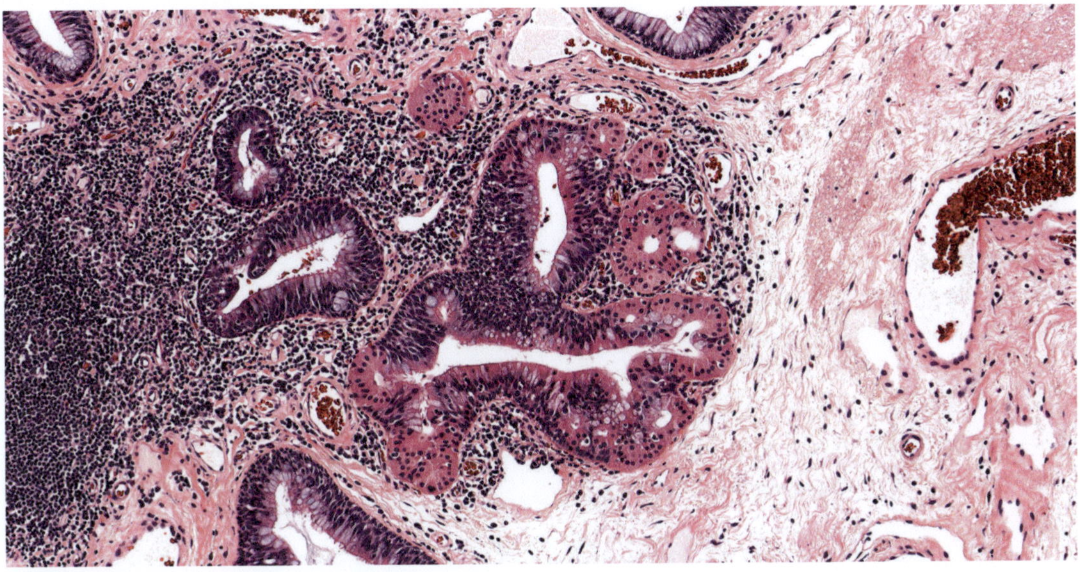

Fig. 1.12 Oncocytic metaplasia of minor salivary ducts is commonly seen as an aging phenomenon

References

1. Sanders I, Mu L. A 3-Dimensional Atlas of human tongue muscles. Anat Rec. 2013;296:1102–14.
2. McDaniel RK. Subepithelial nerve plexus (with ganglion cells) associated with taste buds. Oral Surg Oral Med Oral Pathol Oral Radiol Endod. 1999;87:605–9.
3. Sancheti SM, Sawaimoon S, Zameer MA. Juxtaoral organ of Chievitz, an obscure anatomical structure masquerading as perineural invasion of mucoepidermoid carcinoma: case report and review of literature. Int J Surg Pathol. 2015;2015(23):461–3.
4. Pantanowitz L, Tschen JA, Balogh K. The juxtaoral organ of Chievitz. Int J Surg Pathol. 2003;11:37.

Oral Cavity: Nonneoplastic and Benign Neoplasia

M. S. Brandwein-Weber, *Textbook of Head and Neck Pathology*,
https://doi.org/10.1007/978-3-319-76106-0_2

2.1 Lichen Planus

Oral lichen planus (OLP) is a relatively common T-cell mediated autoimmune inflammatory disease that usually affects individuals over 40 years old, however it may also develop in younger individuals. There is a slight female predominance and association with other autoimmune illnesses (alopecia areata, dermatomyositis, myasthenia gravis, primary biliary cirrhosis, ulcerative colitis) and hepatitis C infection. OLP may be triggered by stress, viral infection, or othe r inducers of cell-mediated immunity. Increased TH1 cytokine production is an important early step OLP pathogenesis, causes activated T cells (Th1, Th17, CD8) to migrate to the oral mucosa. Upregulation of intercellular adhesion molecules (ICAM-1 and VCAM), basement membrane proteins (collagen types IV and VII, laminin and integrins) and lymphocyte chemotactic cytokines (TNF-α and IL-1,IL-8, IL-10, and IL-12) further potentiate the process [1]

OLP most commonly presents as either reticular or erosive disease [2]. **Reticular OLP** is most common, and can be asymptomatic or accompanied by mild symptoms; it's characterized by lacy, bilateral, white buccal mucosal streaks referred to as Wickham's striae (◘ Fig. 2.1). These striae may also be seen on the gingiva, tongue, palate and lips. The plaque-like variant of reticular OLP resembles multifocal leukoplakia, with flat to elevated broad white lesions of the tongue dorsum and buccal mucosa. **Erosive OLP** is the second most common oral variant, and associated with erythematous, ulcerated lesions that can be multifocal, or restricted to one site such as gingiva. Patients with erosive OLP complain of sensitivity to hot or spicy foods, pain, and ulcerations. Erosive OLP presents with erythematous ulcers adjacent to Wickham's striae. **Gingival erosive OLP** (previously referred to as desquamative gingivitis) causes intense, diffuse gingival erythema. Oral **bullous lichen planus** presents as fluid-filled vesicles projecting from the oral mucosa which can rupture [3]. **Atrophic OLP** presents as diffuse, symptomatic erythematous patches surrounded by Wickham's striae. Many patients with OLP may also have mucosal involvement (vulva, vagina, esophagus, larynx, conjunctiva) and skin involvement, with pruritic, purple papules and plaques on the flexor wrists and ankles, and the extensor surfaces of the lower legs, the lower back, and the natal cleft.

The term "lichenoid reaction" refers to OLP-*like* hypersensitivity process which may be caused by contact with dental amalgam, or composite resin dental restoration materials, denture components, and drugs such as nonsteroidal anti-inflammatory drugs, beta-blockers, sulfonylureas, antimalarials, lithium, imatimib, and some angiotensin-converting enzyme inhibitors [4].

OLP can be treated with topical or systemic corticosteroids. Treatment options for individuals with steroid resistance include calcineurin

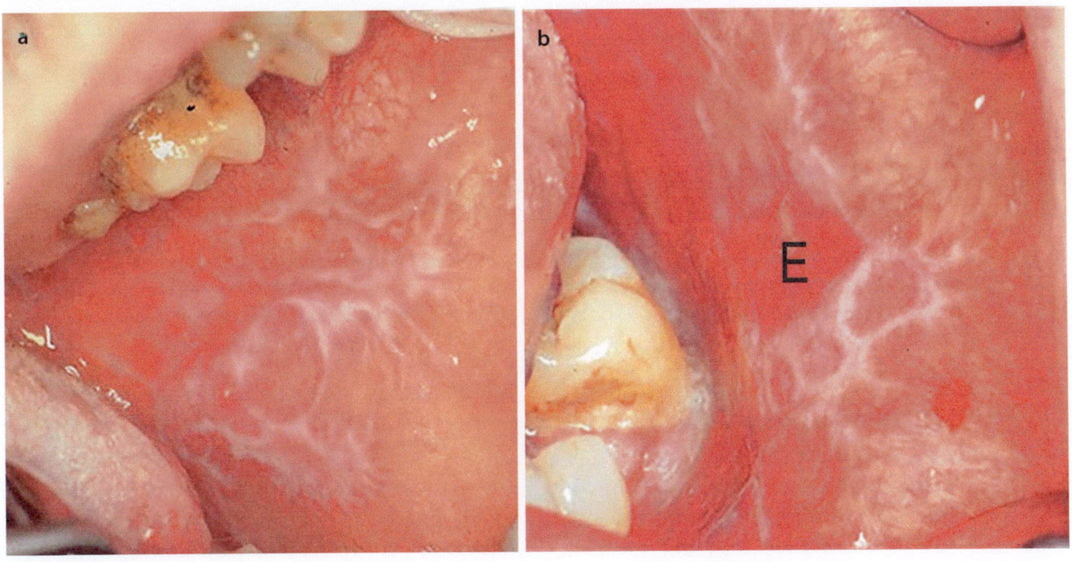

◘ **Fig. 2.1** **a** The most common presentation of lichen planus (LP) is the reticular form, which describes a fine network of white lines (Wickham's stria). **b** Superficial erosion (E) (erosive LP) surrounded by Wickham's stria

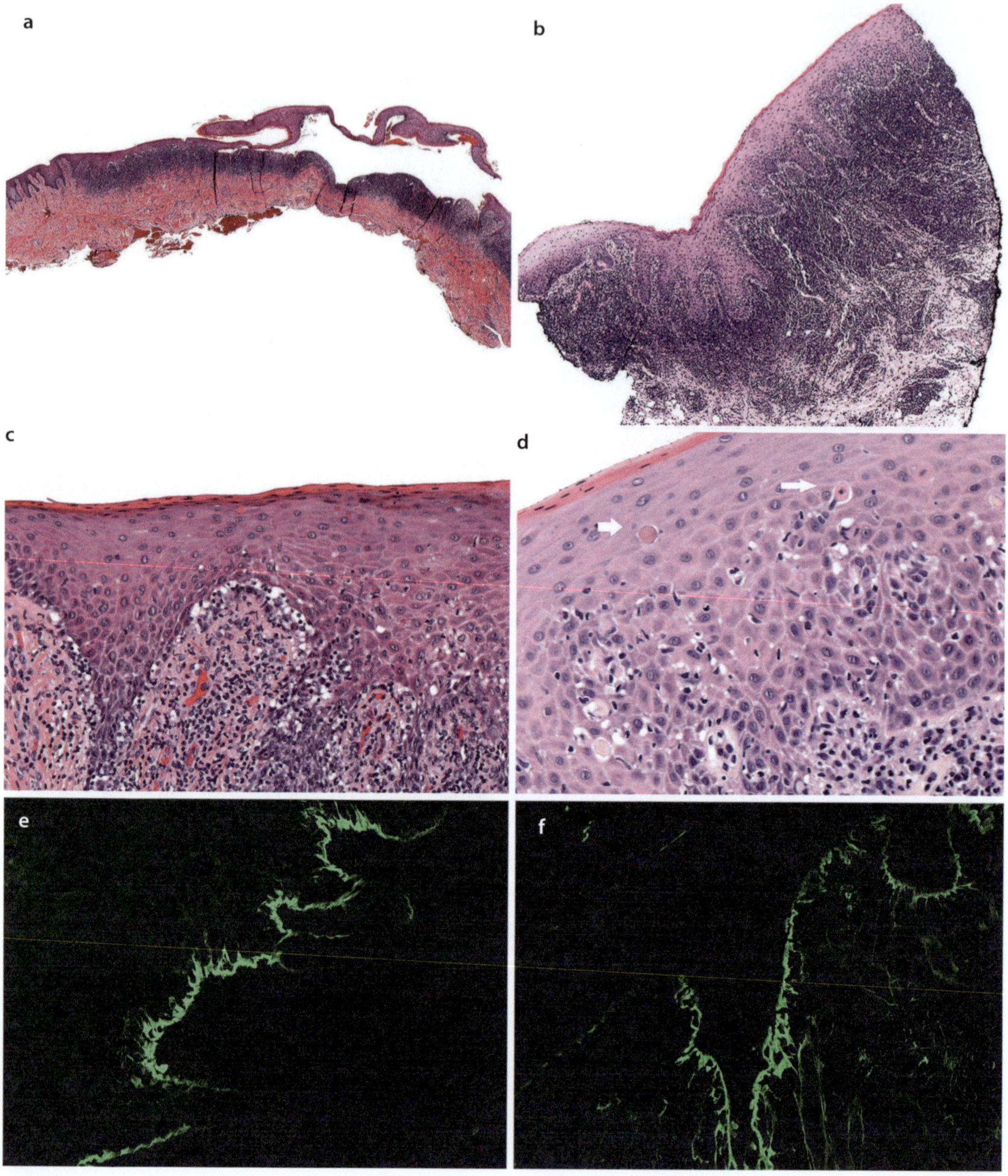

Fig. 2.2 **a**, **b** Dense band of inflammatory cells characteristic of LP. **c** Basal layer degeneration seen at low-power as vacuolar change. **d** Intraepithelial inflammation and Civatte bodies (*arrows*) representing apoptotic epithelial cells. **e**, **f** Immunofluorescence demonstration of dense and ***shaggy*** fibrin deposition at the basement membrane zone

inhibitors, such as tacrolimus and cyclosporine, which block T cell activation, and biologics which target specific cytokines or their receptors [5].

The histopathologic features of OLP include a dense band-like subepithelial infiltrate of T cells and histiocytes (Fig. 2.2) and liquefactive degeneration commencing at the level of basal cells. This degeneration and disruption of the anchoring elements of the basement membrane and basal cells causes submucosal clefts (Max-Joseph spaces). *Intraepithelial* lymphocytes (predominantly T cells) are seen. The squamous mucosa may be acanthotic with saw-tooth rete pegs (Fig. 2.3), or thin and atrophic. The degenerating epithelial cells form colloid bodies (Civatte, hyaline, cytoid bodies – homogenous

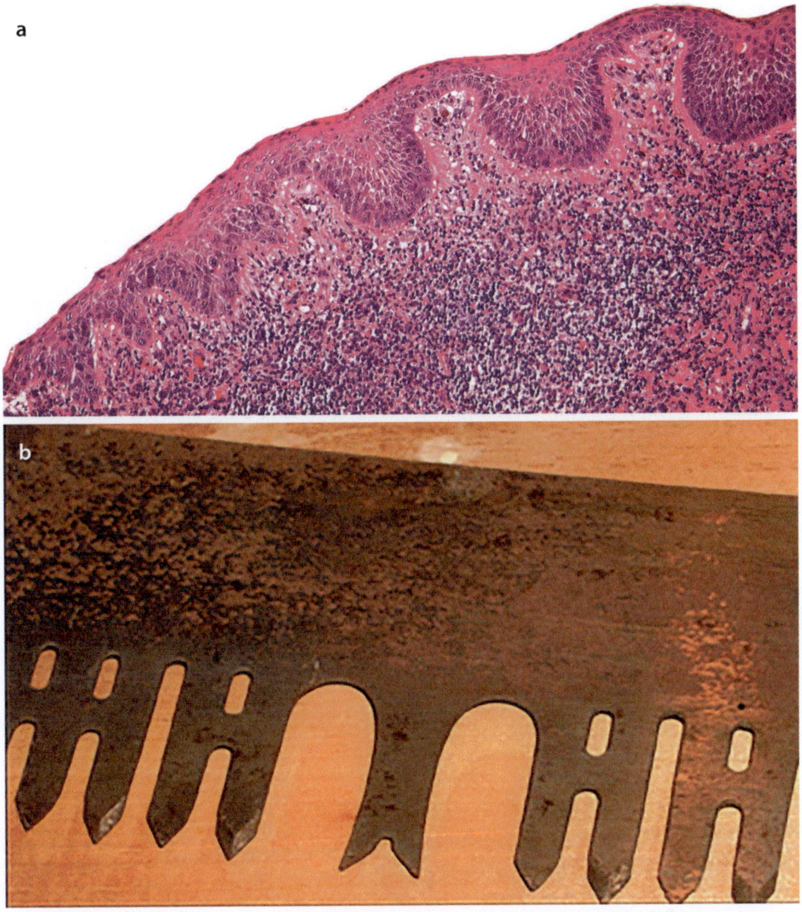

Fig. 2.3 **a** Epithelial acanthosis with "saw tooth" rete pegs. **b** Saw teeth

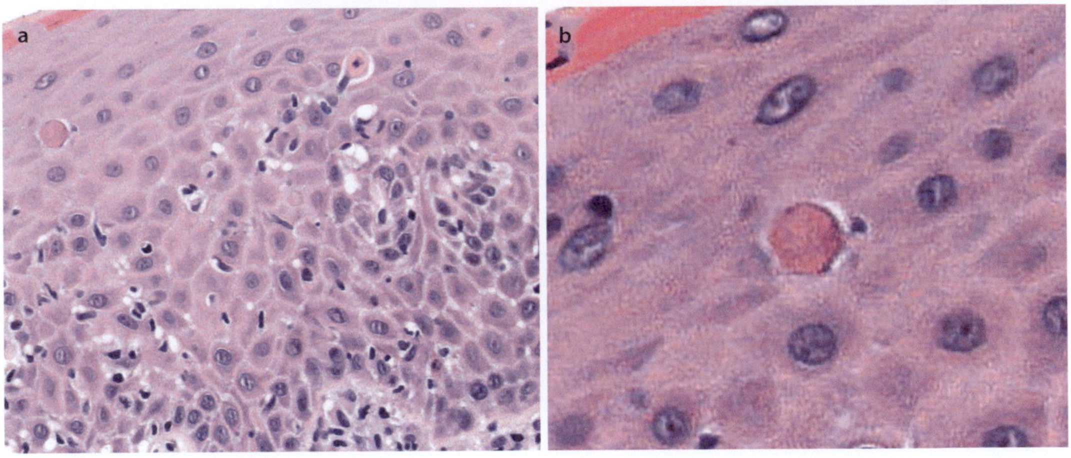

Fig. 2.4 **a, b** Civatte bodies

eosinophilic globules) (Fig. 2.4). *Candida albicans* can be an incidental finding.

Histologically, a lichenoid reaction includes other inflammatory cells such as eosinophils and plasma cells. Liquifactive degeneration can be present but no Civatte bodies are seen (Fig. 2.5).

Direct immunofluorescence (DIF) can be useful in distinguishing OLP from a lichenoid reaction. OLP DIF reveals specific dense and shaggy fibrinogen deposition at the basement membrane zone. Negative DIF can support a clinical impression of lichenoid hypersensitivity reaction.

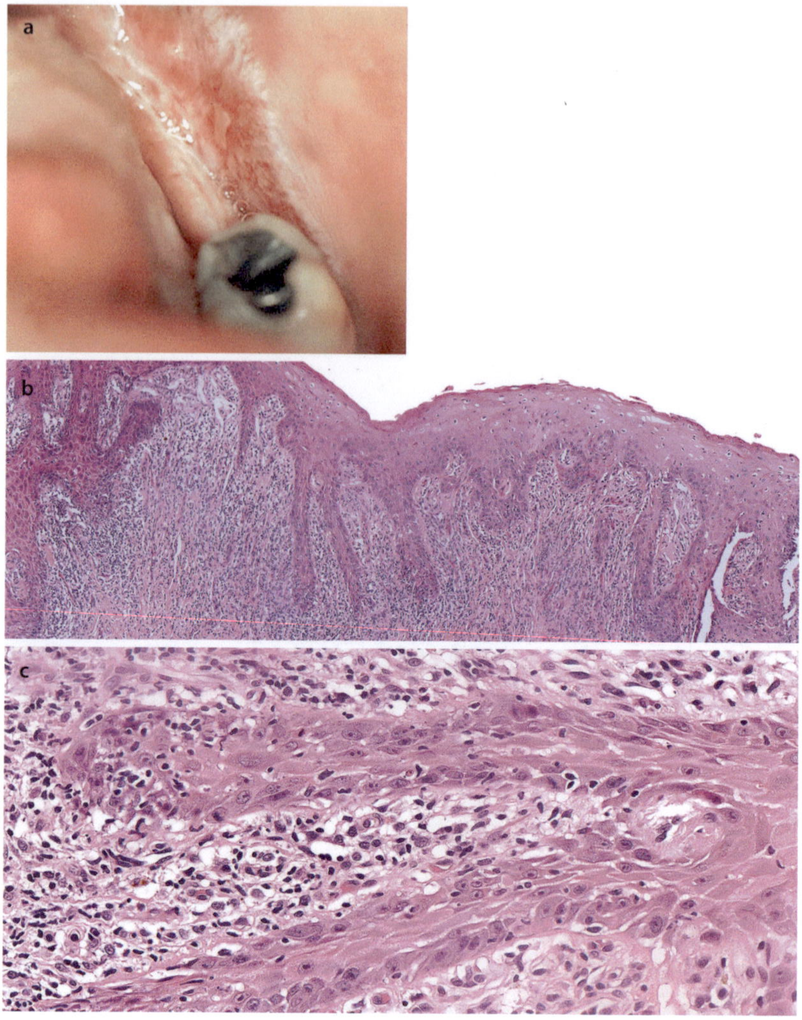

Fig. 2.5 **a** Clinical appearance of a retromolar lichenoid reaction presenting with superficial erosion, erythroplasia, with a halo of white stria. **b** At low-power, a dense inflammatory band is seen. **c** Liquifactive degeneration and intraepithelial inflammation is present. The lack of Civatte bodies, and the presence of eosinophils are histological hints that this is an "-oid", and not the real deal. This must be correlated with the clinical presentation, which would also be atypical for LP

2.2 Vesiculobullous Diseases

Pemphigus represents a blistering disorder caused by autoantibodies against keratinocyte adhesion proteins; it is diagnosed most commonly in the fourth and fifth decades of life, and there is a predisposition for Jewish and Mediterranean individuals. **Pemphigus vulgaris** and **paraneoplastic pemphigus** typically cause intraoral disease. Patients present with painful oral erosions, commonly involving the labial and buccal mucosa (Fig. 2.6). Mucosal pemphigus can also involve the oropharynx and esophagus. Intact oral vesicles are often not observed because they rupture early. These ulcers are usually not serosanguinous, and they *crust readily*. The Nikolsky sign is indicative of the general mucosal fragility. A small amount of applied mucosal pressure (finger, pencil erasure, air blast) will result in shearing and ulceration. This test is non-specific and is positive in pemphigus vulgaris, erythema multiforme, bullous lichen planus, and benign mucosal pemphigoid. **Desquamative** refers to intramucosal blistering which results after slight mucosal rubbing over intact mucosa. A positive Nikolsky test favors pemphigus vulgaris over **benign mucosal pemphigoid gingivitis;** this descriptor refers to painful hemorrhagic process which involves the full width of the gingiva. Dermal involvement may follow mucosal involvement, with a predilection for trunk, groin, axillae, scalp and face.

Other forms of pemphigus which typically spare the oral cavity include **pemphigus foliaceous**, an extensive dermal exfoliation, and **pemphigus erythematosis** (Senear Usher syndrome), which mimics lupus erythematosis with malar distribution of the erythematous, scaling, *crusting* lesions. **Pemphigus vegetans** is characterized by

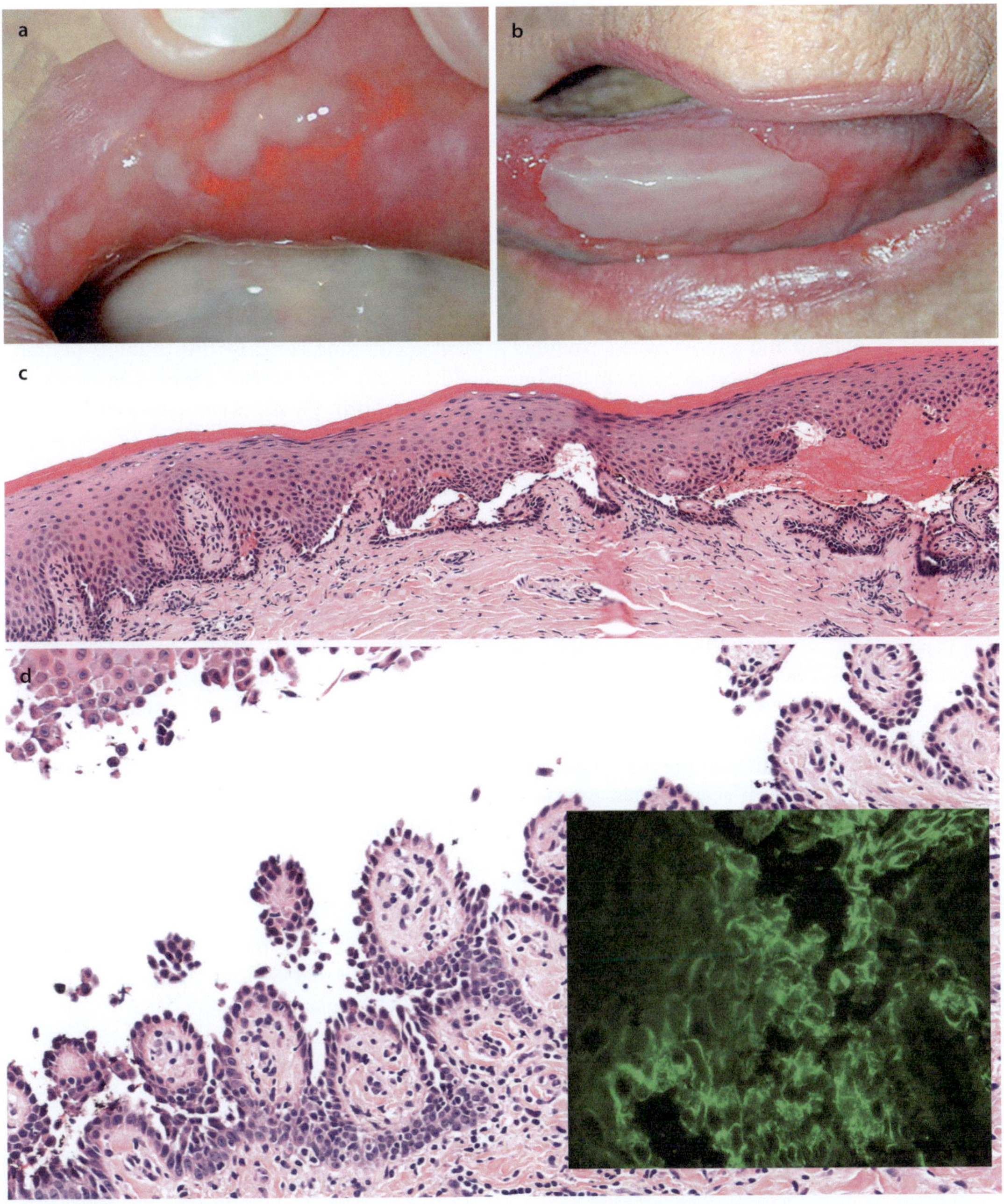

Fig. 2.6 Bullous pemphigus vulgaris: Flaccid bullae on upper lip **a** and lateral tongue **b**. **c** Low power view of acantholysis and intramucosal clefting. **d** At higher power, appreciate the tombstone cells which remain adherent to the basement membrane. Inset: Direct immunofluorescence, IgG, 40X, demonstrating intramucosal IgG with a membraneous staining pattern

eroded bullae which develop hypertrophic crusting granulation tissue producing hyperplastic lesions in the skin and vermillion border of the lips.

Pemphigus is caused by autoantibodies to desmosomal glycoproteins (desmogleins) which disrupt cellular adhesions and cause acantholysis. In skin, desmoglein-1 (Dsg-1) is expressed throughout, with greater concentrations in the more superficial layers; desmoglein-3 (Dsg-3) is expressed in the parabasal and basal layers. In the mucosa, Dsg-1 and Dsg-3 are expressed throughout, with Dsg-1 is present in lower concentrations. Patients with **mucocutaneous pemphigus** vulgaris have autoantibodies to **Dsg-1** and **Dsg-3**, whereas **mucosal pemphigus** patients have only antibodies to **Dsg-3** [6]. Pemphigus may also be drug induced usually by thiol containing drugs such as penicillin and laryngeal involvement has been reported in drug-induced pemphigus.

Histopathologically, **pemphigus vulgaris** is characterized by epithelial cell separation (acantholysis) and intraepithelial clefting. The basal reserve layer remains intact and attached to lamina propria. The cells below the intramucosal cleft have a "tombstone" like effect – irregular, with decreased cytoplasm and almost naked, rounded nuclei, which protrude into the clefts resembling tombstones on a hill (Fig. 2.6). Individual spherical acantholytic cells, referred to as Tzanck cells, can be seen floating within the intraepithelial clefts; they are rounded, enlarged, and have large hyperchromatic nuclei. Direct immunofluorescence (DIF) reveals pronounced intraepithelial IgG and complement deposition with a membranous pattern, especially concentrated in the "prickle layer," corresponding to deposition of autoantibodies against Dsg-1.

Histologically, **paraneoplastic pemphigus** can overlap with pemphigus vulgaris, lichen planus, and erythema multiforme, with intraepithelial blisters, suprabasal acantholysis, interface inflammation, dyskeratotic keratinocytes, and intraepithelial lymphocytes. DIF shows diffuse IgG deposition in all layers of the mucosa and C3 in the basement membrane zone. In contrast to pemphigus vulgaris, intercellular IgG staining is often focal or faint.

Patients with pemphigus are advised to avoid inciting foods or drink (spicy, hot). First line therapy includes systemic steroids and adjuvants such as calcineurin inhibitors (block T cell activation), Rituximab, a monoclonal CD30 antibody, plasmapheresis pulsed with conventional steroids, or immunosuppressants to prevent rebound, or extracorporal immunadsorption of Dsg-3 [6–8].

Cicatricial pemphigoid {benign mucosal pemphigoid, bullous pemphigoid} is a chronic, progressive, autoimmune subepithelial blistering disease with a female to male ratio of 2:1. **Bullous pemphigoid** is a more intense variant of **cicatricial pemphigoid** with a predilection for the skin rather than mucosa. The incidence of cicatricial pemphigoid increases with advancing age. Mucosa is primarily affected, usually oral (88%) and ocular (60%); additionally, 18% of patients have mild skin lesions usually of the limb flexor surfaces. The larynx, oropharynx/hypopharynx are involved in 10% and 8% of patients respectively and usually in the setting of disseminated disease. Benign mucosal pemphigoid causes erythematous, *non-crusting* lesions. Pemphigoid lesions heal by intense scarring hence the appellation "cicatricial". Ocular involvement and scarring leads to conjunctival symblepharon, corneal ulceration and opacification.

Pemphigoid is caused by autoantibodies against hemidesmosomal proteins in the basement membrane zone: **BP180** (bullous pemphigoid antigen 180), **BP230**, **alpha 6 integrin** and **beta 4 integrin** [9, 10]. Rarely, autoantibodies to **laminin 5 (epiligrin)** are produced, this is referred to as antiepiligrin cicatricial pemphigoid.

Histopathologically, pemphigoid is characterized by mucosal separation or clefting ***at the level of the basement membrane*** away from the lamina propria. In distinction to pemphigus, ***no intramucosal clefting*** or intramucosal acantholysis (Tzanck cells, tombstone cells) are seen. The lamina propria has a chronic inflammation and increased vascularity. Direct immunofluorescence (DIF) reveals a linear deposition of IgG and/or IgM and complement directed against the basement membrane. Indirect immunofluorescence using patient serum against control skin reveals the same pattern of deposition of IgG and complement against basement membrane.

The differential diagnosis of pemphigoid includes artifactual clefting, pemphigus vulgaris, erosive lichen planus, herpetic vesicles, and epidermolysis bullosa acquisita. Artifactual clefting may be difficult to distinguish from pemphigoid by light microscopy, especially if the lamina propria is inflamed. Clinical history and immunofluorescence can distinguish between pemphigoid and artifact. Re-epithelization of the floor of the blister in pemphigoid may be confused with the intramucosal clefting of pemphigus.

2.3 Herpes

HSV-1 is ubiquitous to humanity. It is transmitted via infectious saliva and by sexual contact. In less developed countries, seroconversion occurs during childhood or adolescence. In more developed countries, or middle- or upper-socioeconomic strata, seroconversion can take place between the

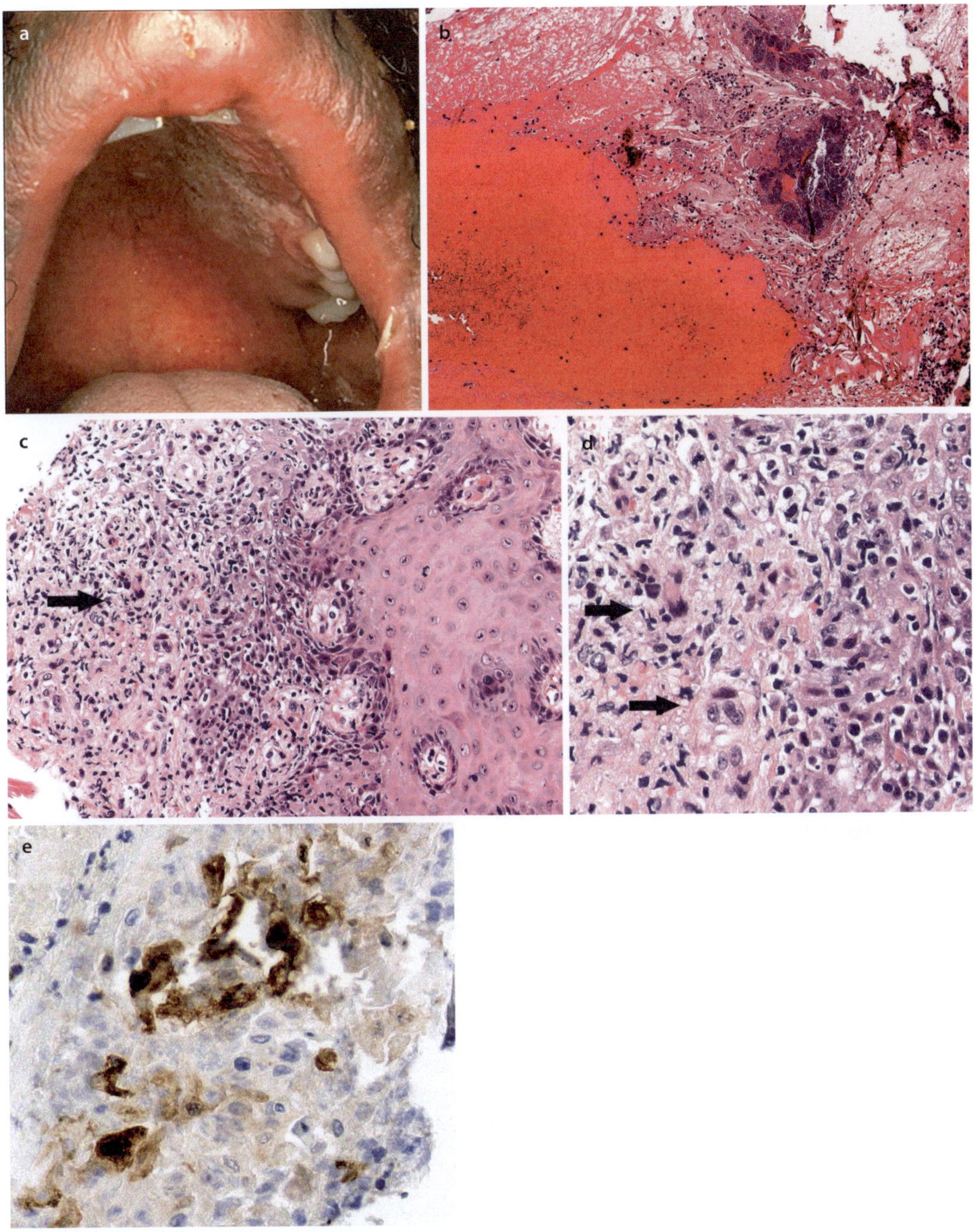

■ **Fig. 2.7** **a** Ulcerating Herpes simplex infection on the left hard palate; the grey white patch represents fibrinopurulent exudate. (Courtesy of Dr. Richard V Smith). **b** Hemorrhagic ulcer bed. **c**, **d** HSV infected cells adjacent to ulcer (*arrows*). **e** IHC for HSV

third and fourth decades of life. Primary childhood HSV-1 exposure usually leads to subclinical seroconversion. Symptomatic primary oropharyngeal infection is characterized by prodromal fever, headache and myalgias, followed by severe gingivostomatitis which may mimic vesiculobullous disease. The gums are red, swollen and friable. Painful vesicles erupt on the inner lip, anterior gingiva, and oral mucosa (■ Fig. 2.7). Tiny vesicles may appear around the nose. The lesions heal within two weeks. Rarely, primary gingivostomatitis can progress to herpetic encephalitis, which is commonly fatal. Both symptomatic and subclinical primary HSV infection result in latent infection of sensory ganglion nuclei. The trigeminal ganglion is the primary site for HSV-1 latency.

HSV-1 can also be sexually transmitted and is an increasing cause for genital herpes. Genital HSV-1 infections are less severe, and less prone to recurrence than genital HSV-2 infections. HSV-2 is usually transmitted sexually; seroconversion occurs after sexual debut.

Reactivation of latent infection, usually in the form of herpes labialis occurs in up to half of infected individuals. It can be stimulated by emotional factors, hormonal changes, excess sunlight, fever, trauma, and dental procedures. Reactivation results in viral replication within nerve ganglia and anterograde translocation to the dermatome. Patients experience tingling and pain, and develop clusters of coalescing vesicles at the labial vermillion ("cold sore"). The vesicles ulcerate and crust within 72–96 h. Immunocompetant individuals tend to have mucocutaneous labial lesions, (herpes labialis) but not intraoral lesions. By contrast, AIDS patients with reactivated HSV-1 infection develop a wider distribution of oral lesions that persist longer. Mucocutaneous herpes lasting more than 1 month was an original defining AIDS criterion prior to serologic testing, and remains a diagnostic criterion.

Histopathologically, HSV infection is characterized by intramucosal/intraepithelial vesicle formation. The infected nuclei are enlarged, with homogeneous basophilic or clear "ground glass" inclusions and peripheral chromatin beading. In early lesions, the nuclear changes are observed in basal and parabasal layers; the nuclear changes extend throughout the epithelium in late lesions. Typically, the multiple nuclei "mold" with each other, rather than overlap. Multinucleated syncytial cells can be seen with both intranuclear and cytoplasmic inclusions. Smear cytology of vesicular fluid can demonstrate Cowdry A type cells with intranuclear eosinophilic viral inclusion bodies. Immunohistochemistry for HSV can be very helpful, positive cases will demonstrate strong nuclear staining.

Immunocompetent patients can benefit from topical antivirals, especially if administered during the prodrome; systemic antiviral therapy (oral or intravenous) are indicated for immunocompromised hosts. Emerging HSV resistance to acyclic guanasine analogues, acyclic nucleotide analogues, and pyrophosphate analogues has lead to new strategies in HSV drug therapies, such as targeting HSV helicase/primase [11, 12].

2.4 Mucocele

A mucocele is an extravasation phenomenon, either from an obstructed duct or paranasal sinus ostium. An oral mucocele can result from an obstruction of a minor salivary gland duct, or the sublingual gland (◘ Fig. 2.8). The rove of minor salivary mucoceles occur on the lower lip, followed by buccal mucosa, retromolar trigone, and palate (◘ Fig. 2.9). Obstruction of the sublingual gland causes a ranula, derived from the word "rana" or frog, which causes a cystic swelling in the floor of mouth. A cervical or plunging ranula is caused by mucus escaping through the mylohyoid muscle; the mucus secretions extend into the cervical fascial planes causing diffuse swelling of the lateral or submental cervical regions.

Histologically, look for a cystically dilated duct. If the cyst has ruptured, there will be granulation tissue, inflammation and neovascularization. Foamy macrophages are invariably seen within the cyst and surrounding soft tissues.

2.5 Oral Focal Mucinosis

Focal mucinosis is an uncommon entity which manifests in the skin of the face, trunk, or extremities. It is even more rare as a submucosal lesion and has been reported in the oral cavity and larynx [13–15]. It presents as a single, discreet, dome-shaped papule and is usually smaller than 1 cm although occasionally it may be larger. Histopathologically, one sees a submucosal localized, lightly basophilic deposition of loose mucinous material (◘ Fig. 2.10). Scattered stellate fibroblasts and capillaries are present within this mucinous material. No inflammation should be seen. Mucicarmine stain will be negative or weakly positive. Alcian blue stain should

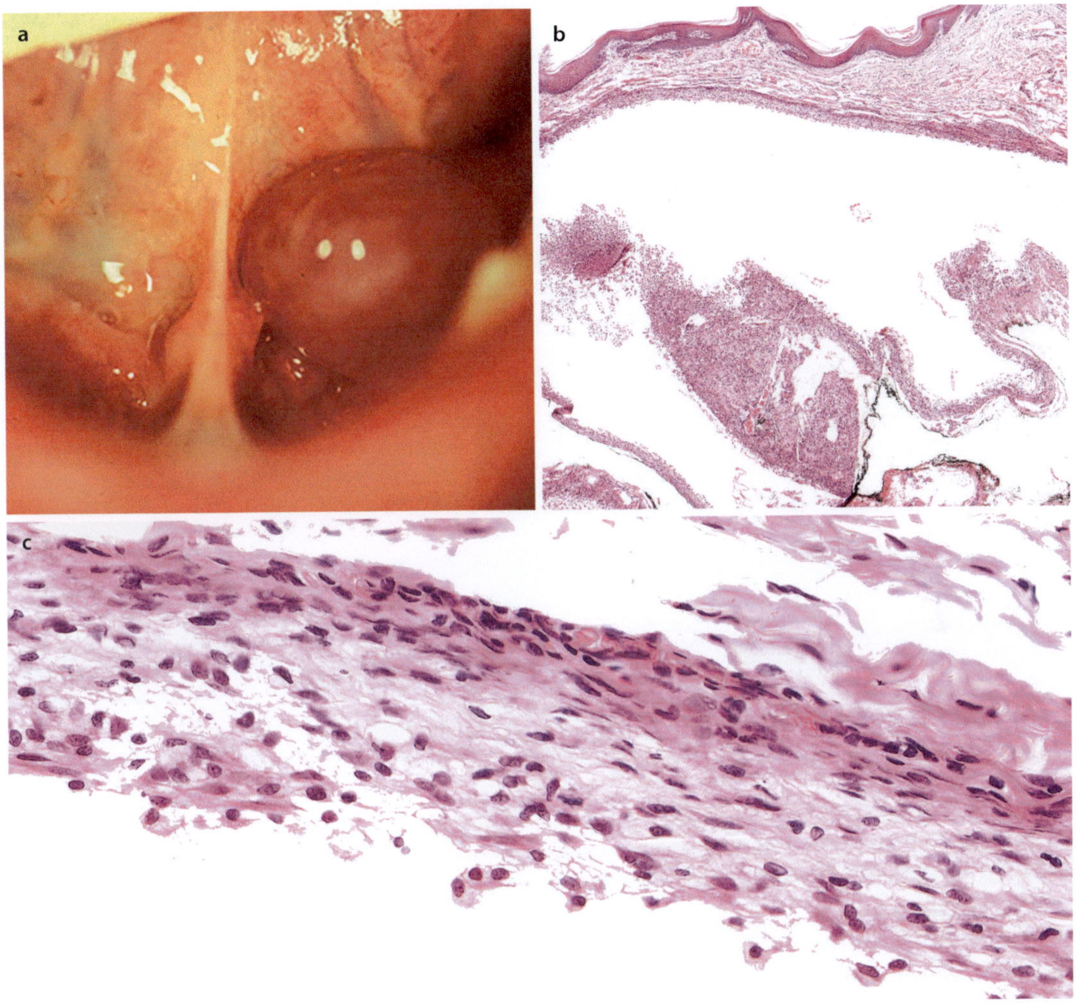

Fig. 2.8 **a** Mucocele in the floor of mouth, also referred to as a ranula. (Courtesy of Dr. Richard V Smith). **b** The cyst wall be show dilated, intact salivary duct, or may be replaced by granulation tissue. **c** Foamy macrophages represent the sine qua non of a ruptured mucocele

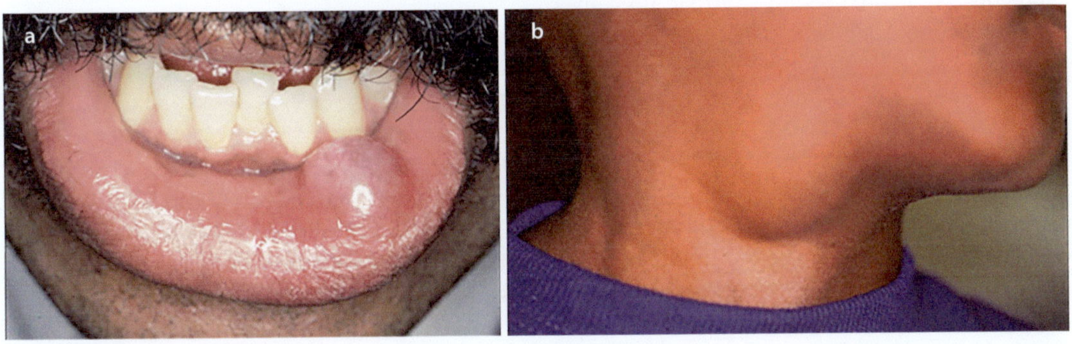

Fig. 2.9 **a** Mucocele lower lip presenting as a blueish, painless cystic swelling, which may fluctuate in size. (Courtesy of Dr. Richard V Smith). **b** Plunging ranula is the result of extravasated sublingual secretions tracking inferiorly. (Courtesy of Dr. Richard V Smith)

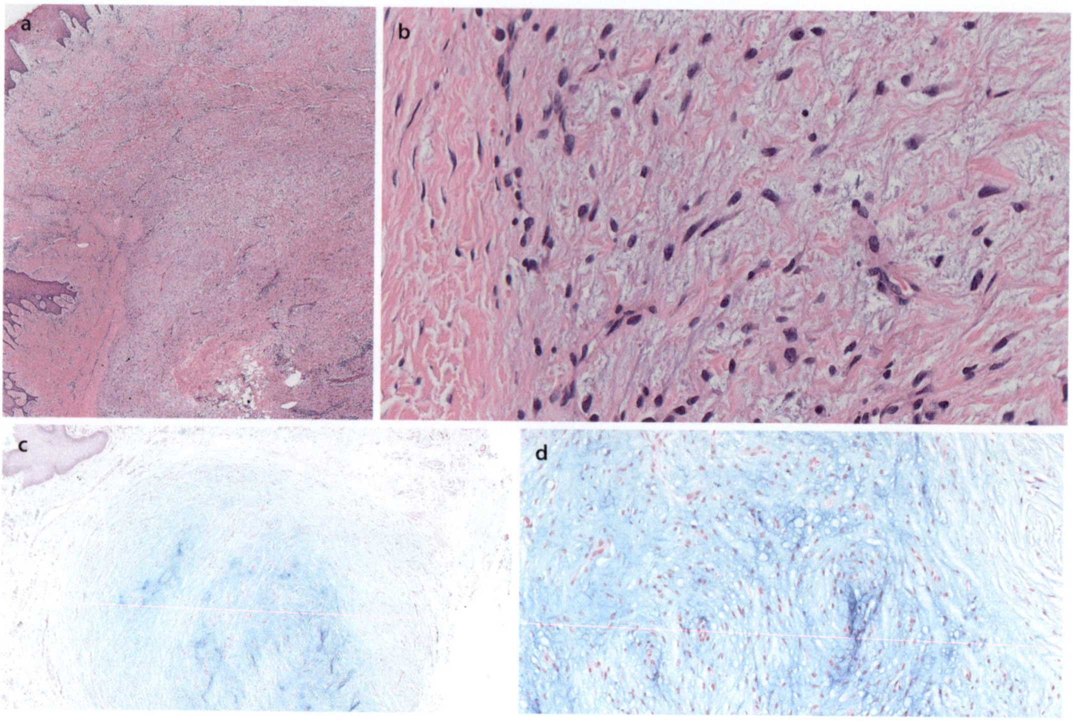

Fig. 2.10 **a, b** Oral focal mucinosis appears as an expansile deposition of myxoid matrix. **c, d** Alcian blue stains these acidic mucins

be positive, and staining is abolished with hyalurinudase treatment. The stellate fibroblasts are S100 negative.

The differential diagnosis includes a ruptured mucocele, which is inflamed and contains foamy macrophages and granulation tissue. A true myxoma is usually a large and infiltrative tumor, with a paucity of capillaries, and abundant collagen deposition. Oral myxomas can be associated with the autosomal dominant syndrome of mucocutaneous pigmented lesions, cardiac myxomas, endocrine abnormalities.

2.6 Amalgam Tattoo

Amalgam tattoo is the most commonly biopsied pigmented oral lesion. It is the result of mechanical implantation or leeching out of dental amalgam. Amalgam tattoos form single or multiple dark, gray, black, or blue, flat macules usually near restored teeth (Fig. 2.11). They are seen most often on the gingiva and alveolar mucosa, followed by buccal mucosa and floor of the mouth. They may be discreet and well-defined, or more irregular and diffuse. Amalgam tattoos are usually small, only millimeters in diameter, but rarely can reach up to 2 cm in size. Most lesions are radiographically negative, although some may demonstrate opaque fragments on X-ray.

Histopathologically, amalgam particles are black on H&E sections; they can be seen as free particles within soft tissues and around vessels and nerves, and within macrophages. There is usually little or no inflammation. Occasionally they may cause foreign body giant cell reaction.

2.7 Melanosis and Melanotic Macules

Oral racial pigmentation can be observed in dark-skinned individuals. These pigmented lesions are usually diffuse, bilateral, involving **gingiva or buccal mucosa** in a ribbon-like or band-like pattern (Fig. 2.12) [16].

Smoker's melanosis can occur in up to a quarter of smokers with a dose-dependent relationship; it is also reversible with the cessation of smoking. Melanin is thought to play a role in detoxifying polycyclic amines, nicotine, and benzopyrene. Smoker's melanosis causes diffuse black brown

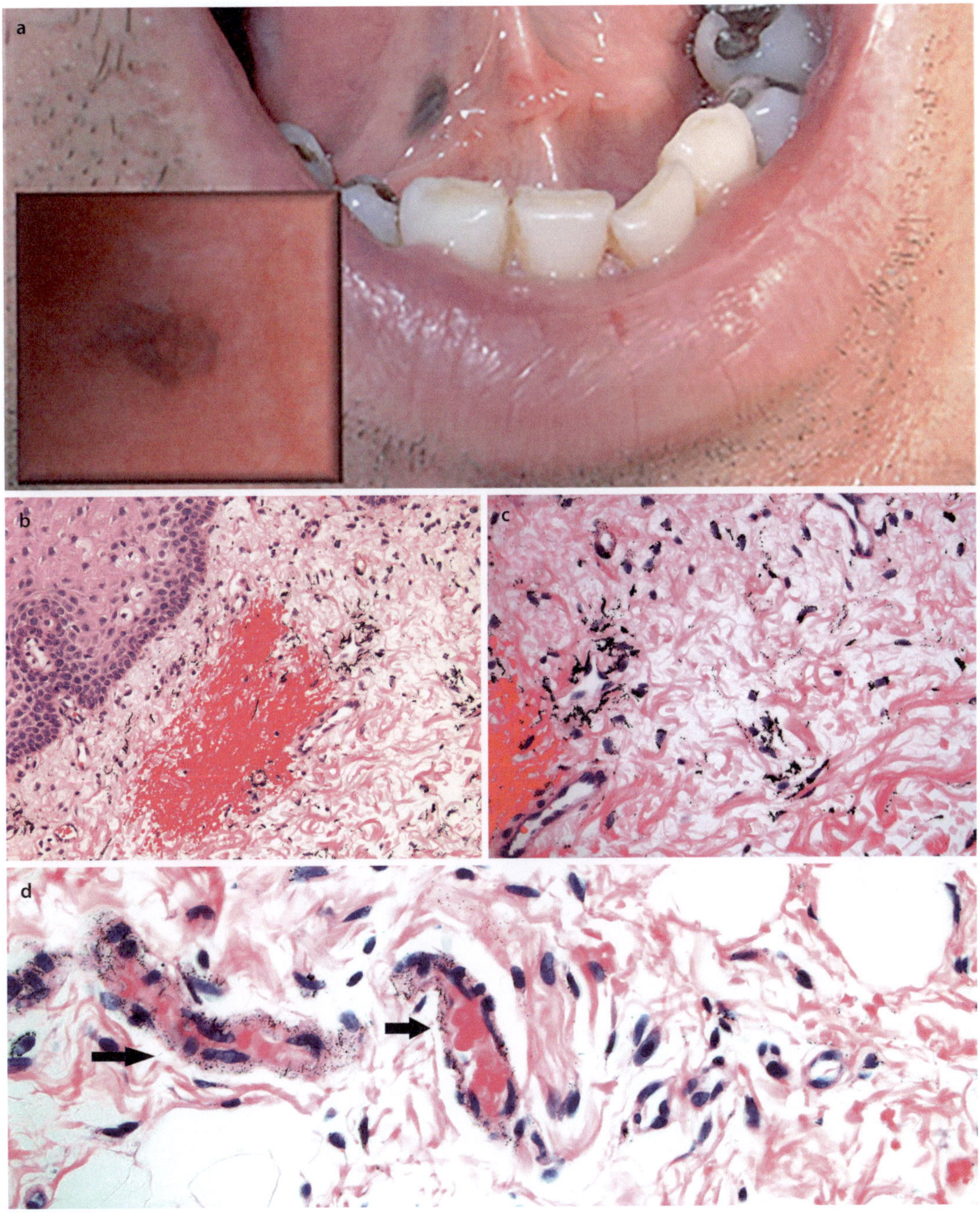

Fig. 2.11 **a** Amalgam tattoos present as dark flat macules (*black, gray, blue*) which are usually adjacent to teeth with dental amalgam. (Courtesy of Drs. Mauricio Wiltz and Robert Kelsch). **b**, **c**, **d** (*arrows*): The amalgam is taken up by macrophages; there is minimal tissue reaction

lesions on the labial gingiva, hard palate, buccal mucosa, lip, commissures, or tongue [17–19].

Melanotic macules are relatively common and seen most often on the **lower lip**, and other subsites such as **vermillion border and anterior gingival** (Fig. 2.13). Melanotic macules are single, well-circumscribed blue, brown to black homogeneous lesions that are usually smaller than 1 cm. Unlike freckles, melanotic macules do not darken with sun exposure. Multiple mucosal melanotic macules may be associated with a number of syndromes:

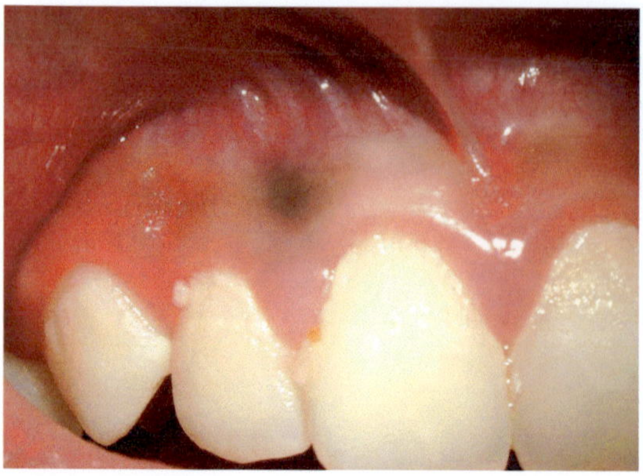

Fig. 2.12 Gingival racial pigmentation

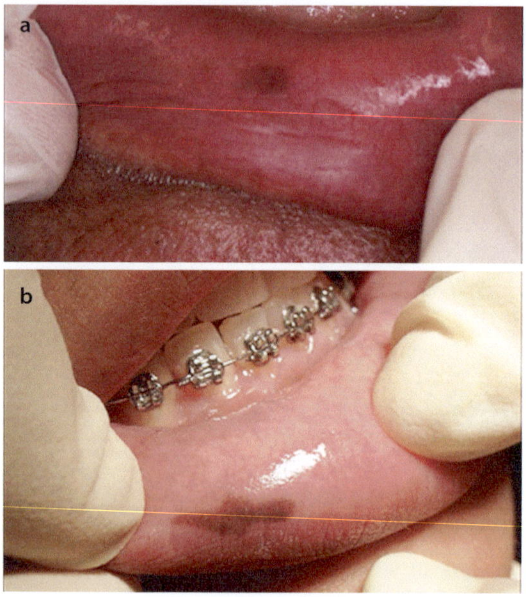

Fig. 2.13 a, b Pigmented melanotic macules. (Courtesy of Drs. Mauricio Wiltz and Robert Kelsch)

Peutz-Jeghers syndrome Mucocutaneous melanotic macules, intestinal hamartomatous polyps, and increased risk of carcinomas of the gastrointestinal tract, pancreas, breast, and thyroid. The mucocutaneous melanotic macules are small and concentrated around the lips.

McCune-Albright syndrome Mono-ostotic or polyostotic fibrous dysplasia and diffuse or discrete melanotic macules of the lips and oral mucosa.

Carney complex Spotty skin pigmentations, occasional oral melanotic macules, myxomas, endocrine overactivity.

Histopathologically, these lesions are characterized by melanin within the basal squamous epithelial cells. Scattered single melanocytes can be seen at the basal epithelium and aggregate at rete ridges, there should be no melanocytic atypia. Melanophages can also be observed in the lamina propria (Fig. 2.14).

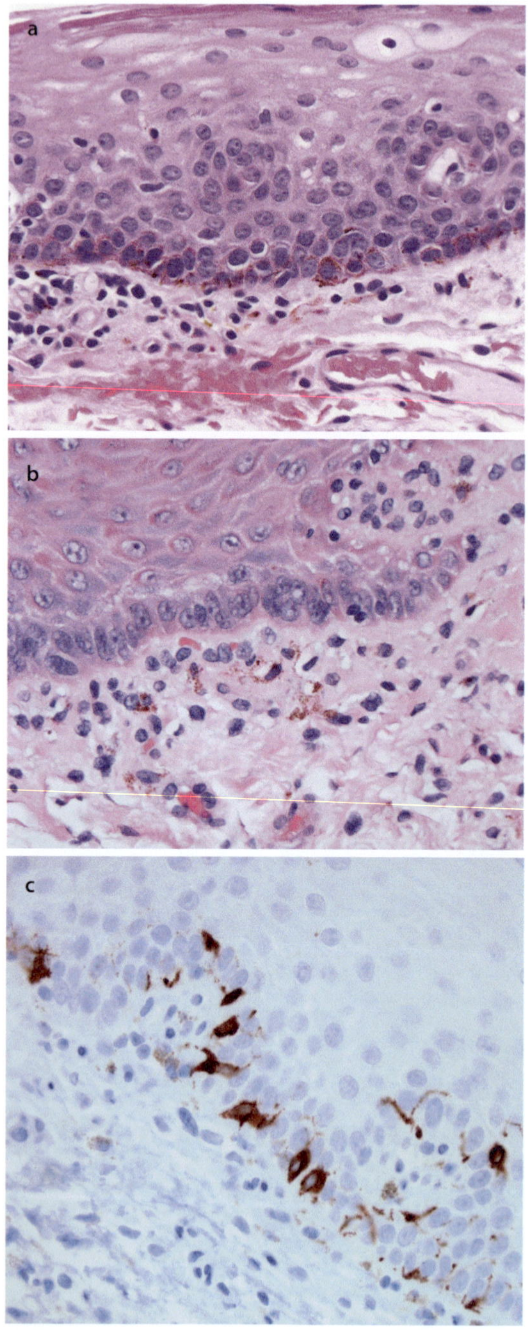

Fig. 2.14 a Benign melanosis of basal cells. b Pigmentary incontinence: melanin uptake by macrophages. c HMB45 highlights intramucosal melanocytes

2.8 Mucosal Melanocytic Nevi

Nevi are common, benign melanocytic proliferations of the skin; they are classified as either **junctional** (melanocytes localized at the epidermal/dermal junction), **intradermal** (entirely within the dermis), or **compound** (within both epidermis and dermis). Oral nevi (also referred to as **mucosal melanocytic nevi, intramucosal nevi**) are extremely rare and their classification is analogous to dermal nevi; they are classified as either **junctional, submucosal,** (also referred to as **intramucosal** or **subepithelial**, analogous to intradermal) or **compound**. More than half of intraoral nevi are classified as **submucosal nevi**, followed by **common blue nevi** [20]. **Junctional** and **compound nevi** comprise only 3–6% of all oral nevi.

Clinically, oral mucosal nevi are typically well-circumscribed; submucosal and compound oral nevi are raised and dome-shaped whereas junctional oral nevi are flat. Oral nevi are usually single, but occasionally may be multiple. About 75% of oral nevi are smaller than 6 mm. The majority of oral nevi are pigmented, varying from brown to black to grey or blue. Nonpigmented nevi can clinically resemble fibromas or papillomas. **Submucosal nevi** are most commonly found on the hard palate (25%), buccal mucosa (25%), gingiva (17%), vermillion border of the lip (12%), and labial mucosa (9%). Two thirds of **common blue nevi** occur in the hard palate and are generally smaller than submucosal nevi, and almost 90% are smaller than 6 mm. **Junctional and compound nevi** are usually diagnosed in individuals under the age of 40. By contrast, there is a wider age range distribution for submucosal nevi with a peak incidence in the fifth decade. This supports the theory that melanocytic nevi go through junctional and compound phases before becoming submucosal. There is no evidence that benign oral nevi may be precursor lesions for melanoma.

Histologically, **junctional oral nevi** are composed of melanocyte nests at the mucosal/submucosal junction, especially at the tips of the rete pegs. **Submucosal oral nevi** are composed of melanocyte nests located entirely within the submucosa (◘ Fig. 2.15). **Compound oral nevi** are composed of melanocytic nests within the submucosa and at the mucosal/submucosal junction (◘ Fig. 2.16). Zones of maturation can be seen in both submucosal and compound nevi starting from the bottom and maturing upwards. **Type A** nevus cells are epithelioid with abundant pink cytoplasm and large round or oval nuclei; they are present in the superficial aspects of nevi. Larger type A cells usually contain melanin. **Type B** cells are smaller, resemble lymphocytes, and are usually found in the mid portion of nevi. **Type C** cells are spindled and resemble fibroblasts; they

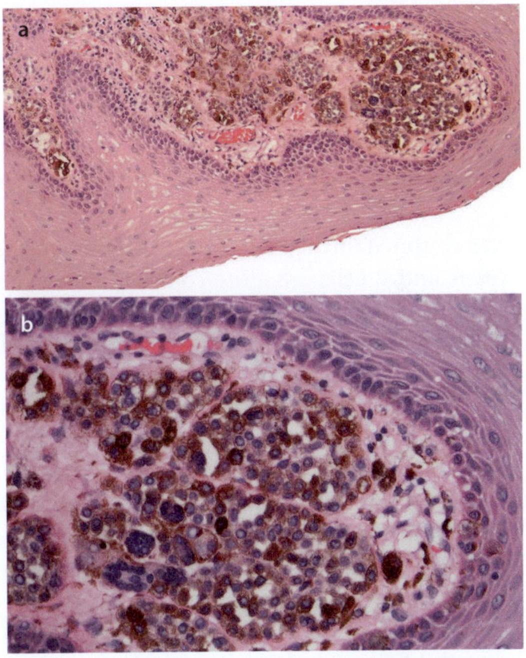

◘ **Fig. 2.15** **a** Intraoral compound nevus: Junctional nests of nevus cells. **b** Typical pigmented nevus cell have viarably sized round dark nuclei with intranuclear holes

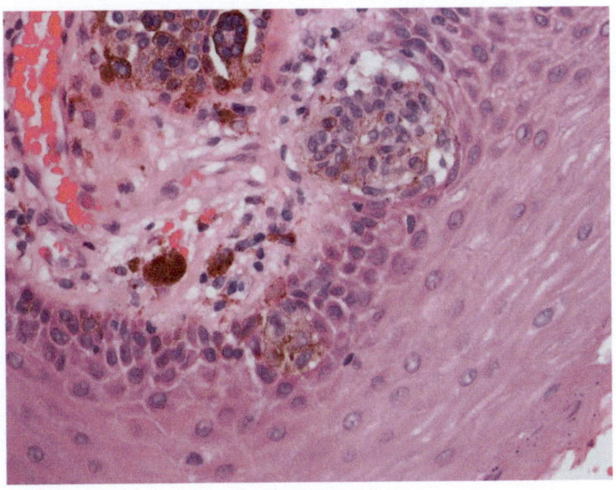

◘ **Fig. 2.16** Intraoral *submucosal* nevus – the mucosal equivalent of an intradermal nevus

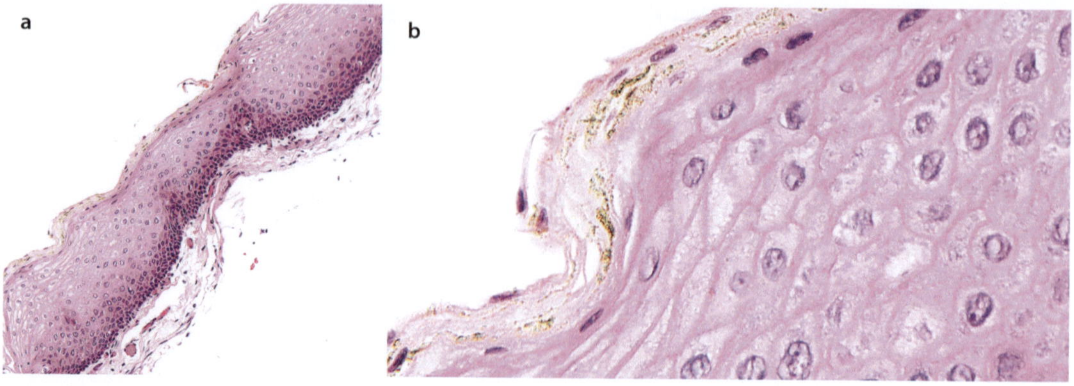

Fig. 2.17 a, b Argyria: Silver nitrate deposition seen in the superficial squamous mucosa

are found in the deeper aspects of nevi. **Type D** cells are multinucleated nevus giant cells and are often scattered throughout the lesion. In oral nevi, type A and B cells are more common than type C cells. In nonpigmented nevi, type A cells are often absent. **Common blue nevi** are composed of submucosal, pigmented, spindled melanocytes (type C cells), stromal fibrosis, pigmented dendritic melanocytes, and melanophages within the deep tissues (in this case submucosa). Variants of blue nevi include epithelioid (cellular) blue nevi and compound blue nevi. **Cellular blue nevi** are composed of densely cellular plump spindled melanocytes within the submucosa.

Other nevus variants are extremely rare in oral cavity. The **combined nevus** is composed of a blue nevus plus another nevus, usually a compound nevus. The **balloon cell nevus** is composed of melanocyte clusters with abundant, finely vacuolated, *clear* cytoplasm, and more typical melanocytes at the periphery of the lesion. Balloon cell change is thought to be due to impairment of melanogenesis. A **Spitz nevus is** usually a compound nevus and is characterized by a mixture of large, spindled and epithelioid melanocytes. The epithelioid melanocytes have bizarre shapes, may be multinucleated and have multiple large nucleoli. Superficial abundant mitotic figures and Pagetoid spread of melanocytes can be seen. Features that distinguish Spitz nevus from melanoma include symmetry, sharp lateral demarcation, absent or rare mitoses, no atypical mitoses, and maturation of cellular elements toward the mucosa. The term congenital nevus is used for either an intramucosal or compound nevus that is present at birth; this represents a very rare entity [21]

Dysplastic nevi are either junctional (mucosal/submucosal junction) or compound (mucosal/submucosal junction plus submucosa) nevi which can harbor the following findings: **Shoulder phenomenon**, which refers to the junctional component extending laterally beyond the beyond the submucosal component, **bridging**, which refers to poorly circumscribed melanocytic nests which form connections between adjacent rete ridges, and melanocyte atypia with respect to nuclear size and intramucosal location [20]

Melanin is recognized in H + E stained sections as fine, dusty brown pigment. The uniform fineness of the granularity distinguishes it from hemosiderin, which is more "chunky" and less uniform. Dermal/mucosal melanin is nonrefractile whereas neuromelanin is refractile. Figure 2.17 is an example of another dark pigment silver nitrate, deposition, seen only in the superficial epithelium.

2.9 Geographic Tongue

Geographic tongue (benign migratory glossitis) is a benign condition seen in up to 3% of the general population. Patients are usually asymptomatic; some patients complain of dysgeusia, or sensitivity to hot and spicy foods [22]. Geographic tongue manifests as an erythematous lesion with atrophic filiform papillae, surrounded by a well-demarcated, serpiginous, yellow- white, hyperkeratotic border (Fig. 2.18). Patients often report spontaneous resolution of the lesion in

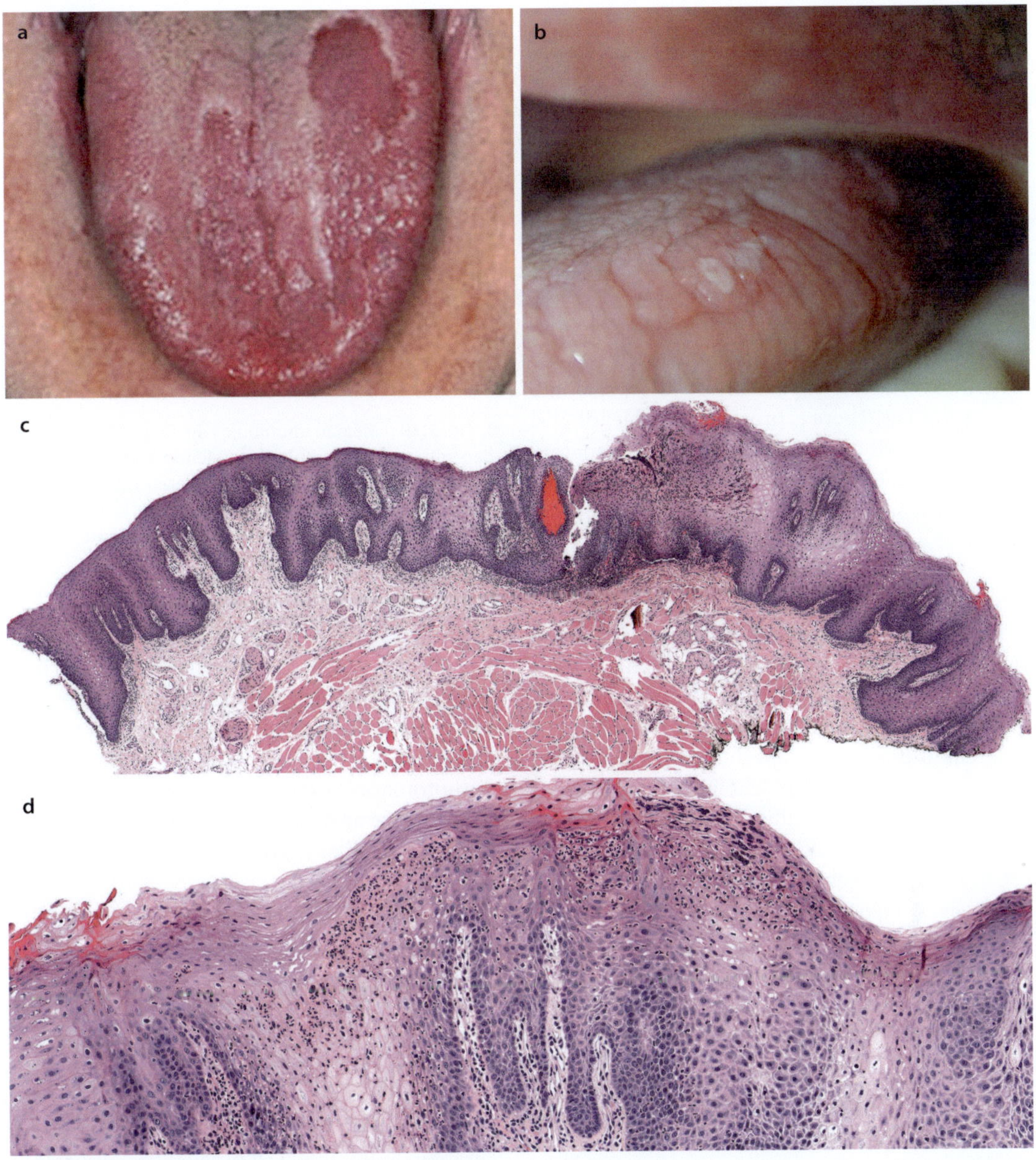

Fig. 2.18 **a** Geographic tongue appears as a well-demarcated atrophic erythematous area with a serpiginous, white border. The lesion occurs on the tongue dorsum and may extend to the lateral tongue. The serpiginous white border results in a map-like "geographic" appearance. **b** Fissured tongue is commonly associated with geographic tongue. (Courtesy of Dr. Robert Kelsch). **c**, **d** Hyperplastic, acanthotic squamous epithelium with long, fused rete pegs and robust intramucosal abscesses

one area, with the return of normal architecture, but the concomitant development of new tongue lesions elsewhere.

The specific etiology of geographic tongue is unknown, although it is thought to be autoimmune or allergic in origin, and triggered by stress. Geographic tongue frequently is associated with fissured tongue, characterized by grooves of variable depth along the dorsal and lateral tongue. A strong association has been noted between geographic tongue and pustular dermal psoriasis [23]. It has also been associated with a number of other conditions such as hypertension [24], Down's syndrome, lichen planus, Reiter syndrome, juvenile diabetes, iron-deficient anemia, celiac disease, and allergy. The dynamic pattern of migrating inflammation, especially the spiral patterns, are quite unique to geographic tongue; a wave-like response to local irritation has been suggested [25]

Histopathologically, the central atrophic region is characterized by loss of filiform papillae and desquamated keratin. The periphery demonstrates variable epithelial acanthosis, hyperplasia and downward expansion of rete pegs, and hyperkeratosis. There is prominent intraepithelial spongiosis with acute and chronic inflammatory exudate and superficial microabscesses (Munroe's microabscesses, pustular mucositis). Rare Candida hyphae may be observed.

Confirmation of the anatomic site as dorsal tongue limits the differential diagnosis to few other entities that can affect this site: median rhomboid glossitis, secondary syphilis, and granular cell tumor. Usually, the possibility of geographic tongue will be included in the clinical differential diagnosis. Superficial microabscesses are not seen in median rhomboid glossitis or lingual secondary syphilis, the latter is characterized by a dense and deep submucosal plasma cell infiltrate which can extend around vessels and nerves. Hyperplastic chronic Candidiasis is associated with superficially invasive Candida hyphae. Superficial biopsy of a dorsal granular cell tumor may reveal pronounced 'pseudoepithelial hyperplasia", however, a submucosal mass will be clinically appreciated. The vast majority of cases of geographic tongue are self-limiting, requiring no treatment.

2.10 Median Rhomboid Glossitis

Median rhomboid glossitis (central papillary atrophy, posterior midline atrophic candidiasis) specifically affects the ***posterior midline dorsal tongue, anterior to the circumvallate papillae.***

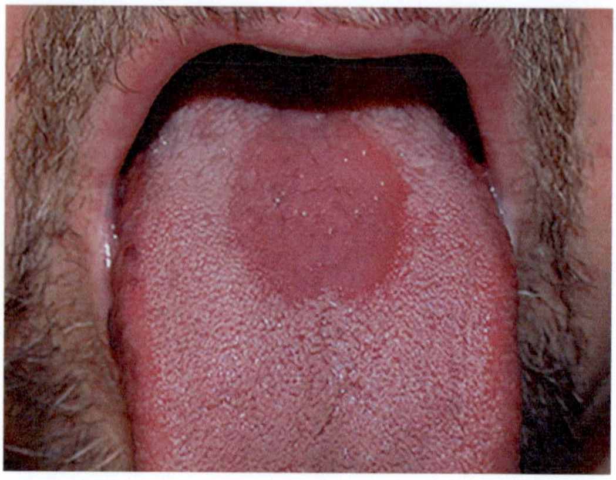

Fig. 2.19 Median Rhomboid Glossitis – 62-year-old man with a pink, atrophic, depapillated lesion of midline dorsum tongue. This is usually associated with poor oral hygiene, tobacco use, and Candidiasis. (Courtesy of Eric Ehrsam, MD, ► www.dermatlas.org/derm, with permission)

(Fig. 2.19) Lesional contact with the palate may result in "kissing lesions". There is a male predilection and most patients are middle aged. An association with diabetes and oral Candida has been noted [26, 27]. Most patients are asymptomatic Lesions are usually smaller than 2 cm. in size and have a smooth, flat red surface reflecting papillary atrophy. Raised mammillary lesions can occur. Occasionally, median rhomboid glossitis can develop more anteriorly but it has not been described posterior to the circumvallate papillae.

Histopathologically, median rhomboid glossitis is an atrophic process characterized by loss of papillae. (Fig. 2.20) The surface mucosa is flattened with elongated, branching, and anastomosing rete pegs. Hyperparakeratosis is variable. Submucosal lymphocytic infiltrate is present. There is intraepithelial inflammation. Fungal hyphae can be found commonly in parakeratin and/or invading the spinous layers, but the absence of *Candida* does not mitigate against the diagnosis in the correct setting.

The differential diagnosis includes geographic tongue and chronic hyperplastic Candidiasis.

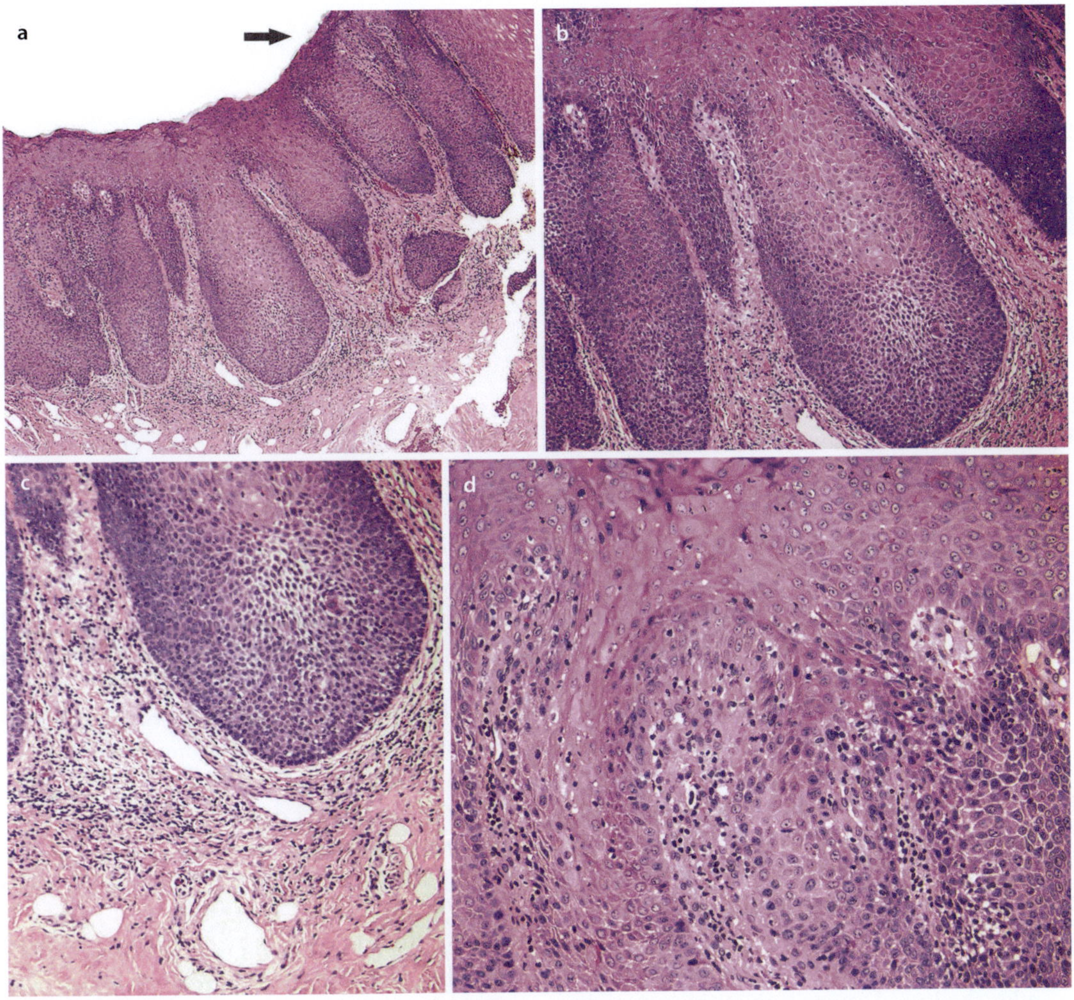

Fig. 2.20 Median Rhomboid Glossitis **a** Flattened atrophic surface (*arrow*). **b**, **c** Hyperplastic rete pegs. **d** Compare this nonspecific intramucosal inflammatory infiltrate to the pustular microabscesses of geographic tongue

Pautrier's microabscesses are characteristic of geographic tongue, and not present in median rhomboid glossitis. Chronic hyperplastic Candidiasis is the opposite of an atrophic process, the epithelial surface demonstrates corrugated to papillary hyperplasia. Atrophic glossitis can also be caused by nutritional deficiencies, alcoholism, and medications.

2.11 Candida

Primary oral candidiasis (thrush) usually affects adults with some predisposing condition such as diabetes, dentures, decreased saliva due to radiation or Sjogren's syndrome, steroid inhalants, or tobacco. Newborn thrush is common in the first months of life and associated with

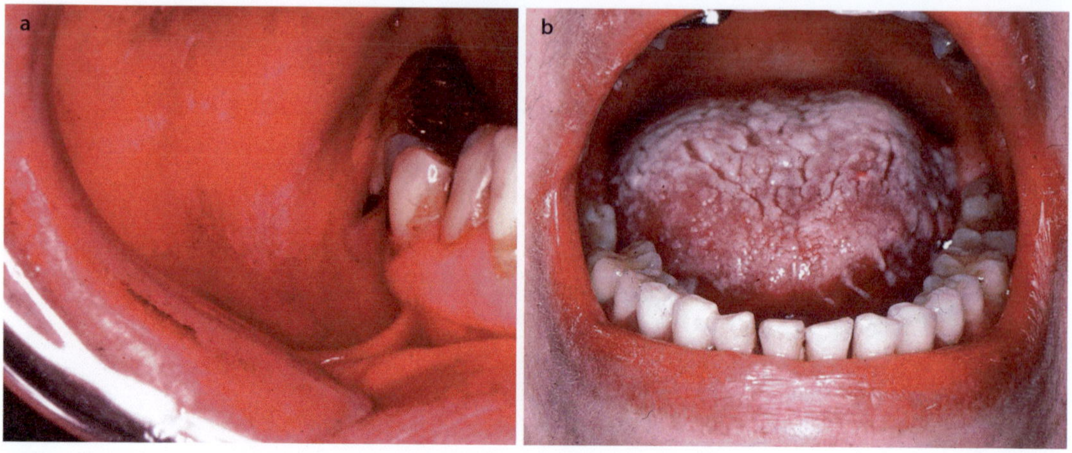

Fig. 2.21 **a** Buccal Chronic Candidiasis results in erythematous mucosa with white to yellow, curd-like (pseudomembranous) exudate. **b** Lingual Chronic Candidiasis with exuberant pseudomembrane

perinatal exposure or concomitant diaper rash. Childhood thrush can be seen with chronic use of steroid inhalants for asthma. **Secondary oral candidiasis** can be due to a number of conditions, such as Familial Chronic Mucocutaneous Candidosis, DiGeorge syndrome, Chronic Granulomatous Disease, Severe Combined Immunedeficiency, Candidosis Endocrinopathy syndrome, organ transplant, and AIDS [28–33]. Oropharyngeal candidiasis is the most common opportunistic infection encountered in HIV-infected patients. Lastly, there is a group of conditions referred to **Candida-associated lesions:** angular cheilitis, denture stomatitis, and median rhomboid glossitis.

Oral thrush commonly involves the buccal commissures, buccal mucosa, palate, and tongue. Patients complain of burning and pain. The oral mucosa is ulcerated with a white, creamy, or milk curd-like pseudomembranous exudate. (Fig. 2.21) Stripping the mucosal pseudomembrane leaves a raw bleeding surface. **Chronic hyperplastic candidiasis** produces leukoplakic lesions of the buccal mucosa, palate, and tongue, which may be homogeneous, or nodular (speckled erythroleukoplakia). The nodular lesions can cause soreness or discomfort whereas homogenous lesions are usually asymptomatic. **Angulitis chielitis** refers to formation of red, swollen crusty patches at the oral commissures which may be painful and itchy. It is associated *C albicans* and *S aureus* infection, usually in conjunction with other predisposing factors such as malnutrition, smoking, impaired immunity. **Denture stomatitis** is a common condition in the elderly causing asymptomatic erythema and petechial in regions in contact with upper dentures.

Candida albicans in the most common pathogenic species, followed by *C glabrata, C tropicalis, C parapsilosis,* and *C krusei.* The ability of *Candida* to adhere to the polymethylacrylate material of dentures promotes colonization and multispecies biofilm formation, allowing for a persistent *Candida* reservoir [34–36]. Fungal virulence is enhanced by secreted aspartyl proteinases, phospholipases, and the production of extracellular matrix which sequesters antifungal agents.

Histopathologically, the oral mucosa is acutely inflamed and microabscesses can be seen. The squamous mucosa shows variable hyperplasia with ortho- or parakeratosis. *Candida* pseudohyphae and abundant small, oval, globose yeasts can be observed on H + E, periodic acid Schiff, or Gomori methanamine silver stains (Fig. 2.22). Hyphal invasion is always limited to the parakeratotic layer. *Candida* pseudohyphae are thin, regular, and "pinched" at the point of pseudoseptation. True branching is not seen.

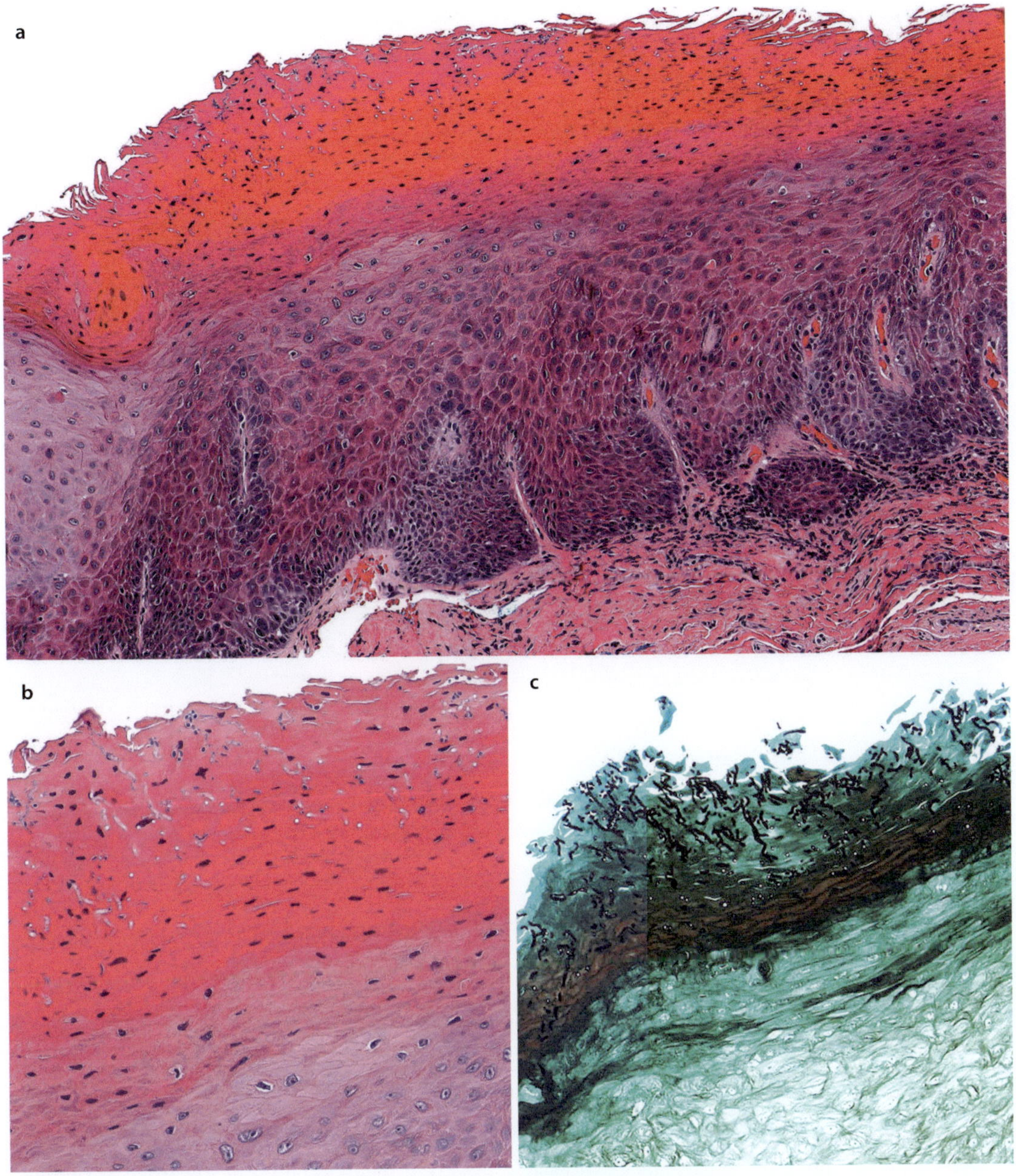

Fig. 2.22 **a** Any intramucosal neutrophils should prompt you to consider Candida infection. Here we see an unusual degree of hyperplasia and hyperkeratosis, due to chronic Candidiasis. **b** Candida pseudohypae can be seen on H + E stain, superficially invading up to the granular layer. **c** GMS

2.12 Heck's Disease (Focal Epithelial Hyperplasia)

Focal epithelial hyperplasia, or Heck's disease, has a strong genetic predisposition and is seen among American Navajo Indians, South American Indians, Greenlandic, Alaskan and Canadian Eskimos, and Laplanders. It is extremely rare, but documented among Caucasians [37–41]. Usually, the diagnosis is made in the first two decades; there is a known female predisposition.

Heck's disease causes lesions on the lower lip, buccal mucosa, tongue and labial commissure. Clinically, they are soft, pale, sharply circumscribed, and elevated, round to oval, papular or plaque-like, and either red, pink, gray or white. Characteristically,

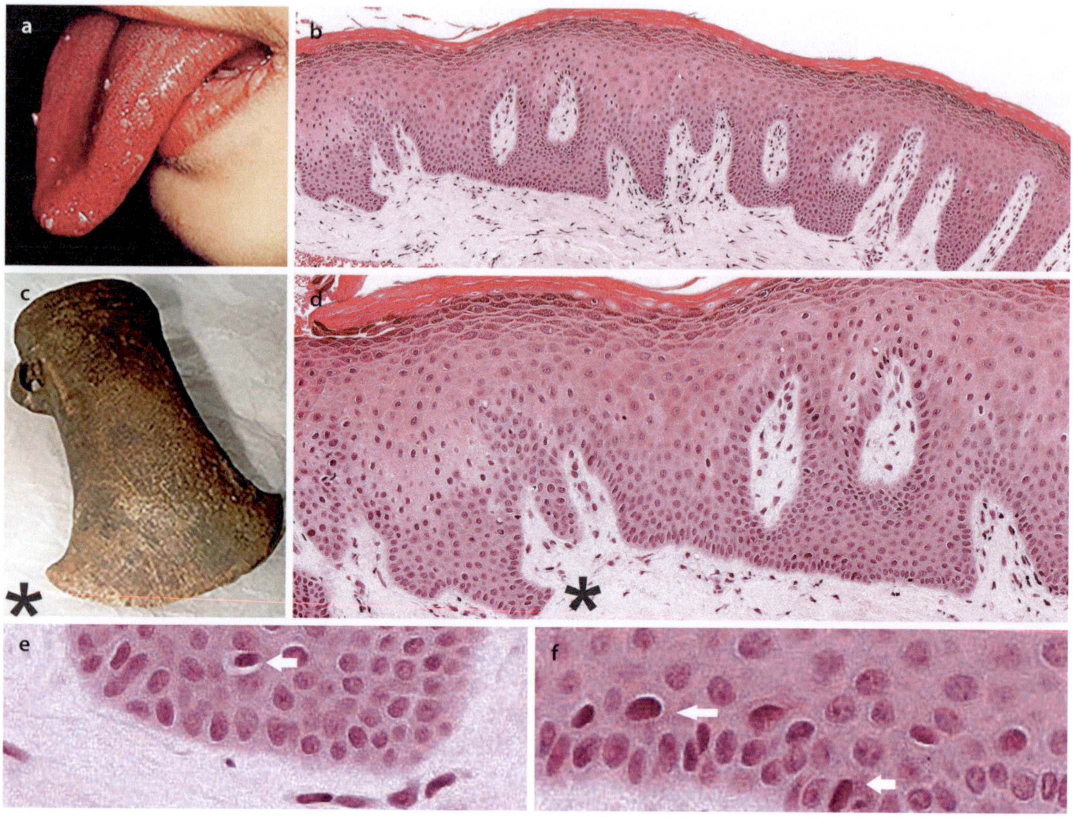

Fig. 2.23 **a** Heck's Disease (Focal Epithelial Hyperplasia): Multiple raised, smooth, lingual and labial papules on 4-year-old child [41]. **b** The silhouette of the broad, hyperplastic rete pegs has been likened to a "Bronze age axe". **c** Notice the flaring out (*) at the working end of a "Bronze age axe". **d** Elongated and fused rete pegs with lateral wings (*). **e**, **f** Brick-shaped "mitosoid" bodies (*arrows*). (Courtesy of Dr. Carla Penner)

the lesions have a smooth pearly surface and "disappear" when the mucosa is stretched. Lesions may be single but are often multiple and clustered; flat-topped or sessile, and in extreme cases the confluent lesions result in a "cobblestone" mucosa. For this reason, the term "multifocal papillomavirus epithelial hyperplasia" has been suggested as a replacement for "Focal epithelial hyperplasia".

HPV13 is usually detected in Heck's disease; [42] HPV32 is detected less frequently. Transmission occurs via routine household contact and it is common for siblings to be affected. The lesions are asymptomatic and may spontaneously regress; there is no potential for malignant progression [43]. Symptomatic lesions may be managed by conservative local means [41]

Histopathologically, FEH is characterized by acanthotic, hyperplastic squamous mucosa, which is hyperkeratotic, parakeratotic, with elongated, anastomosing rete pegs. (Fig. 2.23) The silhouette of some rete pegs has been likened to a "**bronze age ax**" because the distal tips expand out laterally. Squamous metaplasia and hyperplasia may continue into underlying minor salivary ducts. Typical koilocytes can be seen. A characteristic finding is "mitosoid" nuclear degeneration; the nuclei are enlarged with clumped chromatin mimicking mitotic figures.

The differential diagnosis includes **exophytic papilloma**, which demonstrates well-defined, exophytic fibrovascular stalks and **condyloma**, which is sessile and broad-based. The thin elongated rete pegs of a condyloma point towards the center of the lesion and the "bronze ax" silhouette is lacking. **Verruca vulgaris** is exophytic lesion with a serrated surface contour composed of hyperplastic, hyperkeratotic epithelium with a pronounced granular layer and serrated spires. The rete pegs of verruca are also elongated and relatively thin, pointing towards the lesion's center.

2.13 Condyloma

Condyloma acuminatum (venereal wart) is a common genitourinary tract epithelial proliferation mediated by Human Papillomavirus (HPV).

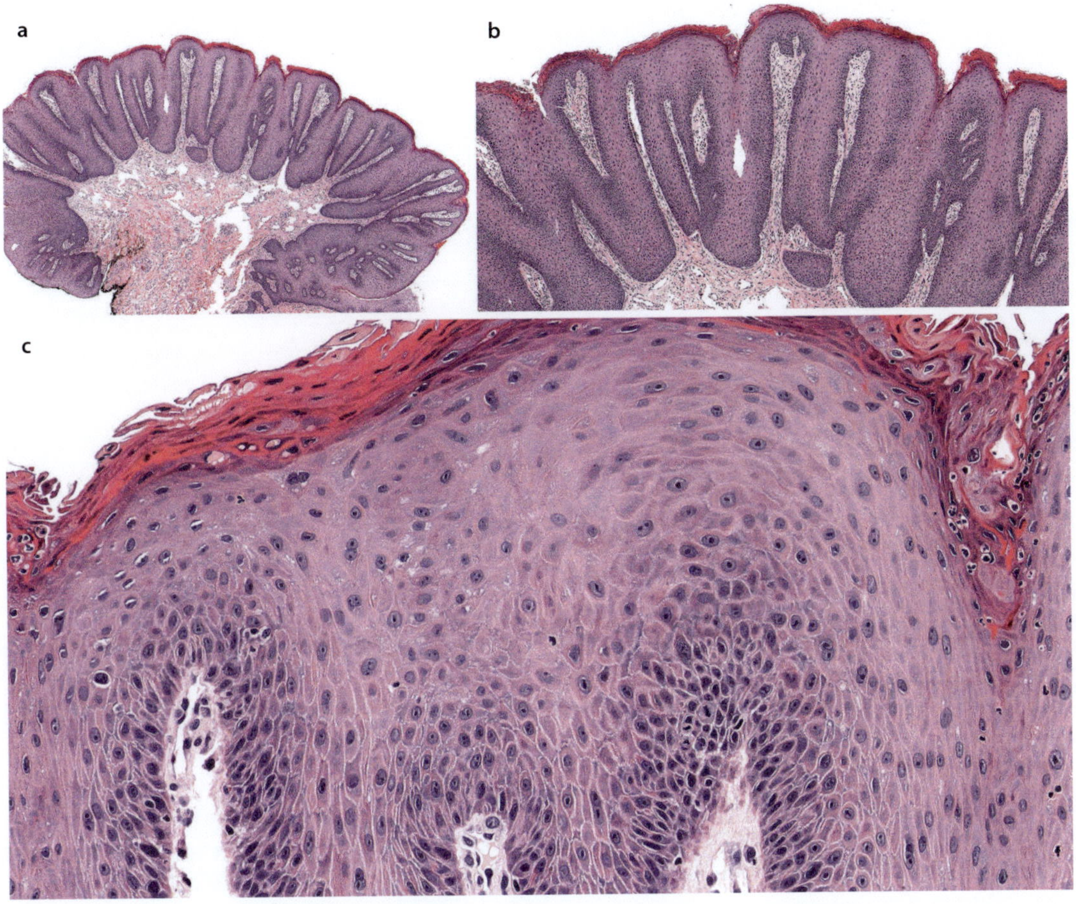

Fig. 2.24 a–c Oral condyloma in an HIV+ patient

Intraoral condyloma can also be encountered (with or without concomitant genital lesions) arising from gingiva, buccal mucosa, lips, and palate [41, 44–47]. The incidence of oral condyloma in the general population is very low; the incidence is higher in HIV+ patients, and higher yet in patients responding to highly active antiretroviral therapy (HAART), likely an immune reconstitution phenomenon [48, 49]. Clinically, condyloma can vary from small, pink, red, sessile growths to larger, grey white pedunculated exophytic lesions. The surface may have a cobblestone appearance or exophytic projections.

Histopathologically, a condyloma demonstrates epithelial hyperplasia with prominent acanthosis and parakeratosis (Fig. 2.24). The papillary projections are blunter compared to exophytic papillomas. Koilocytic change (irregular shrunken nuclei and perinuclear halo) may be seen in the spinous layer but are not requisite for the diagnosis. Dysplastic oral condylomas are more likely associated with high-risk HPV and impaired immune status.

2.14 Hairy Leukoplakia

The two most common oral lesions seen in HIV+ patients in the post-HAART (highly active antiretroviral therapy) era are oral hairy leukoplakia and Candidiasis. Oral hairy leukoplakia presents as a white plaque on the lateral tongue with ill-defined borders, and a raised, corrugated or "hairy" like appearance. Other intraoral sites include ventral tongue and the junction of hard and soft palate. Oral hairy leukoplakia is caused by an active, productive (lytic) EBV infection [50]. The presence of oral hairy leukoplakia has been significantly associated with high HIV viral loads (>3000 copies/ul), oral Candida, lack of HAART therapy, and the presence of antifungal therapy. Development of oral hairy leukoplakia is not limited to HIV+ patients and may also occur in solid organ transplant recipients, patients with hematologic malignancies, and those receiving steroid therapy (either systemic or inhalant) [51–53].

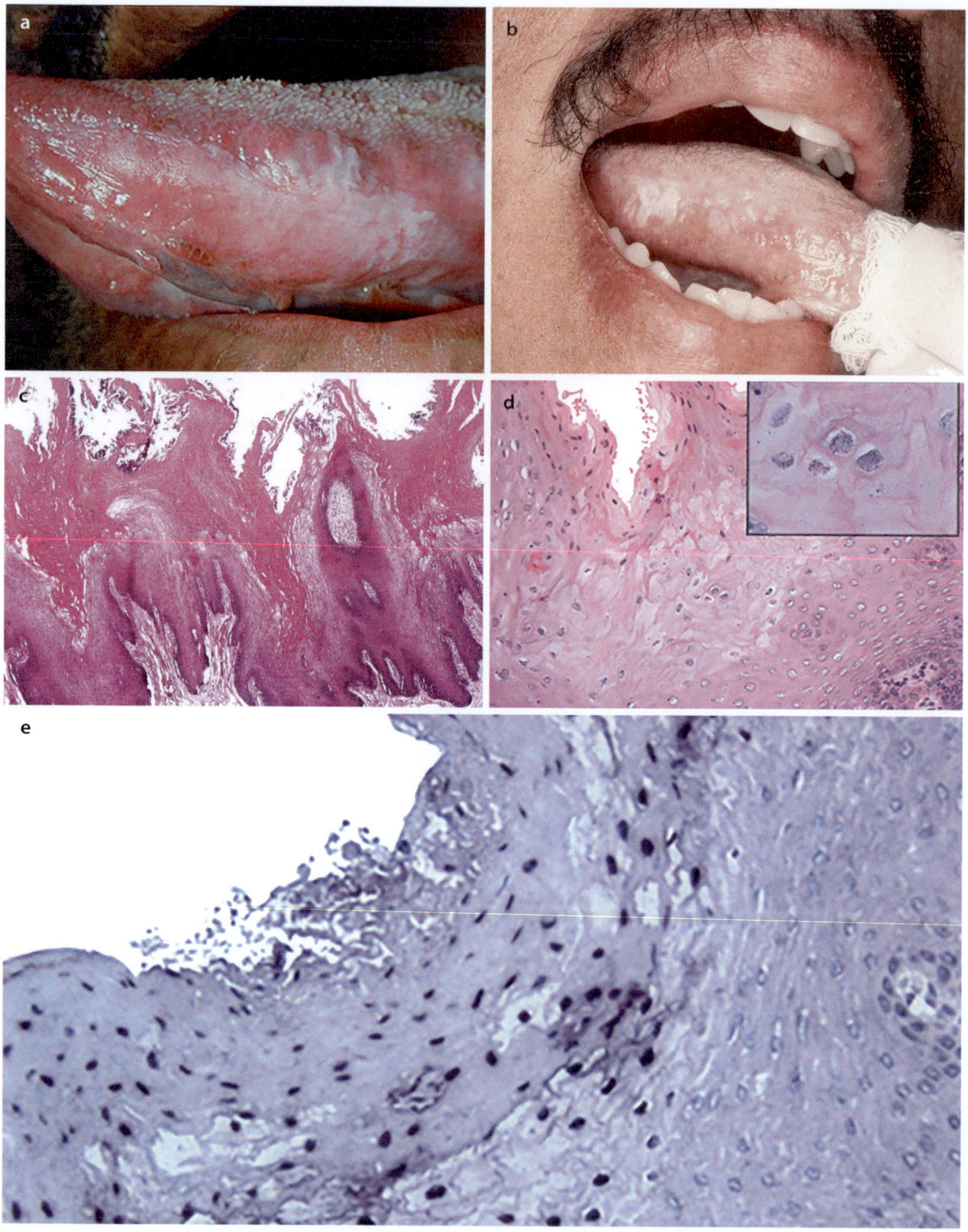

Fig. 2.25 **a**, **b** Hairy Leukoplakia – Corrugated leukoplakia on the lateral tongue. (Courtesy of Dr. Marie Ramer). **c** Spikey hyperkeratosis **d** Viral infected nuclei show chromatin margination and beading, thus mimicking a string of pearls. **e** EBER

Histopathologically, the mucosal surface of oral hairy leukoplakia is irregular, with ridges and "hair-like" keratin projections. The squamous epithelium is hyperplastic, acanthotic, and hyperparakeratotic. Characteristic intranuclear Cowdry A type "ground glass" inclusions are seen in the upper stratum spinosum. "Beads" of marginalized chromatin surround these intranuclear inclusions. The presence of intranuclear EBER (EBV untranslated RNAs) in these cells is diagnostic (Fig. 2.25). Koilocytes and *Candida* may also be present.

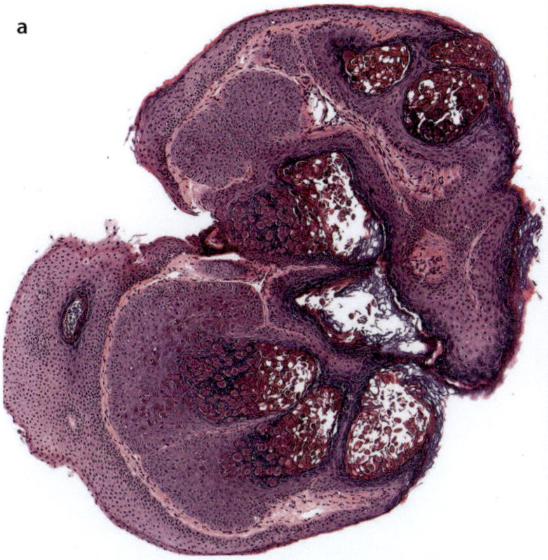

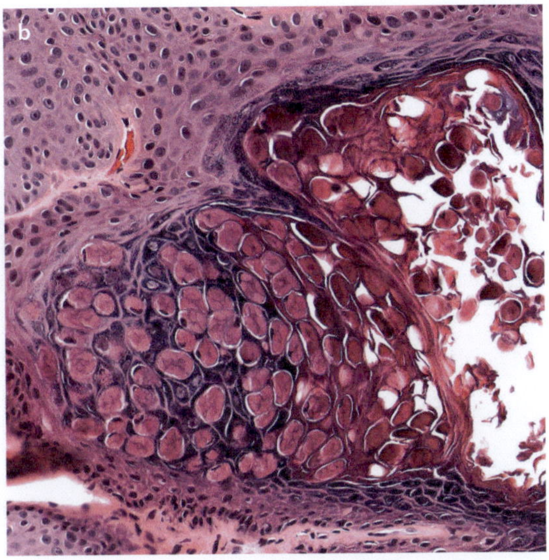

Fig. 2.26 **a, b** Labial molluscum contageosum – Molluscum bodies refer to infected cells. Infection causes umbilicated papules. The cytoplasmic viral inclusions enlarge and transition from eosinophilic to basophilic. Keratinous debris and infectious mollluscum bodies are discharged from the center of these papules

2.15 Molluscum Contagiosum

Molluscum contagiosum is a common eruptive lesion caused by the MC virus, a DNA poxvirus, which is transmitted by direct contact. It is usually seen in the first two decades of life. MC infection results in eruption of asymptomatic, single or multiple small, pink waxy *dermal* papules with central umbilication. *Intraoral mucosal* molluscum contagiosum is extremely uncommon [54, 55].

Histopathologically, the infected epithelium forms a cup-like crater. Enlarging cytoplasmic viral inclusions transition from eosinophilic to basophilic (mollluscum bodies). Keratinous debris and infectious mollluscum bodies are discharged from the center of these papules (Fig. 2.26).

2.16 Histoplasmosis

Histoplasma capsulatum is endemic to North America and South America, and is associated with bird and bat droppings. The severity of infection after exposure is dependent upon inoculum dose, host immunity, pulmonary status, and fungal virulence. The range of manifestations in oral histoplasmosis includes a localized lesion in an immune competent patient to the initial manifestation of disseminated infection in HIV+ individuals [56–61]. The oral lesions form red, ulcerated, painful nodules with a pseudomembranous exudate. Histopathologically, there is a dense granulomatous inflammatory infiltrate with multinucleated giant cells (Fig. 2.27). The tiny intracytoplasmic yeast forms (1–4 microns)

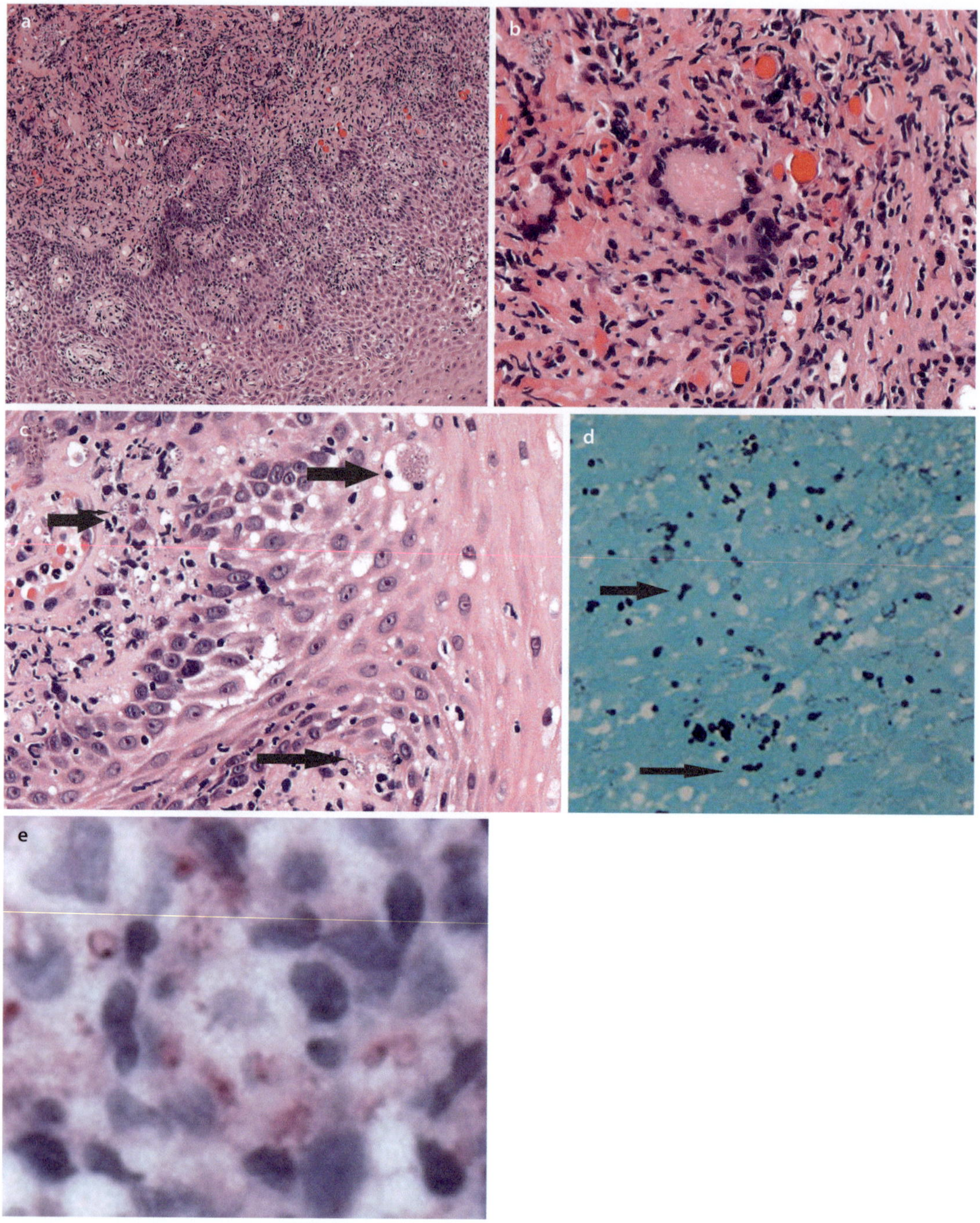

Fig. 2.27 **a**, **b** Oral Histoplasma infection – intense, mixed inflammatory infiltrate and occasional multinucleated giant cells. **c** You can see the tiny intracytoplasmic amphophilic organisms on H + E (*arrows*). **d** GMS stain – Look for budding yeast forms (*arrows*). **e** Histoplasma is also positive on PAS stain

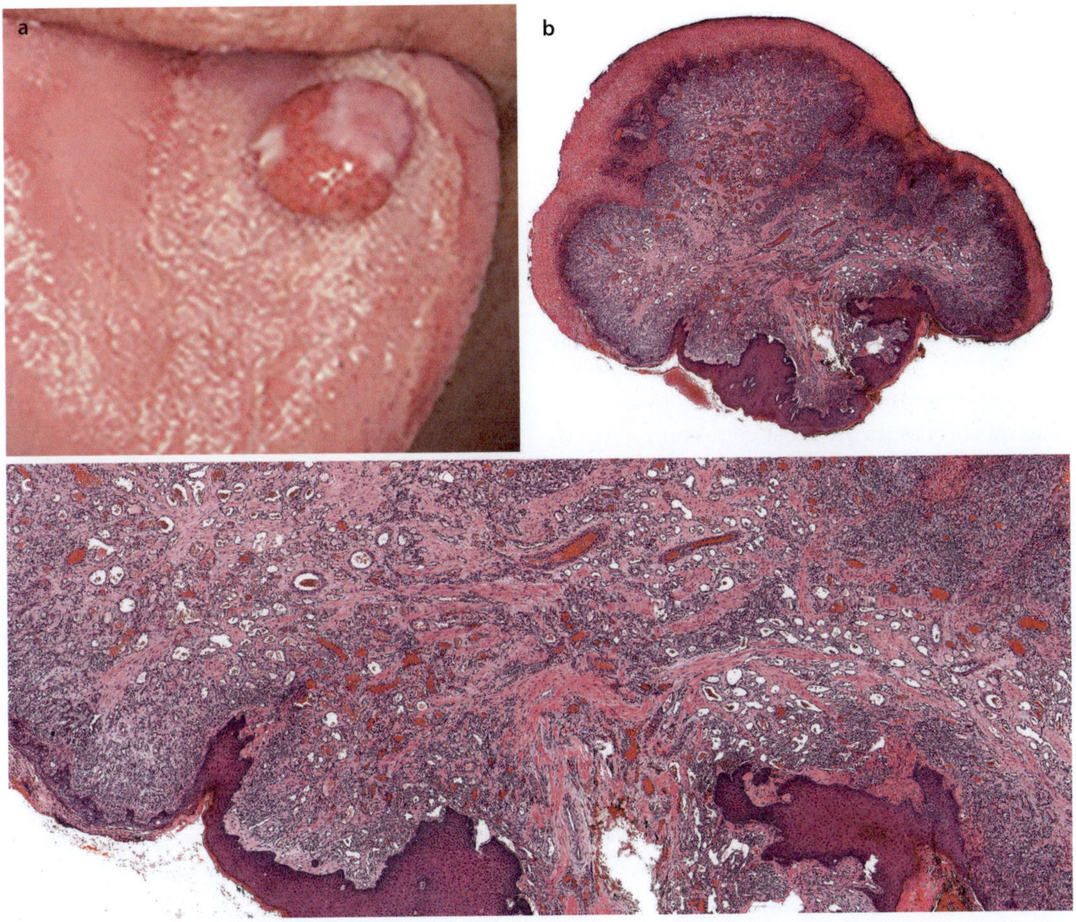

■ **Fig. 2.28** Pyogenic granuloma **a** Discreet raised lesion on dorsal tongue. (Courtesy of Dr. Richard V Smith). **b** Polypoid lesion forming vascular lobules with a distinctive collarette of squamous mucosa. **c**: Inset: Inflamed granulation tissue. **c** Pyogenic granuloma is nothing more than vascular granulation tissue

are observed in macrophages and giant cells. They stain with Gomori silver and periodic acid-Schiff stains. Budding yeasts are diagnostic and elevated serum antibody titers are confirmatory.

2.17 Pyogenic Granuloma

Pyogenic granuloma describes a common, reactive vascular proliferation which occurs with a female predominance. A history of prior trauma is common [62–64]. Pyogenic granulomas have been reported secondary to dental implants [65, 66]. They can present as rapidly enlarging smooth, pedunculated or sessile, tan/white or red/purple lesions which tends to bleed. They may enlarge during puberty, pregnancy (pregnancy tumor), or menopause. Spontaneous post-partum regression has been known to occur. There is a striking predisposition for gingival involvement, either marginal or interdental; anterior maxillary gingival involvement is more common than mandibular gingiva. Other oral sites include lips, tongue dorsum and buccal mucosa. Pyogenic granulomas range from millimeters to several centimeters in size and may mimic malignancy [67]. In fact, this diagnosis can be very gratifying to make in the face of a clinical impression of cancer. Pyogenic granulomas are cured by local excision. However, local recurrence has been associated with satellitosis, which should not cast doubt on the original diagnosis [68, 69]

Histopathologically, there is no "granuloma" in pyogenic granuloma. Pyogenic granuloma is composed of vascularized granulation tissue that forms lobular clusters of proliferating new blood vessels. (Hence the synonym capillary hemangioma.) (■ Fig. 2.28). The endothelium is plump and mitotically active. There is a prominent acute and chronic inflammatory component. The mucosal surface is usually ulcerated and a "collarette" of intact mucosa may be seen at the periphery.

2.18 Peripheral Giant Cell Granuloma (Giant Cell Epulis)

Peripheral giant cell granuloma is an uncommon reactive lesion that may arise within the jaw bone (central), or peripherally from the periodontal ligament, periosteum, or mucosal tissue. The gingival soft tissues are most commonly affected, usually in the premolar, canine, or incisor regions. There is a slight mandibular predisposition as compared to maxillary sites. Most patients are in the fourth to sixth decades of life, but a wide age range is reported. There is a slight female predilection. The typical presentation is that of a rapidly growing red/pink/purple, sessile/pedunculated, smooth papule or nodule which may be ulcerated. Peripheral giant cell granulomas can reach impressive, considerable sizes, leaving bony destruction in their wake; they have been associated with poor dentition, periodontal disease, poor dental restorations, dental extractions, ill-fitting dentures, and dental implants [70–74]. Peripheral giant cell granuloma are cured by local excision or curettage. However, local recurrence can occur [75].

Histopathologically, this lesion contains numerous osteoclast-like multinucleated giant cells with pale vesicular nuclei, embedded within a background of spindled mesenchymal stromal cells with similar pale vesicular nuclei and eosinophilic cytoplasm (■ Fig. 2.29). Mitotic activity is common in these stromal cells. There is variable inflammation and a fibroblastic/collagenized background. Blood vessels are numerous with plump endothelial nuclei, scattered extravasated erythrocytes, and hemosiderin deposition. Mineralization, cementum-like deposition, and bone formation can be seen.

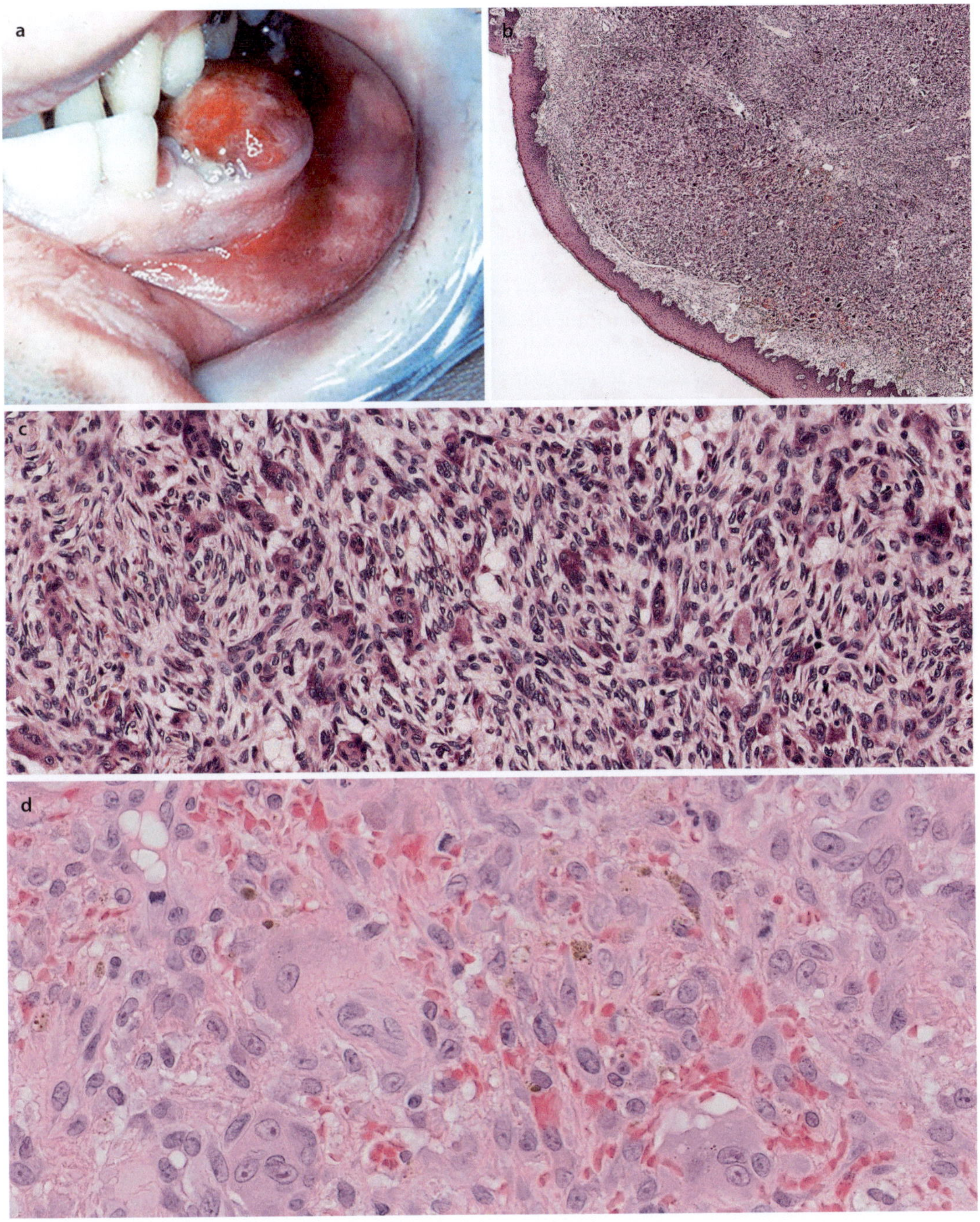

Fig. 2.29 **a** "Epulis" is a general term for a reactive gingival lesion. A giant cell epulis is synonymous with peripheral reparative (giant cell) granuloma. Here we see a smooth bulging polypoid lesion. **b** Low-power view of a well-vascularized process. **c, d** Osteoclastic giant cells are scattered throughout a background of reactive fibroblasts and hemorrhage

2.19 Traumatic Ulcerative Granuloma with Stromal Eosinophilia (TUGSE)

Traumatic ulcerative granuloma with stromal eosinophilia represents an uncommon reactive lesion. There is a known male predominance. The majority of reported cases affect the tongue, followed by buccal mucosa, retromolar trigone, floor of mouth, and lip [76–81]. Patients complain of a slowly enlarging ulcer which may be painful. Ulcers may have rolled margins and reach considerable sizes. In many cases clinicians are convinced that these lesions are malignant. In other cases, an association with a ragged tooth edge or ill-fitting dentures is noted. Traumatic ulcerative granuloma with stromal eosinophilia is self-limited and heals on its own. However, recurrence have been known to happen [76].

Histopathologically, traumatic ulcerative granuloma with stromal eosinophilia is comprised of the requisite ulceration, fibrinopurulent ulcer bed, mixed inflammatory infiltrate, and a variable degree of eosinophils in a scattered clustered pattern (◘ Figs. 2.30, 2.31, and 2.32). Like many a misnomer, no granulomas are seen. The eosinophils become less dense further from the ulcer bed. The entire process may extend deep into skeletal muscle. Inflammatory epithleiotropism is observed. Interestingly, clusters of CD30+ cells have been described in traumatic ulcerative granuloma with stromal eosinophilia which are map to mature lymphocytes and large atypical, reactive mononuclear cells with irregular nuclear contours [81]. These atypical mononuclear cells may also be mitotically active and angiocentricity has been noted [79]. However, necrosis has not been described, and no data to date support the concept that represents a pre-lymphomatous condition.

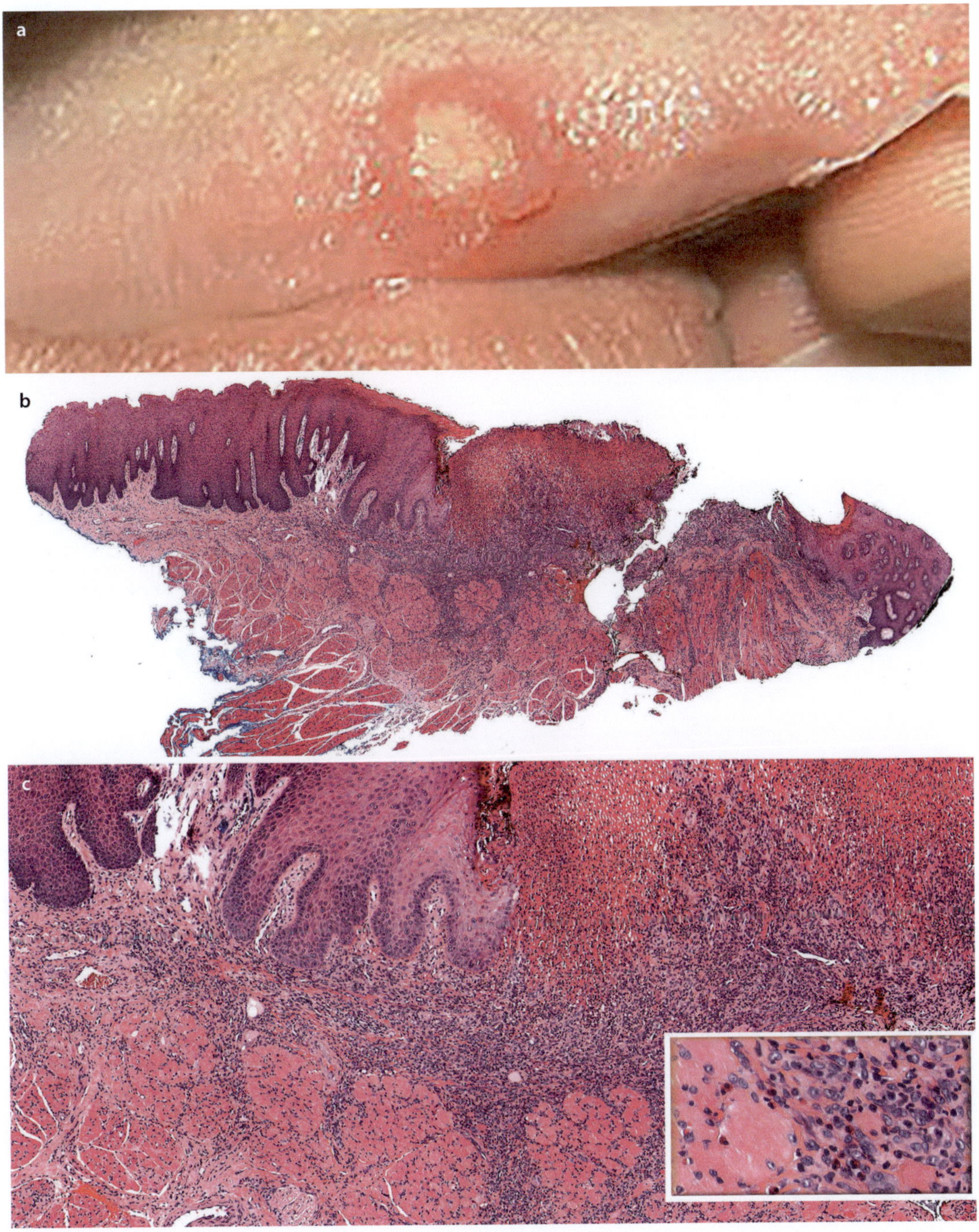

Fig. 2.30 **a** TUGSE: Traumatic ulceration granuloma with stromal eosinophilia. **b**, **c** Sharply demarcated ulcer with inflammatory infiltrate extending into musculature. **Inset:** Eosinophils

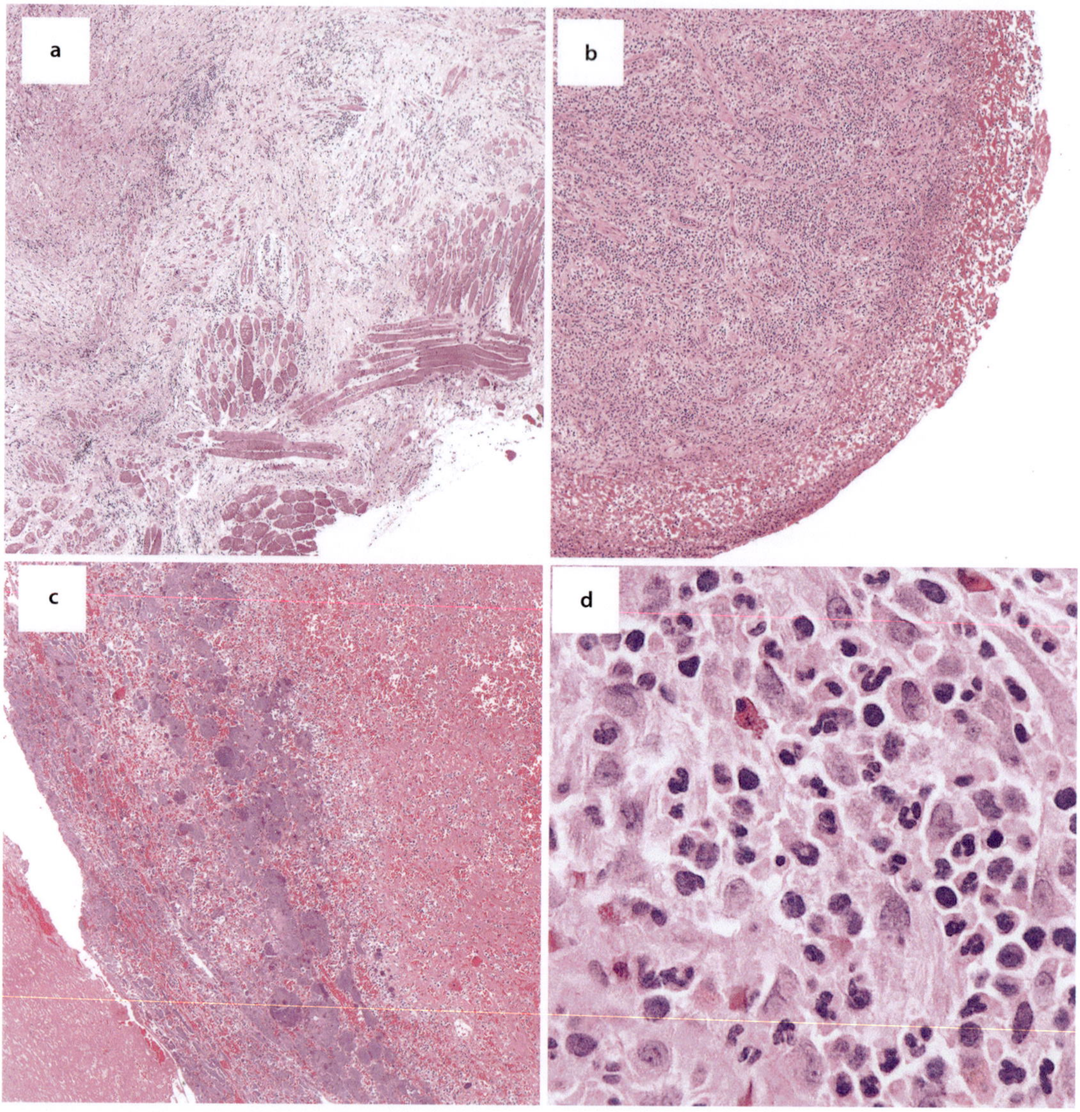

Fig. 2.31 TUGSE clinically mimicking cancer – This 50-year-old woman developed a dramatically enlarging, painful, ulcerated lesion of the left lateral oral tongue. There was a history of two prior oral carcinomas; the clinical impression was that of a new oral malignancy. **a** Inflammation extended deep into lingual musculature. **b**, **c** Beyond the fibrinopurulent exudate and bacterial colonies, this lesion was merely a matter of inflamed granulation tissue with eosinophils **d**

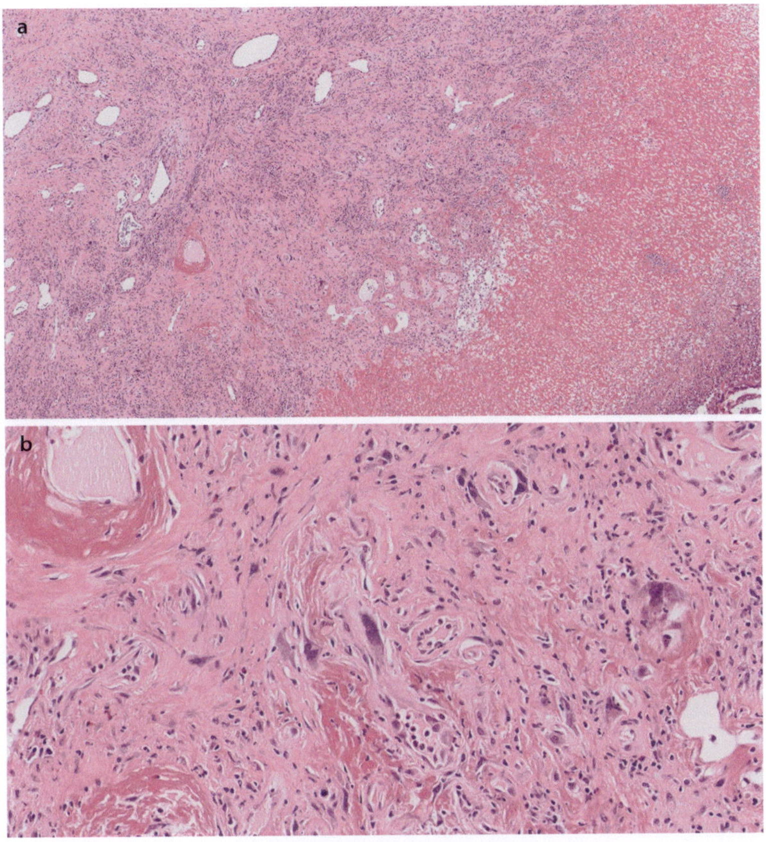

Fig. 2.32 **a** Post chemotherapy TUGSE: This patient was treated with neoadjuvant chemotherapy and resection for oropharyngeal carcinoma. **b** The lingual lesion reveals typical bizarre "chemotherapy" fibroblasts with smudged watercolor chromatin

2.20 Necrotizing Sialometaplasia

Necrotizing sialometaplasia represents a rare, self-limiting reactive process, notorious in its ability to mimic squamous carcinoma [82–85] (Figs. 2.33, 2.34, 2.35, and 2.36). There is a male predominance and the majority of cases affect the hard palate. The typical presentation is that of a painful, crateriform ulceration and adjacent submucosal mass. There may also be systemic complaints such as fever, chills, malaise. Alternatively, any mucosal site that has experienced radiation or recent surgery can also histologically manifest sialometaplasia, minus the necrosis. Factors responsible in the etiology of this process include local ischemia, trauma, ill-fitting dentures, smoking, alcohol, and chronic vomiting secondary to eating disorders [86]. The majority of cases resolve without therapy.

Histopathologically, necrotizing sialometaplasia is characterized by broad zones of coagulative necrosis of the palatal mucinous glands rimmed by waves of acute inflammation

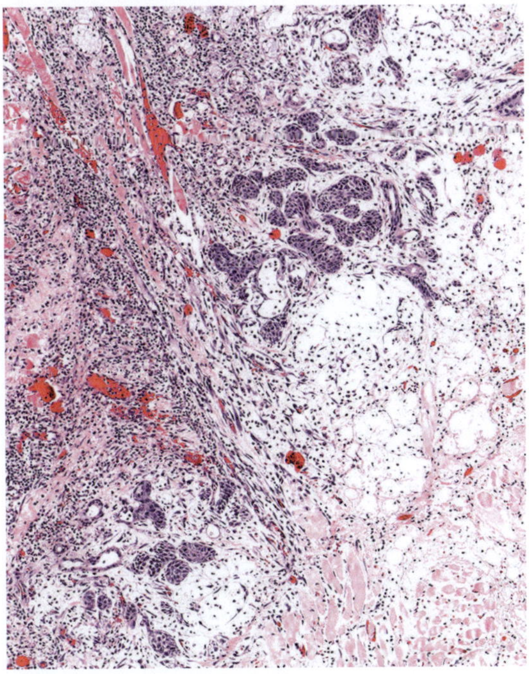

Fig. 2.33 Histological cancer mimics **a** Why *wouldn't* you call this invasive squamous carcinoma? Nothing sets your heart beating like sialometaplasia! This mimicker is often present after radiotherapy or re-excision for inadequate margins

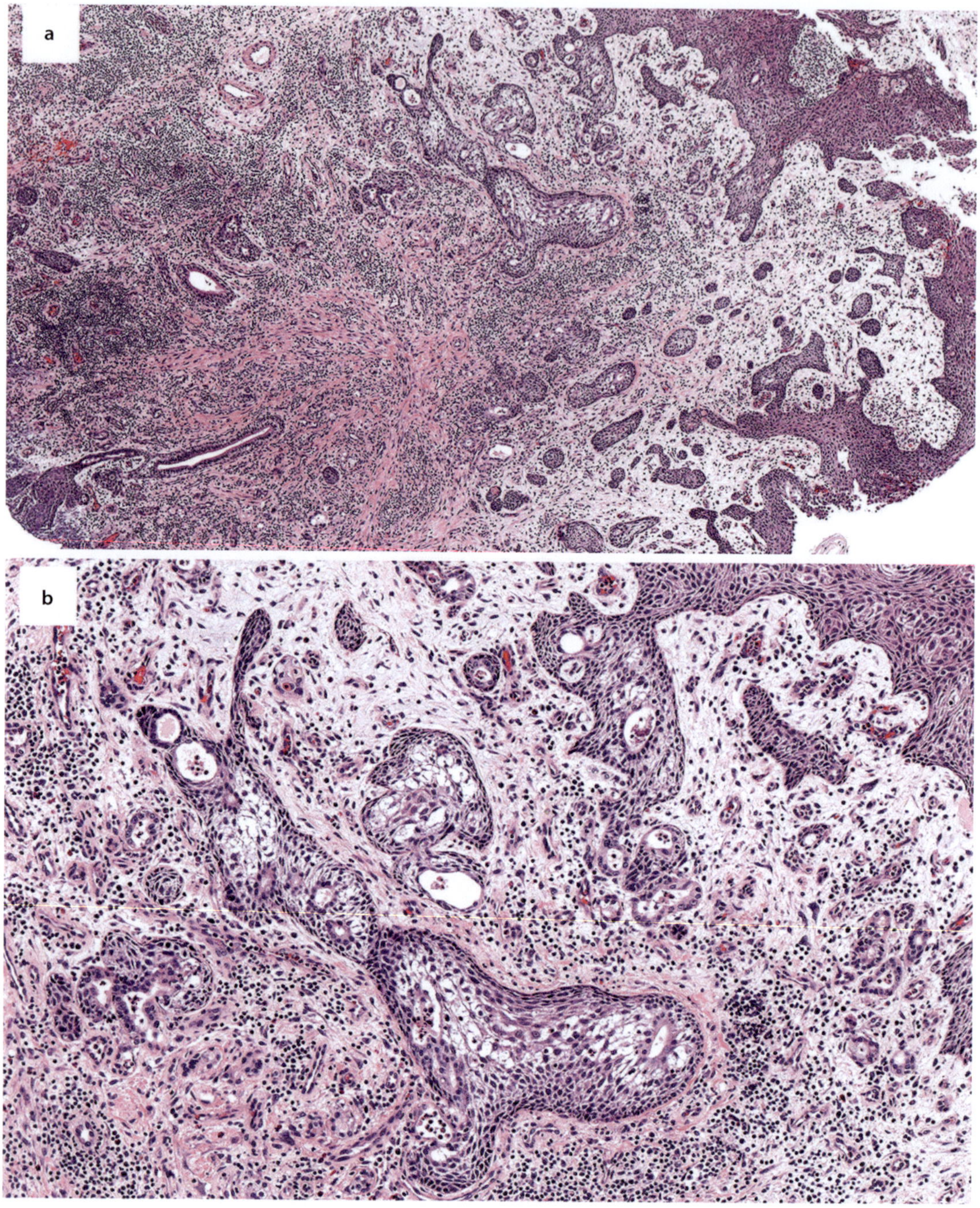

Fig. 2.34 a, b Finding ductal lumena in the context of acute inflammation is one hint to recognize sialometaplasia

with nuclear debris (Fig. 2.37). The mummified silhouettes of the non-vital cells can still be discerned. Mucin extravasation with attendant inflammation may be seen. The process of mucosal re-epithelialization includes squamous metaplasia and hyperplasia of minor salivary ducts. These ducts become dilated and filled with glycogenated squamous cells and traversed by acute inflammatory cells. These are the ducts that can be confused with nests of well-differentiated squamous carcinoma if viewed out of context. The "kinked tube" appearance is a great hint that the process is sialometaplasia, as is the acute inflammation and finding ductal lumena.

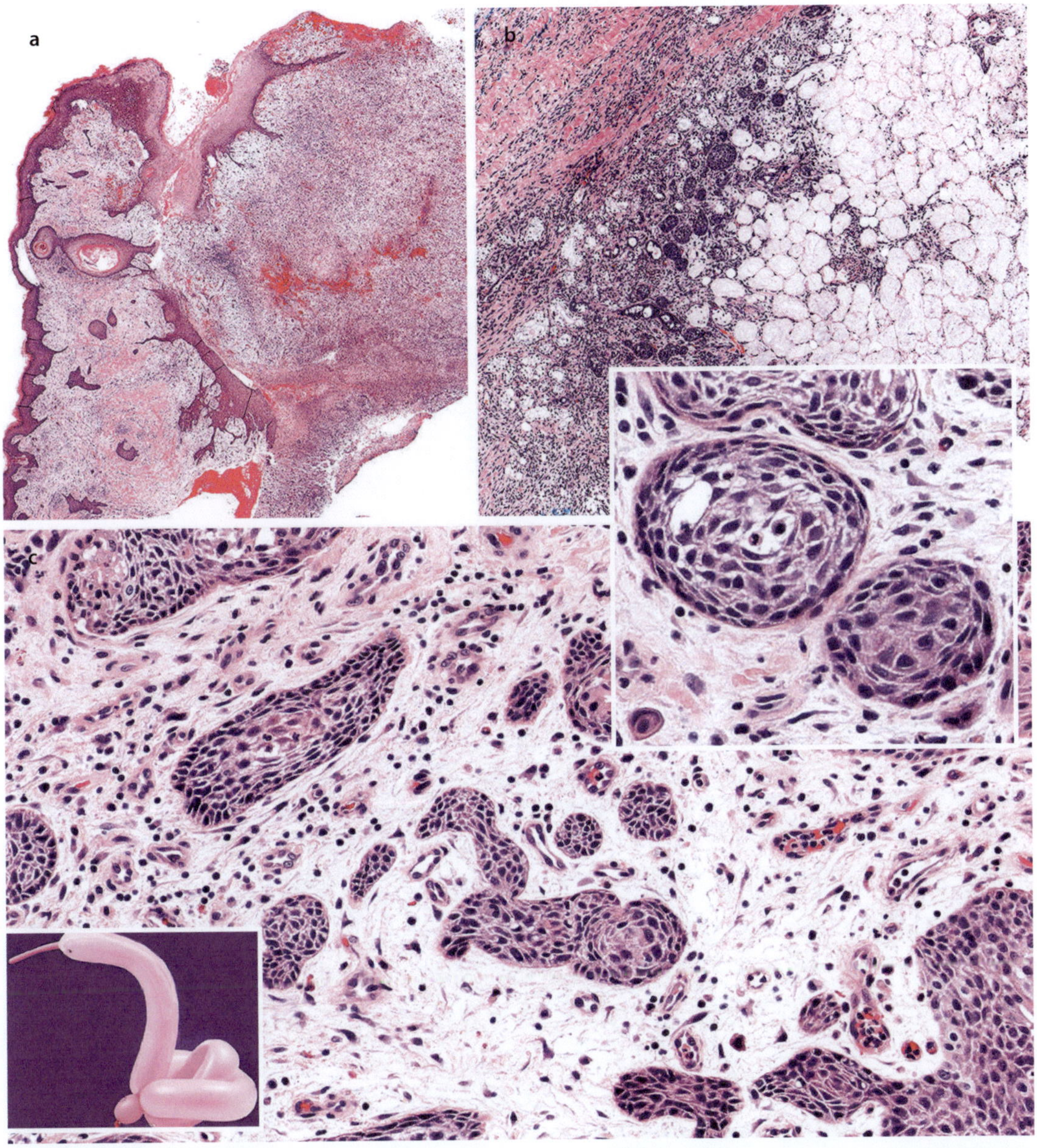

Fig. 2.35 **a–c** Notice the "kinked" tube appearance of the distended minor salivary ducts. Imagine bending a partially expanded long twisting balloon (**Inset c**). Most often, sialometaplasia is a benign, reactive phenomenon. The proliferating cells are histologically benign. (**Inset**)

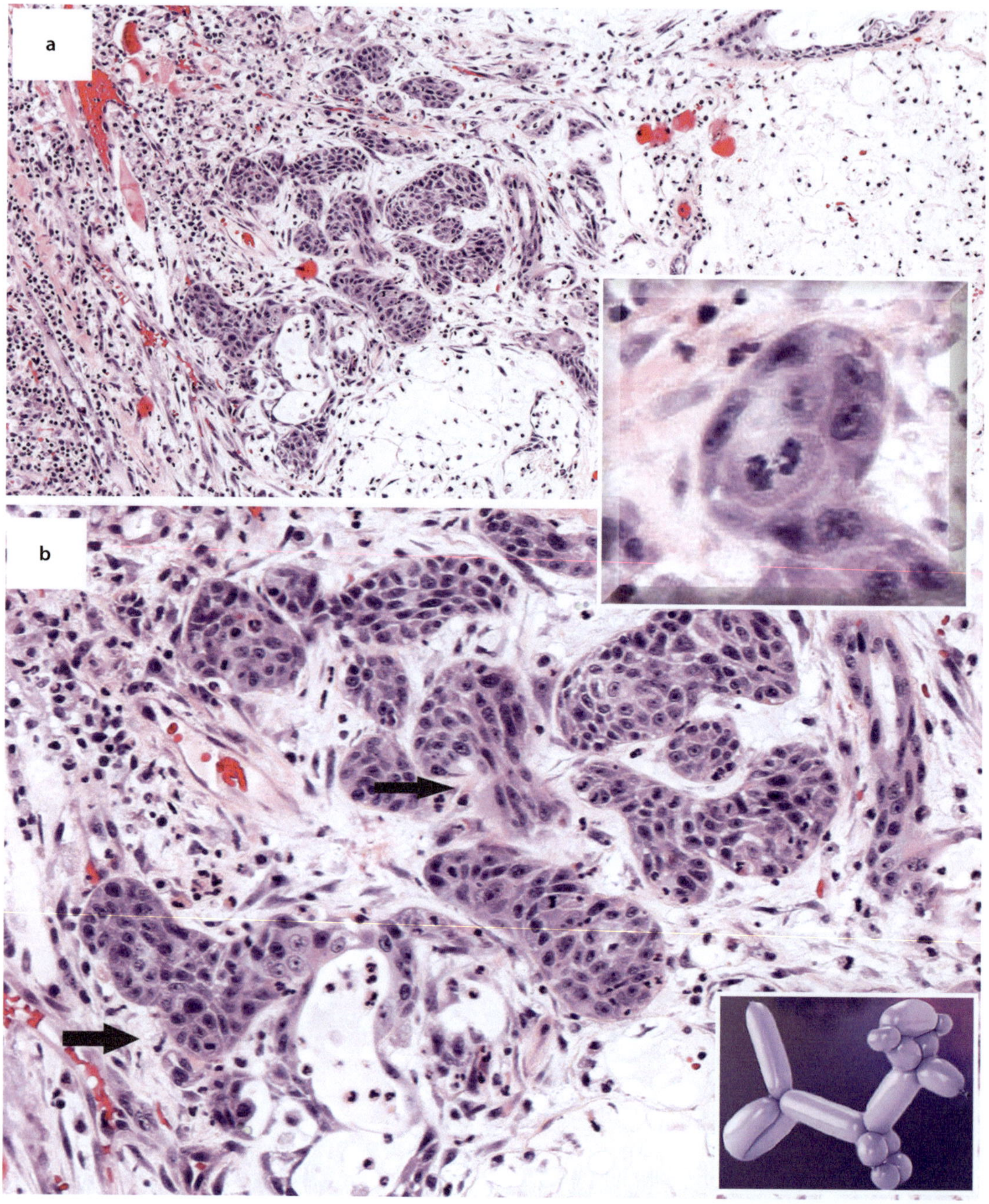

▣ **Fig. 2.36** Dysplastic sialometaplasia. Let's return to the case illustrated in ▣ Fig. 2.33. It stands to reason if you can see sialometaplasia in re-excisions for inadequate margins, then you may also encounter dysplastic sialometaplasia as a field effect, which might be mistaken for invasive carcinoma. **a** Notice that the distended ducts still "respect" a lobular architecture. **Inset**: Atypical mitotic figure indicative of dysplasia. **b** "Kinked tubes" (*arrows*)

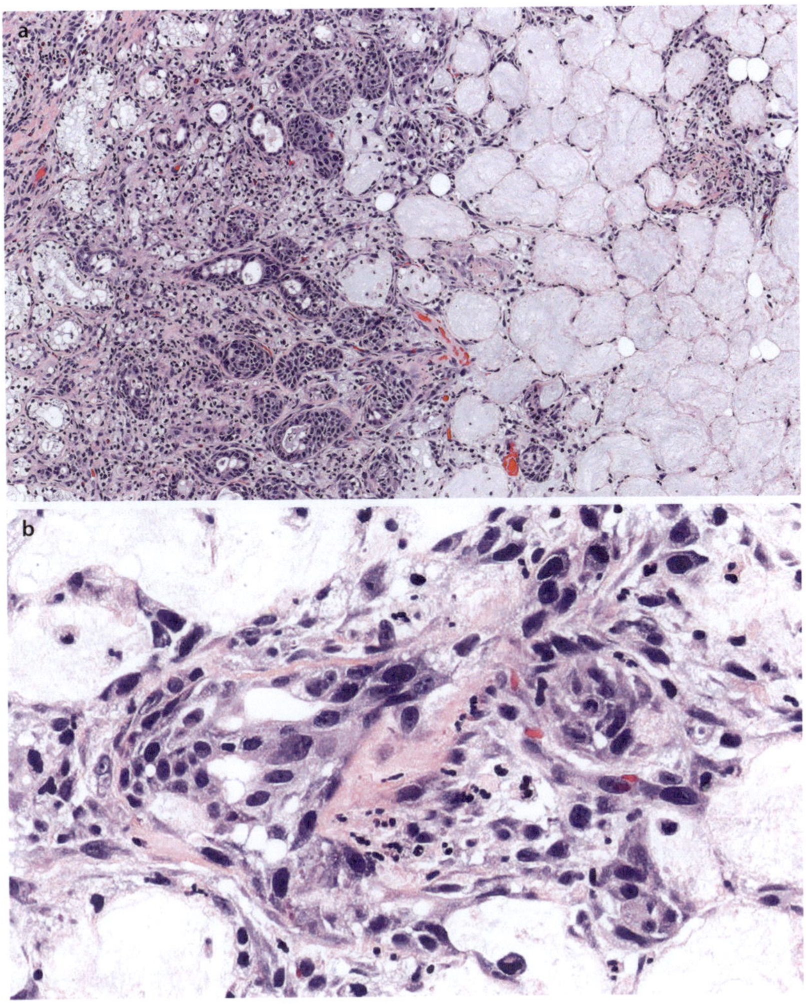

■ **Fig. 2.37** Necrotizing sialometaplasia represents a specific clinical entity of a painful, sharply demarcated enlarging hard palate ulcer which clinically mimics malignancy. **a** The mucinous glands (right) are entirely necrotic, the adjacent viable tissue is acutely inflamed with sialometaplasia. **b** You can recognize reactive cells by their enlarged single nucleolus, fine chromatin pattern, and basophilic cytoplasm

2.21 Fibromas

The pedestrian fibroma is the most commonly biopsied oral lesion, and is taken to result from trauma or repeated local irritation, hence the synonym irritation fibroma. Intraoral fibromas most commonly develop in the buccal mucosa along the occlusion line. Fibromas appear as round, smooth, firm, sessile or pedunculated masses and range from millimeters to up to 2 cm. in size. Having framed the above, there are a few interesting intraoral variants, namely: **peripheral ossifying fibroma, giant cell fibroma, sclerotic fibroma, collageneous fibroma, elastofibroma,** and **myofibroma,** which are discussed below.

Histopathologically, think of a **fibroma** as a "peninsula", a "thing that sticks out" (■ Fig. 2.38). You should be able to discern "three mucosal covered surfaces" and a base. The submucosal

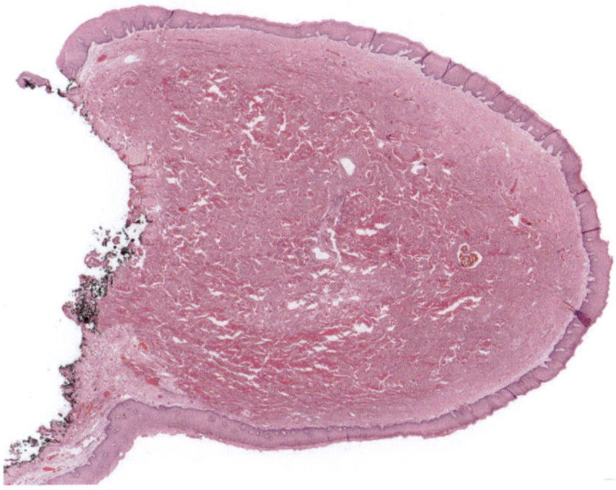

■ **Fig. 2.38** Fibroma – this represents the most commonly excised oral lesion. A fibroma is three-sided, like a peninsula

component is composed of dense fibroconnective tissue which may be hyalinized. The overlying squamous mucosa is hyperplastic and hyperkeratotic, or atrophic, or ulcerated. Inflammation is variable.

Peripheral ossifying fibroma (peripheral cemento-ossifying fibroma, calcifying fibrous epulis) is a reactive gingival lesion which arises from the periodontal ligament or periosteum. The term "peripheral" refers to an intraoral lesion that arises from the extraosseous soft tissues; by contrast the term "central" refers to an intraoral lesion that arises from the jaw bones. Peripheral ossifying fibromas are most often encountered during the second decade of life, but may occur at any age; there is a female predisposition. The typical presentation is that of a sessile or pedunculated mass growing in the anterior gingival papilla; the maxillary gingiva is more often involved than the mandibular gingival. Peripheral ossifying fibromas can reach considerable size. The underlying alveolar bone is usually intact, occasionally there may be superficial cortical erosion. Multifocal involvement is rare [87].

Histopathologically, one sees similar to a fibroma, a discreet, polypoid, dense fibroblastic proliferation, but with increased plump, immature fibroblasts (myofibroblasts). The defining feature here is the variable calcified osteoid and/or cementoid, and/or mature ossification (◘ Fig. 2.39). If you confuse the mature bone for native alveolar bone, your credibility will diminish.

Histopathologically, a **giant cell fibroma** contains numerous large, plump, spindle-shaped, stellate, and multinucleated fibroblasts (◘ Fig. 2.39). The rete pegs are thin and elongated.

Histopathologically, a **sclerotic fibroma** appears as a discreet mass of densely collagenized, hypocellular fibrous tissue with a prominent storiform pattern. Characteristically, there are prominent clefts between the collagen bundles. Of note, sclerotic fibromas may be sporadic or associated with **Cowden syndrome.**

Collagenous fibroma (desmoplastic fibroblastoma) is a rare, benign lesion affecting subcutaneous and deep soft tissues. It can rarely develop in the oral cavity (◘ Figs. 2.40 and 2.41) and has been described in the palate, buccal mucosa, gingiva and tongue [88, 89]. Histopathologically, collagenous fibroma is characterized by an expansile, circumscribed mass composed of paucicellular densely collagenized stroma, which can be keloid-like, densely hyalinized, and sclerotic. Collagenous stroma can be confirmed with a trichrome stain. Fibromyxoid degeneration can be present. Commonly, fat and or muscle may become entrapped in the expanding lesion, which should not be misconstrued as invasion. The cellular component is composed of bland spindled and stellate cells which are **vimentin +,** and can express **smooth muscle actin.** They are **CD34/S100 negative.** Binucleate and multinucleated cells may be seen.

Intraoral **elastofibromas** represent another rare fibroma variant reported in the palate, buccal mucosa, floor of mouth, and lip [90]. Elastofibromas are distinguished from all other fibromas by dense elastic fiber deposition, confirmed by histochemistry for elastic fibers. H&E stained section will reveal swollen eosinophilic collagen and beaded elastic fibers which form "flower-like" (petaloid) forms [90].

Lastly, intraoral **myofibromas** represent rare, benign, expansile growth of myofibroblasts, which are modified fibroblasts with contractile fibers. Myofibromas can occur at all ages but most commonly develop within the first few years of years of life. The most commonly affected site is the mandible, followed by gingiva, tongue, buccal mucosa, palate and lip [91–96]. Histologically, myofibromas are composed of uniform dense proliferation of interlacing fascicles and whorls of plump, bland, spindled myofibroblasts, which are **smooth muscle actin +, muscle specific actin +** and **CD34/desmin/S100/caldesmon negative** (◘ Fig. 2.42). The myofibroblasts have tapered and/or cigar-shaped nuclei and eosinophilic cytoplasm. Hemangiopericytoma-like "stag-horn" vessels may be present. Collagenous stroma can be confirmed with a trichrome stain. Necrosis and calcifications can be seen, which may actually relate to regression. Patients are cured with conservative resection.

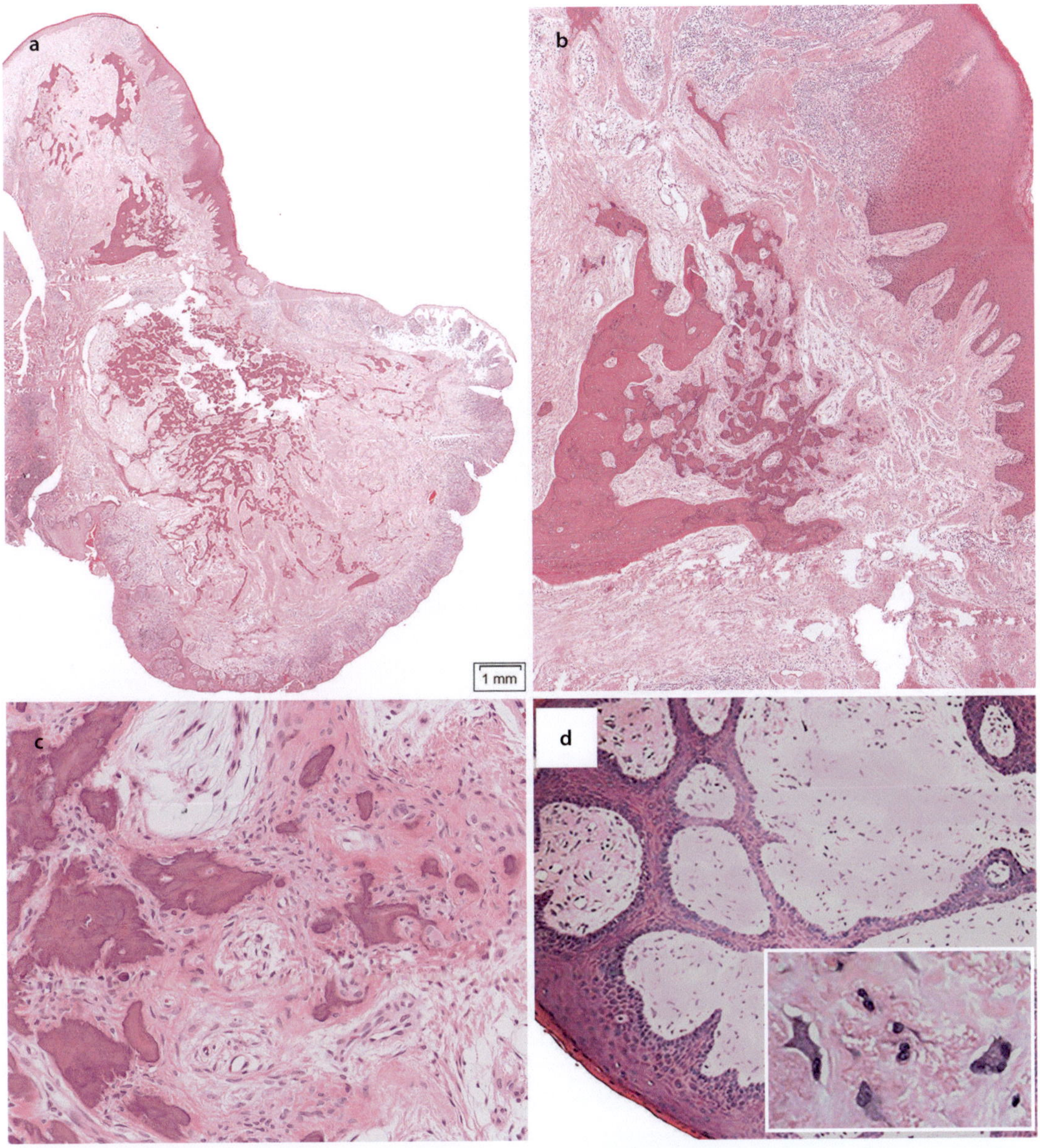

Fig. 2.39 **a** Peripheral ossifying fibroma represents a fancy fibroma which commonly arises in the gingiva. Given the scale bar, you could imagine that this was a rather sizable polypoid gingival lesion. **b** You can also imagine that if you were to initially focus on the ossification, you'd become lost in the differential diagnosis of benign fibroosseous lesions. Take a step back and recognize gingival mucosa and fibroconnective tissue. This is a "peripheral", not a "central" lesion. **c** The fibroblastic stroma is more cellular than in the usual fibroma, and composed of myofibroblasts which produce osseous matrix. **d** Giant cell fibroma is the rarest variant

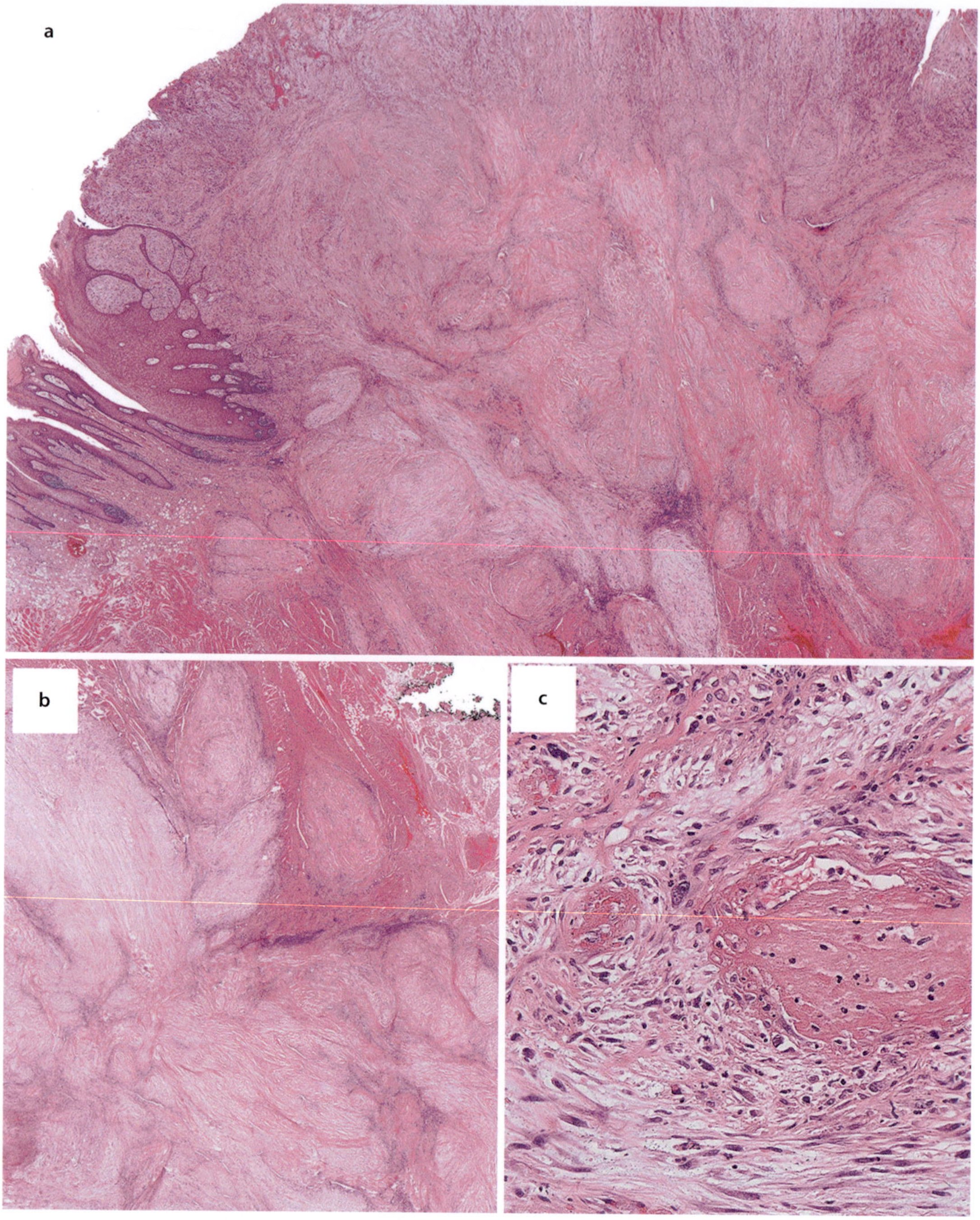

Fig. 2.40 Collagenous fibroma a, b Here is an exophytic, mushroom-like growth, with superficial erosion. This patient was status post resection and irradiation for oral cavity carcinoma. The light blue regions represent whorls of myxofibrous nodules which extended deep into the tongue musculature. Keloid-like maturation with dense collagen and decreasing cellularity is seen in the nodules deeper in the lesion. **c** Myxoid inflammatory component and neovascularization

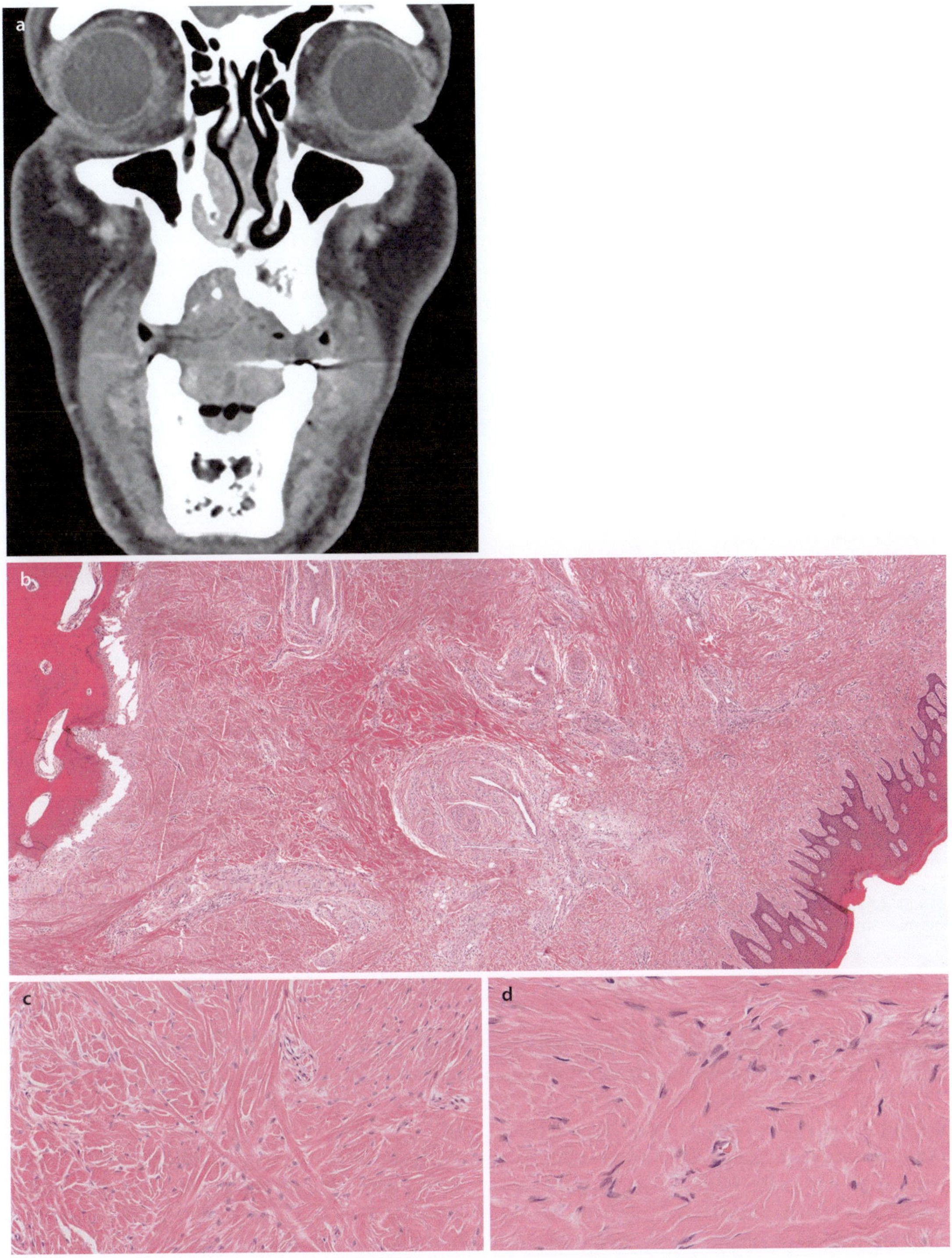

Fig. 2.41 **Collagenous fibroma a** The radiograph demonstrates a large, right-sided palatal mass eroding bone. **b** Submucosal keloid-like lesion with glassy pink collagen deposition. **c**, **d** The lesion is paucicellular, lacks inflammation, and is characterized by dense keloidal collagen deposition

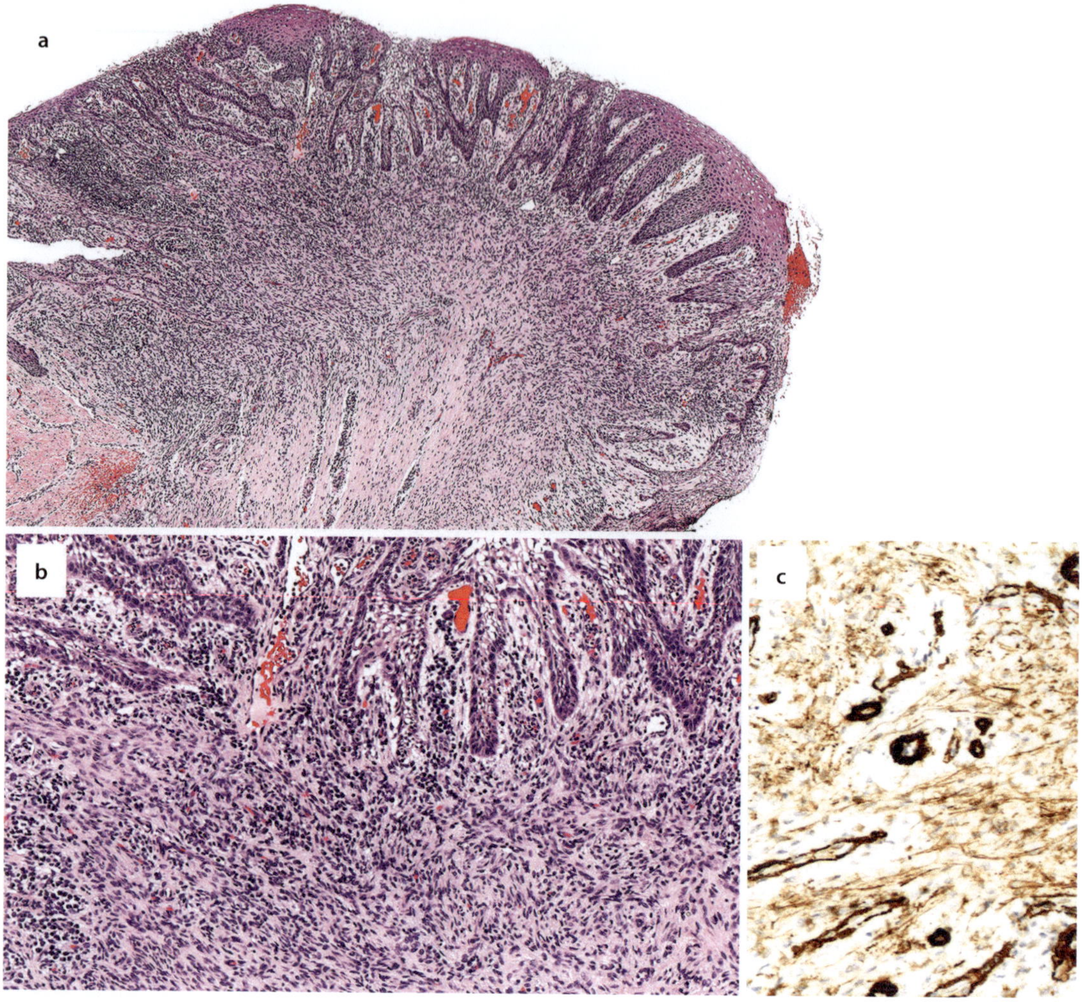

Fig. 2.42 Gingival myofibroma a, b Polypoid submucosal lesion comprised of densely packed bland myofibroblasts. **c** Smooth muscle actin

2.22 Tori

Tori (plural of *torus*, Latin, "to stand out) are nodular benign protuberances of mature bone. They are not considered pathological entities, but rather are anatomic variations. **Tori palatinus** occur on the hard palate and **tori mandibularis** occur adjacent to the lingual aspect of the mandible [97–99]. A third, rare variant warrants mention: **torus maxillaris**. Tori palatinus is most commonly encountered. Generally, women are twice more likely to be affected than are men. Women are more likely to have tori palatinus, whereas men are more likely to have tori mandibularis. Coexisting tori palatinus and tori mandibularis are seen in up to one quarter of patients. Tori are frequently observed in young adults and middle-aged persons and are more common in Asians and Eskimos populations. Tori are associated with an autosomal dominant inheritance pattern with variable penetrance: 85% of children with tori also have parents with tori. Tori are not part of the Gardener syndrome.

Tori have a typical, diagnostic clinical appearance. They manifest as submucosal protuberances may be asymmetrical, lobulated or nodular, or smooth and spindle shaped. Most tori mandibularis are bilateral, and in the region of the canine or incisor teeth. Tori maxillaris are exostoses from either the buccal or palatal aspect of the maxillary alveolar processes. In general, tori rarely require biopsy but may be excised if they interfere with dentures, or cause symptoms. Histopathologically, one sees a dense expansion

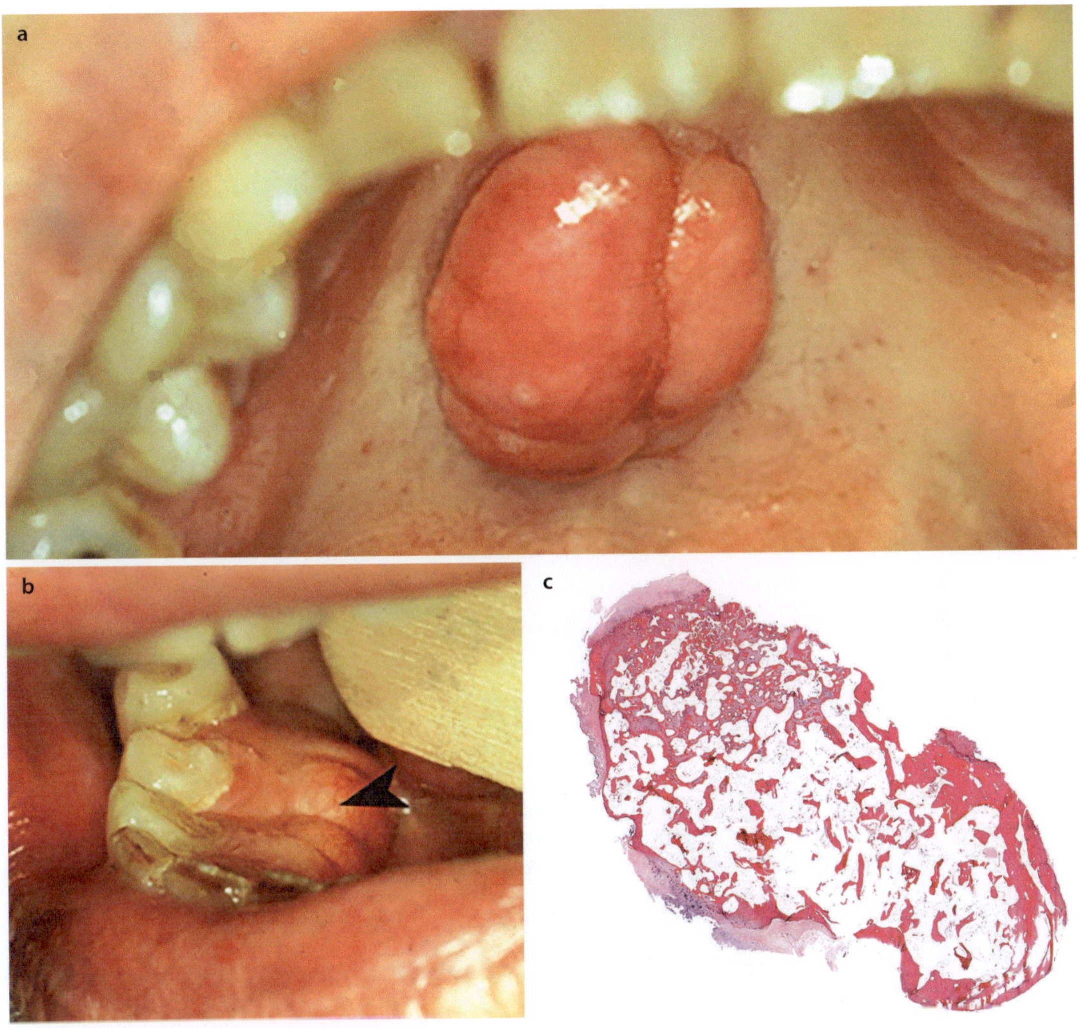

◘ **Fig. 2.43** **a** Torus palatini – exophytic boney growth on palate. **b** Torus mandibularis (*arrow*) protruding from lingual aspect of mandible. **c** Tori are composed of mature cortical and trabecular bone

of mature, lamellar cortical bone (◘ Fig. 2.43). There is a variable subcortical component of mature, lamellar trabecular bone.

2.23 Sialadenoma Papilliferum

Sialadenoma papilliferum is an extraordinarily rare benign salivary tumor which is considered the mucosal analogue of syringocystadenoma papilliferum. Sialadenoma papilliferum may arise from either the minor or major salivary glands, but the single most common site is the palate [100–104]. A male predominance and a wide age range at diagnosis have been reported. Clinically, these lesions have a papillary surface. Histopathologically, sialadenoma papilliferum is a well-circumscribed lesion with **biphasic pattern**. The **exophytic** component is composed broad papillary projections lined by stratified, acanthotic, nonkeratinized squamous epithelium, similar to an exophytic papilloma (◘ Fig. 2.44). The **base** of the lesion is composed of elongated, dilated, **proliferating glands** which retain a bilayer pattern of columnar, ciliated, and goblet luminal cells, over cuboidal basal cells. Continuity between the squamous and glandular elements is seen. The glandular elements may form a complex micropapillary branching pattern with "star-like" spaces. Atypia and mitotic activity are minimal.

The differential diagnosis includes **ductal papilloma** and **inverted papilloma**; both of

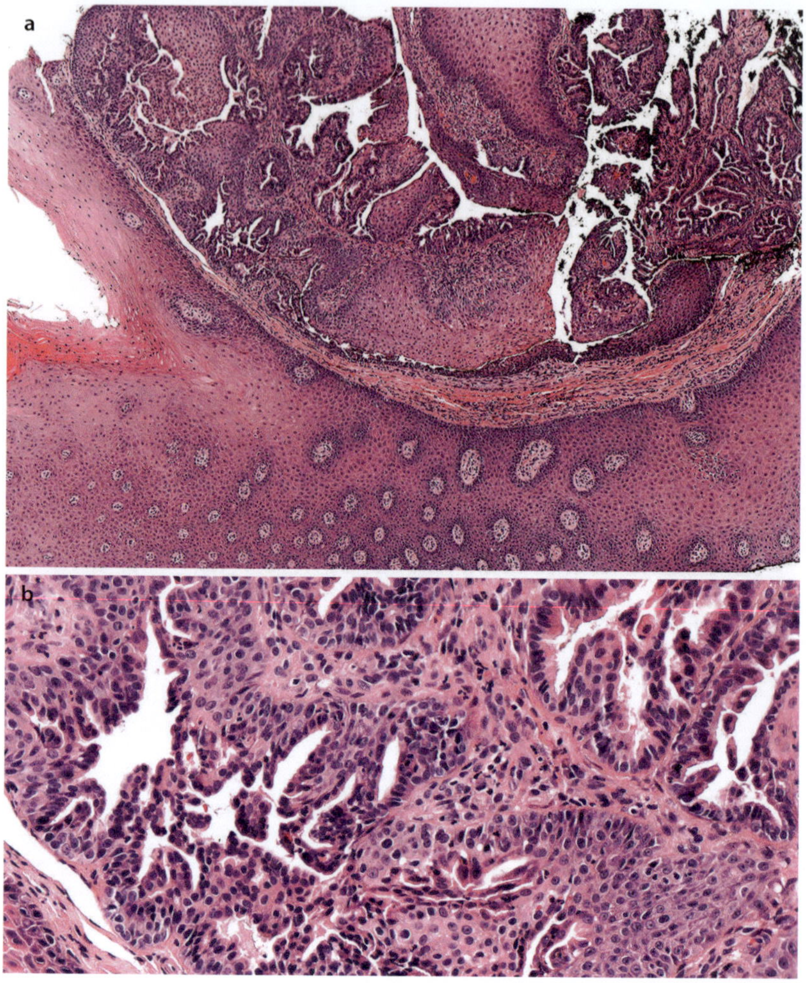

Fig. 2.44 **a** Sialoadenoma papilliferum represents a complex intraductal proliferation of metaplastic seromucinous glands to form squamous papillae and squamoglandular elements. **b** Cleft-like glands lined by columnar cells +/– squamous metaplasia

these lesions are predominantly submucosal. An inverted papilloma demonstrates endophytic broad papillary fronds, pushing growth pattern, and terminates with a mucosal pore-like component. Inverted papilloma is predominantly a proliferation of squamous epithelium; some goblet cell differentiation is retained but a prominent glandular component is absent. An **intraductal papilloma** is entirely contained within a cystically dilated duct, and is composed of proliferating papillary structures covered by glandular and squamous epithelium. Inverted papillomas and ductal papillomas lack the mucosal exophytic component of sialadenoma papilliferum.

Sialadenoma papilliferum is usually cured by conservative excision. There are rare reports of highly unusual cases that manifest aggressive behavior, local recurrences, and/or histologic malignant progression [105–108].

2.24 Granular Cell Tumor

Granular cell tumor (granular myoblastoma) is a benign tumor of Schwannian or pre-Schwannnian origin. A wide age range is seen with a peak incidence in the third to fifth decades of life. Generally, granular cell tumors occurs with a female preponderance and a predilection for African-Americans. It may develop at any soft tissue site or organ, however the head and neck is the most common site, most often the oral cavity. Intraoral granular cell tumors have no gender predilection. The majority of intraoral tumors occur on the lingual dorsum followed by lingual border; other intraoral sites include soft palate, uvula, lip, floor of mouth, gingiva, and buccal mucosa [109–115]. The usual clinical appearance for GCT is that of a sessile, painless, firm nodule, under 2 cm which is smooth with a yellow mucosal discoloration. For lingual GCT, the surface papillae are distinctly separated from one another. **Multiple synchronous** or **metachronous GCT at various sites occur in approximately 5% of patients.**

Histopathology, the tumor cells form small nests and cords with an infiltrative growth pattern (Figs. 2.45 and 2.46). The tumor cells have a syncytial "histiocytoid" appearance with small eccentric nuclei, abundant, granular cytoplasm

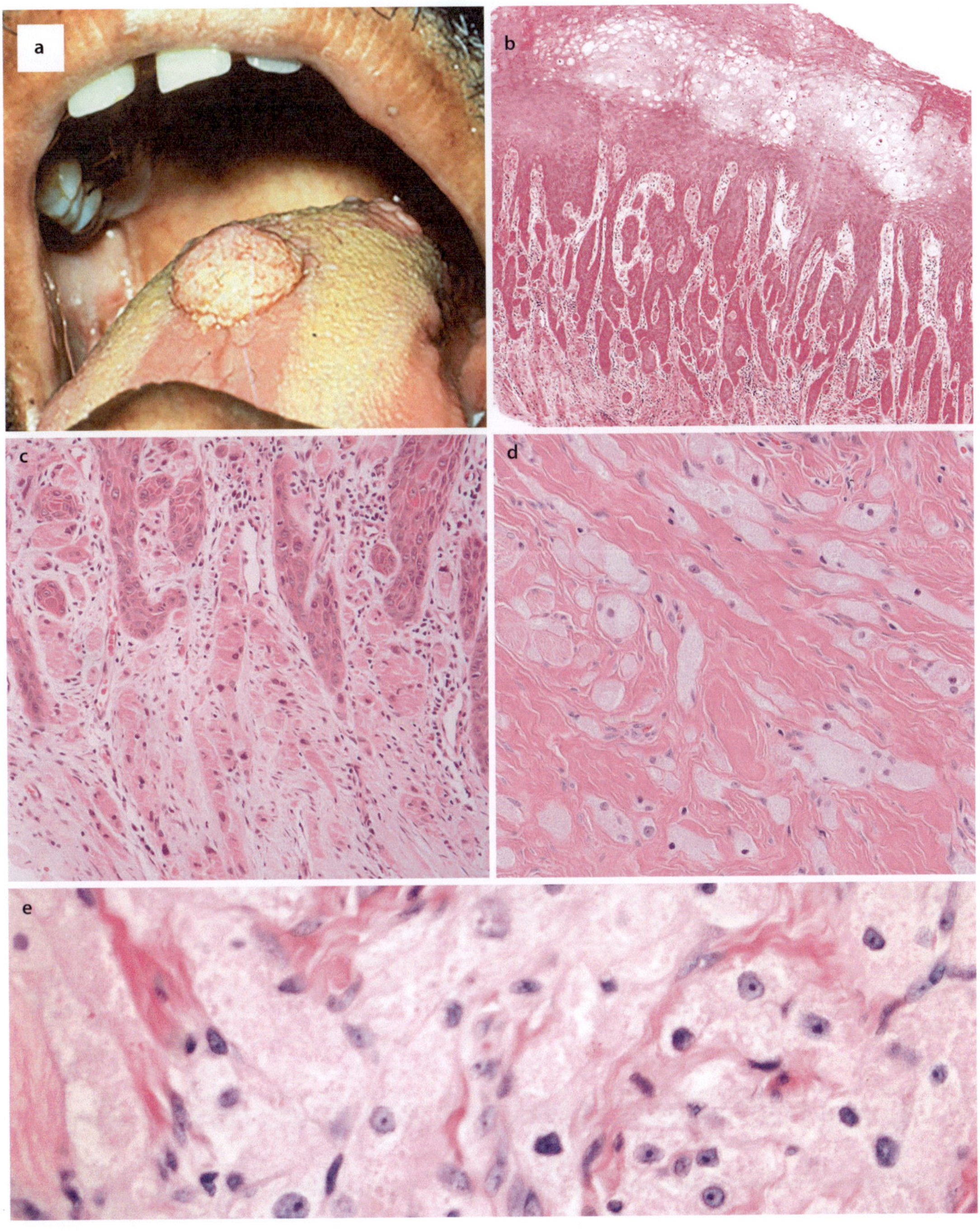

Fig. 2.45 **a** Granular cell tumor is one of the few lesions responsible for a mass on the dorsal tongue. **b, c** Dramatic pseudoepitheliomatous hyperplasia. **d** Strap-like granular cells **e** Nest of granular cells with bland eccentric nuclei and eosinophilic "fluffy" cytoplasm

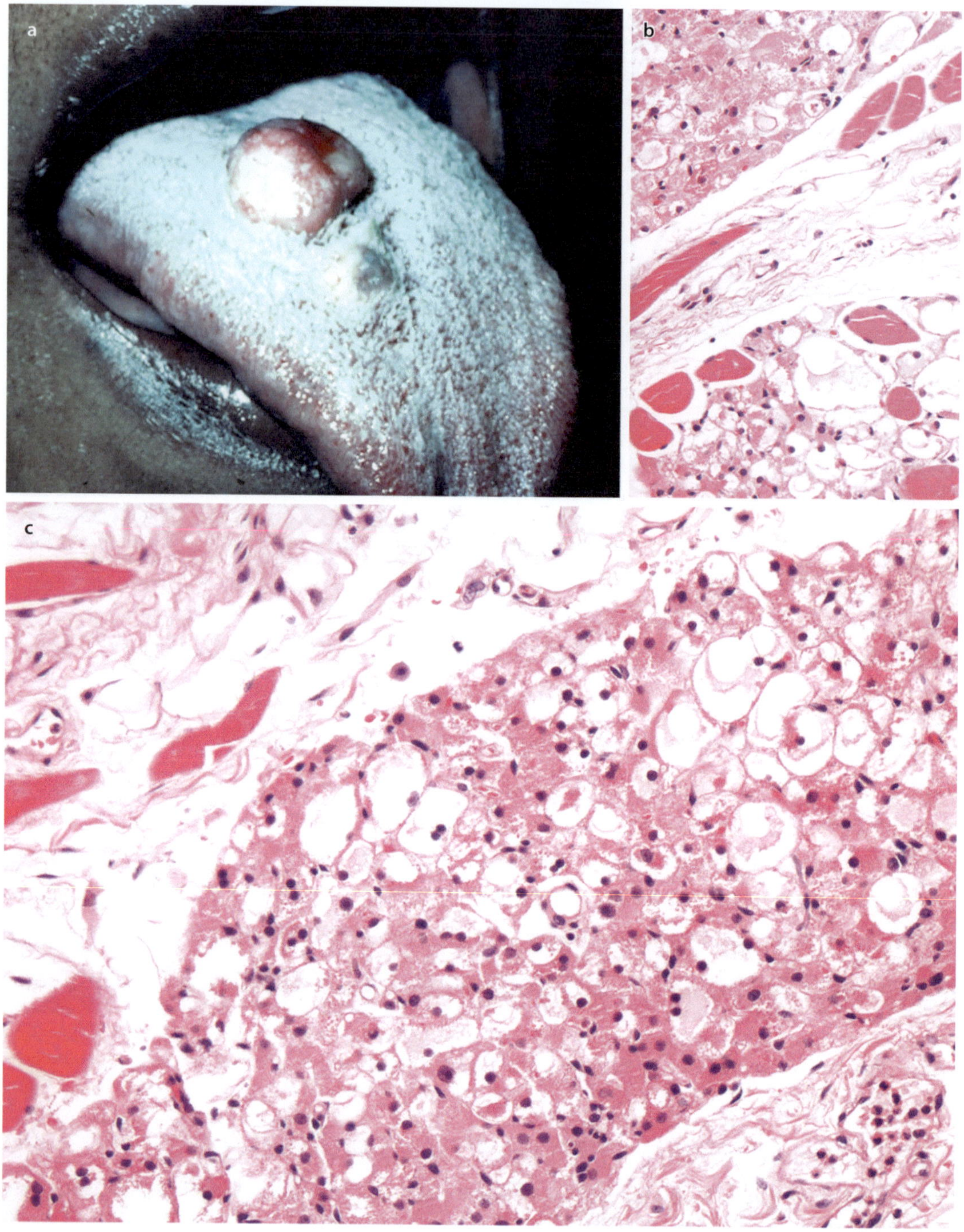

Fig. 2.46 **a** The smaller mass anterior to the dominant mass represents multifocality, **b**, **c** Here we cell granular cells originating from, and distending, skeletal muscle fascicles, thus the older nosology of "granular cell myoblastoma"

and indistinct cytoplasmic membranes. Origin from skeletal muscle bundles may be observed (hence the term granular myoblastoma). Nuclear pleomorphism and mitotic figures are usually absent. Marked desmoplasia may be seen within older or larger tumors; the typical, recognizable granular cells are concentrated at the periphery. The cytoplasmic granules are PAS positive, and diastase resistant. **S-100 is usually strongly positive**. However, **S100 negative** non-congenital

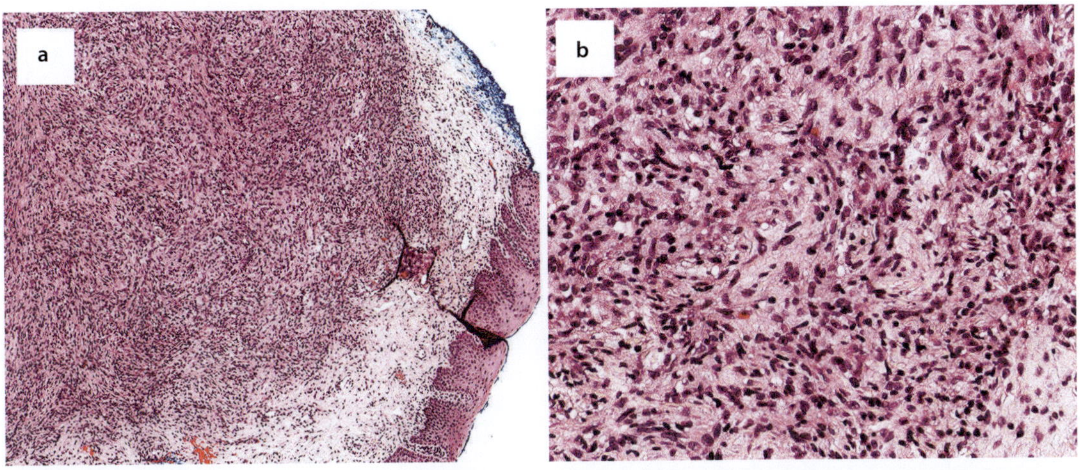

Fig. 2.47 a, b Oral fibrous histiocytoma – Proliferation of fibroblasts and foamy macrophages with inflammatory background

granular cell tumors have been reported, thus emphasizing the adage that H + E trumps IHC [116]. Histiocytic differentiation (KP-1+, CD68+) can be seen. Vimentin is negative. True histiocytic processes such as fibrous histiocytoma usually do not form nests and cords as does granular cell tumor (Fig. 2.47). An exception to this rule is the lipidized variant of fibrous histiocytoma which can form nests and cords.

Multiple tumor satellites are commonly observed and resection margins can often be positive. A well-known series of 110 patients reported that tumors were incompletely excised in 24 of 56 patients with adequate follow-up; only five of these 24 patients experienced local tumor recurrence [109].

Pseudoepitheliomatous hyperplasia is present in half of granular cell tumors. When extreme, it's known as a potential mimicker of squamous carcinoma [117]. Conversely, the coexistence of lingual squamous carcinoma and granular cell tumor has been reported [118].

The **congenital granular cell tumor (congenital epulis of newborn, Neuman's tumor)** warrants separate mention here. This is an extremely neoplasm present at birth, restricted to the anterior gingiva [119–125]. These tumors are presumed to arise from **odontogenic epithelium** of the dental lamina. Maxillary tumors are more common than mandibular tumors; rare multifocal tumors have been reported. There is a female predisposition. Congenital granular cell tumors have been reported in association with XXX syndrome, neurofibromatosis, maxillary hypoplasia, polydactyly, congenital goiter, facial cleft, and polyhydramnios. Histologically, it is similar to the congenital granular cell tumor is to the usual, non-congenital granular cell tumor; it's composed of the same polyhedral cells with abundant eosinophilic granular cytoplasm. Pseudoepitheliomatous hyperplasia is usually absent. Of note, congenital granular cell tumor is **vimentin + and S-100/CD 68 negative.** Excision of congenital granular cell tumor is curative, and spontaneous regression is known to occur.

True malignant granular cell tumor is a rarity [126–128]. It may be either histologically benign yet very large (>9 cm) with evidence of metastases at presentation, or it may be overtly histologically malignant. This latter scenario is marked by spindled tumor cells with nuclear pleomorphism, vesicular nuclei, large nucleoli, irregular infiltrative pattern, increased mitoses (2 mitoses/10 fields at 200x) and necrosis. The nosology of "atypical granular cell tumor" can be used for those tumors demonstrating pleomorphism, but no evidence of metastases [129].

2.25 Rhabdomyoma

Rhabdomyoma is a benign and uncommon mesenchymal tumor with skeletal myogenic differentiation which is classified as either cardiac or extracardiac; 90% of extracardiac rhabdomyomas occur in the head and neck, followed by the genitourinary tract [130–136]. Interestingly, rhabdomyomas represent an exception to the rule that benign soft tissue tumors are more common than their malignant counterparts. Extracardiac rhabdomyomas is classified as either **adult type** or **fetal type**. **Adult rhabdomyomas** are more common and demonstrate mature skeletal differentiation whereas **fetal rhabdomyomas** are less common and exhibits immature skeletal muscle differentiation. In contrast to cardiac tumors, extracardiac tumors are not associated with tuberous sclerosis.

Adult rhabdomyoma The median age is 60 years (range, 33–80 years) with a male predominance. The oral cavity is the most common mucosal site for this tumor, followed by the pharynx and larynx; the neck is the most common soft tissue site. Adult-type rhabdomyomas are usually solitary, but may be **multinodular (25% of cases)** in the same anatomic location; they can rarely involve separate sites, such as the larynx and the neck. Conservative excision is curative.

Histopathologically, an adult rhabdomyoma is a well-demarcated, unencapsulated tumor composed of a sheet-like proliferation of large polygonal cells with abundant, eosinophilic, granular or vacuolated cytoplasm ("spider" cells) (◘ Fig. 2.48). Tumor nuclei are small, round, central or peripherally located with vesicular chromatin. Characteristic "spider cells" may be seen, although they are more prevalent in cardiac rhabdomyomas. These cells have a central eosinophilic cytoplasmic inclusion, which radiates to the cell membrane by thin strands. Haphazard, rod-like cytoplasmic striations can be accentuated with phosphotungstic acid-hematoxylin-stain. Rhabdomyomas are **strongly muscle specific actin +, desmin +, myogenin +**, and **myo-D1** +. Variable rare or weak staining is seen with vimentin, smooth muscle actin, and S-100.

Fetal rhabdomyoma The median age of 4 years (range, 3 days-58 years.) with a male to female ratio of 2:1. Approximately half of fetal-type rhabdomyomas present in babies. Classic fetal-type rhabdomyoma is most likely found as posterior auricular soft tissue masses during infancy. Interestingly, fetal rhabdomyomas have been reported in basal cell nevoid syndrome, which is associated with constitutive activation of the Hedgehog pathway [137]. Mutations in *PTCH1,* which encodes a transmembrane protein that normally suppresses *Smoothened,* have been reported in fetal rhabdomyomas [138].

Histopathologically, fetal rhabdomyomas can display a spectrum of differentiation. The classic immature fetal-type rhabdomyoma shows bland, primitive strap-like spindled cells with delicate fetal myotubules haphazardly arranged in a myxoid stroma. Intermediate (or juvenile) fetal-type rhabdomyoma shows a variety of components including interlacing large strap-like cells with striated cytoplasm and fascicles of spindled leiomyoma-like rhabdomyoblasts, and ganglion cell-like rhabdomyoblasts. The tumor is **strongly muscle specific actin +, desmin +, myogenin +**, and **myo-D1** +. Variable rare or weak staining is seen with vimentin, smooth muscle actin, S-100 and GFAP. The most important criterion in distinguishing fetal-type rhabdomyoma from rhabdomyosarcoma is the absence of prominent nuclear atypia. Fetal-type rhabdomyomas are well-circumscribed, superficial, and noninvasive. They lack the "cambium" layer and hypercellularity seen in rhabdomyosarcoma Necrosis and mitoses are very rare in fetal-type RM.

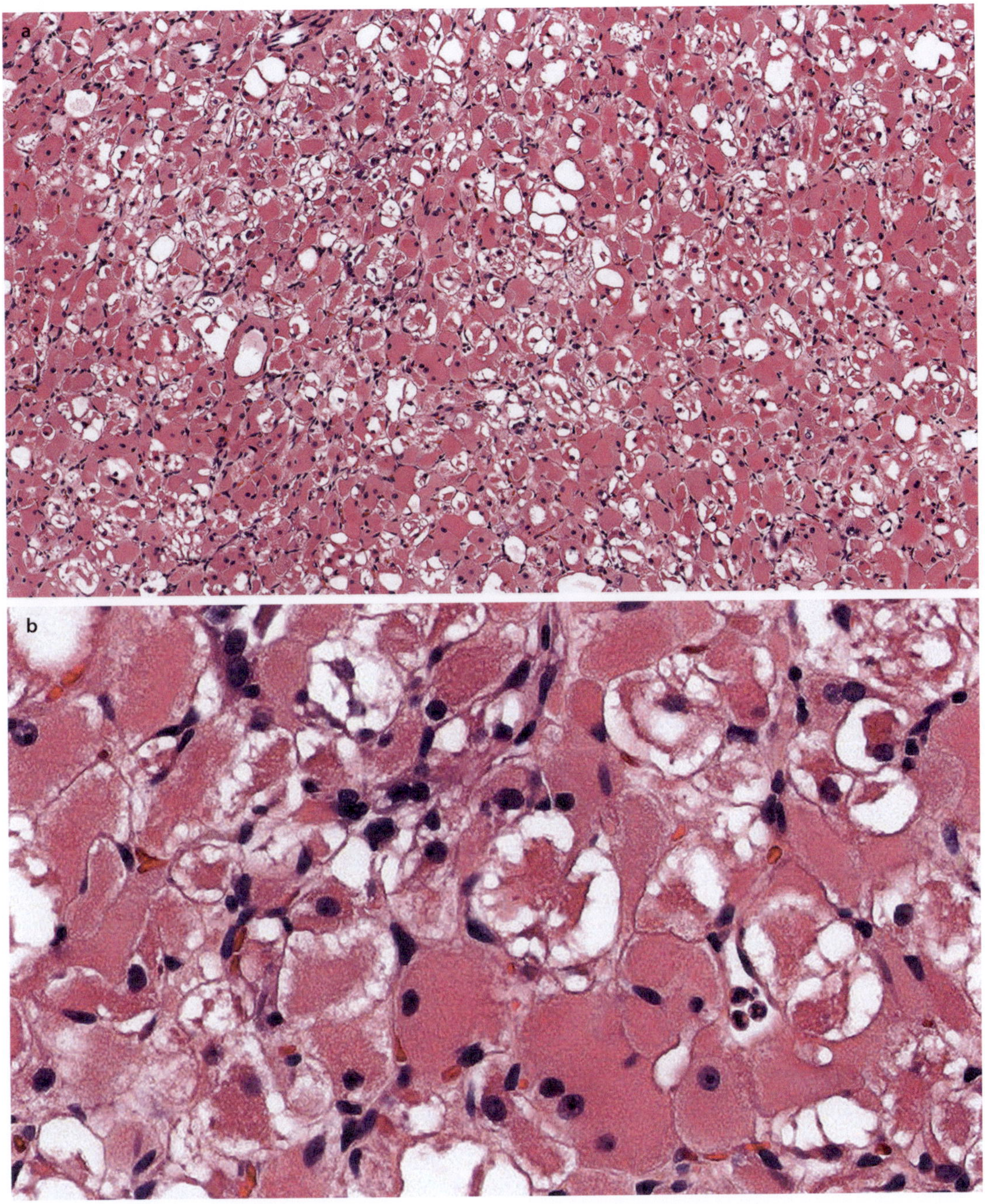

Fig. 2.48 Rhabdomyoma **a** Solid proliferation of polygonal cells with dense, deeply eosinophilic cytoplasm. **b** Retraction of cytoplasm from the cell membranes produces a star-like appearance. The rhabdomyocyte nuclei are condensed and peripheral

Self Study: Look sharp!

1. Which of the following statements is false?
   A. Wickham's striae are observed in erosive oral lichen planus.
   B. Liquefactive degeneration of basal cells in oral lichen planus leads to Max-Joseph spaces.
   C. Lichenoid reaction may be induced by dental amalgam.
   D. Lichenoid reaction is characterized by shaggy fibrinogen deposition at the basement membrane zone.
2. Which of the following statements is/are false?
   A. Pemphigus is a subepithelial vesicular bullous disease caused by antibodies to desmogleins.
   B. A positive Nikolsky is specific for pemphigus vulgaris.
   C. Patients with mucosal pemphigus have only Dsg-1 autoantibodies.
   D. Tzanck cells can be seen in benign mucosal pemphigoid.
   E. A and C false.
   F. All are false.
3. Regarding ▣ Fig. 2.49, which statement is true?
   A. Often observed in dark-skinned individuals.
   B. Reversible with smoking cessation.
   C. This represents the second most common type of intraoral nevus.
   D. May be observed in the hard palate.

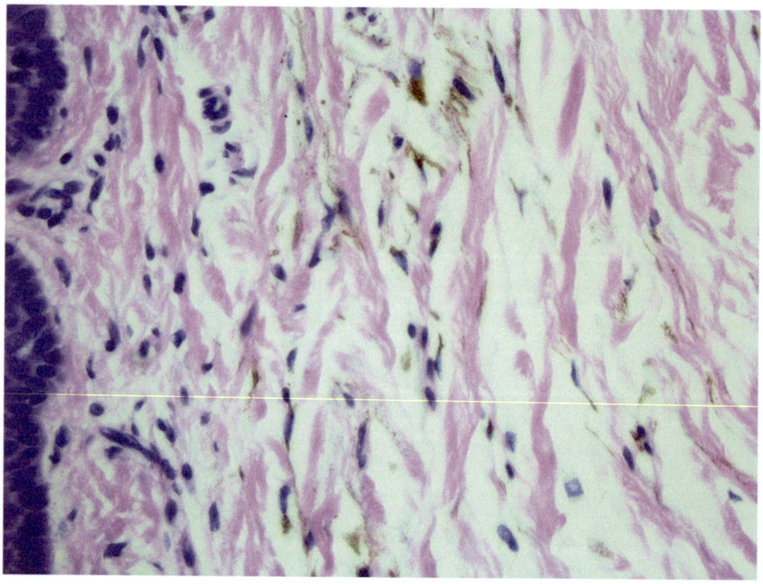

▣ **Fig. 2.49** Self study #3

4. Regarding ◘ Fig. 2.50, which statement is true?
   A. It is usually accompanied by some predisposing condition (diabetes, radiation, steroid inhalants).
   B. This process can be caused by caused by nutritional deficiencies, alcoholism, or medications.
   C. This is mediated by HPV13.
   D. This represents a lytic cycle of EBV infection.
   E. This may be associated with fissured tongue.

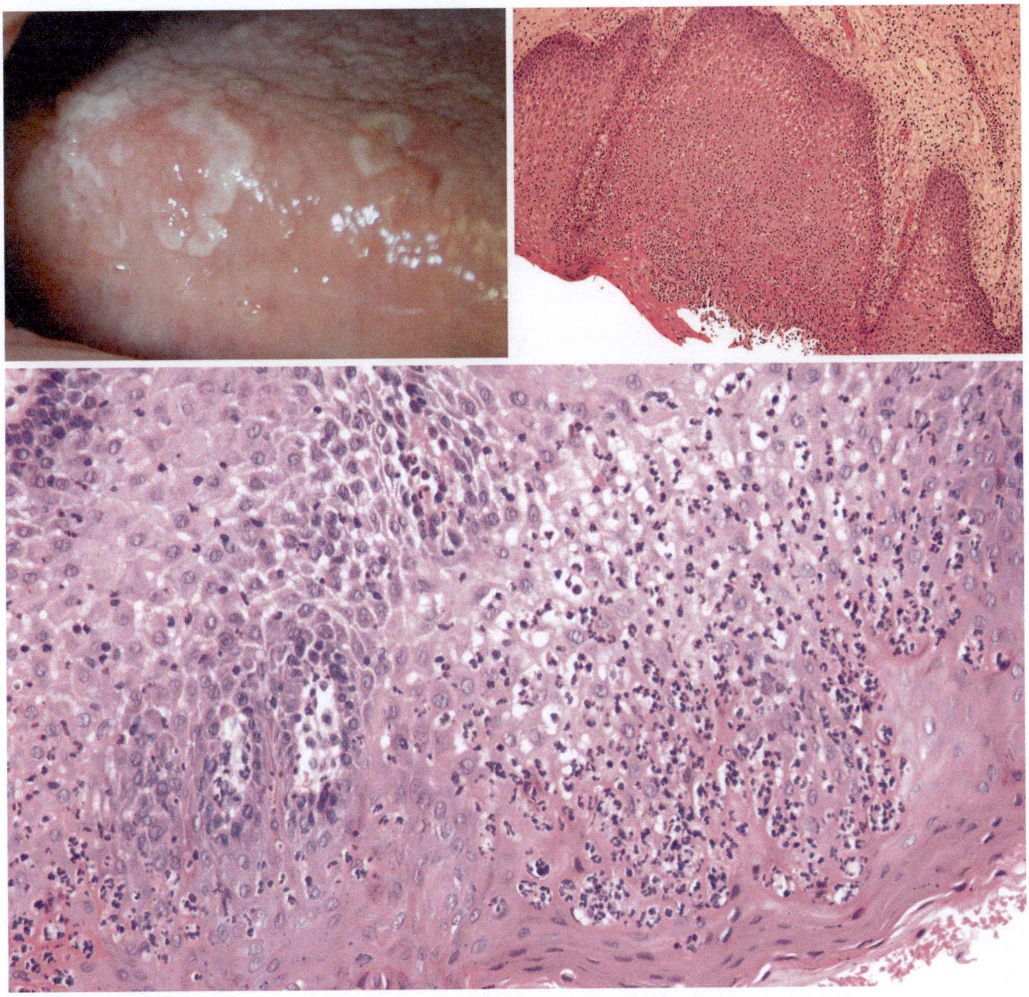

◘ **Fig. 2.50** Self study #4

5. Which of the following statements regarding these intraoral entities is false?
   A. Sclerotic fibroma may be associated with Cowden's syndrome.
   B. Desmoplastic fibroma has a dense keloid-like collagenized component.
   C. Myofibromas are more common in pediatric patients.
   D. Sialadenoma papilliferum may be distinguished from inverted and ductal papillomas by their exophytic component.
   E. Tori maxillaris presents as a midline palatal mass.

6. Figure 2.51: Which of the following statements are true?
   A. Autoantibodies desmoglien are positive
   B. Autoantibodies BP180 and epiligrin positive
   C. Shaggy fibrinogen deposition at the basement membrane zone
   D. This is a hypersensitivity reaction to amalgam

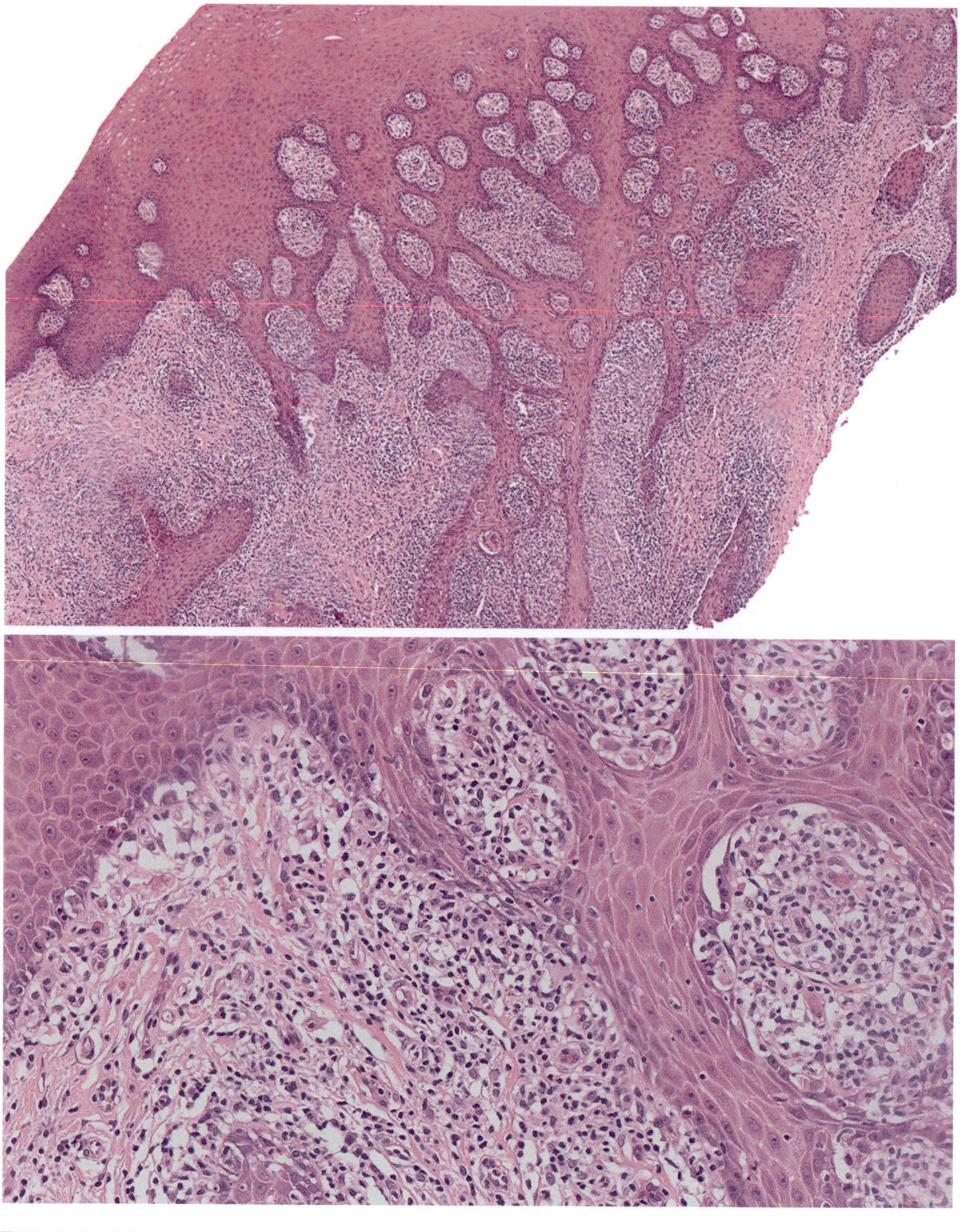

Fig. 2.51 Self study #6

7. Figure 2.52: What is the causative agent here?
   A. EBV
   B. HHV-8
   C. HPV 32
   D. Candida
   E. Other

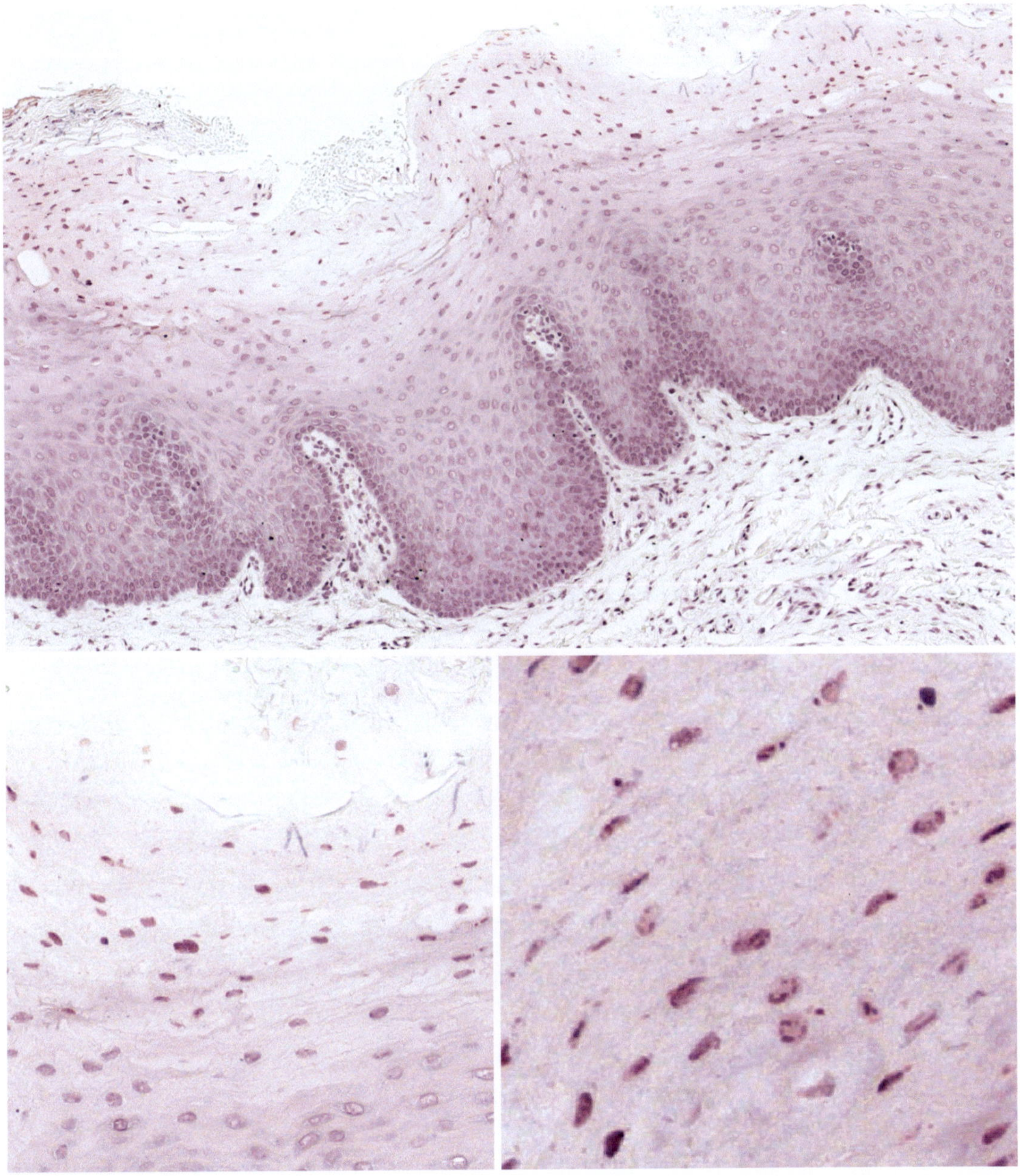

Fig. 2.52 Self study #7

8. ◘ Figure 2.53: Which statement is true?
   A. This is caused by bisphosphate intake
   B. This is a benign neonatal tumor
   C. This has a predilection for older men with Paget's disease of bone
   D. This is a reparative process
   E. This is responsible for phosphauria

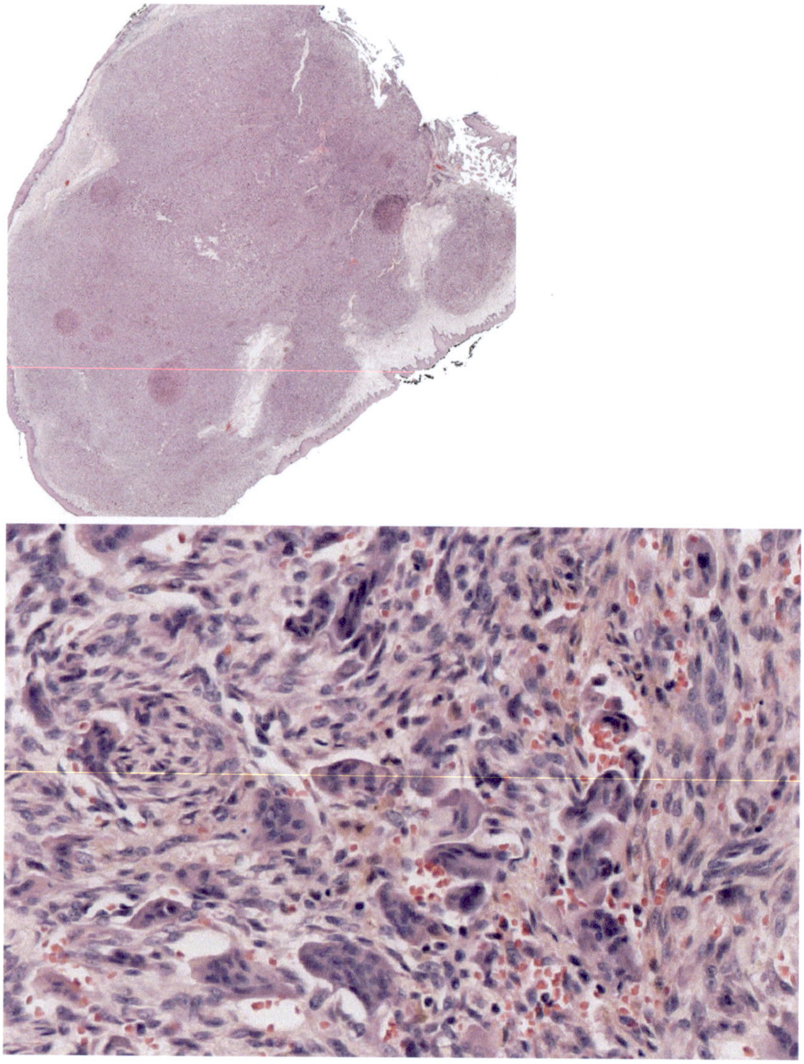

◘ **Fig. 2.53** Self study #8

9. ■ Figure 2.54: What's your diagnosis?
   A. Hairy leukoplakia
   B. Hairy tongue
   C. Geographic tongue
   D. Median rhomboid glossitis
   E. Other

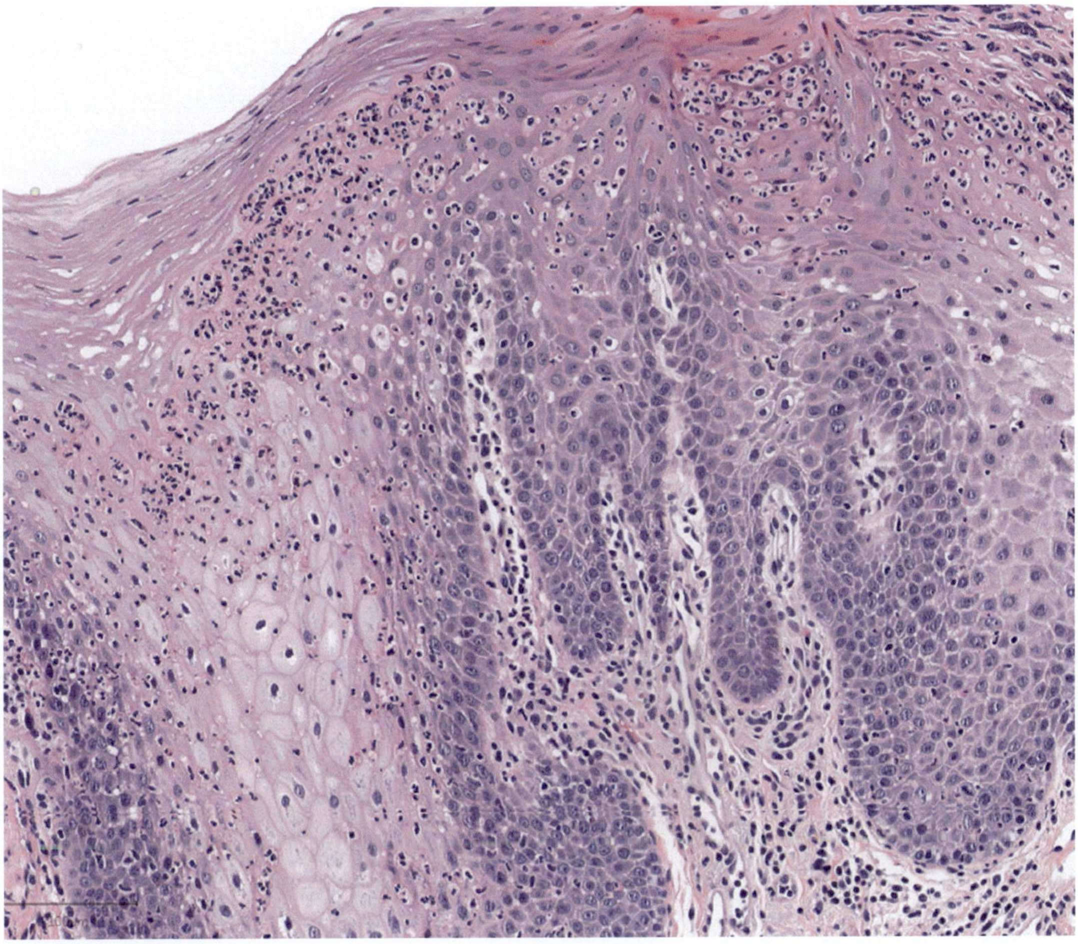

■ **Fig. 2.54** Self study #9

10. Figure 2.55: What is the causative agent here?
    A. EBV
    B. HHV-8
    C. HPV 32
    D. Candida
    E. Other

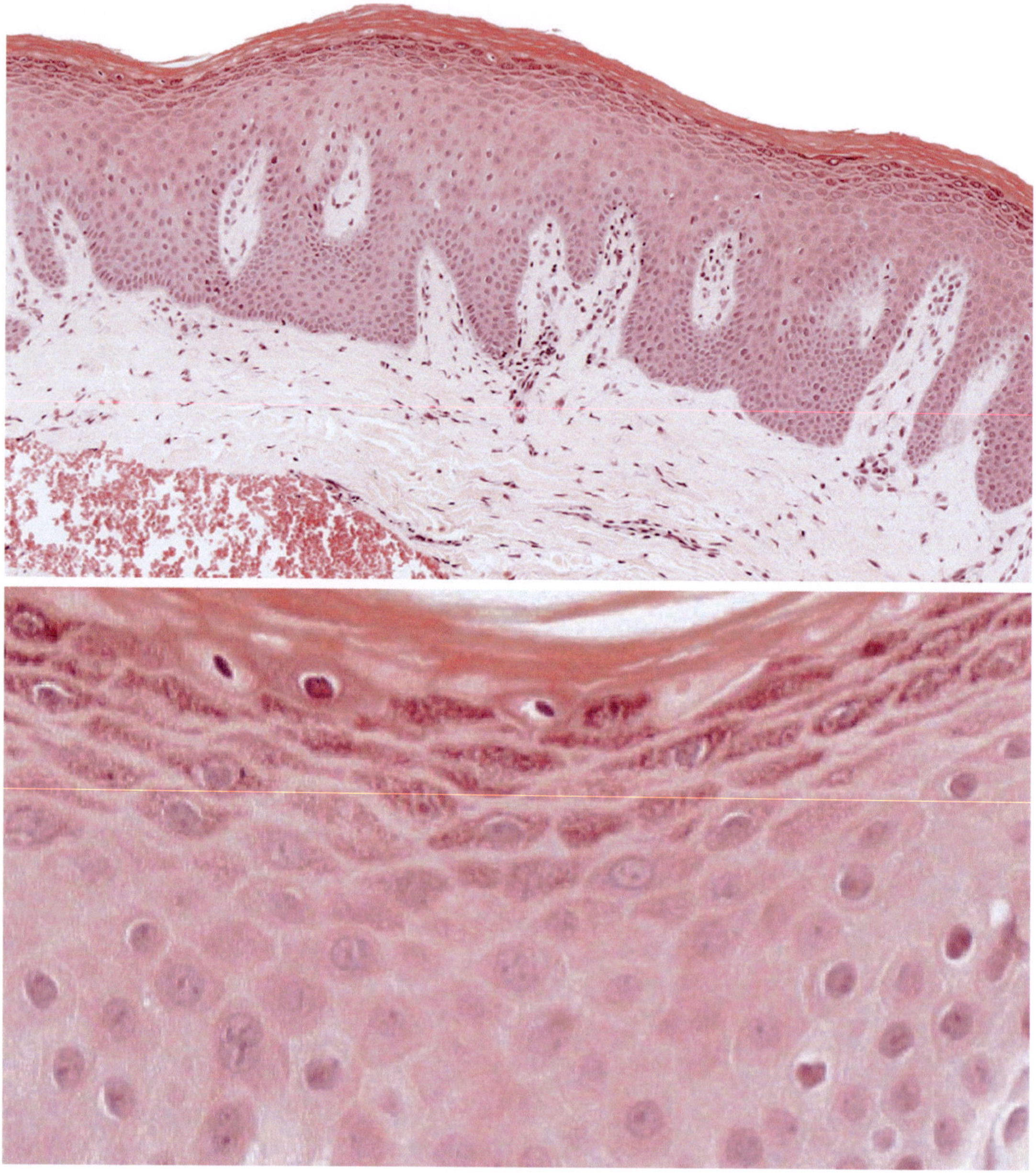

Fig. 2.55 Self study #10

11. Figure 2.56: Causation please
    A. EBV
    B. Trauma
    C. HPV 32
    D. Candida
    E. Other

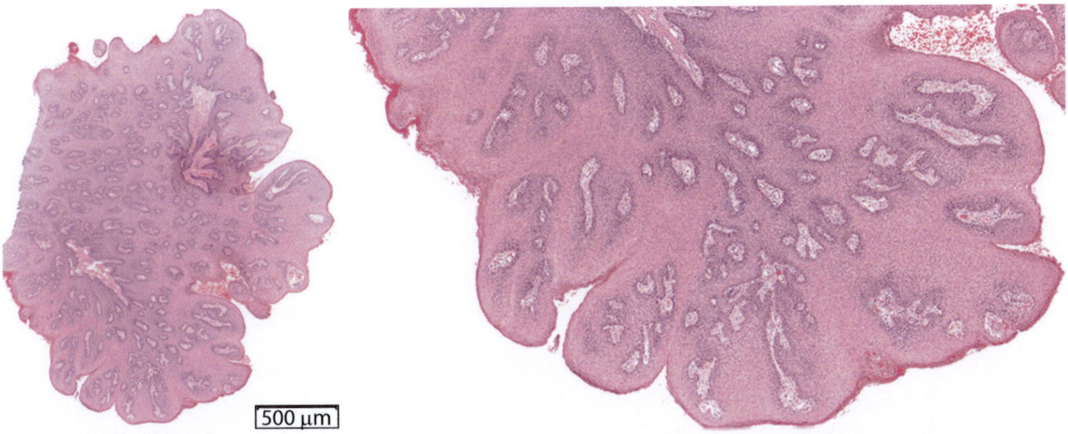

Fig. 2.56 Self study #11

12. Figure 2.57: Which test would you order?
    A. IHC for HSV
    B. IHC for CMV
    C. ISH for EBER
    D. DIF for fibrinogen, C3, IgA, IgG
    E. GMS

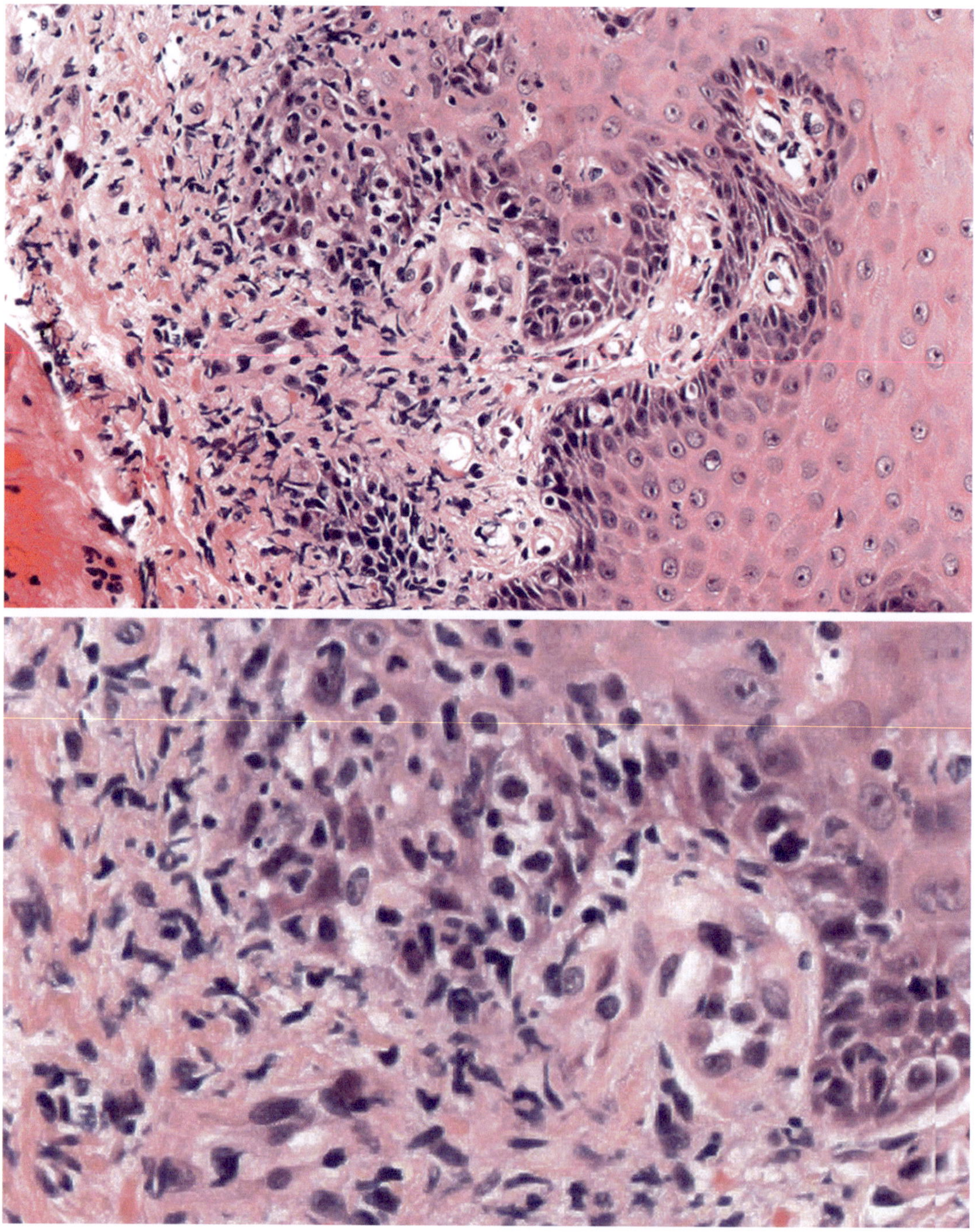

Fig. 2.57 Self study #12

Answers

1. Which of the following statements is false?
   A. Wickham's striae are observed in erosive oral lichen planus.
   TRUE. While striae are characteristic of reticular variant oral lichen planus, they can also be present adjacent to mucosal erosions in the erosive lichen planus.
   B. Liquefactive degeneration of basal cells in oral lichen planus leads to Max-Joseph spaces. **TRUE.**
   C. Lichenoid reaction may be induced by dental amalgam. **TRUE.**
   D. Lichenoid reaction is characterized by shaggy fibrinogen deposition at the basement membrane zone.
   FALSE. The bright "shaggy" signal, (also described as "stalagmites") distinguishes a true immunofluorescence signal from background immunofluorescence. A lichenoid reaction lacks this finding.
2. Which of the following statements is/are false?
   A. Pemphigus is a subepithelial vesicular bullous disease caused by antibodies to desmogleins. **FALSE.** Pemphigus refers to ***intraepithelial*** bullous formation, secondary to desmoglien autoantibodies.
   B. A positive Nikolsky is specific for pemphigus vulgaris. **FALSE.** This clinical sign refers to mucosal fragility, which may be present in other entities.
   C. Patients with mucosal pemphigus have only Dsg-1 autoantibodies. **FALSE.** These patients have excess autoantibodies to Dsg-3.
   D. Tzanck cells can be seen in benign mucosal pemphigoid. **FALSE.** Tzanck cells reflect *intramucosal* blistering, which is indicative of pemphigus.
   E. A and C false. **TRUE**, but not limited to…
   F. **All are false. TRUE, all are FALSE**
3. Regarding Fig. 2.49, which statement is true?
   A. Often observed in dark-skinned individuals. **FALSE.** Racial pigmentation and smokers melanosis are associated with epithelial melanosis and pigment incontinence. **Here we see pigment in spindled dendritic cells.**
   B. Reversible with smoking cessation. **FALSE.** – see above.
   C. This represents the second most common type of intraoral nevus. **FALSE.** These are not spindled (Type C) melanocytes.
   D. May be observed in the hard palate. **TRUE** Amalgam tattoo may clinically raise the suspicion for mucosal melanoma if the tattoo is not adjacent to the restored tooth.
4. Regarding Fig. 2.50, which statement is true?
   A. It is usually accompanied by some predisposing condition (diabetes, radiation, steroid inhalants). **FALSE.** This is an example of **geographic tongue**, which may be autoimmune or allergic in origin. The diagnostic hint here is the serpiginous white borders. The above-mentioned conditions predispose one to chronic candidiasis.
   B. This process can also be caused by caused by nutritional deficiencies, alcoholism, or medications. **FALSE.** The above-mentioned conditions predispose one to atrophic glossitis.
   C. This is mediated by HPV13. **FALSE.** HPV13 is associated with focal epithelial hyperplasia (Heck's disease).
   D. This represents a lytic cycle of EBV infection. **FALSE.** Hairy leukoplakia represents lytic EBV infection.
   E. This may be associated with fissured tongue. **TRUE.** Geographic tongue may be concurrent with fissured tongue. It is quite common in Down's syndrome, and also part of the rare Melkersson-Rosenthal syndrome, which also includes orofacial swelling and transient Bell's palsy.
5. Which of the following statements regarding these intraoral entities is false?
   A. Sclerotic fibroma may be associated with Cowden's syndrome **TRUE.**
   B. Desmoplastic fibroma has a dense keloid-like collagenized component. **TRUE.**

C. Myofibromas are more common in pediatric patients. **TRUE.**
D. Sialadenoma papilliferum may be distinguished from inverted and ductal papillomas by their exophytic component. **TRUE.**
E. Tori maxillaris presents as a midline palatal mass. **FALSE.** Tori maxillaris arise from the buccal or palatal aspect of the maxillary alveolar processes.

6. Figure 2.51: Which of the following statements are true?
You are looking at a lichenoid reaction.
A. Autoantibodies desmoglien are positive. **FALSE.** Desmoglien-1 and desmoglien-3 autoantibodies are seen in mucocutaneous pemphigus. If only desmoglien-3 autoantibodies are present – this supports the diagnosis of mucosal pemphigus.
B. Autoantibodies BP180 and epiligrin positive. **FALSE.** BP180 and epiligrin autoantibodies relate to pemphigoid.
C. Shaggy fibrinogen deposition at the basement membrane zone. **FALSE.** "Shaggy" fibrinogen deposition is a true immunofluorescence finding, as compared to a linear and non-bright signal due to background signal. This can be found in lichen planus, as well as other autoimmune diseases.
D. This is a hypersensitivity reaction to amalgam. **CORRECT.** How can you tell this is a lichenoid reaction? This stratified squamous mucosa with from the gingiva, a site which could be involved by either lichen planus or a lichenoid reaction. The top view shows a broader inflammatory distribution than the dense band-like infiltrate of lichen planus. The bottom view does not reveal any Civatte bodies, or liquifactive degeneration of the basal cells.

7. Figure 2.52**:** What is the causative agent here?
A. EBV. **CORRECT. You are looking at hairy leukoplakia,** caused by lytic EBV infection. The top panel reveals a hyperplastic process. You might spy some Candida in the top panel. You definitely should have noticed it in the bottom left panel. The diagnosis is confirmed by EBER ISH. But you should think about hairy leukoplakia when you see the "beads" of marginalized nuclear chromatin, displaced by nuclear viral inclusion (Bottom right).
B. HHV-8. **FALSE.**
C. HPV 32. **FALSE.**
D. Candida. **FALSE.** Candida is frequently present in hairy leukoplakia, which has a proclivity for the immunosuppressed. But it is caused by EBV!
E. Other. **FALSE.**

8. Figure 2.53**:** Which statement is true?
A. This is caused by bisphosphate intake. **FALSE. You happen to be looking at a giant cell reparative granuloma.** Bisphosphate therapy is associated with an avascular osteonecrosis, which will be covered in Volume 4.
B. This is a benign neonatal tumor. **FALSE.** *I'm just trying to confuse you!* See the section on congenital granular cell tumor (congenital epulis of newborn, Neuman's tumor).
C. This has a predilection for older men with Paget's disease of bone. **FALSE.** True giant cell tumors of the jaws are pretty rare! They can be seen in Paget's disease of bone, with a genetic clustering of men with jaw giant cell tumors and Paget's disease in Southern Italy [139]
D. This is a reparative process. **CORRECT.** The features that distinguish a "true" giant cell tumor from among the legions of entities which can be accompanied by giant cells are: (1) The number of nuclei in the giant cells are greater, up to hundreds of nuclei. (2) The nuclei are identical to those within the stroma. (3) Hemorrhage and a reactive stromal background are lacking. The bottom panel is typical of a reactive process.
E. This is responsible for phosphauria. **FALSE**. Phosphaturic mesenchymal tumor will be covered in Volume 4.

9. Figure 2.54**:** What's your diagnosis?
A. Hairy leukoplakia. **FALSE**. You are looking at benign migratory glossitis (geographic tongue). The intraepithelial polys are not characteristic of hairy leukoplakia.

B. Hairy tongue. **FALSE.**
C. Geographic tongue. **CORRECT.** How can you tell this is geographic tongue? Collections of high intraepithelial polys (Pautrier's microabscesses) are characteristic of geographic tongue.
D. Median rhomboid glossitis. **FALSE.** Median rhomboid glossitis occurs solely in the dorsal midline tongue; but I give you no site clues. Histologically, this is associated with submucosal lymphocytic infiltrate and mixed intraepithelial inflammation. Pautrier's microabscesses are not present in median rhomboid tongue but are characteristic of geographic tongue.
E. Other. **FALSE.**

10. ◘ Figure 2.55: What is the causative agent here?
    A. EBV. **FALSE.** You are looking at Heck's disease (focal epithelial hyperplasia). EBV causes hairy leukoplakia.
    B. HHV-8 causes Kaposi's sarcoma.
    C. HPV 32. **CORRECT.** Heck's disease is caused by HPV13, and less often HPV32. How can you tell this is Heck's disease? The top panel shows you "clubbed" disfigured rete pegs, some with "Bronze Age ax" configuration (See ◘ Fig. 2.23). The lower panel shows you "mitusoid" bodies. These are the diagnostic findings for focal epithelial hyperplasia.
    D. Candida. **FALSE.** No inflammation. It would be highly unusual to see Candida in the absence of inflammation.
    E. Other. **FALSE.**
11. ◘ Figure 2.56: Causation please
    A. EBV. **FALSE.** You are looking at a condyloma.
    B. Trauma. **FALSE.**
    C. HPV 32. **FALSE.**
    D. Candida. **FALSE.**
    E. Other. **CORRECT.** Yes, oral condyloma accuminatum happen. HPV 6 is most commonly responsible followed by HPV 16 [140]. How can you tell this is condyloma accuminatum? A condyloma is basically a broad based sessile papilloma.
12. ◘ Figure 2.57: Which test would you order?
    A. IHC for HSV. **CORRECT.** You are looking at HSV infection. The top panel shows you non-specific inflammation and blood and fibrin. The bottom panel shows you larger cells a "smudgy" chromatin which actually represents intranuclear virus.
    B. IHC for CMV. **FALSE.** The cytomegalic cells show prominent nuclear and cytoplasmic inclusions.
    C. ISH for EBER. **FALSE.** Hairy leukoplakia is not inflamed.
    D. DIF for fibrinogen, C3, IgA, IgG. **FALSE.**
    E. GMS. **FALSE.** Candida is seen in the upper squamous mucosa. I'm deliberately not showing you that region.

References

1. Kurago ZB. Etiology and pathogenesis of oral lichen planus: an overview. Oral Surg Oral Med Oral Pathol Oral Radiol. 2016;122:72–80.
2. Edwards PC, Kelsch R. Oral lichen planus: clinical presentation and management. J Can Dent Assoc. 2002;68:494–9.
3. Patil A, Prasad S, Ashok L, Sujatha GP. Oral bullous lichen planus: case report and review of management. Contemp Clin Dent. 2012;3:344–8.
4. Garouhi F, Davari P, Fazel N. Cutaneous and mucosal lichen planus: a comprehensive review of clinical subtypes, risk factors, diagnosis, and prognosis. Sci World J. 2014;2014:22. 742826 https://doi.org/10.1155/2014/742826.
5. Gupta S, Ghosh S, Gupta S. Interventions for the management of oral lichen planus: a review of the conventional and novel therapies. Oral Dis. 2017. https://doi.org/10.1111/odi.12634.
6. Santoro FA, Stoopler ET, Werth VP. Pemphigus. Dent Clin N Am. 2013;57:597–610.
7. Ruocco E, Wolf R, Ruocco V, Brunetti G, Romano F, Lo Schiavo A. Pemphigus: associations and management guidelines: facts and controversies. Clin Dermatol. 2013;31:382–90.
8. Atzmony L, Hodak E, Leshem YA, Rosenbaum O, Gdalevich M, Anhalt GJ, Mimouni D. The role of adjuvant therapy in pemphigus: a systematic review and meta-analysis. J Am Acad Dermatol. 2015;73:264–71.
9. Yasukochi A, Teye K, Ishii N, Hashimoto T. Clinical and immunological studies of 332 Japanese patients tentatively diagnosed as anti-BP180-type mucous membrane pemphigoid: a novel BP180 C-terminal domain enzyme-linked immunosorbent assay. Acta Derm Venereol. 2016;96:762–7.
10. Amber KT, Bloom R, Hertl M. A systematic review with pooled analysis of clinical presentation and

immunodiagnostic testing in mucous membrane pemphigoid: association of anti-laminin-332 IgG with oropharyngeal involvement and the usefulness of ELISA. J Eur Acad Dermatol Venereol. 2016;30:72–7.
11. Balasubramaniam R, Kuperstein AS, Stoopler ET. Update on oral herpes virus infections. Dent Clin N Am. 2014;58:265–80.
12. Jiang YC, Feng H, Lin YC, Guo XR. New strategies against drug resistance to herpes simplex virus. Int J Oral Sci. 2016;8:1–6.
13. Yadav S, Malik S, Mittal HC, Singh G, Kamra H. Bimaxillary oral focal mucinosis. J Craniofac Surg. 2016;27:e665–7.
14. Joshi CP, Dani NH, Mahale SA, Patel NR. A case of oral focal mucinosis of gingiva: lesion in disguise. J Indian Soc Periodontol. 2015;19:586–8.
15. Rambhia KD, Khopkar US. Verrucous oral focal mucinosis. Indian J Dermatol Venereol Leprol. 2016;82:330–2.
16. Kauzman A, Pavone M, Blanas N, Bradley G. Pigmented lesions of the oral cavity: review, differential diagnosis, and case presentations. J Can Dent Assoc. 2004;70:682–3.
17. Marakoğlu K, Gürsoy UK, Toker HC, Demirer S, Sezer RE, Marakoğlu I. Smoking status and smoke-related gingival melanin pigmentation in army recruitments. Mil Med. 2007;172:110–3.
18. Sarswathi TR, Kumar SN, Kavitha KM. Oral melanin pigmentation in smoked and smokeless tobacco users in India. Clinico-pathological study. Indian J Dent Res. 2003;14:101–6.
19. Gondak RO, da Silva-Jorge R, Jorge J, Lopes MA, Vargas PA. Oral pigmented lesions: clinicopathologic features and review of the literature. Med Oral Patol Oral Cir Bucal. 2012;17:e919–24.
20. Ferreira L, Jham B, Assi R, Readinger A, Kessler HP. Oral melanocytic nevi: a clinicopathologic study of 100 cases. Oral Surg Oral Med Oral Pathol Oral Radiol. 2015;120:358–67.
21. Marangon Júnior H, Souza PE, Soares RV, de Andrade BA, de Almeida OP, Horta MC. Oral congenital melanocytic nevus: a rare case report and review of the literature. Head Neck Pathol. 2015;9:481–7.
22. Magliocca KR, Fitzpatrick SG. Autoimmune disease manifestations in the oral cavity. Surg Pathol Clin. 2017;10:57–88.
23. Nandini DB, Bhavana SB, Deepak BS, Ashwini R. Paediatric geographic tongue: a case report, review and recent updates. J Clin Diagn Res. 2016;31. https://doi.org/10.7860/JCDR/2016/16452.7191.
24. Dafar A, Bankvall M, Garsjö V, Jontell M, Çevik-Aras H. Salivary levels of interleukin-8 and growth factors are modulated in patients with geographic tongue. Oral Dis. 2017. https://doi.org/10.1111/odi.12654.
25. Seiden G, Curland S. The tongue as an excitable medium. New J Phys. 2015;31:1–8.
26. Goregen M, Miloglu O, Buyukkurt MC, Caglayan F, Aktas AE. Median rhomboid glossitis: a clinical and microbiological study. Eur J Dent. 2011;5:367–72.
27. Ghabanchi J, Tadbir A, Darafshi R, Sadegholvad M. The prevalence of median rhomboid glossitis in diabetic patients: a case-control study. Iran Red Crescent Med J. 2011;13:503–6.
28. Williams D, Lewis M. Pathogenesis and treatment of oral candidosis. J Oral Microbiol. 2011;3. https://doi.org/10.3402/jom.v3i0.5771.
29. Singh A, Verma R, Murari A, Agrawal A. Oral candidiasis: an overview. J Oral Maxillofac Pathol. 2014;18:S81–5.
30. Junqueira JC, Fuchs BB, Muhammed M, Coleman JJ, Suleiman JMAH, Vilela SFG, Costa ACB, Rasteiro VMC, Jorge AOC, Mylonakis E. Oral Candida albicans isolates from HIV-positive individuals have similar in vitro biofilm-forming ability and pathogenicity as invasive Candida isolates. BMC Microbiol. 2011;11:247–56.
31. Dongari-Bagtzoglou A, Dwivedi P, Ioannidou E, Shaqman M, Hull D, Burleson J. Oral Candida infection and colonization in solid organ transplant recipients. Oral Microbiol Immunol. 2009;24:249–54.
32. Choudhary S, McLeod M, Torchia D, Romanelli P. Autoimmune polyendocrinopathy-candidiasis-ectodermal dystrophy. J Clin Aesthet Dermatol. 2012;5:18–22.
33. Ferre EMN, Rose RS, Rosenzweig SD, Burbelo PD, Romito KR, Niemela JE, Rosen LB, Break TJ, Gu W, Hunsberger S, Browne SK, Hsu AP, Rampertaap S, Swamydas M, Collar AL, Kong HH, Chyi-Chia RL, Chascsa D, Simcox T, Pham A, Bondici A, Natarajan M, Monsale J, Kleiner DE, Quezado M, Alevizos I, Moutsopoulos NM, Yockey L, Frein C, Soldatos A, Calvo KR, Adjemian J, Similuk MN, Lang DM, Stone KD, Uzel G, Kopp JB, Bishop RJ, Holland SM, Olivier KN, Fleisher TA, Heller T, Winer KK, Lionakis MS. Redefined clinical features and diagnostic criteria in autoimmune polyendocrinopathy-candidiasis-ectodermal dystrophy. JCI Insight. 2016;1(13):e88782. Published online 2016 Aug 18. https://doi.org/10.1172/jci.insight.88782.
34. O'Donnell LE, Robertson D, Nile CJ, Cross LJ, Riggio M, Sherriff A, Bradshaw D, Lambert M, Malcolm J, Buijs MJ, Zaura E, Crielaard W, Brandt BW, Ramage G. The oral microbiome of denture wearers is influenced by levels of natural dentition. PLoS One. 2015;10(9):e0137717. https://doi.org/10.1371/journal.pone.0137717.
35. Chandra J, Mukherjee PK. Candida biofilms: development, architecture, and resistance. Microbiol Spectr. 2015;3. https://doi.org/10.1128/microbiolspec.MB-0020-2015.
36. Taff HT, Mitchell KF, Edward JA, Andes DR. Mechanisms of Candida biofilm drug resistance. Future Microbiol. 2013;8. https://doi.org/10.2217/fmb.13.101.
37. Castro LA, Castro JGLE, Cruz ADL, Barbosa BHDS, Spindula-Filho JV, Costa MB. Focal epithelial hyperplasia (Heck's disease) in a 57-year-old Brazilian patient: a case report and literature review. J Clin Med Res. 2016;8:346–50.
38. Ozden B, Gunduz K, Gunhan O, Ozden FO. A case report of focal epithelial hyperplasia (Heck's disease) with PCR detection of human papillomavirus. J Maxillofac Oral Surg. 2011;10:357–60.
39. Mansouri Z, Bakhtiari S, Noormohamadi R. Extensive focal epithelial hyperplasia: a case report. Iran J Pathol. 2015;10:300–5.
40. Galanakis A, Palaia G, Tenore G, Del Vecchio A, Romeo U. Focal epithelial hyperplasia in a human immunodeficiency virus patient treated with laser surgery. World J Clin Cases. 2014;2:293–6.

41. Steinhoff M, Metze D, Stockfleth E, Luger TA. Successful topical treatment of focal epithelial hyperplasia (Heck's disease) with interferon-beta. Brit J Dermatol. 2001;144:1067–9.
42. Pfister H, Hettich I, Runne U, Gissmann L, Chilf GN. Characterization of human papillomavirus type 13 from focal epithelial hyperplasia Heck lesions. J Virol. 1983;47:363–6.
43. Bascones-Martinez A, Cok S, Bascones-Ilundain C, Arias-Herrera S, Gomez-Font R, Bascones-Ilundain J. Multifocal epithelial hyperplasia: a potentially precancerous disease? Oncol Lett. 2012;3:255–8.
44. Gupta RR, Puri UP, Mahajan BB, Sahni SS, Garg G. Intraoral giant condyloma accuminatum. Indian J Dermatol Venerol Leprol. 2001;67:264–5.
45. Ozdamar SS, Ozdamar O, Kucukodaci Z. Giant intraoral condyloma accuminatum lesion coexisting with genital condyloma. Pak J Med Sci. 2014;30:1143–6.
46. McNamara K, Allen C, Kalmar J. Multiple papillary lesions of the gingival. J Am Dent Assoc. 2013;144:279–82.
47. Percinoto AC, Danelon M, Crivelini MM, Cunha RF, Percinoto C. Condyloma acuminata in the tongue and palate of a sexually abused child: a case report. BMC Res Notes. 2014;7:467–74.
48. King MD, Reznik DA, O'Daniels CM, Larsen NM, Osterholt D, Blumberg HM. Human papillomavirus-associated oral warts among human immunodeficiency virus-seropositive patients in the era of highly active antiretroviral therapy: an emerging infection. Clin Infect Dis. 2002;34:641–8.
49. Curi DS, Leite-Ribeiro PM, Torregrossa VR, Vieira VC, Sarmento VA. Efficacy of imidazolquinoline on treatment of condyloma acuminatum of the buccal mucosa. Spec Care Dentist. 2017;37:51–4.
50. Braz-Silva PH, Rezende NPM, Ortega KL, Santos RTM, Magalhães MHCG. Detection of the Epstein–Barr Virus (EBV) by in-situ hybridization as definitive diagnosis of hairy leukoplakia. Head Neck Pathol. 2008;2:19–24.
51. Zakrzewska JM, Aly Z, Speight PM. Oral hairy leukoplakia in a HIV-negative asthmatic patient on systemic steroids. J Oral Pathol Med. 1995;24:282–4.
52. Piperi E, Omlie J, Koutlas IG, Pambuccian S. Oral hairy leukoplakia in HIV-negative patients: report of 10 cases. Int J Surg Pathol. 2010;18:177–83.
53. Chambers AE, Conn B, Pemberton M, Robinson M, Banks R, Sloan P. Twenty-first-century oral hairy leukoplakia--a non-HIV-associated entity. Oral Surg Oral Med Oral Pathol Oral Radiol. 2015;119:326–32.
54. Fornatora ML, Reich RF, Gray RG, Freedman PD. Intraoral molluscum contagiosum: a report of a case and a review of the literature. Oral Surg Oral Med Oral Pathol Oral Radiol Endod. 2001;92:318–20.
55. de Carvalho CH, de Andrade AL, de Oliveira DH, de Araújo Lima ED, da Silveira EJ, de Medeiros AM. Intraoral molluscum contagiosum in a young immunocompetent patient. Oral Surg Oral Med Oral Pathol Oral Radiol. 2012;114:e57–60.
56. Sharma D, McKendry A, Nageshwaran S, Cartledge J. A case of oral ulceration and disseminated histoplasmosis in HIV infection. Int J STD AIDS. 2012;23:522–3.
57. Mohammed S, Sinha M, Chavan P, Premalata C, Shivaprakash M, Chakrabarti A, Jayshree RS. Oral histoplasmosis masquerading as oral cancer in HIV-infected patient: a case report. Med Mycol Case Rep. 2012;18:85–7.
58. Vidyanath S, Shameena P, Sudha S, Nair RG. Disseminated histoplasmosis with oral and cutaneous manifestations. J Oral Maxillofac Pathol. 2013;17:139–42.
59. de Paulo LF, Rosa RR, Durighetto Júnior AF. Primary localized histoplasmosis: oral manifestations in immunocompetent patients. Int J Infect Dis. 2013;17:e139–40.
60. Klein IP, Martins MA, Martins MD, Carrard VC. Diagnosis of HIV infection on the basis of histoplasmosis-related oral ulceration. Spec Care Dentist. 2016;36:99–103.
61. Folk GA, Nelson BL. Oral histoplasmosis. Head Neck Pathol. 2017. https://doi.org/10.1007/s12105-017-0797-y.
62. Marla V, Shrestha A, Goel K, Shrestha S. The histopathological spectrum of pyogenic granuloma: a case series. Case Rep Dent. 2016;2016:1323798. https://doi.org/10.1155/2016/1323798.
63. Gomes SR, Shakir QJ, Thaker PV, Tavadia JK. Pyogenic granuloma of the gingiva: a misnomer? – a case report and review of literature. J Indian Soc Periodontol. 2013;17:514–9.
64. Sachdeva SK. Extragingival pyogenic granuloma: an unusual clinical presentation. J Dent (Shiraz). 2015;16:282–5.
65. Anitua E, Pinas L. Pyogenic granuloma in relation to dental implants: clinical and histopathological findings. J Clin Exp Dent. 2015;7:e447–50.
66. Kang YH, Byun JH, Choi MJ, Lee JS, Jang JH, Kim YI, Park BW. Co-development of pyogenic granuloma and capillary hemangioma on the alveolar ridge associated with a dental implant: a case report. J Med Case Rep. 2014;8:192. https://doi.org/10.1186/1752-1947-8-192.
67. Thada SR, Pai KM, Agarwal P. A huge oral pyogenic granuloma with extensive alveolar bone loss and 'sunray' appearance mimicking a malignant tumour. BMJ Case Rep. 2014. https://doi.org/10.1136/bcr-2013-20236.
68. George SMC, Gossain SR, Morrison IK, Coburn PR. Recurrent pyogenic granuloma with satellitosis. BMJ Case Rep. 2012. https://doi.org/10.1136/bcr.11.2011.5162.
69. Erbasar GNH, Senguven B, Gultekin SE, Cetiner S. Management of a recurrent pyogenic granuloma of the hard palate with diode laser: a case report. J Lasers Med Sci. 2016;7:56–61.
70. Shadman N, Ebrahimi SF, Jafari S, Eslami M. Peripheral giant cell granuloma: a review of 123 cases. Dent Res J. 2009;6:47–50.
71. Ogbureke EI, Vigneswaran N, Seals M, Frey G, Johnson CD, Ogbureke KUE. A peripheral giant cell granuloma with extensive osseous metaplasia or a hybrid peripheral giant cell granuloma-peripheral ossifying fibroma: a case report. J Med Case Rep. 2015. https://doi.org/10.1186/1752-1947-9-14.

2

72. Gupta M, Gupta M, Singh S, Kaur R. Central giant cell granuloma of the maxilla. BMJ Case Rep. 2013. https://doi.org/10.1136/bcr-2013-009102.
73. Ishinaga H, Otsu K, Mouri G, Takeuchi K. Aggressive giant cell reparative granuloma of the nasal cavity. Case Rep Otolaryngol. 2013. https://doi.org/10.1155/2013/690194.
74. Jadu FM, Pharoah MJ, Lee L, Baker GI, Allidina A. Central giant cell granuloma of the mandibular condyle: a case report and review of the literature. Dentomaxillofac Radiol. 2011;40:60–4.
75. Yadav S, Singh A, Kumar P, Tyagi S. Recurrent case of central giant cell granuloma with multiple soft tissue involvement. Natl J Maxillofac Surg. 2014;5:60–6.
76. Shen WR, Chang JY, Wu YC, Cheng SJ, Chen HM, Wang YP. Oral traumatic ulcerative granuloma with stromal eosinophilia: a clinicopathological study of 34 cases. J Formos Med Assoc. 2015;114:881–5.
77. Sharma B, Koshy G, Kapoor S. Traumatic ulcerative granuloma with stromal eosinophila: a case report and review of pathogenesis. J Clin Diagn Res. 2016;10:ZD07–9.
78. Sarangarajan R, Vaishnavi Vedam VK, Sivadas G, Sarangarajan A, Meera S. Traumatic ulcerative granuloma with stromal eosinophilia – mystery of pathogenesis revisited. J Pharm Bioallied Sci. 2015;7:S420–3.
79. Brasileiro BF, Alves DB, Andrade BA, Vargas PA, León JE, Almeida OP. Traumatic ulcerative granuloma with stromal eosinophilia of the palate showing an angiocentric/angiodestructive growth pattern. Contemp Clin Dent. 2012;3:S109–11.
80. Gagari E, Stathopoulos P, Katsambas A, Avgerinou G. Traumatic ulcerative granuloma with stromal eosinophilia: a lesion with alarming histopathologic presentation and benign clinical course. Am J Dermatopathol. 2011;33:192–4.
81. Hirshberg A, Amariglio N, Akrish S, Yahalom R, Rosenbaum H, Okon E, Kaplan I. Traumatic ulcerative granuloma with stromal eosinophilia: a reactive lesion of the oral mucosa. Am J Clin Pathol. 2006;126:522–9.
82. Alves MGO, Kitakawa D, Carvalho YR, Cabral LAG, Almeida JD. Necrotizing sialometaplasia as a cause of a non-ulcerated nodule in the hard palate: a case report. J Med Case Rep. 2011. https://doi.org/10.1186/1752-1947-5-406.
83. Gatti A, Broccardo E, Poglio G, Benech A. Necrotizing sialometaplasia of the hard palate in a patient treated with topical nonsteroidal anti-inflammatory drug. Case Rep Dent. 2016. https://doi.org/10.1155/2016/9545861.
84. Samir A, Joshi SA, Rajshekhar Halli R, Vaishali Koranne V, Sarita Singh S. Necrotizing sialometaplasia: a diagnostic dilemma! J Oral Maxillofac Pathol. 2014;18:420–2.
85. Krishna S, S Ramnarayan BK. Necrotizing sialometaplasia of palate: a case report. Imaging Sci Dent. 2011;41:35–8.
86. Yagi T, Ueda H, Amitani H, Asakawa A, Miyawaki S, Inui A. The role of ghrelin, salivary secretions, and dental care in eating disorders. Forum Nutr. 2012;4:967–89.
87. Khan FY, Jan SM, Mushtaq M. Multicentric peripheral ossifying fibroma: a case report and review of the literature. J Indian Soc Periodontol. 2013;17:648–52.
88. Sousa SF, Caldeira PC, Grossmann SMC, de Aguiar MCF, Mesquita RA. Desmoplastic fibroblastoma (Collagenous fibroma): a case identified in the buccal mucosa. Head Neck Pathol. 2011;5:175–9.
89. Bhagalia S, Jain M, Pardhe N, Sireesha SK. Collagenous fibroma (desmoplastic fibroblastoma) of the oral cavity. J Oral Maxillofac Pathol. 2012;16:277–9.
90. Darling MR, Kutalowski M, MacPherson DG, Jackson-Boeters L, Wysocki GP. Oral elastofibromatous lesions: a review and case series. Head Neck Pathol. 2011;5:254–8.
91. Narayen V, Ahmed SA, Suri C, Tanveer S. Myofibroma of the gingiva: a rare case report and literature review. Case Rep Dent. 2015. https://doi.org/10.1155/2015/243894.
92. Lee YM, Son SM, Kim KW, Lee OJ. Solitary myofibroma of the adult mandible: a case report and review of literature. Korean J Pathol. 2014;48:307–10.
93. Satomi T, Kohno M, Enomoto A, Abukawa H, Fujikawa K, Koizumi T, Chikazu D, Matsubayashi J, Nagao T. Solitary myofibroma of the mandible: an immunohistochemical and ultrastructural study with a review of the literature. Med Mol Morphol. 2014;47:176–83.
94. Aiki M, Yoshimura H, Ohba S, Kimura S, Imamura Y, Sano K. Rapid growing myofibroma of the gingiva: report of a case and review of the literature. J Oral Maxillofac Surg. 2014;72:99–105.
95. Haspel AC, Coviello VF, Stevens M, Robinson PG. Myofibroma of the mandible in an infant: case report, review of the literature, and discussion. J Oral Maxillofac Surg. 2012;70:1599–604.
96. Foss RD, Ellis GL. Myofibromas and myofibromatosis of the oral region: a clinicopathologic analysis of 79 cases. Oral Surg Oral Med Oral Pathol Oral Radiol Endod. 2000;89:57–65.
97. Loukas M, Hulsberg P, Tubbs RS, Kapos T, Wartmann CT, Shaffer K, Moxham BJ. The tori of the mouth and ear: a review. Clin Anat. 2013;26:953–60.
98. García-García AS, Martínez-González JM, Gómez-Font R, Soto-Rivadeneira A, Oviedo-Roldán L. Current status of the torus palatinus and torus mandibularis. Med Oral Patol Oral Cir Bucal. 2010;15:e353–60.
99. Gonsalves WC, Chi AC, Neville BW. Common oral lesions: Part II. Masses and neoplasia. Am Fam Physician. 2007;75:509–12.
100. Mahajan D, Khurana N, Setia N. Sialadenoma papilliferum in a young patient: a case report and review of the literature. Oral Surg Oral Med Oral Pathol Oral Radiol Endod. 2007;103:e51–4.
101. Gomes AP, Sobral AP, Loducca SV, de Araújo VC. Sialadenoma papilliferum: immunohistochemical study. Int J Oral Maxillofac Surg. 2004;33:621–4.
102. Brannon RB, Sciubba JJ, Giulani M. Ductal papillomas of salivary gland origin: a report of 19 cases and a review of the literature. Oral Surg Oral Med Oral Pathol Oral Radiol Endod. 2001;92:68–77.

103. Argyres MI, Golitz LE. Sialadenoma papilliferum of the palate: case report and literature review. J Cutan Pathol. 1999;26:259–62.
104. Markopoulos A, Kayavis I, Papanayotou P. Sialadenoma papilliferum of the oral cavity: report of a case and literature review. J Oral Maxillofac Surg. 1997;55:1181–4.
105. Liu W, Gnepp DR, de Vries E, Bibawy H, Solomon M, Gloster ES. Mucoepidermoid carcinoma arising in a background of sialadenoma papilliferum: a case report. Head Neck Pathol. 2009;3:59–62.
106. Solomon MP, Rosen Y, Alfonso A. Intraoral papillary squamous cell tumor of the soft palate with features of sialadenoma papilliferum-? malignant sialadenoma papilliferum. Cancer. 1978;42:1859–69.
107. Shimoda M, Kameyama K, Morinaga S, Tanaka Y, Hashiguchi K, Shimada M, Okada Y. Malignant transformation of sialadenoma papilliferum of the palate: a case report. Virchows Arch. 2004;445:641–6.
108. Ponniah I. A rare case of sialadenoma papilliferum with epithelial dysplasia and carcinoma in situ. Oral Surg Oral Med Oral Pathol Oral Radiol Endod. 2007;104:e27–9.
109. Lack EE, Worsham GF, Callihan MD, Crawford BE, Klappenbach S, Rowden G, Chun B. Granular cell tumor: a clinicopathologic study of 110 patients. J Surg Oncol. 1980;13:301–16.
110. Van de Loo S, Thunnissen E, Postmus P, Van der Waal I. Granular cell tumor of the oral cavity; a case series including a case of metachronous occurrence in the tongue and the lung. Med Oral Patol Oral Cir Bucal. 2015;20:e30–3.
111. Barbieri M, Musizzano Y, Boggio M, Carcuscua C. Granular cell tumour of the tongue in a 14-year-old boy: case report. Acta Otorhinolaryngol Ital. 2011;31:186–9.
112. Cole E, Rahman N, Webb R. Case series: two cases of an atypical presentation of oral granular cell tumour. Case Rep Med. 2012. https://doi.org/10.1155/2012/159803.
113. Vera-Sirera B, Zabala P, Aviño-Mira C, Vera-Sempere FJ. Multiple granular cell tumors with metachronous occurrence in tongue and vulva. Clinicopathological and immunohistochemical study. J Oral Maxillofac Pathol. 2014;18:437–41.
114. Tobouti PL, Pigatti FM, Martins-Mussi MC, Sedassari BT. Orsini-Machado de Sousa SC: extra-tongue oral granular cell tumor: Histological and immunohistochemical aspect. Med Oral Patol Oral Cir Bucal. 2017;22:e31–5.
115. Li X, Parke RB, Rushton JR, Sienko AS, Zhai QJ. An unusually large granular cell tumor of the pharynx: a case report and literature review. Int J Clin Exp Pathol. 2009;2:300–2.
116. Solomon LW, Velez I. S-100 negative granular cell tumor of the oral cavity. Head Neck Pathol. 2016;10:367–73.
117. Ferreira JCB, Oton-Leite AF, Guidi R, Mendonça EF. Granular cell tumor mimicking a squamous cell carcinoma of the tongue: a case report. BMC Res Notes. 2017. https://doi.org/10.1186/s13104-016-2325-7.
118. Said-Al-Naief N, Brandwein M, Lawson W, Gordon R, Lumerman H. Synchronous lingual granular cell tumor and squamous cell carcinoma: a case report and review of literature. Arch Otolaryngol Head Neck Surg. 1997;123:543–7.
119. Tucker MC, Rusnock EJ, Azumi N, Hoy GR, Lack EE. Gingival granular cell tumors of the newborn. An ultrastructural and immunohistochemical study. Arch Pathol Lab Med. 1990;114:895–8.
120. Lack EE, Perez-Atayde AR, McGill TJ, Vawter GF. Gingival granular cell tumor of the newborn (congenital "epulis"): ultrastructural observations relating to histogenesis. Hum Pathol. 1982;13:686–9.
121. Bang KO, Bodhade AS, Dive AM. Congenital granular cell epulis of a newborn. Dent Res J (Isfahan). 2012;9(Suppl 1):S136–8.
122. Aparna HG, Jayanth BS, Shashidara R, Jaishankar P. Congenital epulis in a newborn: a case report, immunoprofiling and review of literature. Ethiop J Health Sci. 2014;24:359–62.
123. Kumar R, Jaiswal S, Singhal A, Garg R. Congenital granular cell lesion: a rare tumor of new born. J Oral Maxillofac Pathol. 2013;17:440–2.
124. Kailash Narasimhan K, Arneja JS, Rabah R. Treatment of congenital epulis (granular cell tumour) with excision and gingivoperiosteoplasty. Can J Plast Surg. 2007;15:215–8.
125. Yuwanati M, Mhaske S, Mhaske A. Congenital granular cell tumor – a rare entity. J Neonatal Surg. 2015;4(2):17. PMCID: PMC4447470
126. McGuire LS, Yakoub D, Möller MG, Rosenberg A, Livingstone A. Malignant granular cell tumor of the back: a case report and review of the literature. Case Rep Med. 2014. https://doi.org/10.1155/2014/794648.
127. Meling TR, Fridrich K, Evensen JF, Nedregaard B. Malignant granular cell tumor of the skull base. Skull Base. 2008;18:59–66.
128. Morita S, Hiramatsu M, Sugishita M, Gyawali B, Shibata T, Shimokata T, Urakawa H, Mitsuma A, Moritani S, Kubota T, Ichihara S, Ando Y. Pazopanib monotherapy in a patient with a malignant granular cell tumor originating from the right orbit: a case report. Oncol Lett. 2015;10:972–4.
129. Brandwein M, Le Benger J, Strauchen J, Biller H. Atypical granular cell tumor of the larynx. Head Neck Surg. 1990;12:154–9.
130. Trey LA, Schmid S, Huber GF. Multifocal adult rhabdomyoma of the head and neck manifestation in 7 locations and review of the literature. Case Rep Otolaryngol. 2013. https://doi.org/10.1155/2013/758416.
131. Souza AA, Araújo VC, Santos FP, Martinez EF, Filho JFM, Araujo NS, Soares AB. Intraoral adult rhabdomyoma: a case report. Case Rep Dent. 2013. https://doi.org/10.1155/2013/741548.
132. Helliwell TR, Sissons MC, Stoney PJ, Ashworth MT. Immunochemistry and electron microscopy of head and neck rhabdomyoma. J Clin Pathol. 1988;41:1058–63.
133. Maglio R, Francesco S, Paolo M, Stefano V, Francesco D, Giovanni R. Voluminous extracardiac adult rhabdomyoma of the neck: a case presentation. Case Rep Surg. 2012. https://doi.org/10.1155/2012/984789.

2

134. Pinho MM, Castro JC, Ramos RG. Adult rhabdomyoma of the larynx. Int Arch Otorhinolaryngol. 2013;17:415–8.
135. Limbach AL, Goyal A. Adult rhabdomyoma: a challenging diagnosis on cytology. Cytojournal. 2012. https://doi.org/10.4103/1742-6413.100124.
136. Wang CP, Chang YH, Chang YT. Fetal rhabdomyoma of the right tonsil with polyp-like appearance. Case Rep Otolaryngol. 2015. https://doi.org/10.1155/2015/713278.
137. Hettmer S, Teot LA, Kozakewich H, Werger AM, Davies KJ, Fletcher CDM, Grier HE, Rodriguez-Galindo C, Wagers AJ. Myogenic tumors in nevoid basal cell carcinoma syndrome. J Pediatr Hematol Oncol. 2015;37:147–9.
138. Hettmer S, Teot LA, van Hummelen P, MacConaill L, Bronson RT, Dall'Osso C, Mao J, McMahon AP, Gruber PJ, Grier HE, Rodriguez-Galindo C, Fletcher CD, Wagers AJ. Mutations in Hedgehog pathway genes in fetal rhabdomyomas. J Pathol. 2013. https://doi.org/10.1002/path.4229.
139. Cosso R, Nuzzo V, Zuccoli A, Brandi ML, Falchetti A. Giant cell tumor in a case of Paget's disease of bone: an aggressive benign tumor exhibiting a quick response to an innovative therapeutic agent. Clin Cases Miner Bone Metab. 2010;7:145–52.
140. Kofoed K, Sand C, Forslund O, Madsen K. Prevalence of human papillomavirus in anal and oral sites among patients with genital warts. Acta Derm Venereol. 2014;94:207–11.

Oral Cavity: Malignancies and Precursors

M. S. Brandwein-Weber, *Textbook of Head and Neck Pathology*,
https://doi.org/10.1007/978-3-319-76106-0_3

Key Points

- The two major phenotypes for mucosal high-grade dysplasia/carcinoma in-situ are:
  1. That which follows uterine cervical dysplasia, in which lack of dysplastic features are full thickness, prior to the development of invasive disease.
  2. The more common phenotype in which there is relatively normal maturation in the superficial mucosa, yet the dysplastic features in the lower mucosa are qualitatively "bad enough" to warrant that diagnosis. How do you recognize this? Experience.
- Dysplasia always looks worst at the time of frozen section.
- Radiation atypia extending into ducts may mimic invasive carcinoma. Look for other changes of radiation, and duct lumena.
- Don't confuse the transitional pattern of invasion with "carcinoma-in-situ". Carcinoma-in-situ is usually limited and flat disease. Abundant "ribbons of epithelium" may represent carcinoma with a non-aggressive pattern of invasion.
- Expect the unexpected: High-grade dysplasia in HIV+ mucosal lesions.
- Resection margin assessment by intraoperative mapping of the resection specimen represents the gold standard for resection adequacy. No parallel (shave) margins! Assess margins perpendicular to the margin plane to allow for measurement in millimeters.
- Drop your condenser when quantifying extranodal extension (ENE). The birefringence of collagen reflects the natural curve of the lymph node hillam. Stretching of the lymph node capsule does not qualify for ENE.
- ENE microscopic or ENE macroscopic upstage nodal N classification.
- Primary oral melanoma is more common in mucosal sites adjacent to bone (hard palate, alveolar process, gingiva) than intraoral soft tissue sites. Maxillary sites are more common than mandibular sites.

3.1 Dysplasia: Epithelial Precursor Lesions

Leukoplakia is a general clinical term which refers to a white mucosal patch that does not rub off on exam (◘ Figs. 3.1, 3.2, and 3.3). Erythroleukoplakia describes heterogeneous, speckled, red and white lesions; it is more often associated with malignant progression than leukoplakic lesions. Leukoplakias/erythroleukoplakias on the lateral/ventral tongue and floor of mouth are particularly worrisome with respect to potential for progression [1, 2]. ◘ Table 3.1 summarizes a number of conditions with the potential for malignant transformation [1]. Mucosal dysplasias may transform into invasive carcinoma usually within 3 years, but progression may develop up to one decade later [3–9]. Features significantly predictive of transformation include grade (high-grade > low-grade), age > 60 years, lateral ventral tongue versus other intraoral sites, and heterogenous clinical appearance (speckled, nodular or verrucous) [4].

Proliferative verrucous leukoplakia represents a rare and distinct entity. Proliferative verrucous leukoplakia is commonly localized to the gingiva and palate and less likely to affect the typical subsites for usual precursor lesions (ventral and lateral tongue, floor of mouth) [10–13]. Typically, proliferative verrucous leukoplakia affects older woman and causes multifocal intraoral lesions. There's a notable absence of the usual risk factors (tobacco and alcohol). A great percentage of lesions (75%) transform into either usual squamous carcinoma or verrucous carci-

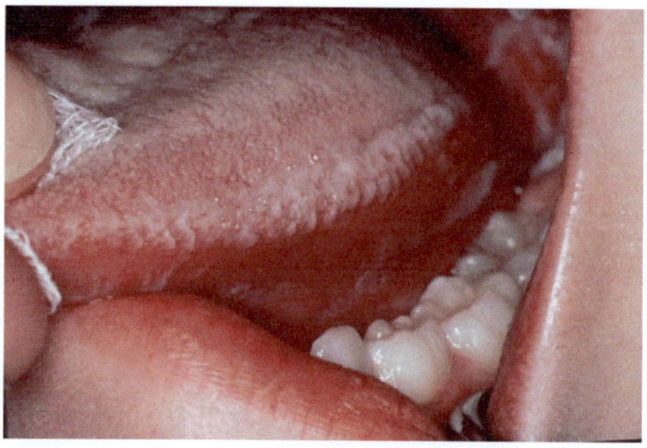

◘ **Fig. 3.1** A corrugated ridge of leukoplakia on the lateral tongue border noma. Importantly, this diagnosis is not based solely on histology but requires clinical correlation (see below); the clinical differential diagnosis includes localized and multifocal leukoplakia. There is no specific treatment for proliferative verrucous leukoplakia; the disease process is controlled by conservative excision or laser ablation of lesions and close surveillance.

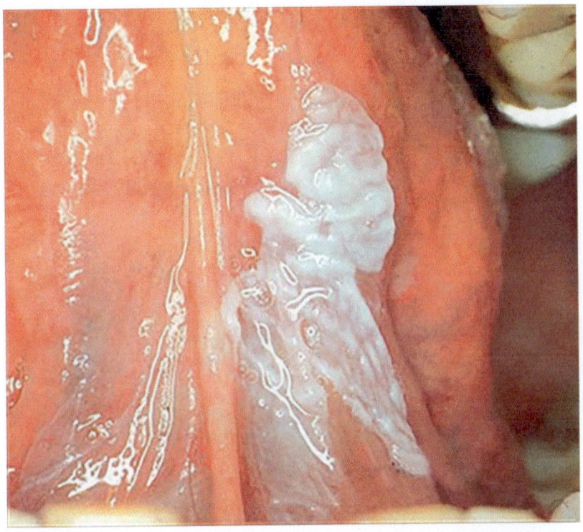

Fig. 3.2 Leukoplakia refers to a white mucosal patch that does not rub off on exam. Leukoplakia in normally nonkeratinizing regions (ventral tongue, floor of mouth) are particularly suspicious for being at risk for malignant progression

- The initial diagnosis of dysplasia increases the clinician's level of surveillance. Failure to recognize low-grade/mild-dysplasia can have critical clinical (and medicolegal) implications.
- Quantify the degree of dysplasia seen (focal, diffuse).
- Ascertain that your clinician is on the "same page" as you! Severe dysplasia and carcinoma-in-situ may have different appearances, but are equally likely to progress to invasive SCC.
- Beware of overcalling radiation-induced atypia.
- If the specimen is too small, do not hesitate to request rebiopsy. Don't compromise the patient, or yourself, with an inadequate biopsy.

It's well established that high-grade displasia/carcinoma-in-situ is more likely to progress to invasive carcinoma than low-grade displasia [39–41]. It's also well-accepted that a two-tiered assessment of dysplasia has greater reproducibility than a three-tiered model. The list of histologic features below is a mere guide which cannot substitute for the one-on-one experience of teaching

Fig. 3.3 Hyperkeratotic lingual mucosa (*arrows*). The small amount of keratinization on the right (*) is within normal limits

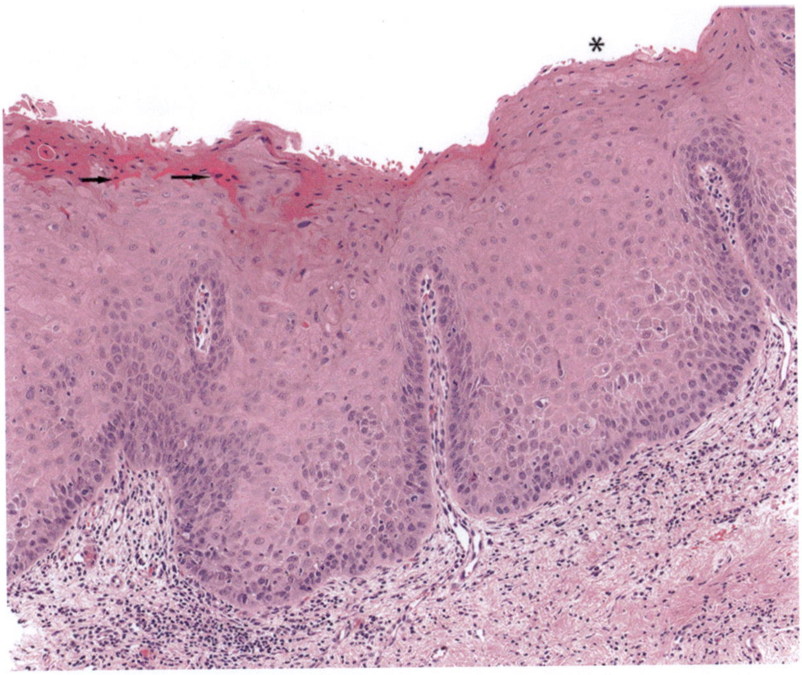

Table 3.1 Oral conditions with the potential for malignant progression [2]

Condition	Definition	Comments
Erythroplakia	Red mucosal patch	Reported progression rates of mucosal dysplasia to invasive carcinoma derived from large clinical studies and metanalyses: 3.5–17.8% [2–9]
Erythroleuko-plakia	Heterogenous red and white mucosal patch	
Leukoplakia	Persistant white mucosal patch	
Proliferative verrucous hyperplasia	Female predominance, multifocal disease, progressive course [10–13]	Unknown etiology, not associated with tobacco or alcohol
Submucous fibrosis	Related to chewing areca nut, gutka, and pan [14–16]. Causes trismus, oral burning, intolerance to spicy food. Increased intraoral fibrosis. Highest incidence in Indian subcontinent, but may be seen in USA and UK Rate of malignant transformation 9.13% [17]	Active metabolite arecoline-N-oxide acts as alkylating agent. Carcinogenic nitrosamines generated by nitrosation of areca alkaloid and persist in saliva **Histology**: Severely atrophic epithelium, submucosal collagen hyalinization, vascular obliteration [18, 19]. IHC for P63 is not restricted to basal and parabasal cells [20]. A series comparing 105 patients with oral squamous carcinoma and oral submucous fibrosis with usual type oral squamous carcinoma has demonstrated a significant skewing towards low-stage, node negative cancers [21]
Smokeless tobacco keratosis	Hyperkeratosis caused by direct contact with smokeless tobacco, most often alveolus/buccal/labial mucosa [22, 23]	Estimated 7 million smokeless tobacco users in USA **Histology**: "Chevrons" or "church spires" of hyperkeratosis, prominent cytoplasmic vaculolation and keratohyaline granules "between the chevrons" [23]
Reverse smokers lesions (bidi or beedi)	Peculiar custom of holding the lit end of this "poor man's cigarette" intraorally. May have been evolved as a means of avoiding the flame going out, or damage caused by falling of hot ash [24–27]	**Histology**: Hyperkeratosis and posible dysplasia of hard palate. Severe chronic inflamation. Melanosis and melanin incontinence
Chronic Candidiasis	Hyperplastic, hyperkeratotic mucosa with superficially invasive hyphae	Prevalence of Candida is greater in dysplastic mucosa. Carcinogenesis is attributed to the production of carcinogenic nitrosamines and cytokine-mediated downregulation of local immunity [28–31]
Lichen planus	A small subset of patients with oral lichen plan can be expected to develop oral squamous carcinoma [32–34]	
Discoid lupus erythematosis	Lupus affecting only skin, causing coin-like (discoid) erythematous-to-violaceous, scaly plaques. Ultra-violet light-induced progression to dysplasia/carcinoma of the lip [35, 36]	
Actinic (solar) keratosis of lip	Ultra-violet light-induced progression to dysplasia/carcinoma of the lip. Malignant transformation of labial solar keratosis is 2.5 times greater than that of skin actinic keratosis [37, 38]	

at the scope. It's important to emphasize that there are two major phenotypes for mucosal high-grade dysplasia/carcinoma in-situ:

1. That which follows uterine cervical dysplasia (classical dysplasia), in which dysplastic features span the full thickness of the mucosa prior to the development of invasive disease.
2. ***The more common phenotype in which there is relatively normal maturation in the superficial mucosa, yet the dysplastic features in the lower mucosa are qualitatively "bad enough" to warrant that diagnosis.*** How do you learn to recognize this? Experience. Experience. Experience.

One final note is that mucosal dysplasia will always looks worst at the time of frozen section. Just as the ***"tear-dropped rete pegs"*** is cause to "***turn the dial up a notch***" for dysplasia, the fact that you are ***evaluating squamous mucosa at the time of frozen section is cause to "dial down a notch for dysplasia"***. Histopathologically, the diagnosis and grading of dysplasia is based on the presence and degree of the following architectural and cytological changes which reflect abnormalities in maturation and proliferation (◻ Table 3.2) (◻ Figs. 3.4, 3.5, 3.6, 3.7, 3.8, 3.9, 3.10, 3.11, 3.12, 3.13, 3.14, and 3.15).

◻ **Table 3.2** Histopathologic variables of dysplasia

Architecture	Cytology
Loss of nuclear polarity	Enlarged nuclei
Increased cellularity, starting with parabasal hyperplasia	Abnormal variation in nuclear size and shape
Dyskeratosis (premature keratinisation)	Increased nuclear/ cytoplasmic ratio
Keratin pearls deep in rete pegs	Hyperchromatic nuclei
Bulbous rete pegs, tear-drop-shaped rete pegs	Coarse chromatin
Mitotic figures at or above the third layer of cells	Increased number and size of nucleoli
	Increased mitotic figures and atypical mitotic figures

Typically, the changes of low-grade displasia reveal abnormalities limited to the lower third of the epithelium, accompanied by a minimal degree of cytological dysplasia. If the cytological changes of mild dysplasia extend into the middle third of the epithelium, the classification of mild-dysplasia may still be warranted. In severe dysplasia/high-grade displasia/carcinoma-in-situ, architectural abnormalities ***can*** extend into the top third of the epithelium, and the degree of cytological dysplasia is markedly greater than that seen in low-grade dysplasia. However, marked cytological dysplasia that does not extend into the top third of the mucosa may still warrant the diagnosis of severe dysplasia/high-grade dysplasia/carcinoma-in-situ. Deep keratin pearls, dyskeratotic cells in the lower third of the epithelium, tear-dropped rete petes, and thin dysplasia are criteria which "bump up" the grade of dysplasia.

The next relevant issue is assessment for microinvasion, that is, tumor satellites clearly separated from overlying diseased mucosa. Epithelial islands which extend to **the same depth as the mucosal rete pegs are likely *not* microinvasive.** Irregular contours at the rete pegs, deep pearls, and loss of basement membrane are features suggestive of microinvasion. However, invasive SCC may produce basement membrane; its presence does not abrogate the possibility of microinvasion. Terminology such as "incipient microinvasion", or "microinvasion cannot be ruled out" are appropriate, if you are suspicious, but cannot definitely substantiate the diagnosis.

Histopathologically, **proliferative verrucoid hyperplasia** demonstrates acanthosis, papillary hyperplasia, hyperkeratosis, wide, bulbous rete pegs and distinctive deep keratin clefts. This last finding is not seen in verrucous carcinoma (◻ Fig. 3.16). Dysplasia may be present, which is also unusual for verrucous carcinoma. Lastly, proliferative verrucoid hyperplasia lacks the degree of pushing broad rete pegs as seen in verrucous carcinoma. As mentioned, the diagnosis of proliferative verrucoid hyperplasia is based on this histology plus correlation with clinical features: older females, multifocal lesions, especially on the gingiva and palate.

Submucous fibrosis due to pan/gutka demonstrated severely atrophic epithelium with only three to four cell layers thick, especially in buccal mucosa [18]. The degree of submucosal collagen hyalinization and vascular obliteration correlates with disease severity [19]. IHC for P63 is

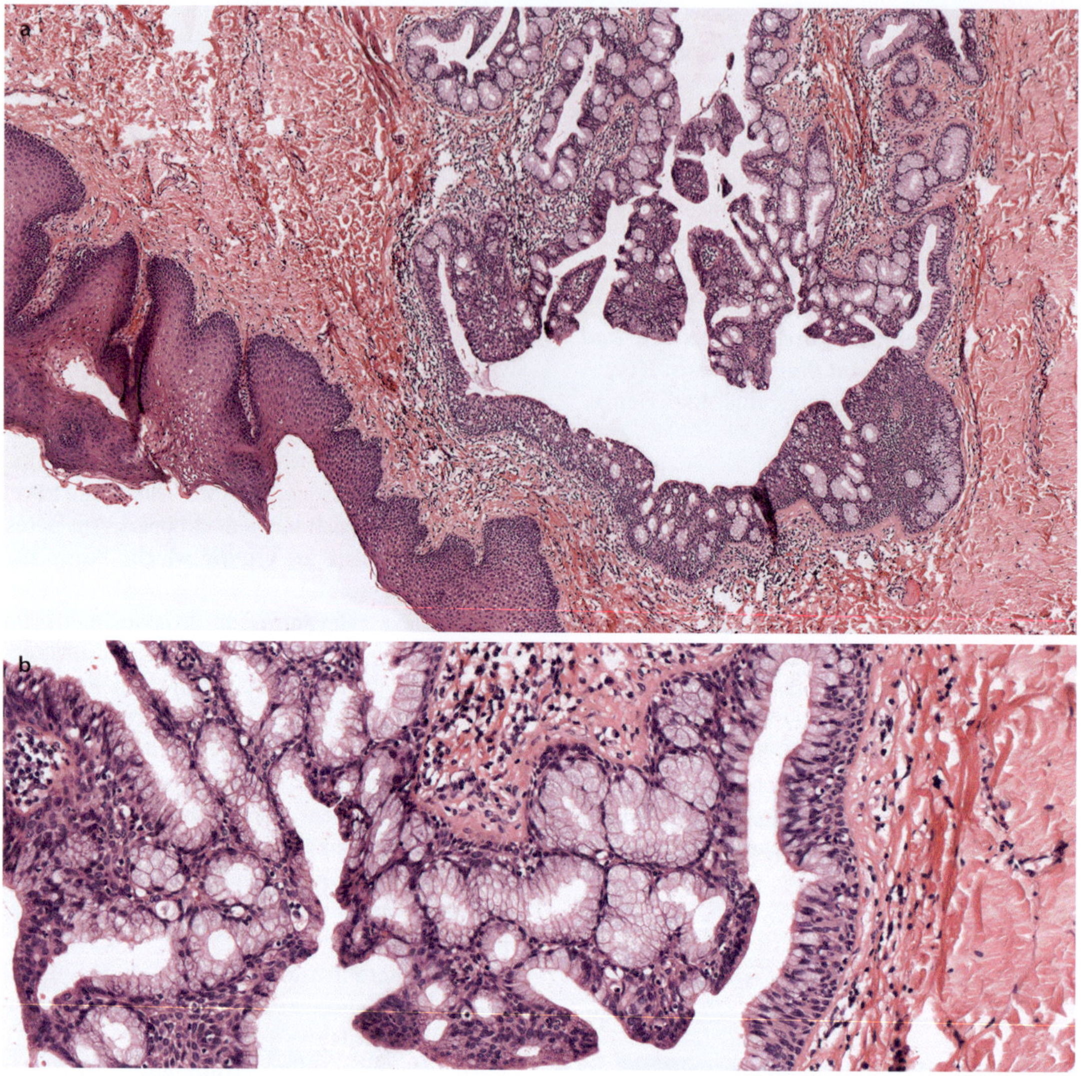

Fig. 3.4 a, b Glandular hyperplasia and squamous metaplasia in a chromate worker

not restricted to basal and parabasal cells but is increased in oral submucous fibrosis [20].

Smokeless tobacco keratosis demonstrates streaks of hyperkeratosis/parakeratosis with a "chevron" or "church spire" appearence. Prominent cytoplasmic vaculolation and keratohyaline granules are present "between the chevrons" [23]. Submucosal deposition of homogenous eosinophilic material, chronic sialadenitis and minor salivary fibrosis are also seen.

The changes of **reverse smoking of bidi** are seen in the **hard palate,** which is normally a protected subsite. Hyperkeratosis, severe chronic inflamation, melanosis, and melanin incontinence of the hard palate are seen. Dysplasia may be present. Reverse smoking may also demonstrate submucosal collagen hyalinization and vascular obliteration.

In the differential diagnosis of dysplasia, one must consider radiation atypia, which can extend into minor salivary ducts and mimic invasive carcinoma. Radiation causes cellular enlargement of both nuclear and cytoplasmic compartments; the nuclear/cytoplasmic ratio is not increased. Nuclear chromatin can have a "water-color" smudged appearence. The presence of submucosal fibrosis, perivascular fibrosis, atrophic minor salivary tissue suggest previous irradiation. It would be wise to confirm this with your clinician.

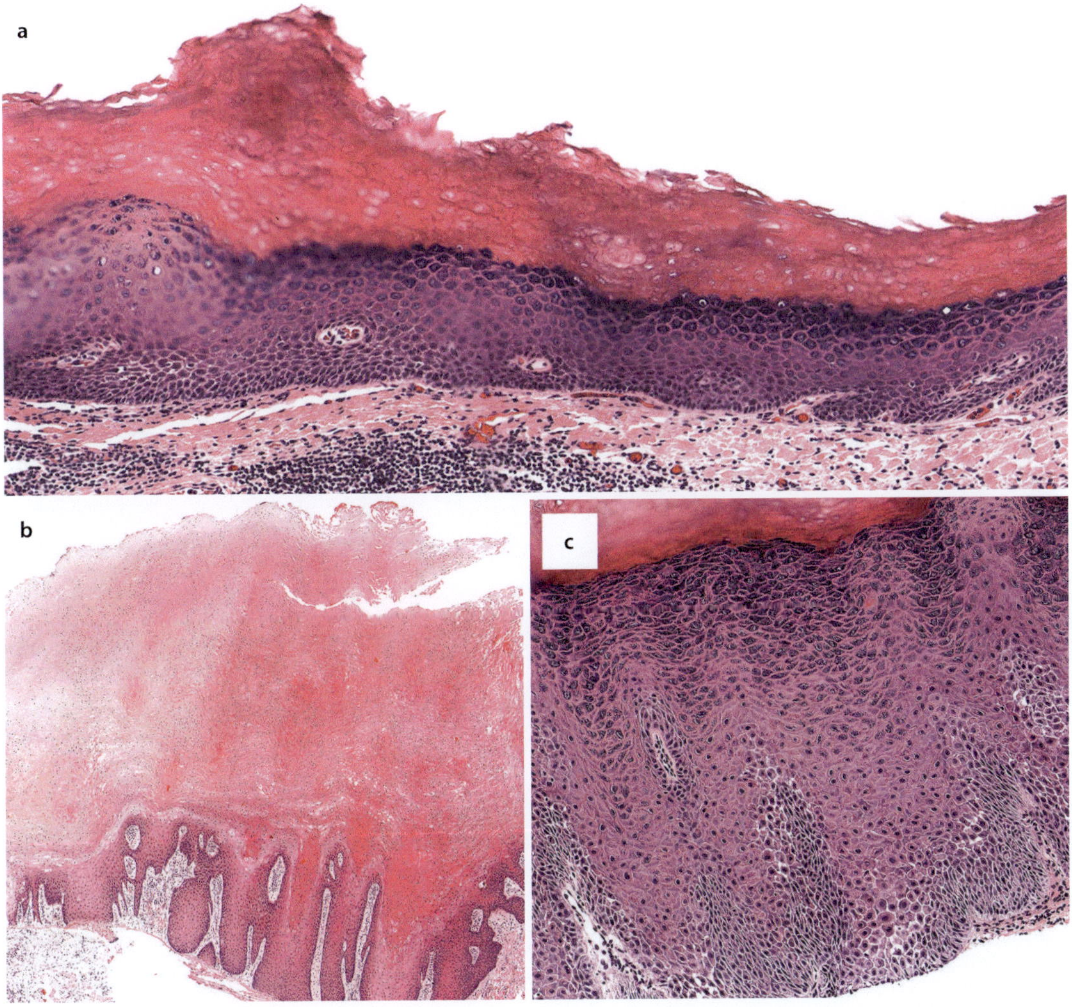

Fig. 3.5 a–c Examples of hyperkeratosis of the floor of mouth. Keratohyaline granules are abnormal to oral mucosa, and are seen in **a** and **c**. Even in the absence of dysplasia these lesions are worrisome

A common problem is mistaking the transitional variant of squamous carcinoma with "diffuse carcinoma-in-situ" on biopsies. This misconception originates from the criteria for recognizing invasive cáncer in the urinary bladder. In the upper aerodigestive tract, carcinoma-in-situ is usually "flat disease". ***Finding ribbons of epithelium with maturation, smooth borders, and intact basement membranes does not negate the possibility of invasive SCC.*** Let the amount of submitted tissue be your guide. Biopsies from *carcinoma-in-situ* rarely yield as much tissue as do transitional variant of squamous carcinoma. Speak to your clinician; the patient may have a mass and a metastatic lymph node.

3.2 Oral Squamous Carcinoma and Variants

3.2.1 Epidemiology

On a global, annual level, almost 200,000 people are diagnosed with oral cavity and lip cancers, and almost 100,000 die from the same [41]. Review of global statistics demonstrates ***declining*** age-standardized incidences for ***oral cavity cancers*** in some regional populations (e.g. Canada, males, U.S. males and females) and ***increasing*** incidences in Eastern and Northern Europe (Belarus, Czech Republic, Denmark, Estonia, Finland, Latvia, United Kingdom, and

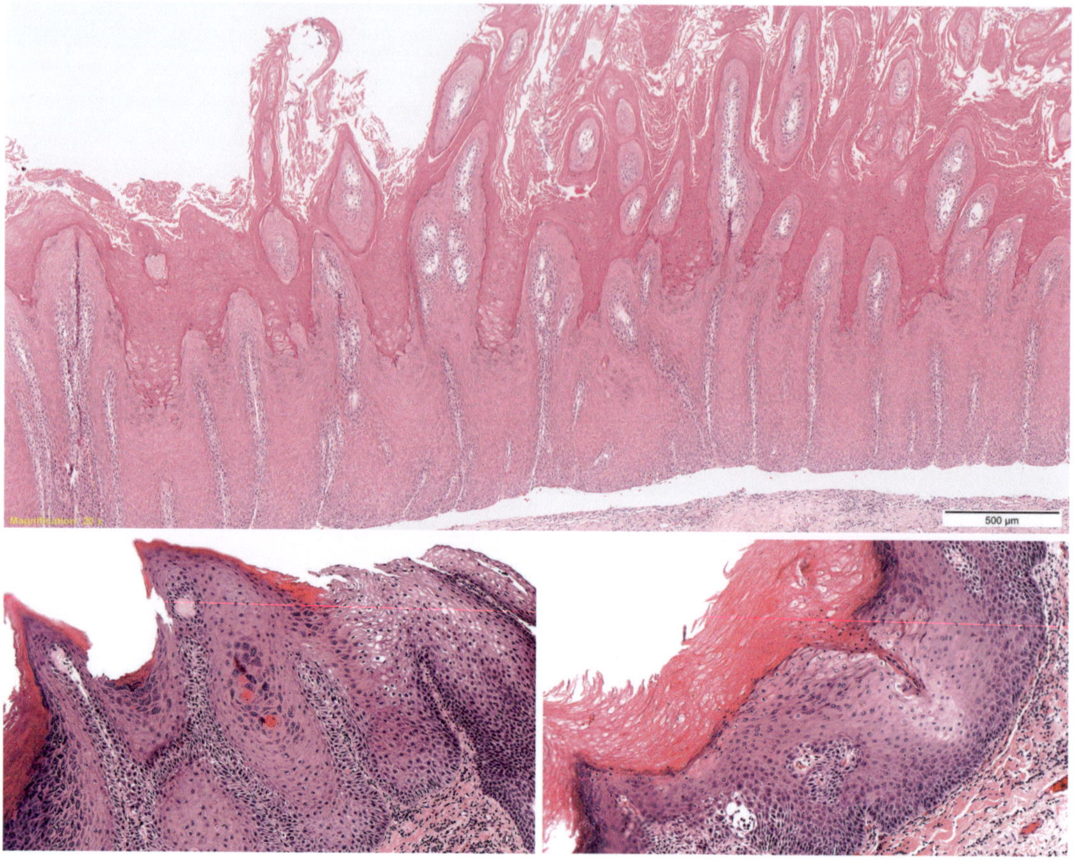

Fig. 3.6 "Spiky" hyperkeratosis of the floor of mouth. **Top**: This papillary, spiky, yet histologically bland lesion was present adjacent to an invasive squamous carcinoma. **Bottom right and left** Other patients with floor of mouth lesions. Again, even in the absence of dysplasia these lesions are worrisome

Scotland) and India, reflecting changing patterns of tobacco and alcohol consumption [42–47]. In the US, the incidences of oral cancers have usually been threefold greater than that of oropharyngeal cancer; one may expect that to change in the future. The estimated age-standardized incidences and mortality rates for oral cancers are higher in more developed countries, as compared to less developed regions: 7.0/2.3 and 2.6/0.6/100,000 per year for males and females, respectively, versus 5.0/2.8 and 2.5/1.4/100,000 per year, for males and females respectively [48]. For oropharyngeal cancers, the greatest increases in age-standardized incidences are seen in Belarus, Czech Republic, Poland, Russia, Denmark, Finland, Latvia, United Kingdom, and Scotland [42]. The estimated age-standardized incidences/mortality rates for oropharyngeal cancers are highest in Western Europe, **reaching similar rates as oral cavity cancer**: 7.5/2.5 and 2.7/0.5/100,000 per annum, for males and females respectively [48].

The floor of mouth and ventrolateral tongue are the anatomic subsites at greatest risk for developing smoking/alcohol mediated cancers (Fig. 3.17). Tobacco smoking and / or alcohol alone are independently causative in a dose-dependent manner [49, 50]. However, tremendous synergy is seen with combined consumption. Data on 689 oral cavity cancer patients from the ICARE (Investigation of occupational and environmental CAuses of

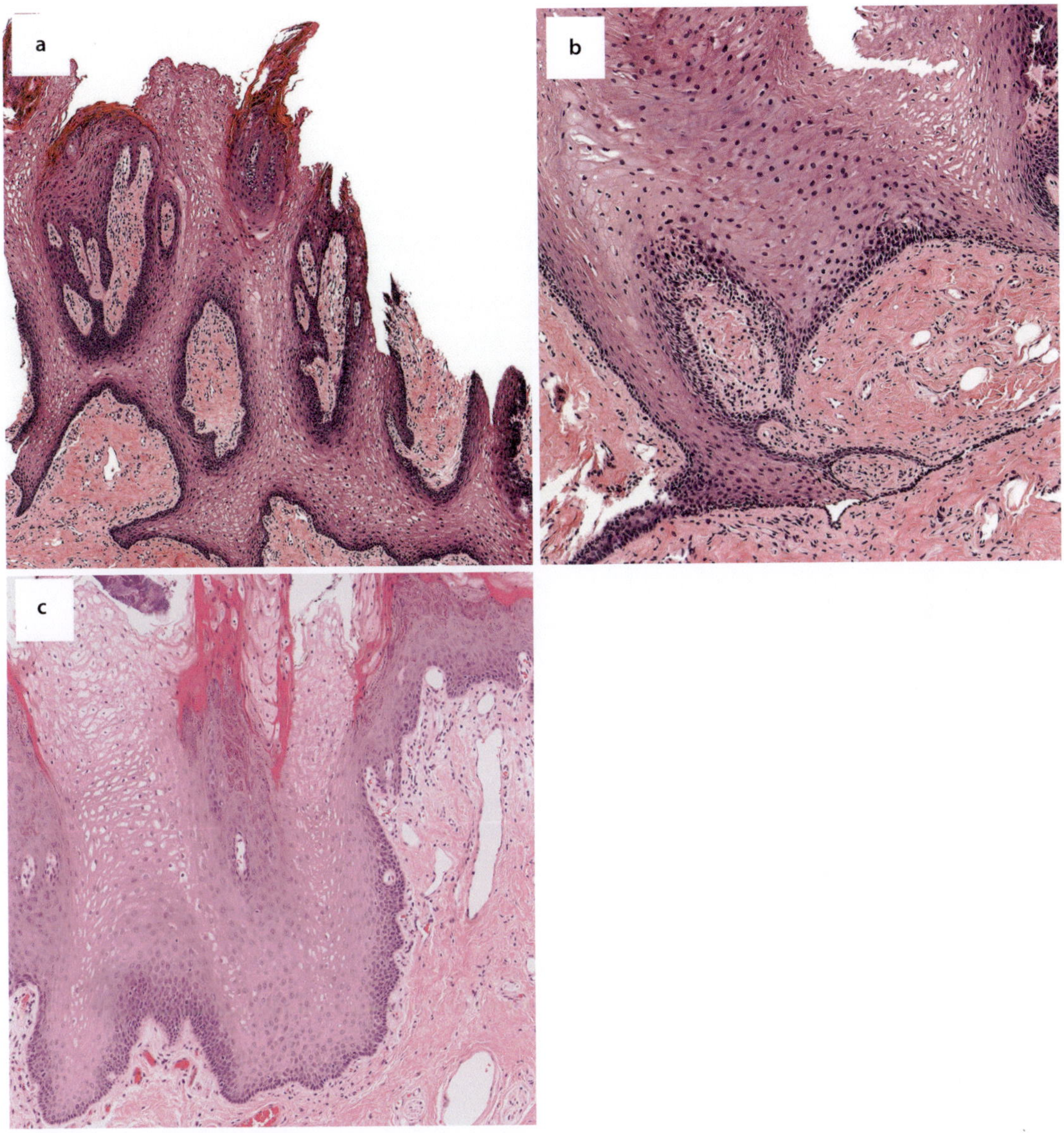

Fig. 3.7 **a–c** "Normal is a low-power diagnosis". One feature common to all three tongue images is the rather abrupt transition from basal/parabasal cells to differentiating epithelium

REspiratory cancers) study demonstrate population attributable risk of 0.3% (95% CI −3.9%; +3.9%) for alcohol alone, 12.7% (6.9–18.0%) for tobacco alone, but at attributable risk of 69.9% (64.4–74.7%). for joint consumption [51]. Interestingly, high-risk HPV seropositivity also significantly increases ***risk*** for ***oral cavity*** cancer [49], but unlike HPV-mediated oropharyngeal cancers, ***no prognostic benefits have been observed*** [49, 52]. In contrast to smoking/alcohol mediated cancers, buccal mucosa is at greatest risk for developing cancers promoted by chewing of tobacco/betel nut/pan [53, 54].

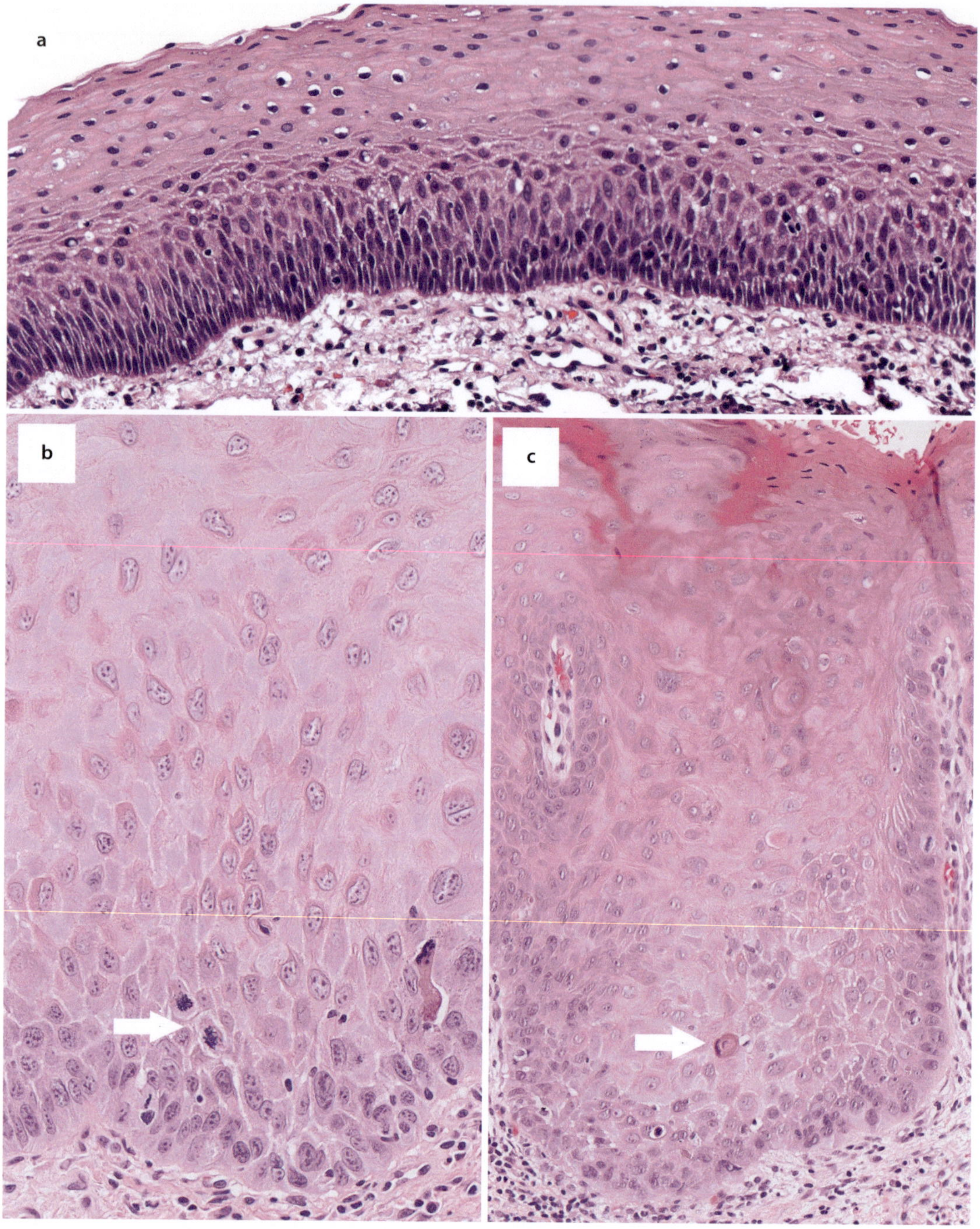

Fig. 3.8 **a** In contrast, see how parabasal cell hyperplasia alters this sharp transition. On low-power, this may be your subconscious queue to investigate the mucosa at higher power. **b** The diagnosis of low-grade dysplasia requires an accumulation of features. The white arrow demonstrates two high atypical mitotic figures. **c** Dyskeratosis can be considered the mirror-image of mitotic figures; low dyskeratotic cells = high mitotic figures. This too is included in the balance of features that weigh towards dysplasia

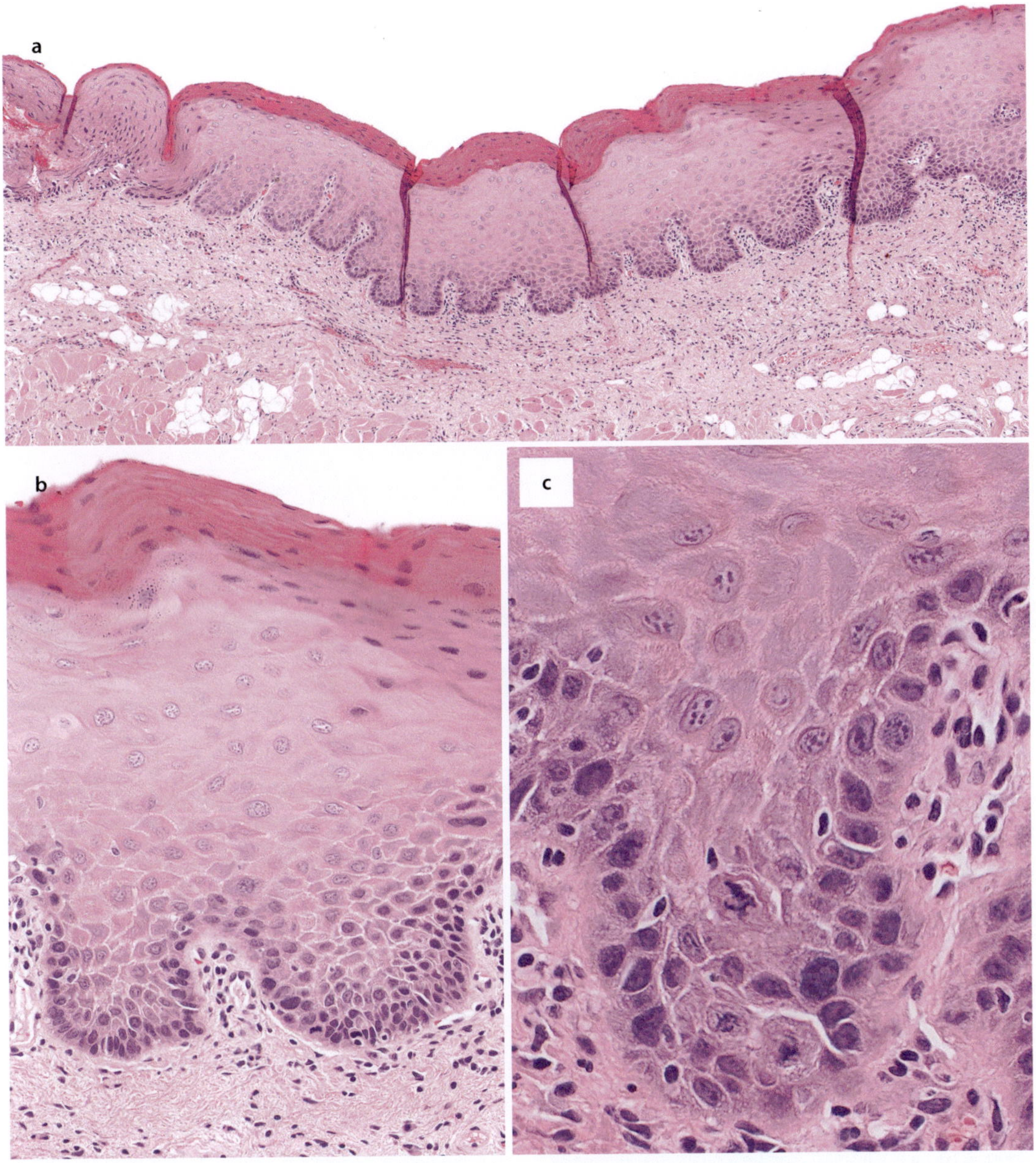

Fig. 3.9 **a**, **b** Tear dropped rete pegs are also a worrisome feature which can "upgrade" dysplasia. Here, the tear dr.opped rete pegs, cytologic pleomorphism of basal/parabasal cells, and atypical mitotic figures **c** allows for a diagnosis of low-grade dysplasia

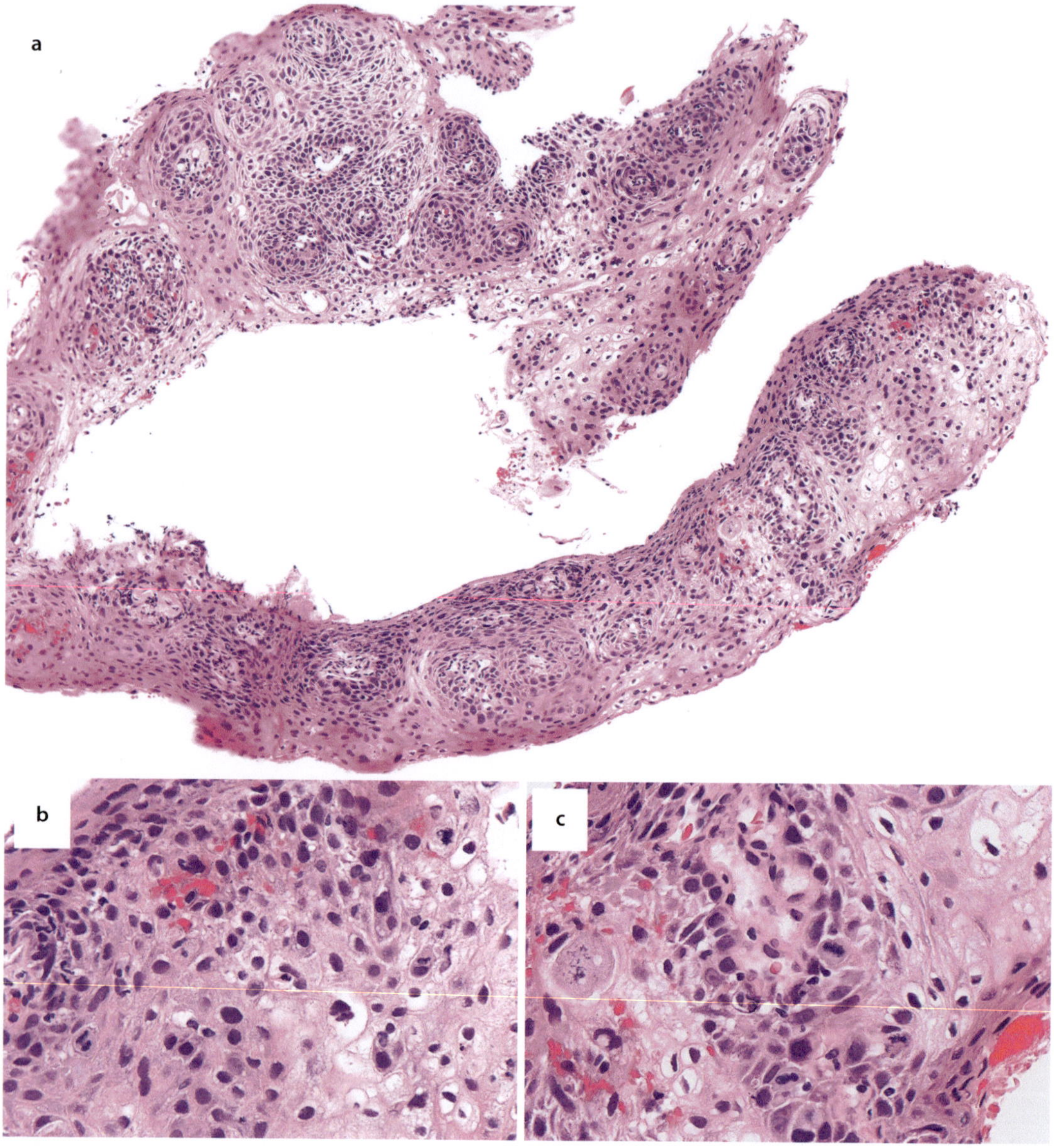

Fig. 3.10 **a–c** "Dysplasia can be a qualitative diagnosis". That is, the diagnosis can be based on the *degree* of a feature, and not necessarily *where* (quantitative) it is situated in the mucosa. In this high-grade dysplasia, pleomorphic epithelial cells and atypical mitotic figures are confined to the bottom half of the mucosa, yet the degree of pleomorphism warrants the high-grade classification. The category "high-grade dysplasia" incorporates histology ranging from moderate-dysplasia to carcinoma-in-situ; the terms high-grade dysplasia and carcinoma-in-situ are used synonymously

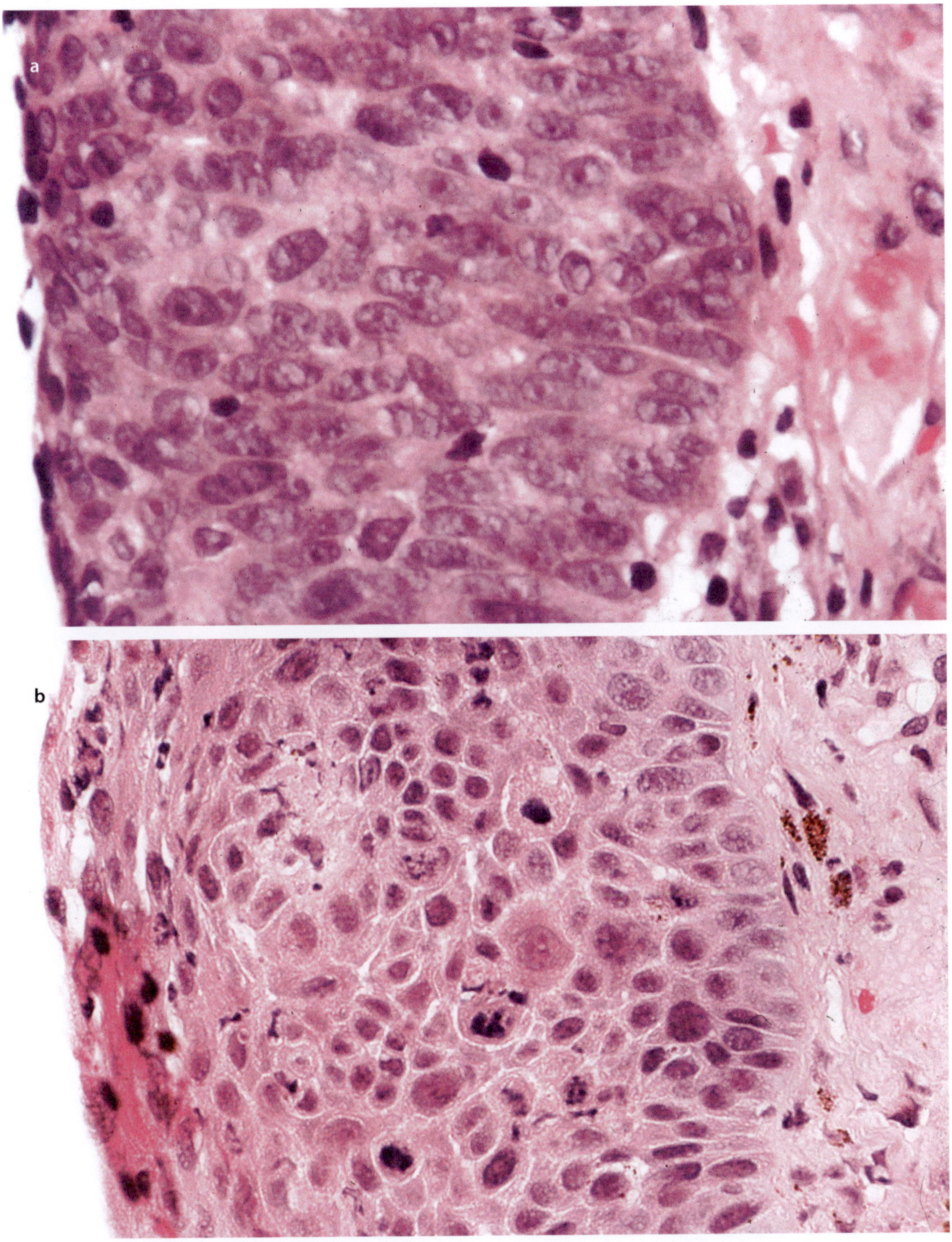

Fig. 3.11 **a**, **b** These are examples of "classical" high-grade dysplasia, where the abnormality extends the full-thickness of the mucosa. **a** The nuclear axis remains perpendicular to the basement membrane from bottom to top, indicating no maturation. **b** Here, the epithelial cells gain cytoplasm (mature) as they move upwards. Full thickness pleomorphism can be appreciated

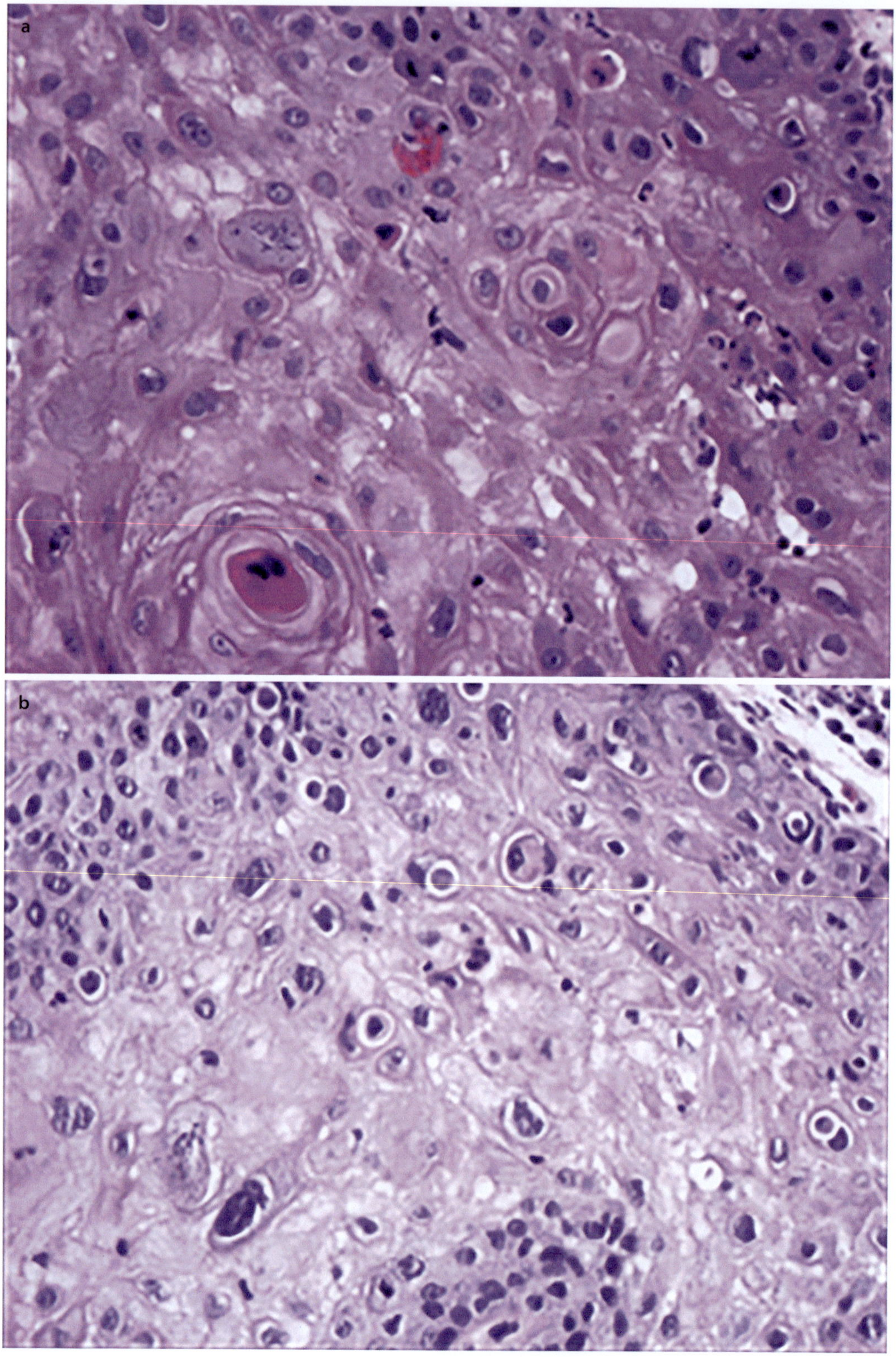

Fig. 3.12 **a**, **b** Mucosal dysplasia associated with vitamin B12 deficiency has an unusual appearance in that both the nuclear and cytoplasmic components are enlarged. The dysplastic cells appear "spread apart" rather than crowded. One can appreciate the numerous atypical mitotic figures in metaphase arrest

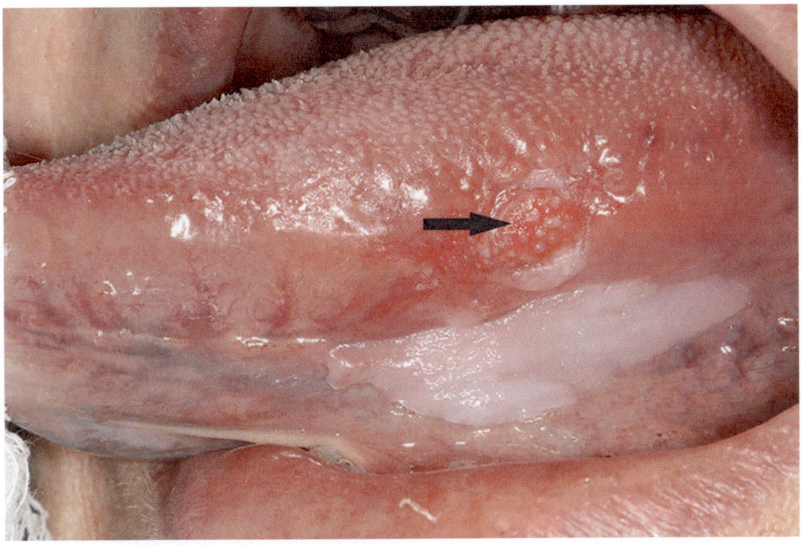

Fig. 3.13 Erythroleukoplakia consists of white mucosal patches alternating with erythematous regions. The arrow demonstrates "checkerboard" erythroleukoplakia. (Courtesy of Dr. Nicole Hinchy. DDS)

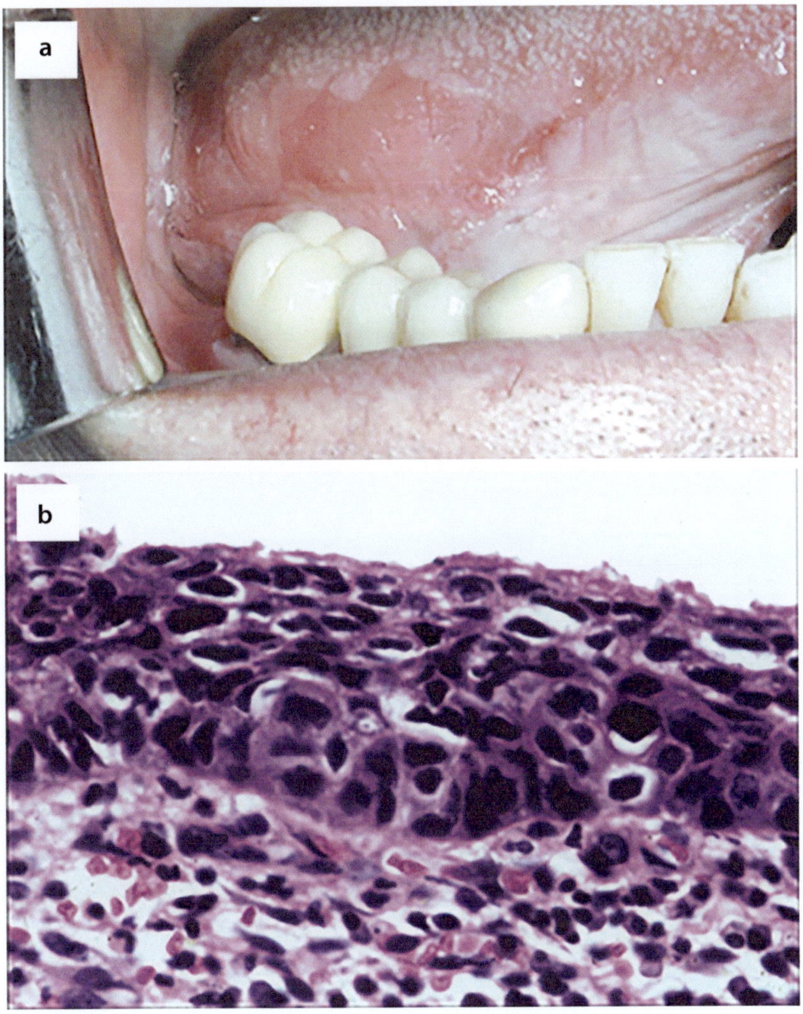

Fig. 3.14 **a** Erythroplakia of the lateral posterior tongue. **b** Microscopically, erythroplakic lesions are usually thin, as seen in this example of high-grade dysplasia/carcinoma-in-situ

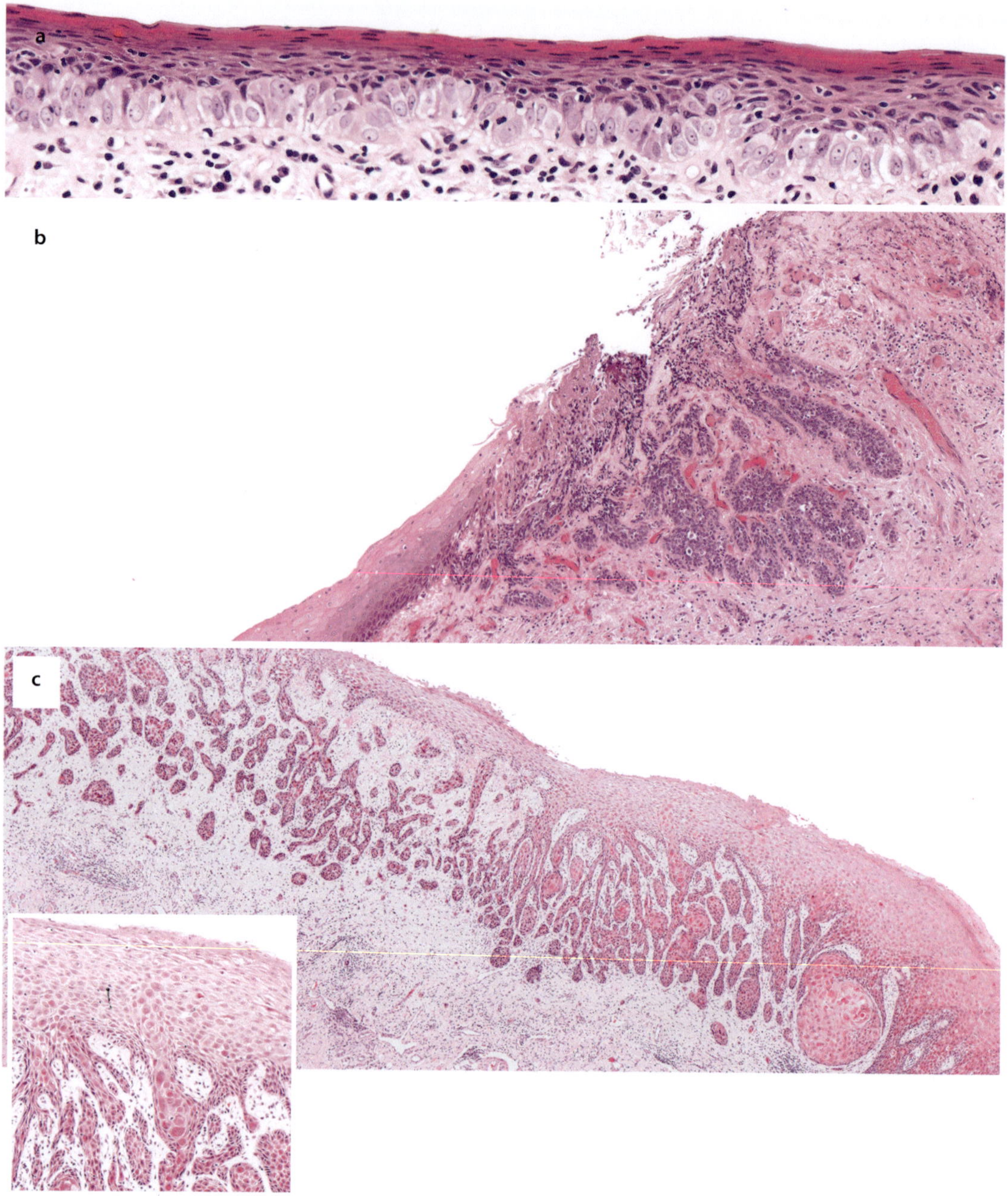

Fig. 3.15 **a** Another example of thin high-grade dysplasia/carcinoma-in-situ. **b**, **c**, **inset** Disconcerting examples of invasive squamous carcinoma which arise directly from rather normal squamous mucosa

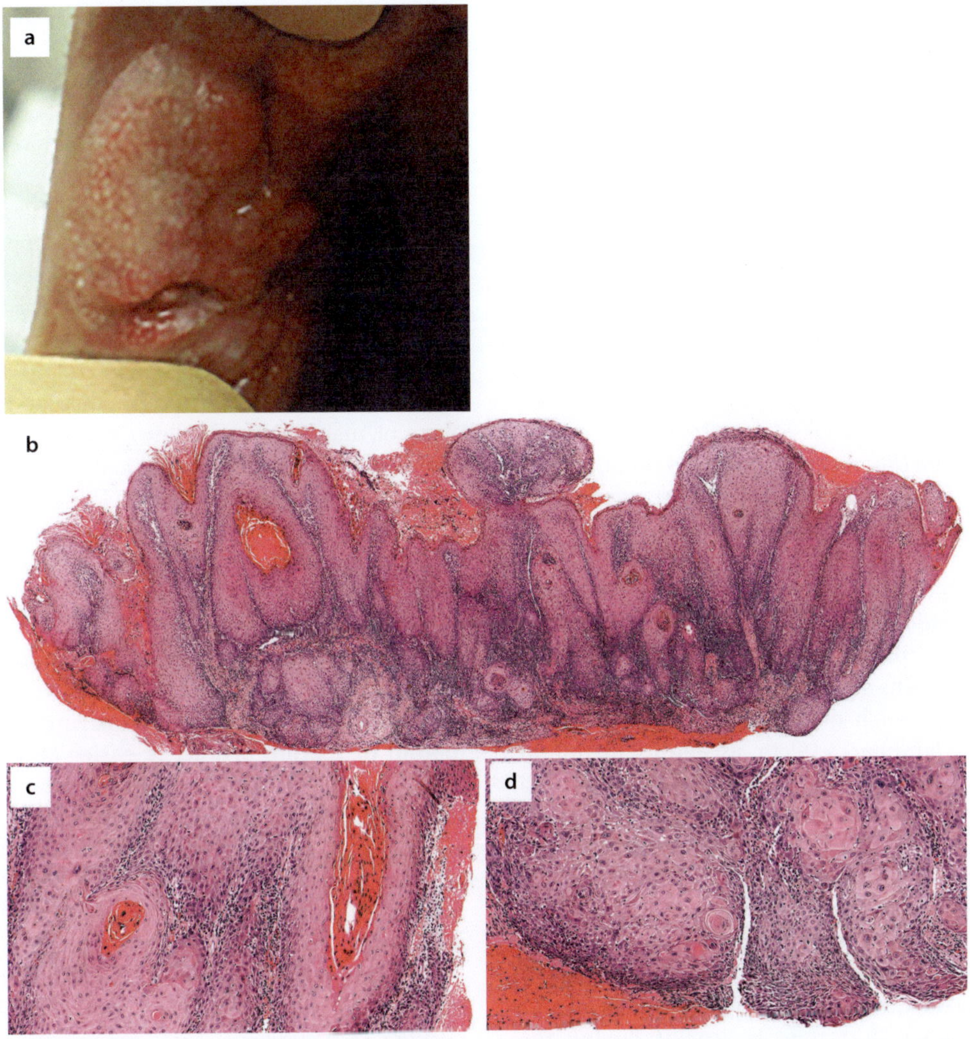

Fig. 3.16 **a** Buccal verrucoid hyperplasia: large speckled white and red mucosal lesion with a cobblestone appearance. (Courtesy of Dr. Randy Owen). **b** Verrucoid hyperplasia is characterized by surface papillations and keratin clefts. It lacks the dense hyperkeratosis and deeply pushing broad rete pegs of verrucous carcinoma. **c**, **d** Cytologic pleomorphism is usually absent

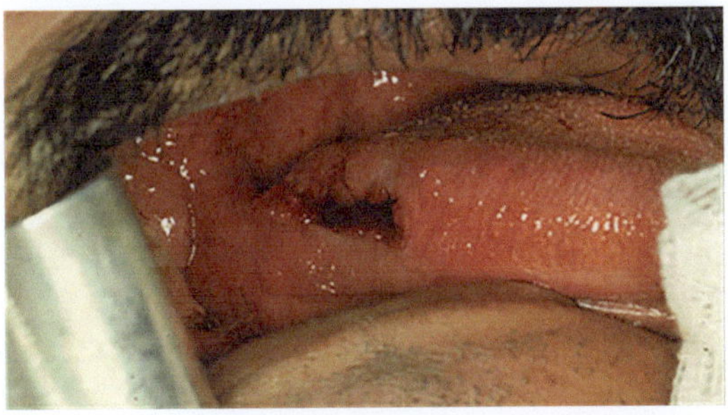

Fig. 3.17 Ulcerated carcinoma of the right lateral tongue

3.2.2 Gross Dissection and Intraoperative Margin Assessment

The gross dissection of oral composite resection specimens is one of the most complicated in surgical pathology. A composite specimen consists of mandible and/or maxilla and contiguous mucosal and soft tissues and neck dissection. Here we explain efficient dissection and analysis of these specimens, which provides adequate information to substantiate a complete report.

Orientation: Grossing starts with a sound foundation in anatomy; if in doubt, a quick gross anatomy reference is a good guide. Surgeons will commonly orient specimens as they see the patients on the operating table; the specimen faces the observer. The observer's right side becomes patient left side. It's easy to lose orientation with this approach. We recommend orienting specimens as congruent to the observer, meaning your right side is the patient's right side. The anterior aspect of the specimen should point away from the dissector.

Margins: The basic principle is that ***each tissue plane that meets the surgeon*** (bone, mucosa, soft tissue, vessels, and nerve) ***represents a resection margin and requires evaluation***. Each specimen can be thought of as a multi-planed manifold; each cut surface from each orthogonal plane represents a margin surface. There are anatomic planes which ***do not*** represent resection margins such as skin and mucosal surfaces. Quickly sketch out specimen and identify orienting landmarks (teeth, ascending mandibular ramus, tongue base, maxillary bone). Identify mucosal cut surfaces: look for where the "gleam" where the mucosa ends. Then begin to paint the different tissue planes with different color (◘ Fig. 3.18). Red dye tends to be a pain in the neck. The purpose of the paint is to correlate orientation on the slide. A second person can write down the designations as you paint the surfaces. ***Remember that time is crucial during these assessments.*** As ink runs, it is not the sole determination of a resection margin (**see below**).

At specimen hand-off, the first 10 min of discussion between surgeon and pathologists yields the most actionable information. After orientation and mapping, ***the pathologist makes multiple perpendicular cuts into the margin planes at 5 mm intervals.*** This gross survey identifies regions of concern requiring histological analysis. Remember, margin assessment is ***not confined to mucosal margins, but should embrace all deep soft tissue resection planes.***

Resection margin assessment by intraoperative mapping of the resection specimen represents the gold standard for resection adequacy. The decision for adjuvant radiotherapy is made postoperatively, based on adverse pathological features. The guiding principal of resection adequacy is to avoid the need for adjuvant radiotherapy based on margin status alone. A "specimen-driven" margin approach has demonstrated superiority to "defect-driven" margins, where the surgeon selects the samples to be evaluated [54, 55]. The defect-driven approach often focuses on mucosal margins whereas the majority of inadequate resection margins occur within deep surgical planes. From a practical point of view, margin assessment requires that tissue sections be taken perpendicular to the plane of margin, which allows for actual measurements. ***Avoid parallel shave margins for mucosal/soft tissue assessment.*** The pitfall with shave margins is that they may be negative, but on permanent sections you find that cancer is present on deeper sections, and you've lost the opportunity for measurements.

Ink is used only for orientation; ink alone does not indicate a resection margin. We have all had the experience of watching ink run. **A "false" margin or tearing artifact is easier addressed by inking it first with a unique color, rather than attempting to avoid that area becoming inked.** Histologically, resection margin status is confirmed by (1) irregular contour, (2) cautery artifact, (3) retracted mucosa, (4) blood and fibrin at the cauterized edge (◘ Fig. 3.19).

The best rule of thumb is: One Cassette One Margin. Don't try to save on cassettes here by pushing many margins into one cassette, hoping for the color coding to sort out the margins. This adds time and effort to the sign-out. Dictate each cassette identity with the orientation of the margin. Thus each margin can be identified by both the cassette label and the ink color.

Remember that **depth of invasion** is now necessary for T staging. Sections for **depth of invasion** and **pattern of invasion** should be separate from margin sections. In the context of intraoperative assessment, the mucosal and soft tissue margins should be processed first, these are actionable steps. Then process sections deliberately aimed to assess depth of invasion, and pattern of invasion, the latter is harvested from the tumor advancing edge at the soft tissue interface. Multiple sections may be necessary.

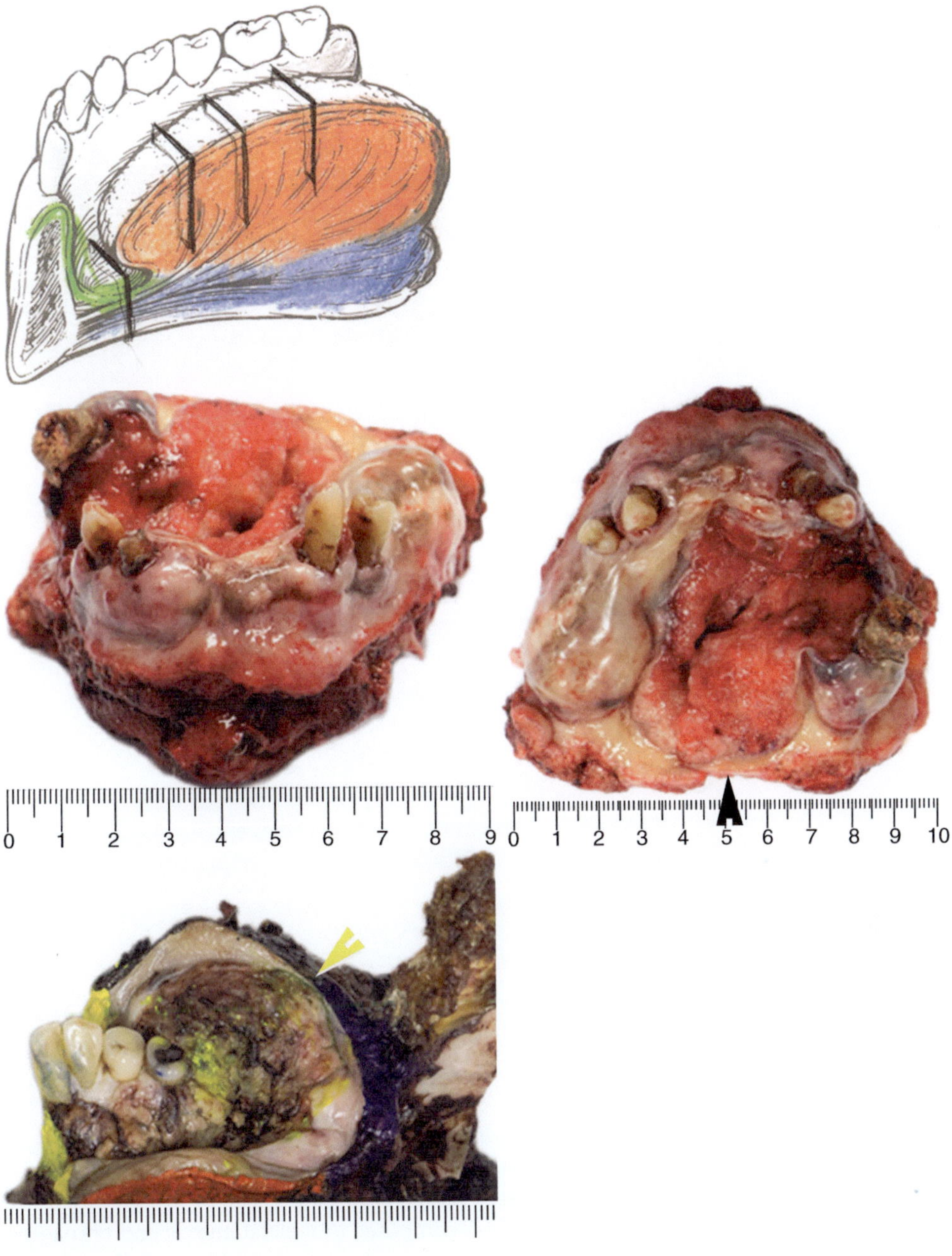

Fig. 3.18 **Top** Specimen driven resection margin analysis – Schematic diagram of right combined hemiglossectomy. Survey the specimen by making multiple cuts, perpendicular to the plane of the resection specimen. Histological assessment should also follow perpendicular alignment. Avoid "shave" "parallel" margins. **Middle** Composite mandibular resection specimen including the anterior mandible with attached 5 teeth (lateral incisors) and 1 premolar. A tan, white, ulcerated tumor with a central crater arises from the floor of mouth, measuring 5.0 × 5.0 cm. No tongue was removed. The middle right image demonstrates that the carcinoma comes to within 0.2 cm of the posterior cauterized margin of resection (*black arrowhead*). **Lower** This is a composite resection of the mandible with identifiable lateral incisors and premolar teeth. At the extreme posterior aspect is the ramus of mandible with retromolar attached soft tissue. In this example the mucosal resection margins and the corresponding attached soft tissue portion are inked in different colors as mentioned earlier (blue posterior, orange medial, yellow anterior and black as lateral). There is a slightly raised and ulcerated lesion on the gingival aspect measuring 3.5 cm which comes to within 1.0 cm of inked posterior margin of resection (*yellow arrowhead*)

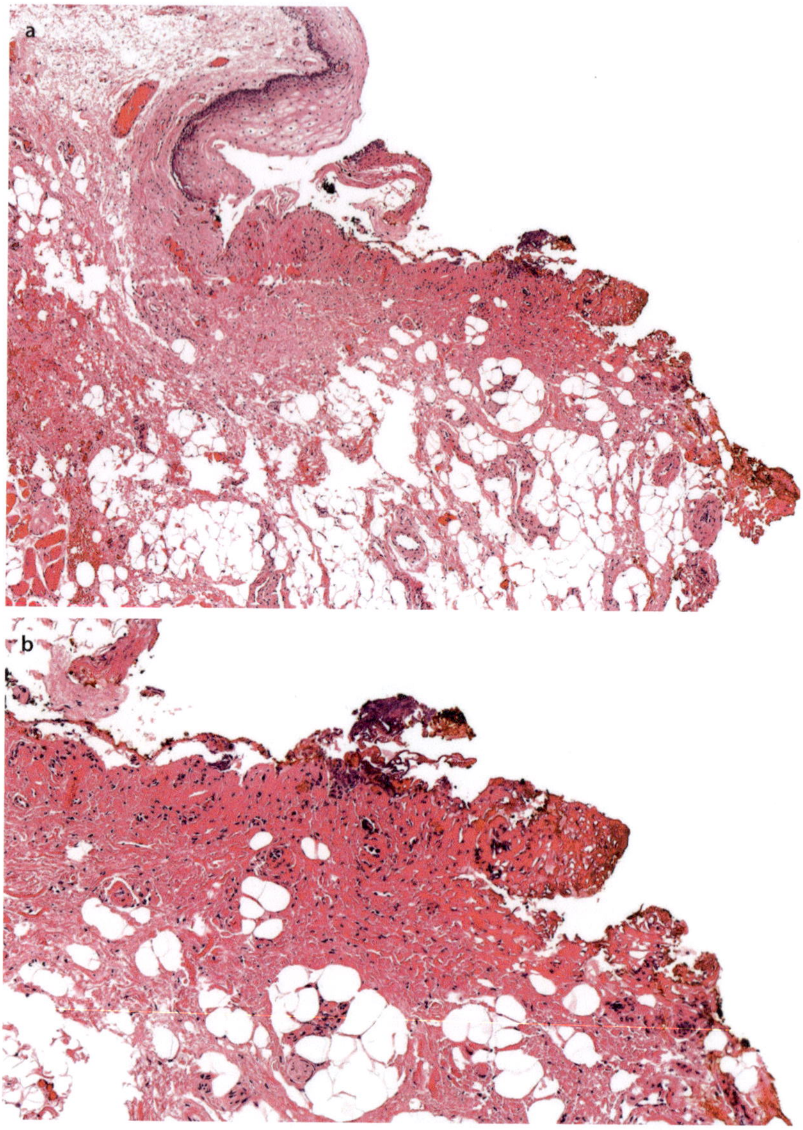

Fig. 3.19 **a, b** Margin assessment requires that tissue sections be taken perpendicular to the plane of margin, which allows for measurements. Ink is used only for orientation; ink alone does not indicate a resection margin. Histologically, resection margin status is confirmed by (1) irregular contour, (2) cautery artifact, (3) retracted mucosa, (4) blood and fibrin at the cautery

Assess the **mucosal margins** along all mucosal cut points including the immediate submucosa. Gingival mucosa has limited submucosal fibroconnective tissue, and should be quite thin. With respect to **soft tissue margins,** there will be potentially five soft tissue planes to consider, in addition to the mucosal and bony margins. These five planes are: **medial** – either floor of mouth or mobile tongue, **anterior** floor of mouth with/without mobile tongue, and **posterior** gingiva with/without tongue base. The **lateral** plane represents the gingiva – it is usually not a significant margin for resections of floor of mouth and tongue cancers. It will be a significant margin for gingival/buccal cancers. Lastly, the **inferior** soft tissue margin is the entire underside of the specimen – usually composed of skeletal muscle and fibroadipose tissue, may or may not include sublingual glands and possibly occasional Level IA/IB lymph nodes. The inferior margin plane is most times not important with respect to the primary tumor. If you encounter carcinoma inferiorly, carefully dissect and ascertain if this is metastasis to the submandibular triangle (more likely) versus inferior extension of primary cancer (less likely). If skin is present, document with your sections where carcinoma extends closest to the subcutaneous tissues. Survey the skin ellipse for the closest regions to sample.

Ideally, after margin assessment, the resection specimen remains in the frozen section lab and is dissected by the same team for permanent sections. This is the most efficient in terms of fewer people handling a specimen, retention of information, and turnaround time. The specimen can be brought back to the gross dissection lab to harvest boney margins at the end of the frozen day.

Specific specimens – Marginal mandibulectomy specimen includes the upper mandibular rim, or alveolus, and mandibular cortex, which represents the inferior margin. This type of specimen is encountered for floor of mouth cancers with no evidence of boney invasion on imaging studies. The **three boney margin planes** are **anterior medial, posterior lateral,** and **inferior mandibular medullary cavity**. If the composite resection extends beyond the anterior midline, then the mandibular margins are designated as right and left. Harvest these margins with a bone saw ***after*** taking soft tissue margins. Use a bone saw to render 3 mm slice shave margins which should reveal a full face of the mandibular margin. Keep the teeth attached to the mandible as an anchor when using the bone saw. After sawing the bony margins, you can manually extract any teeth to shorten decal time.

Segmental mandibulectomy specimen contains only two cut mandibular planes: **anterior/medial** and **posterior/lateral**. This type of specimen is more common than marginal mandibulectomy specimen, and is used for larger cancers. Often there is also attached skin of the chin or cheek, as well as buccal mucosa or a portion of the tongue. As with the marginal mandibulectomy, the first step is to orient the specimen and identify margins. If the resection includes the midline anterior mandible, then the bony margins are designated as right and left lateral (◘ Fig. 3.18). Harvest the bony margins after the mucosal and soft tissue margins, using a bone saw to render 3 mm slice shave margins. As above, you can extract teeth after cutting the boney sections to decrease decalcification time.

Some authors recommend that if the tumor is up to 0.3 cm of the bone margin then a perpendicular section should be taken, which is ideal if feasible. In the case of gingival carcinomas, teeth should not be extracted from the specimens, as this may impact assessment of bony invasion.

3.2.3 The Impact of Resection Margins

Recent studies have challenged the convention of the 5 mm resection margin distance. The largest study involved 827 consecutive oral cavity cancer patients of all stages; resection margin distance was examined as a continuous variable. An optimal resection margin distance of 7 mm was found [57]. In contrast, two other studies of 432 and 381 oral cavity cancer patients, found optimal resection margin cut-points of 1 mm and 2.2 mm, respectively [58, 59]. It is difficult to resolve such contradictory conclusions. Future studies need to also correlate worst pattern of invasion with resection margin distances.

3.2.4 Staging

The 8th AJCC staging for oral cavity and lips cancers is presented in ◘ Table 3.3. The newly introduced elements are tumor depth of invasion and extranodal extension. Happily, involvement of tongue root (extrinsic muscles), which could only be assessed clinicoradiographically, is no longer criteria for T4. The depth of invasion criteria are based on an international multicenter retrospective review of massive proportion, reviewing 3149 patients treated with curative intent by primary surgery +/− adjuvant therapy [60]. Primary depth of invasion (DOI) was examined as a continuous variable. It was significantly associated with disease specific survival ($p < 0.001$, HR 1.31 (1.13–1.52) when adjusted for confounders in multivariate analysis. The optimized cut-points for stage stratification were found to be 5 and 10 mm.

The inclusion of extranodal extension in the new staging schema has formalized that which has always been appreciated: fixed palpable positive lymph nodes predict poor outcome. The clinicopathologic studies which serve as the basis for the new staging criteria examined 595 patients in total with oral cavity and laryngeal carcinomas; one study looked at ENE as a continuous variable, the other as categorical [61, 62]. Both studies demonstrate pathologically confirmed and quantified ENE is significantly predictive of outcome in multivariate analysis.

Table 3.3 8th American Joint Committee on Cancer Staging System – Oral Cavity and Lips

T stage	Greatest dimension	Depth of invasion
T1	≤2 cm	≤5 mm
T2	≤2 cm	>5 mm but ≤10 mm
	>2 cm but ≤4 cm	≤10 mm
T3	>4 cm	Or any >10 mm
T4a	Moderately advanced local disease invading through cortical bone, or involving the inferior alveolar nerve, floor of mouth, or skin of face Invades adjacent structures (e.g., through cortical bone of the mandible or maxilla, or involves the maxillary sinus or skin of the face) Note: Superficial erosion of bone/tooth socket (alone) by a gingival primary is not sufficient to classify a tumor as T4	
T4b	Very advanced local disease, invading masticator space, pterygoid plates, or skull base and/or encases the internal carotid artery	

N category	Number and size	ENE
N0	No metastases	None
N1	One ipsilateral lymph node ≤3 cm	None
N2a	One ipsilateral lymph node ≤3 cm	Yes
N2b	One ipsilateral lymph node >3 cm but ≤6 cm	No
N2c	Multiple ipsilateral, bilateral or contralateral lymph nodes ≤6 cm	No
N3a	One lymph node >6 cm	No
N3b	One ipsilateral lymph node >6 cm, or any multiple ipsilateral, contralateral or bilateral lymph nodes	Yes

Stage grouping

If T…	And N…	And M…	Then stage
T1	No	M0	I
T2	No	M0	II
T3	No	M0	III
T1, T2, T3	N1	M0	III
T4a	N0, N1	M0	IVA
T1, T2, T3, T4a	N2	M0	IVA
Any T	N3	M0	IVB
T4b	Any N	M0	IVB
Any T	Any N	M1	IVC

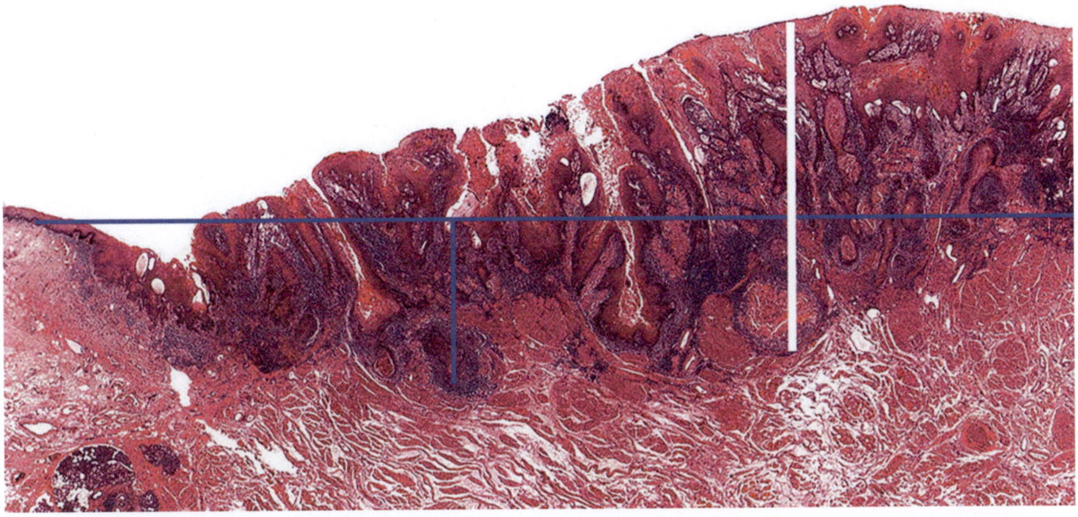

Fig. 3.20 The terms "depth of invasion (DOI)" and "tumor thickness" have been used interchangeably, which is incorrect. The white bar represents maximum tumor thickness. The blue bar is DOI. The horizon is established at the level of the basement membrane relative to the closest intact squamous mucosa. The greatest DOI is measured by dr.opping a "plumb line" from the horizon. For printable rulers, see ▶ http://www.vendian.org/mncharity/dir3/paper_rulers/UnstableURL/rules_cm_narrow_20cm.pdf

Histopathologically, tumor depth of invasion is measured from the level of the basal reserve cells relative to the closest normal mucosa (Fig. 3.20). Determine your horizon, and then drop a plumb line to the deepest region of infiltration. The carcinomas illustrated in Figs. 3.21 and 3.22, are now staged as T2, provided they are ≤4 cm in greatest dimension.

Extranodal tumor extension now upstages N classification for cancers of the oral cavity, hypopharynx, p16-negative oropharynx, and larynx. Of note, while further stratification into microscopic (ENE_{mi}, ≤ 2 mm) versus macroscopic or gross (ENE_{ma}, > 2 mm) is requested for staging, any ENE is criteria for upstaging. Figure 3.23 illustrates lymph node expansion with stretching of the capsule. This does not represent ENE. ENE is demonstrated in Fig. 3.24; carcinoma has breached the lymph node capsule and extends into the parahilar soft tissue. Dropping the microscope condenser is helpful in determining the natural contour of the lymph node, and sets a boundary for quantifying extranodal extension.

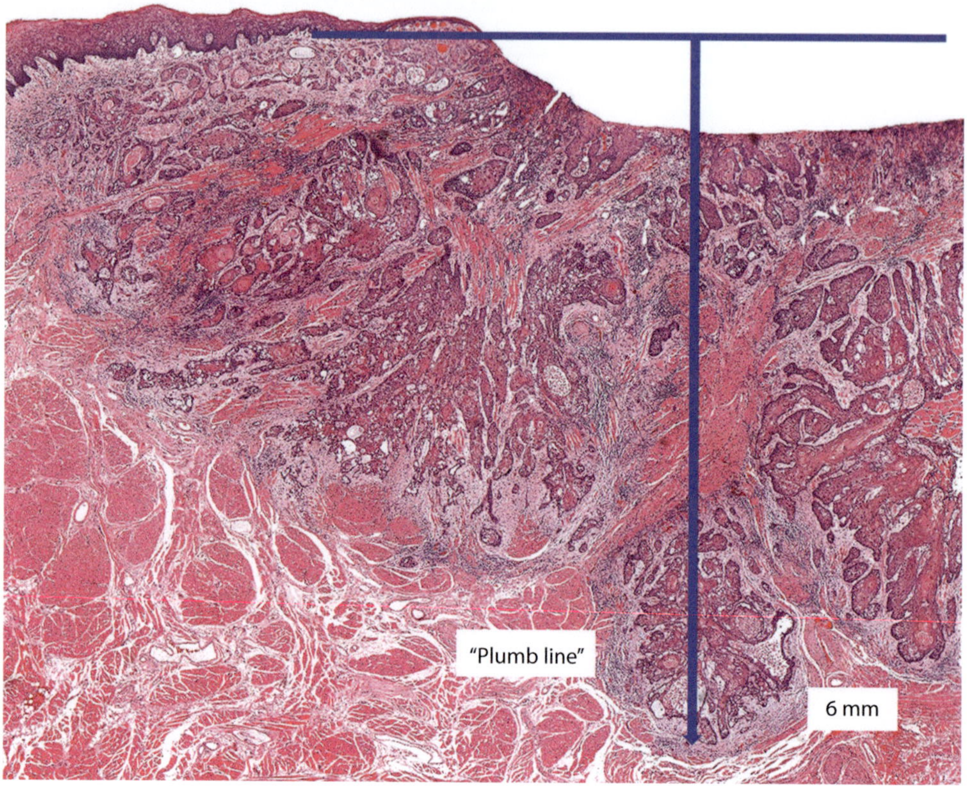

Fig. 3.21 DOI in an ulcerated carcinoma. Notice how "tumor thickness" would be deceptively thinner than DOI

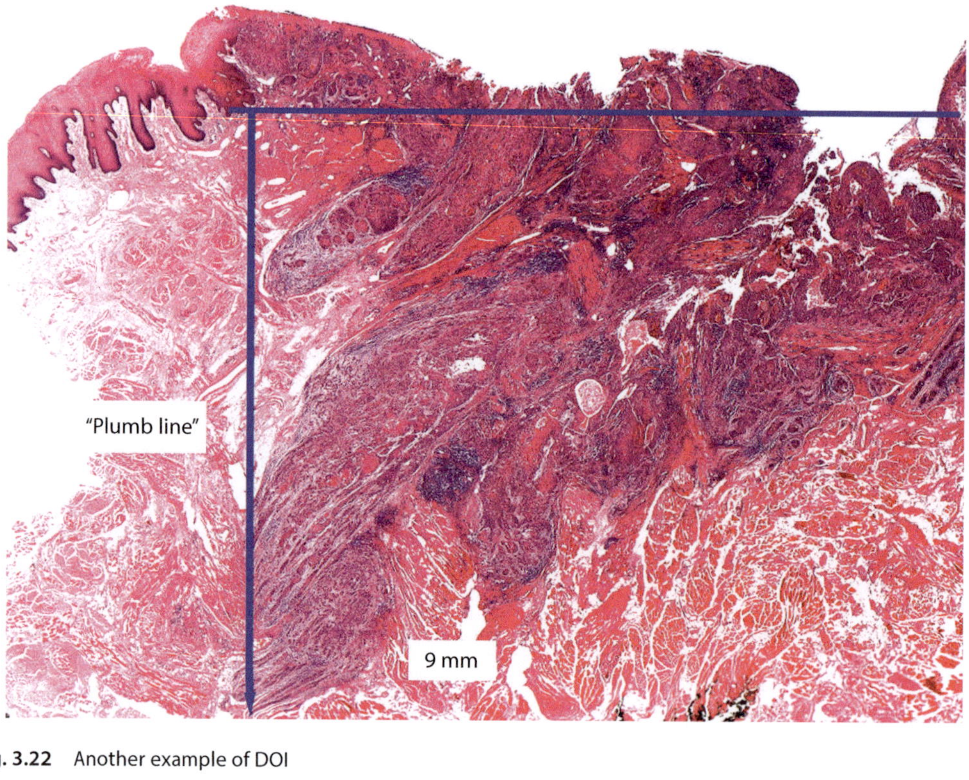

Fig. 3.22 Another example of DOI

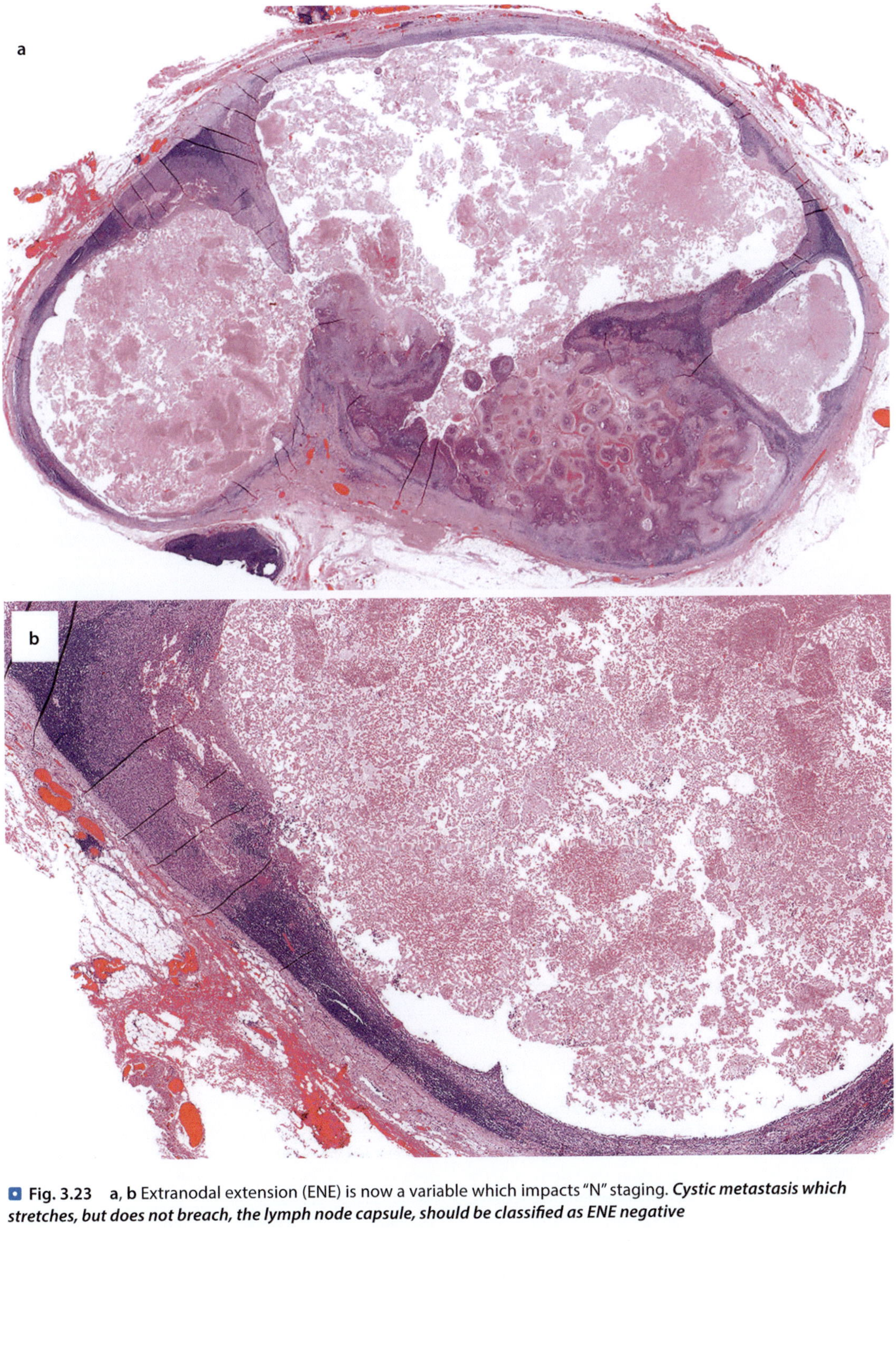

Fig. 3.23 **a**, **b** Extranodal extension (ENE) is now a variable which impacts "N" staging. ***Cystic metastasis which stretches, but does not breach, the lymph node capsule, should be classified as ENE negative***

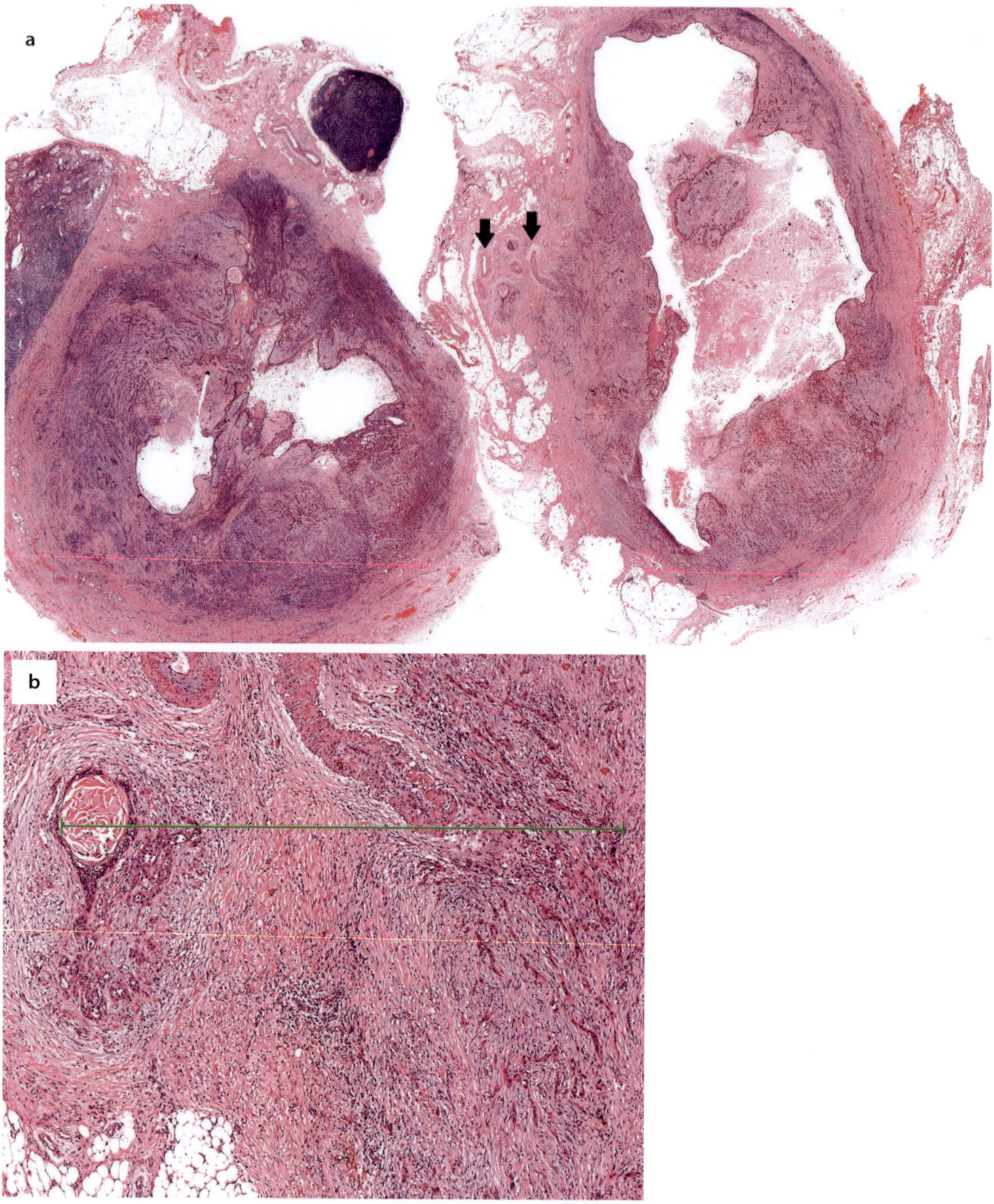

Fig. 3.24 **a** ENE, low-power. The large extranodal vessels (*black arrows*) are good microscopic landmarks. **ENE$_{mi}$** is defined as microscopic ENE ≤ 2 mm. Macroscopic (gross) ENE (**ENE$_{ma}$**) is defined as either extranodal extension apparent to the naked eye at the time of dissection, or extension >2 mm beyond the lymph node capsule microscopically. ENE$_{ma}$ includes obliterated lymph node architecture with carcinoma in soft tissues. Either ENE$_{mi}$ or ENE$_{ma}$ are considered ENE+ for pN staging. **b** If the lymph node capsule is obliterated by desmoplasia, where is the reference point for measurement? Drop the microscope condenser and look for the refraction of residual capsular collagen to estimate its position. Here, the green line is >2 mm from the estimated lymph node boundary and should be classified as ENE$_g$

3.2.5 The Risk Model and WPOI-5

The biologic complexity of oral squamous carcinoma has defied efforts at prognostication using traditional single histological indicators (nuclear grade, mitotic rate, keratinization, necrosis, etc.). Having said that, **perineural invasion** (PNI) has traditionally been used as an adverse pathologic feature with respect to the recommendation of adjuvant radiotherapy (◘ Figs. 3.25 and 3.26) [63–65]. The Risk Model [66–68] represents an extension and simplification of models pub-

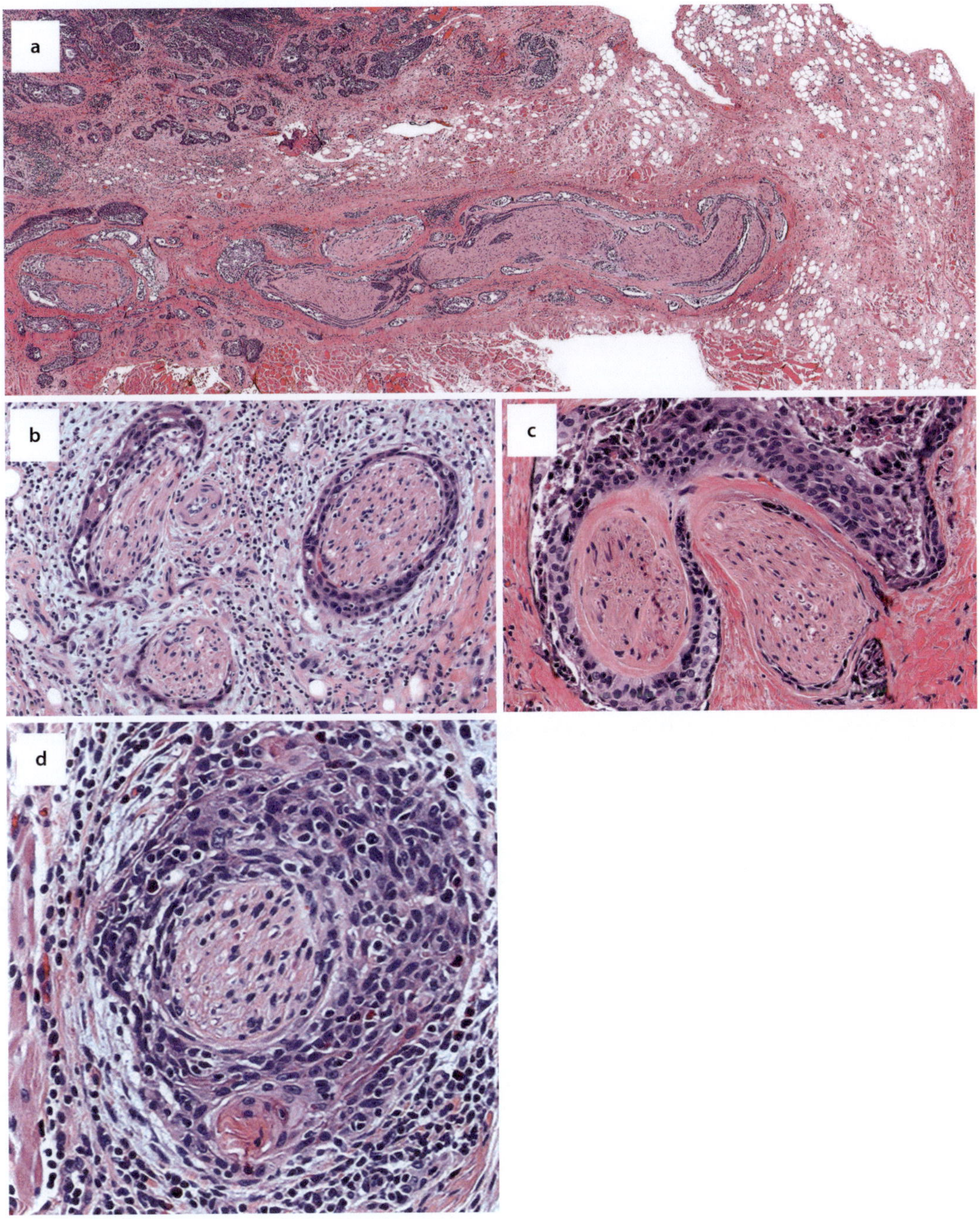

◘ **Fig. 3.25** **a–d** WPOI-5 secondary to extratumoral perineural invasion (PNI). Carcinoma should demonstrate a specific architectural relationship with nerve, such as wrapping around nerves, in order to be classified as PNI

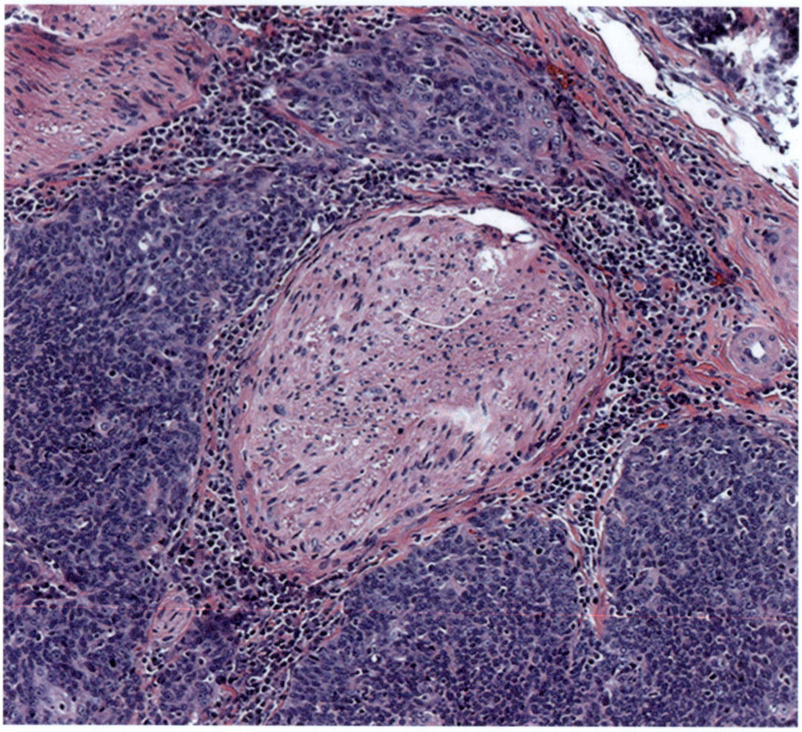

Fig. 3.26 Merely "bumping" into a nerve does not constitute PNI

lished by Jakobsson, and later by Bryne; these models never gained widespread application by pathologists for a number of reasons [69–71]. Jakobsson's model required the evaluation of eight variables in a four-tiered scoring system; its extreme complexity begged for a simplified version. The Bryne model was not always significantly associated with outcome for head and neck cancers in subsequent validation studies. The Bryne and Jakobssen scoring systems are linear (i.e. +1, +2, +3...), assuming equal impact with the progression from one category to the next. The Risk Model is nonlinear and gives greater weight to unique, more aggressive features such as WPOI-5 and PNI of large nerves. The elements of the Risk Model are presented in Table 3.4.

Human nature, being what it is, craves simplification. Therefore, to assure transportability, the recommended **"low-hanging fruit" of prognostication is the cut-point: "WPOI-5 versus not WPOI-5".** Receiver operator curves in the validation study show the positive predictive value for WPOI-5 is 41.7%; that is to say that ***patients with low-stage oral cavity cancer and WPOI-5 have a 42% percent likelihood of developing locoregional recurrence*** [68]. Furthermore, WPOI-5 is associated with occult cervical metastases ($p < 0.0001$, positive predictive value of 68%, negative predictive value 78%) [68]. Examples of WPOI-5 are illustrated in Figs. 3.27, 3.28, and 3.29. The usual phenotype for dispersed carcinoma is a generalized scatter throughout soft tissues. Extratumoral lymphatic emboli or extratumoral perineural invasion are less common phenotypes of WPOI-5, and recognized on their own as poor prognosticators [72].

"Tumor budding" has also been evaluated by an indicator of pattern of invasion [73–75]. High-grade budding is defined as <5 cells at the invasive front. A significant limitation in evaluating budding is the failure to recognize tumor dispersion, an important and validated prognostication.

Table 3.4 The Elements of the Risk Model: Assessment of Worst Pattern of Invasion (WPOI), evaluated at tumor/host interface

		Definition	Score
Non-aggressive	WPOI 1	Broad pushing tumor front	–
	WPOI 2	Finger-like pushing tumor	–
	WPOI 3	Large tumor islands >15 cells	–
Aggressive	WPOI 4	Small tumor islands ≤15 cells or strands of tumor (regardless of size)	+1
	WPOI 5	≥ 1 mm of normal tissue between tumor satellites at the invasive front, regardless of the size of the satellites	+3
Lymphocytic Host Response (LHR), evaluated at tumor/host interface			
LHR type 1	The greatest response. At least one lymphoid nodule per low-power 4x field at the interface.		–
LHR type 2	Intermediate response, defined as lymphoid nodules in at least one, but not all low-power 4 x fields		+1
LHR type 3	Limited response, defined as little or no lymphoid reaction, no single "lymphoid nodule" seen.		+3
Perineural Invasion (PNI), evaluated throughout tumor			
None			–
PNI, small nerves	Tumor must be specially associated with nerve (wrapping around, perineurium, intraneural)		+1
PNI large nerves	Large nerve involvement = ≥ 1 mm		+3
Score tally and risk category assignment			
Total score = 0		Low-risk	
Total score = 1–2		Intermediate risk	
Total score ≥ 3		High-risk	

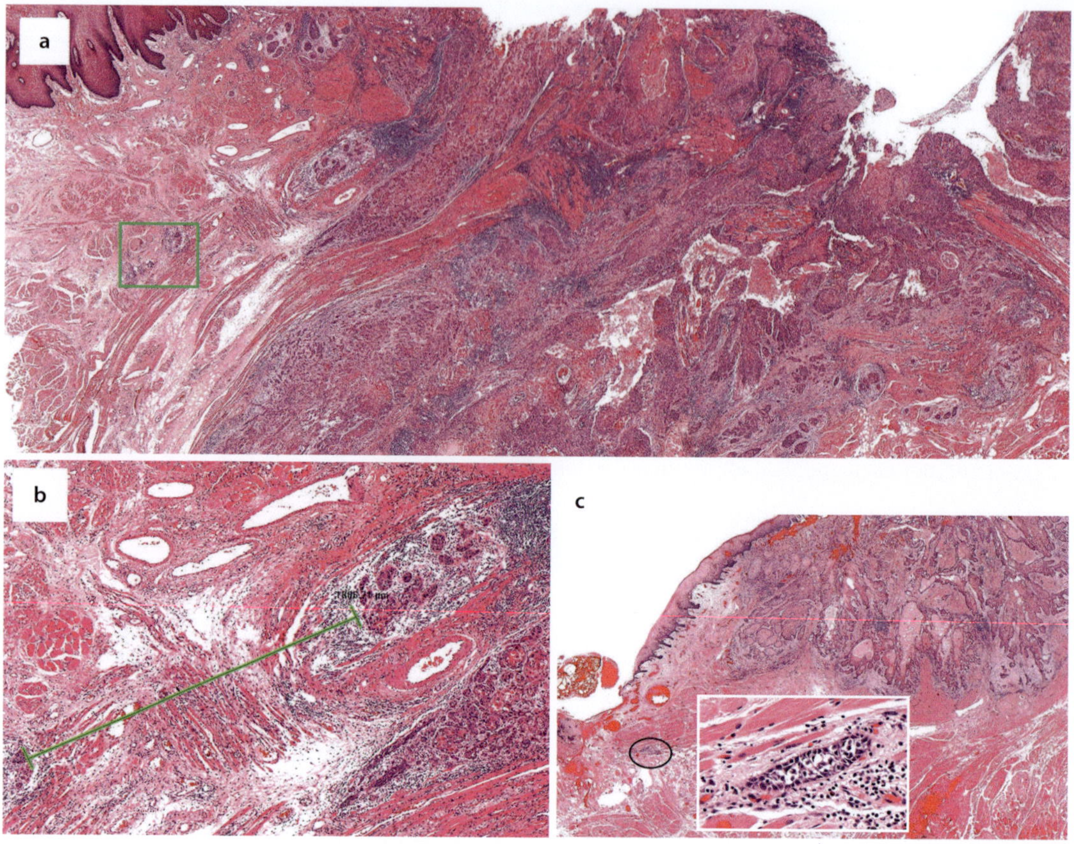

Fig. 3.27 "WPOI-5" describes a dispersed tumor pattern of invasion which is significantly predictive of worst outcome. Carcinomas are classifiable as WPOI-5 when satellite dispersion is ≥1 mm from neighboring satellites. **a** Low-power overview demonstrating a context of generalized tumor dispersion. Tumor dispersion is measured at the advancing tumor edge. Carcinoma satellites in the green box are shown in **b**, lower edge. The green line measures dispersion of almost 2 mm. **c** This carcinoma reveals only few dispersed satellites fulfilling this criteria, likely due to extratumoral lymphovascular emboli

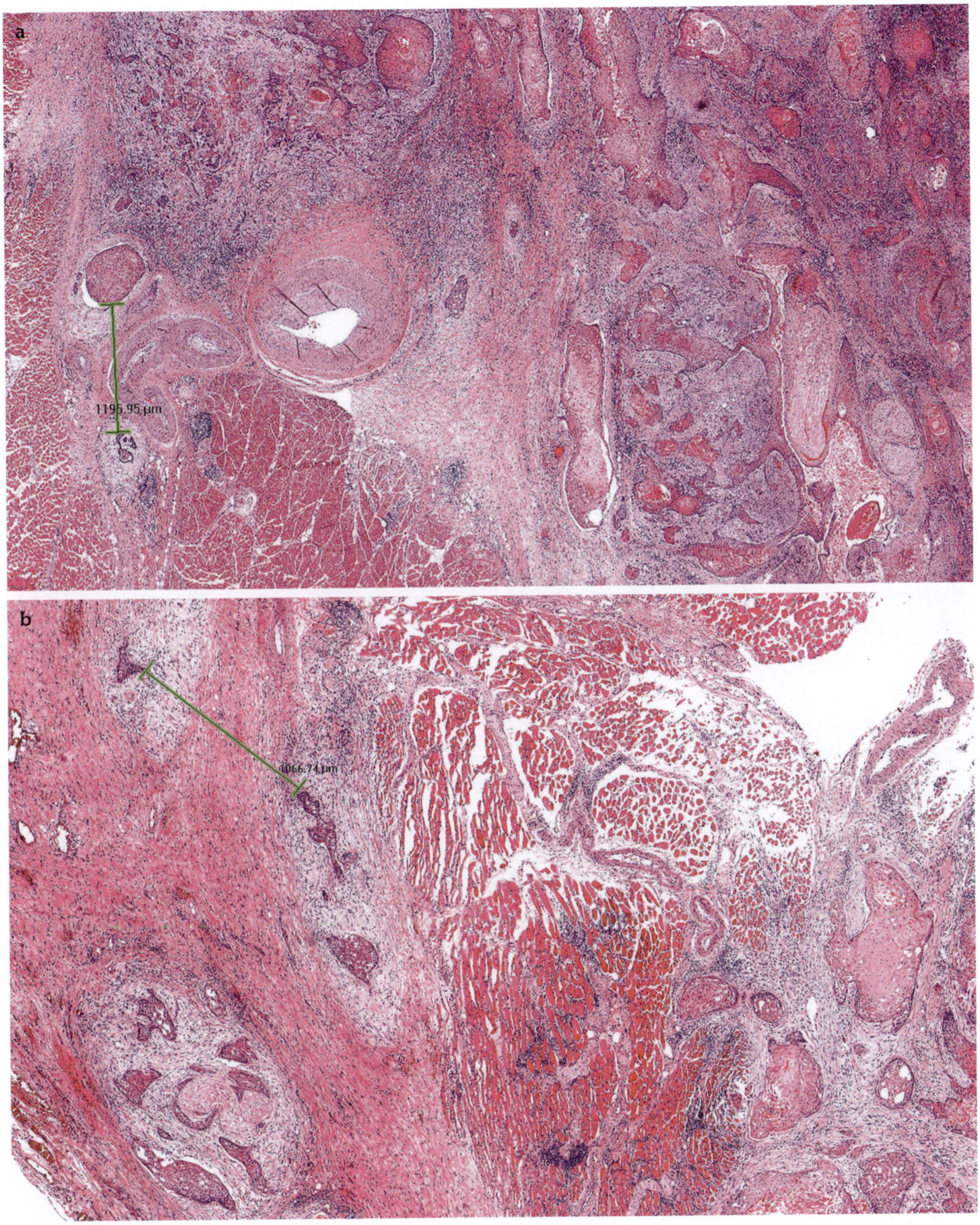

Fig. 3.28 WPOI-5. The context of tumor dispersion can be recognized by the abundance of skeletal muscle between tumor islands. **a**, **b** Both green lines measure a distance of >.1 mm between satellites

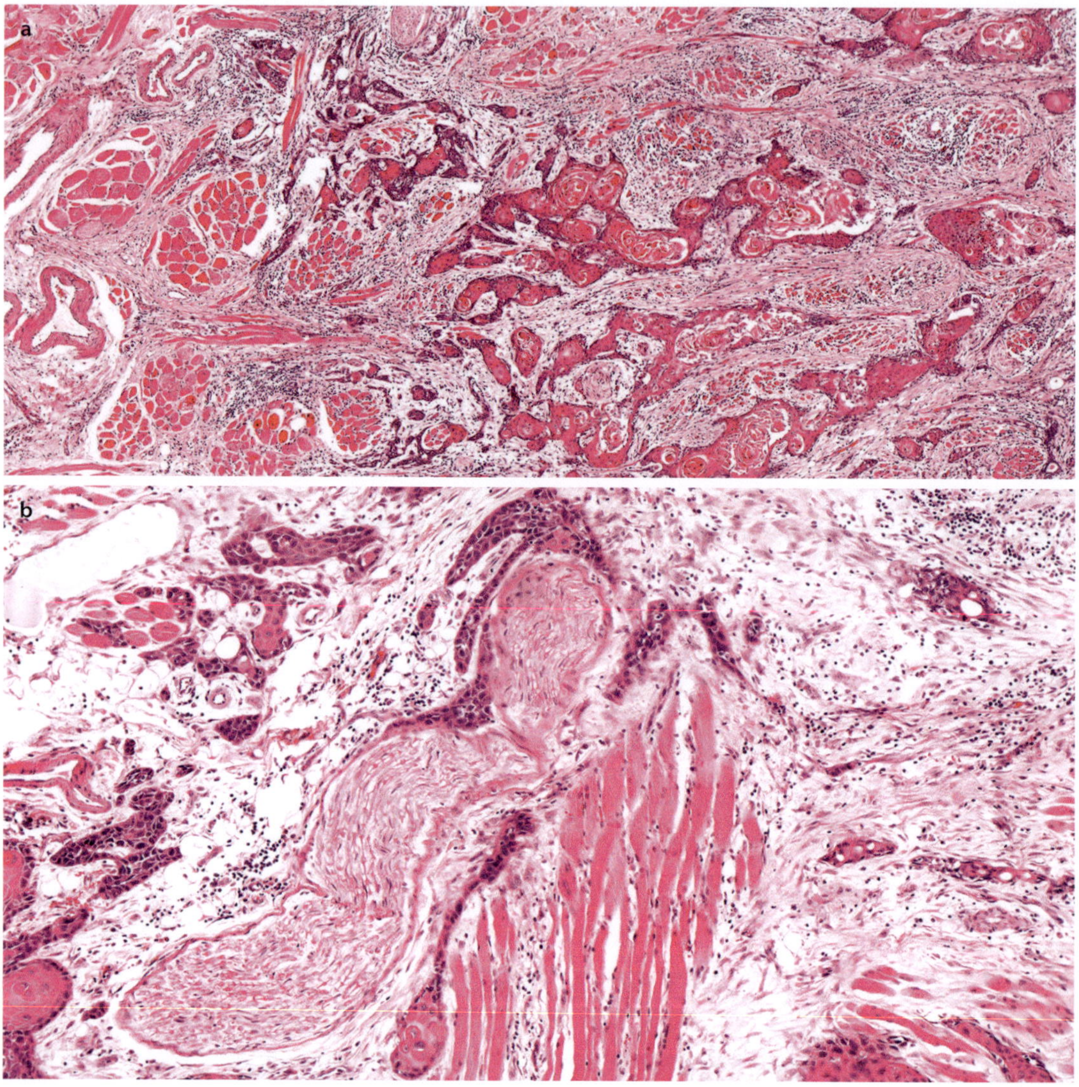

Fig. 3.29 **a** WPOI-5. "Strandy" pattern of invasion is often classifiable as WPOI-5. **b** This strandy pattern is also often associated with perineural invasion

3.2.6 The Surgical Pathology Report

This may be a good a place to discuss writing up a surgical pathology report. Consider the fact you have two audiences: your surgeon, and the next pathologist to review your case. Let's think about your surgeon. Your report is fighting, literally in hand to hand combat, with ten thousand other things, for that brief window of opportunity called, "attention span." Do you want to lose this opportunity in a sea of words? **Think "poem". Think "haiku". Think "news headlines"**. Your report should be accurate descriptive yet terse, and also pleasing to the eye. In broad strokes, these are the steps to consider when reviewing your written report:

1. Is it complete? Now is the time to avoid silly omissions like a specimen part, or necessary reporting element. Each specimen part should contain 1) Anatomic site, procedure (biopsy, excision, resection, etc), and the diagnosis. Resections should specify the tumor origin (squamous carcinoma ***of*** lateral tongue, ***of*** retromolar trigone, etc.)
2. Is it accurate? Is the diagnosis really what you state? Does it *feel* right? Does anything ***bother you*** about this case? Listen to your gut instinct. Seek out sage advice, and listen to it.
3. Does it paint the correct picture? Think of the inherent limitations of the descriptors "well-differentiated" and "poorly differentiated". Let your terse words paint a picture for your surgeon that individualizes this patient's pathology.
4. Is it internally consistent? This is an easy step, requiring you to just scan through your report. Not only should the facts be internally consistent, but your reporting style should also reflect your consistency.

   Don't forget to reconcile frozen section and permanent section findings.
5. Scrub your report:
   1. Look for wordiness. Be stingy with your words. Save them for reports where they're really necessary. Wouldn't "Negative" convey the same idea as, "Squamous mucosa, skeletal muscle and fibroadipose tissue negative for carcinoma?" Do you really need to say, "Squamous ***cell*** carcinoma?"
   2. Look for potential pitfalls of misunderstanding. It is our ethical and medicolegal obligation that the reader of our reports really understand what we are saying. For example, I had signed out an excisional biopsy of a grade I laryngeal chondrosarcoma. In the comment, I noted that although Grade I laryngeal chondrosarcomas require conservative re-excision, this was probably not indicated for this particular case, as the excisional biopsy was quite generous. Imagine my surprise when I saw the (negative) laryngectomy specimen. I discretely inquired the surgeon, who was generally a careful, humble sort. He told me he read my report, but missed my comment! From that time on, if there is an important piece I want my surgeon to note, I give it pride of place within the body of the report.

How then should we consider our pathology audience? As professional nerds, we take the time to read reports carefully. Consider the future of your report. I like to specify which slide demonstrates perineural invasion or a margin of 2 mm. The next busy pathologist reviewing your case will be grateful.

3.2.7 New Therapies

The advent of the Cetuximab era (adjuvant anti-EGFR therapy as a radiosensitizer, in combination with platinum and flurouracil) over one decade ago, represented the first major advance in the treatment of head and neck cancers over the prior 50 years [76]. Cetuximab was found to improve locoregional control but not overall survival suggesting a local radio-sensitizing effect. The response rate to EGFR targeted therapies is around 20–35% and associated with skin rash. Unfortunately, this skin reaction remains the most consistent predictor of drug response. Protein expression of the EGF-receptor (immunohistochemistry) does not correlate with clinical drug response, although strong diffuse EGFR expression predicts poor outcome [77, 78]. EGFR mutations are extremely uncommon in head and neck cancers and lack predictive value [79]. Functional labeled cetuximab uptake studies could potentially yield new insights into predicting response [80, 81]. MAPKs (mitogen-activated protein kinases) represent a family of serine/threonine protein kinases involved in proliferation, differentiation, motility, stress response, apoptosis, and survival; this pathway is upregulated by EGFR activation and pMAPK expression may be predictive of anti-EGFR response [82]. EGFR also interacts with the Src pathway and activates STAT3 signalling; Src inhibitors such as dasatinib are also being evaluated in conjuction with EGFR inhibitors [82]. Clinical trials evaluating monoclonal antibodies that block the suppression of local cytotoxic T-cells through the PD-1/PD-L1 pathway will hopefully lead to new immunomodulating adjuvant therapies [83, 84].

3.2.8 Variants of Squamous Carcinoma

Acantholytic Variant

This rare variant is most often found on sun exposed skin, but has also been reported in various head and neck sites including the oral cavity [86–88]. The decreased cohesiveness that characterizes this variant results in significant intratumoral clefting (acantholysis). These spaces may contain keratin, keratinized tumor cells, necrotic debris, or may be empty; these spaces suggest glandular or vascular spaces (◘ Fig. 3.30). Cytologically, tumor nuclei are usually pleomorphic; the cytoplasm is eosinophilic, glassy and keratinizing. This variant is so uncommon that no conclusions about outcome can be drawn.

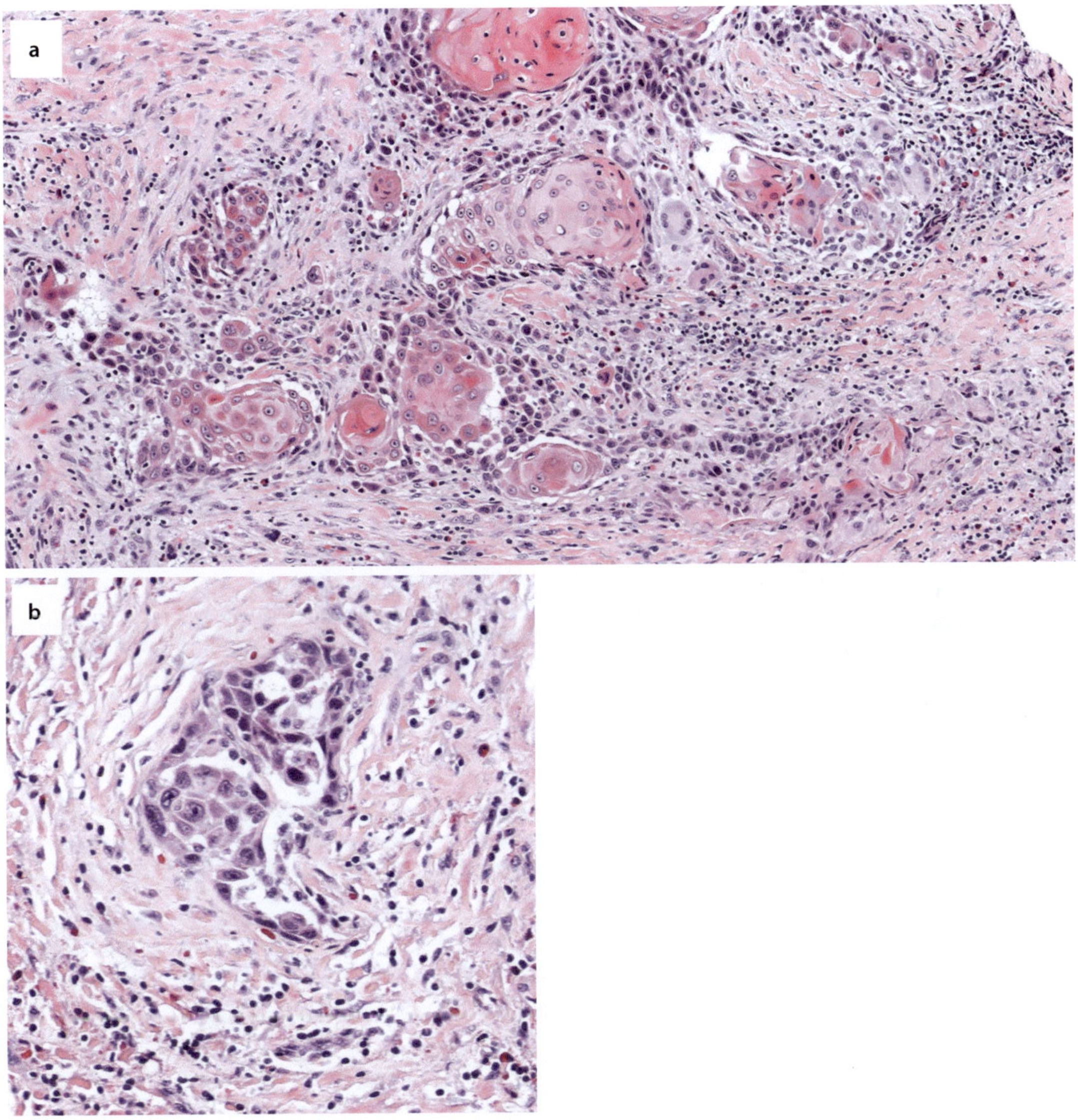

Fig. 3.30 **a, b** "When cancer has a come-apart" – Acantholytic variant of squamous carcinoma: The inherent discohesion between keratinizing tumor cells results in gland-like spaces

Adenosquamous Variant

This is another rare variant which can involve the oral cavity [85–92]. It is comprised of squamous carcinoma elements plus separate, distinct true adenocarcinoma elements (◘ Fig. 3.31). This variant is also so uncommon that no conclusions about outcome can be drawn.

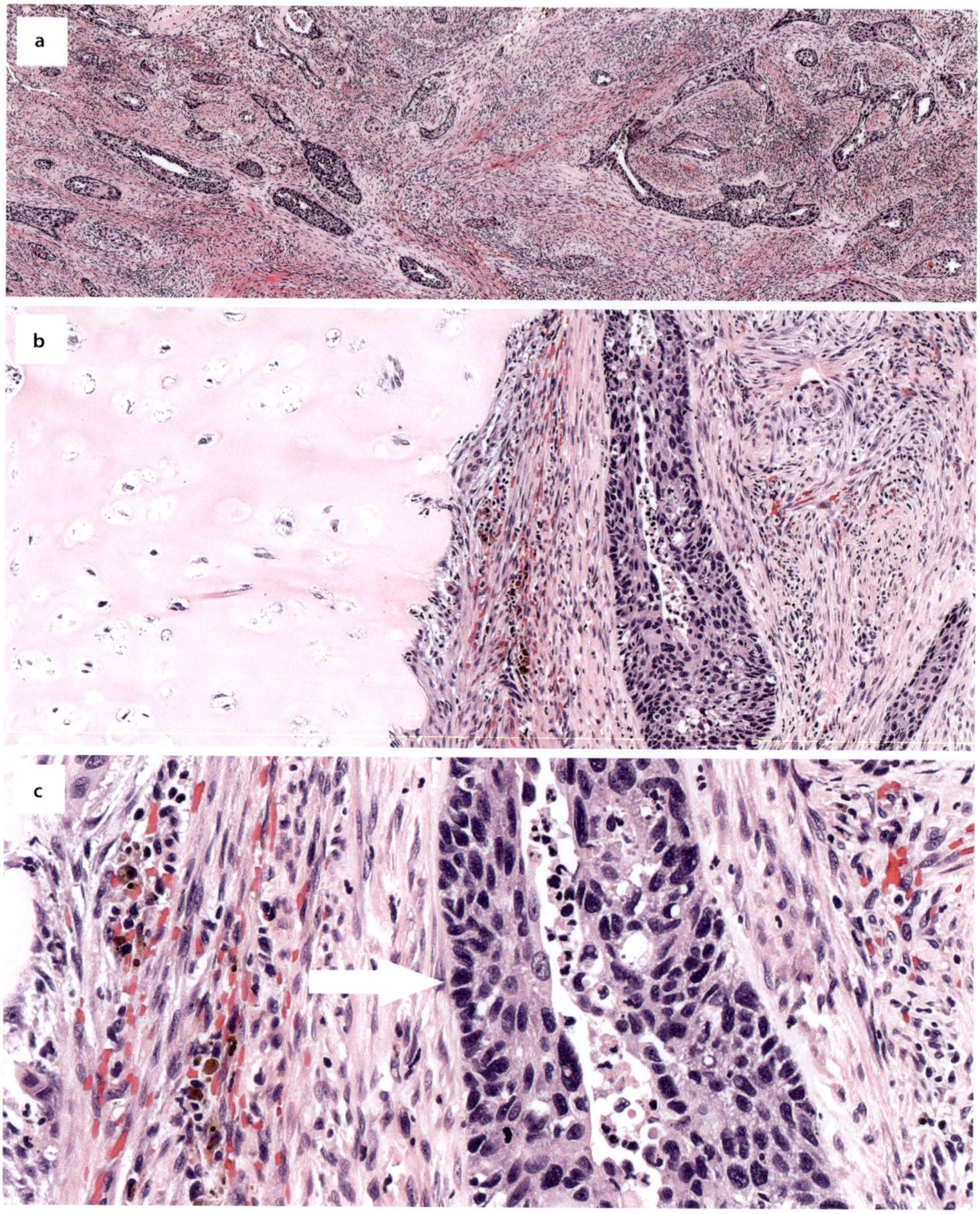

◘ **Fig. 3.31** **a, b** Adenosquamous variant of squamous carcinoma represents another variation on pseudoglandular formation. **c** Notice the polarity of maturation ("down side and up side"). One side of the ribbon recapitulates the basal reserve layer (*arrow*) while the opposite end demonstrates maturation as the tumor cells flatten. This "down and up" morphology confirms squamous differentiation and excludes a true adenocarcinoma

Basaloid Variant

Basaloid squamous carcinoma may present as a polypoid submucousal neoplasm, or may be indistinguishable from the usual SCC. Intraoral basaloid squamous carcinomas are not uncommon [93–95]. This variant is composed of basaloid tumor cells with high nuclear/cytoplasmic ratio. Prominent pallisading of tumor cells can be seen at the periphery of tumor islands (◘ Figs. 3.32 and 3.33). Necrosis is common; keratinization usually

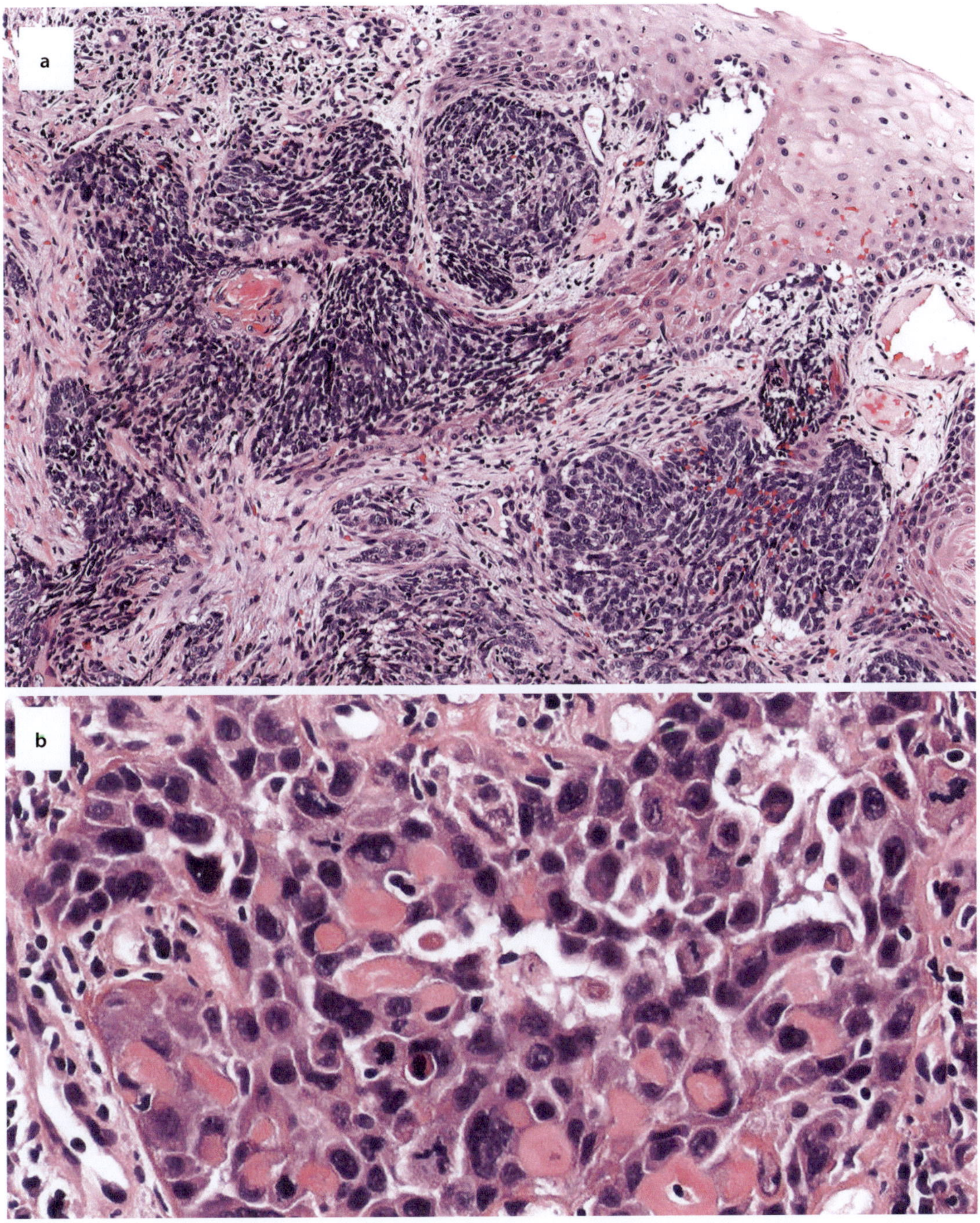

◘ **Fig. 3.32** **a** Basaloid variant of squamous carcinoma is composed of tumor cells with dark oval nuclei and little cytoplasm. Here we see the *in-situ* component arising from mucosal rete pegs. **b** Tumor cells produce a variable amount of basement membrane material, which can be seen dissecting between tumor cells. In contrast, the basement membrane material elaborated by adenoid cystic carcinoma is confines within the pseudoglandular cribriform spaces limited. There is variable elaboration of basement membrane material, which may mimic salivary neoplasia such as adenoid cystic carcinoma. ***The basement membrane material dissects between tumor cells forming microcystic, cribriform-like areas, rather than the sharply punched out cribriform spaces of adenoid cystic carcinoma.*** *In-situ* squamous carcinoma can also be helpful in distinguishing basaloid squamous carcinoma from adenoid cystic carcinoma. The prognosis of oral cavity basaloid squamous carcinoma is comparable to conventional squamous carcinoma [95].

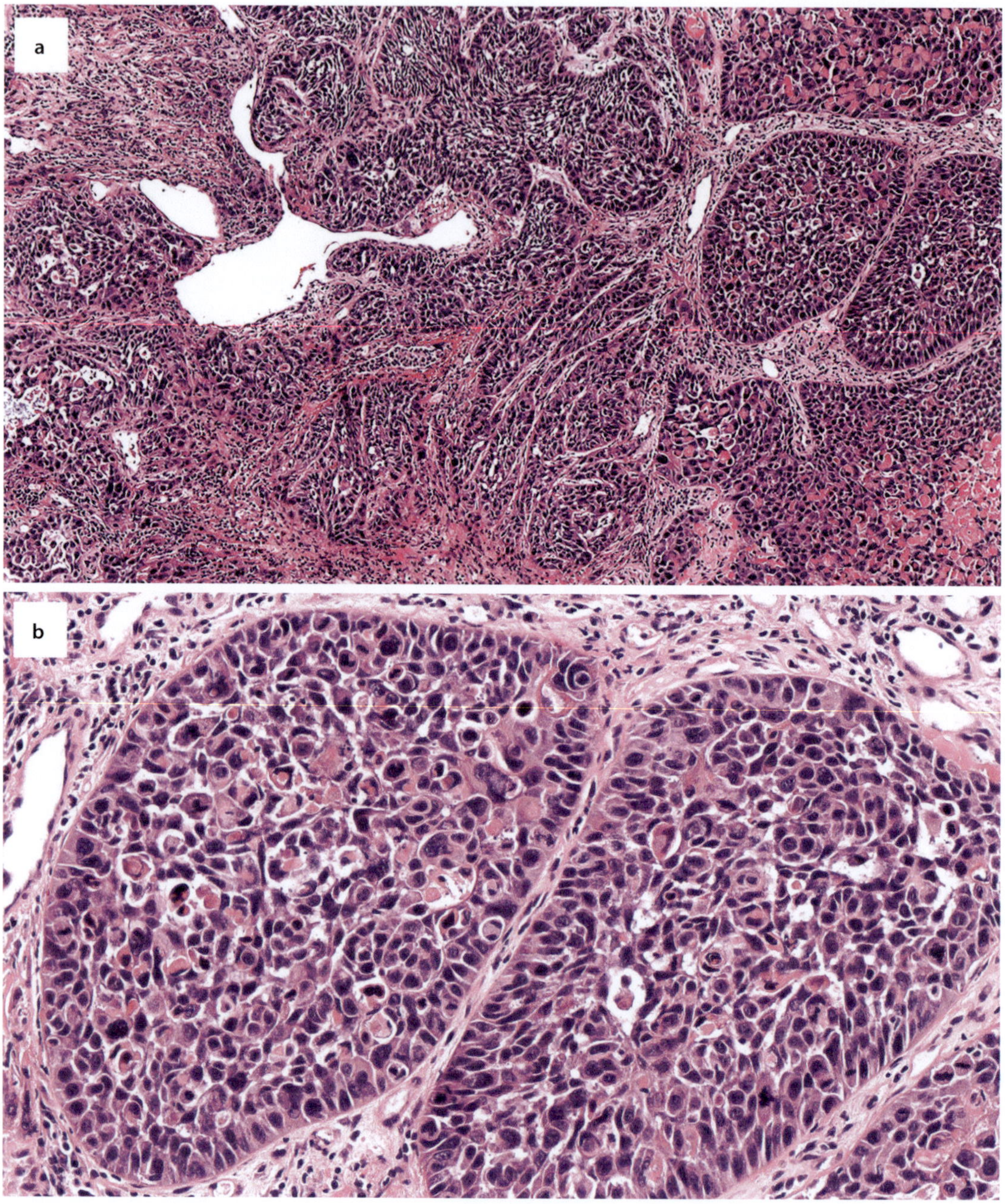

Fig. 3.33 **a, b** Basaloid variant of squamous carcinoma: palisading tumor cells at satellite periphery

Clear Cell Variant

This is another rare variant, first described in the skin, which has also been described in the oral cavity and characterized by tumor cells with abundant cytoplasm with extensive clear cell change [96–99] which may be due to cytoplasmic glycogen (◘ Fig. 3.34). No cytoplasmic mucin or goblet cells should be found, distinguishing this variant from mucoepidermoid carcinoma.

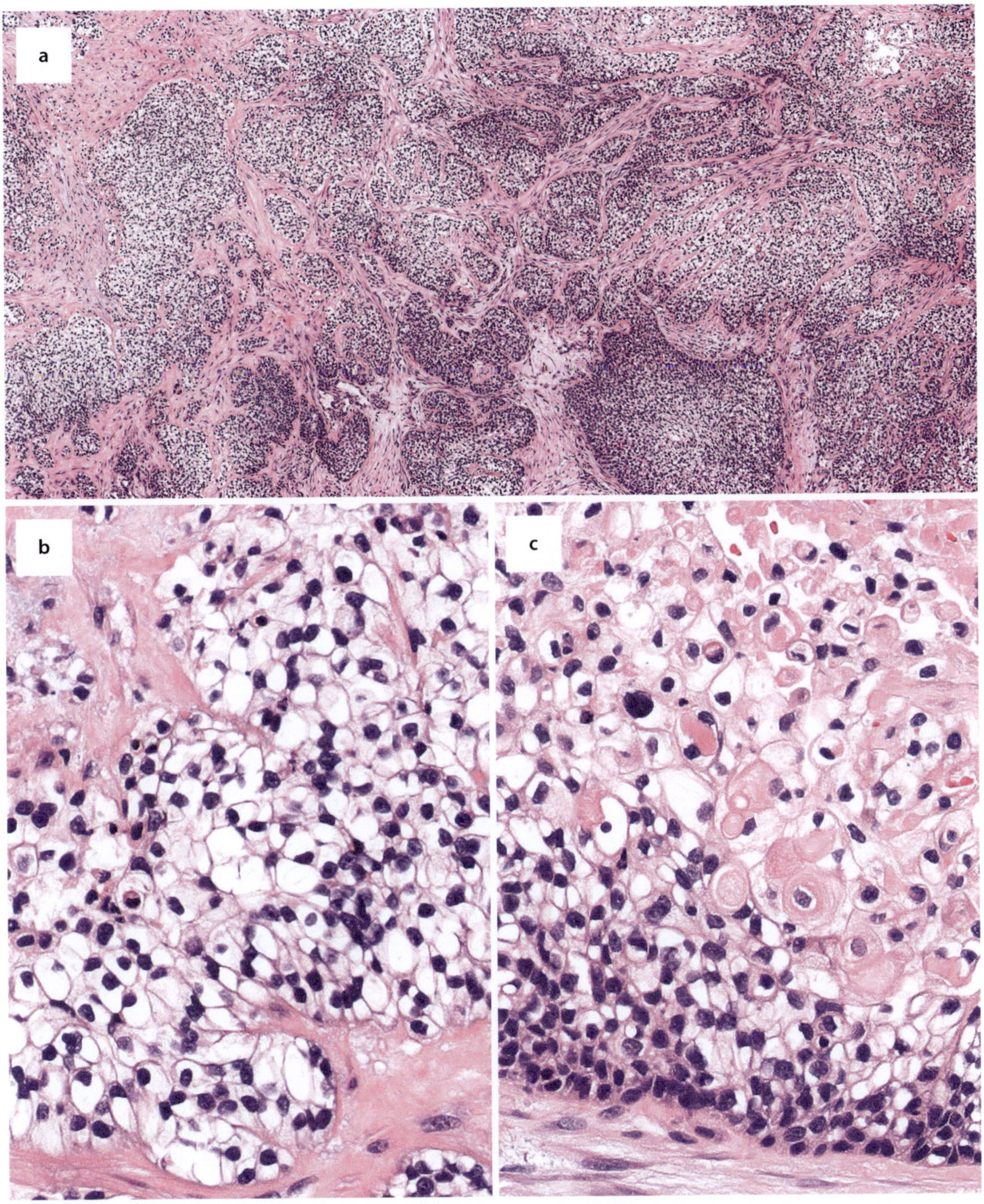

◘ **Fig. 3.34** **a, b** Clear cell variant of squamous carcinoma: The differential diagnosis includes clear cell predominant mucoepidermoid carcinoma and salivary hyalinizing clear cell carcinoma. **c** Tumor cell keratinization

Carcinoma Cuneiform (Cuniculatum)

This uncommon variant has also been called inverted verrucous carcinoma. Most commonly, carcinoma cuneiform occurs on the foot. ***Oral carcinoma cuneiform has a predilection for the gingiva and palate.*** It can have an exophytic papillary granular surface or present as an endophytic crateform growth. The "cuneiform" descriptor refers to the writing instrument used on clay tablets, a writing system invented by the Sumerians at least 3000 years ago. The inverted nature of this tumor is not unlike the impression the instrument leaves on the clay.

Histologically, these tumors are uniformly bland; architecturally, the tumor forms deep burrowing "rabbit warren"-like (cuniculatum) complex branching tunnels and cysts with abundant keratinization [100–102]. Similar to verrucous carcinoma, the diagnosis of carcinoma cuneiform requires clinical correlation, or else patients may suffer delay (◘ Figs. 3.35, 3.36, and 3.37). Locoregional or distant metastases are rare events for this tumor.

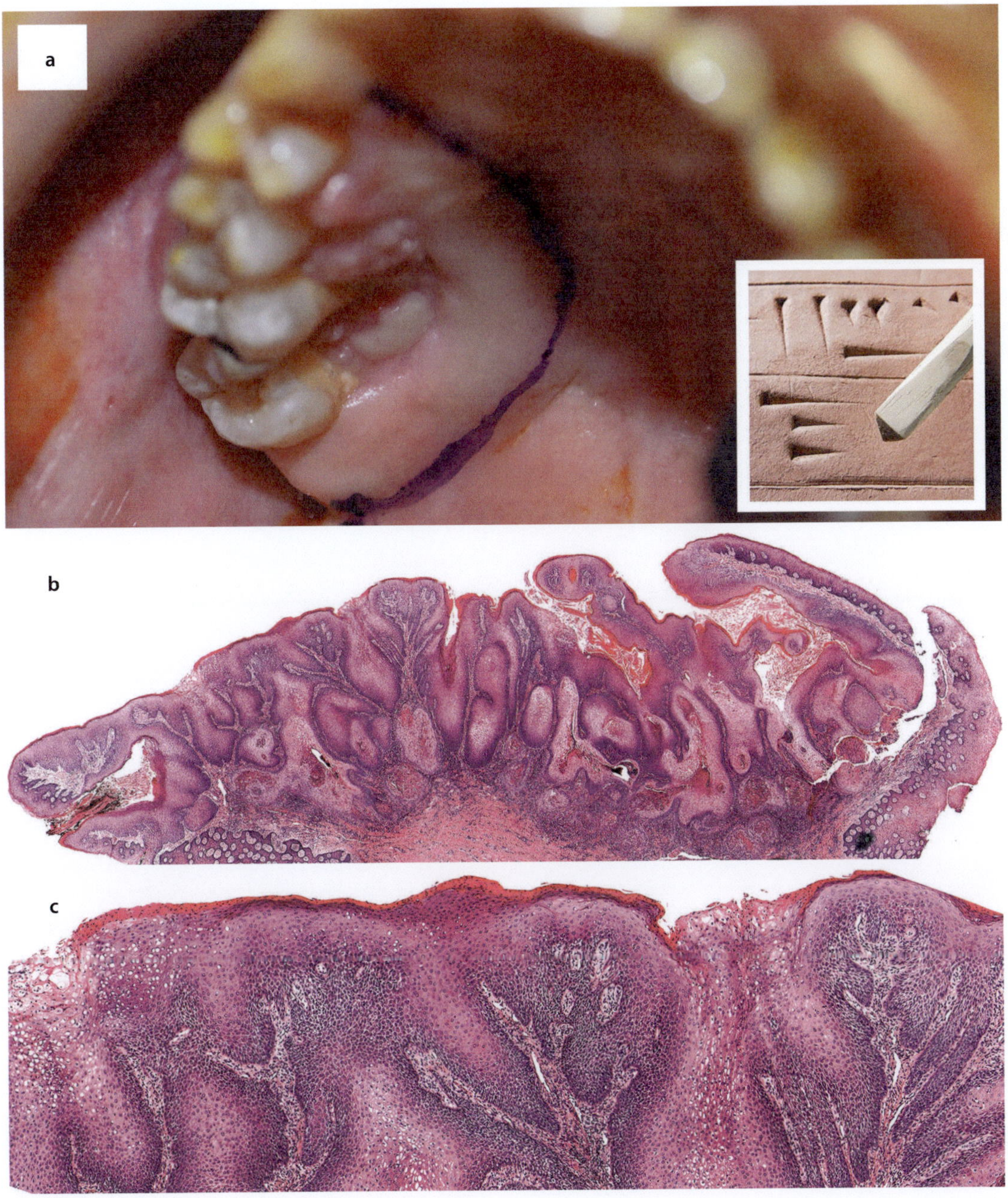

Fig. 3.35 **a** Cuneiform variant of squamous carcinoma presenting as an ulcerating lesion which eroded maxillary bone. Cuneiform is derived from the Latin term "cuneus" meaning "wedge". Cuneiform script was produced using a wedge shaped stylus impressed upon clay tablets (Inset). In the context of neoplasia, "cuneiform" is meant to describe the burrowing nature despite the flat surface. (Courtesy of Dr. Anthony Morland). **b**, **c** This diagnosis requires clinicopathologic correlation as pleomorphism is usually lacking

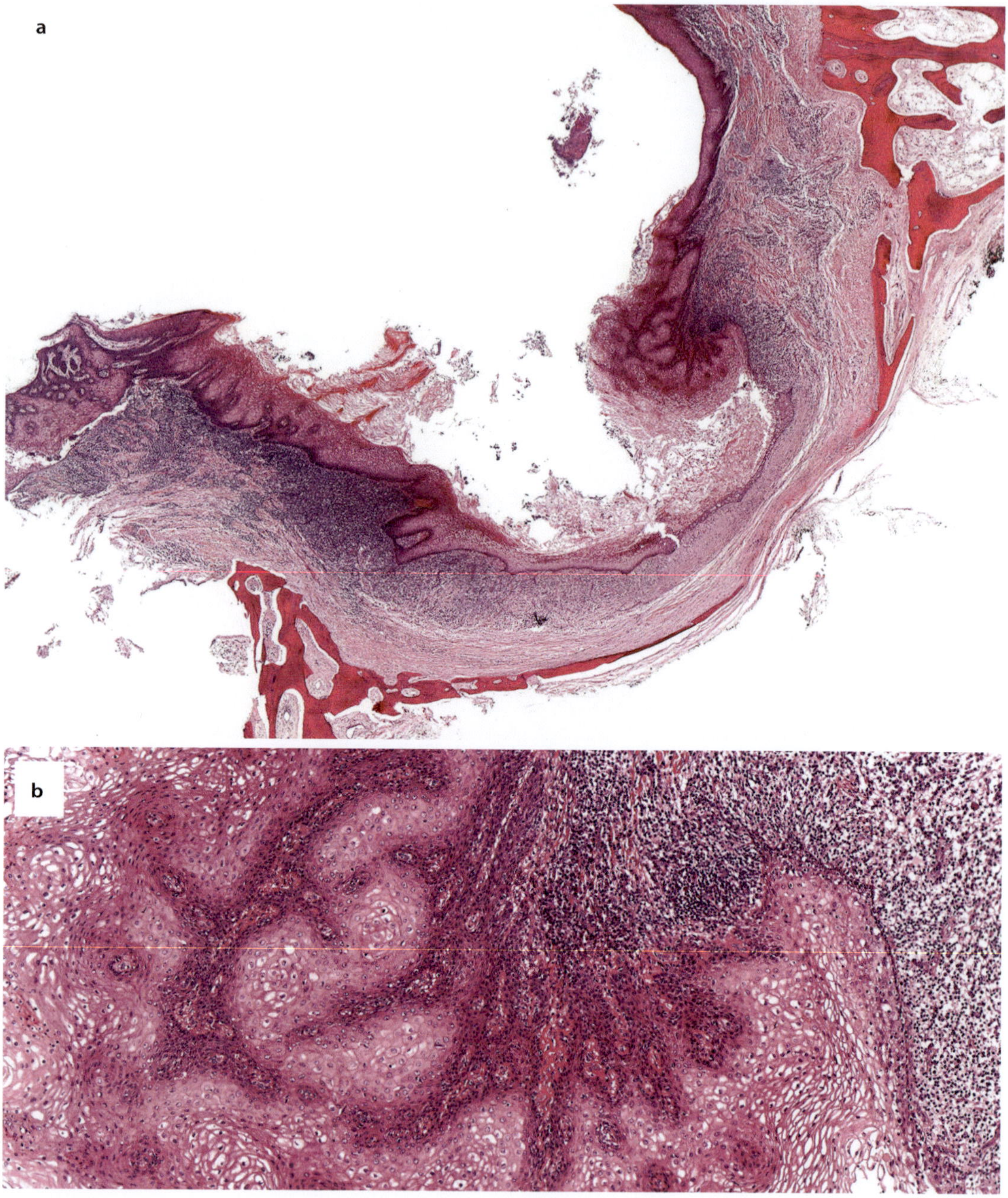

Fig. 3.36 **a**, **b** Cuneiform variant of squamous carcinoma with an expansile cystic component that destroyed the mandible

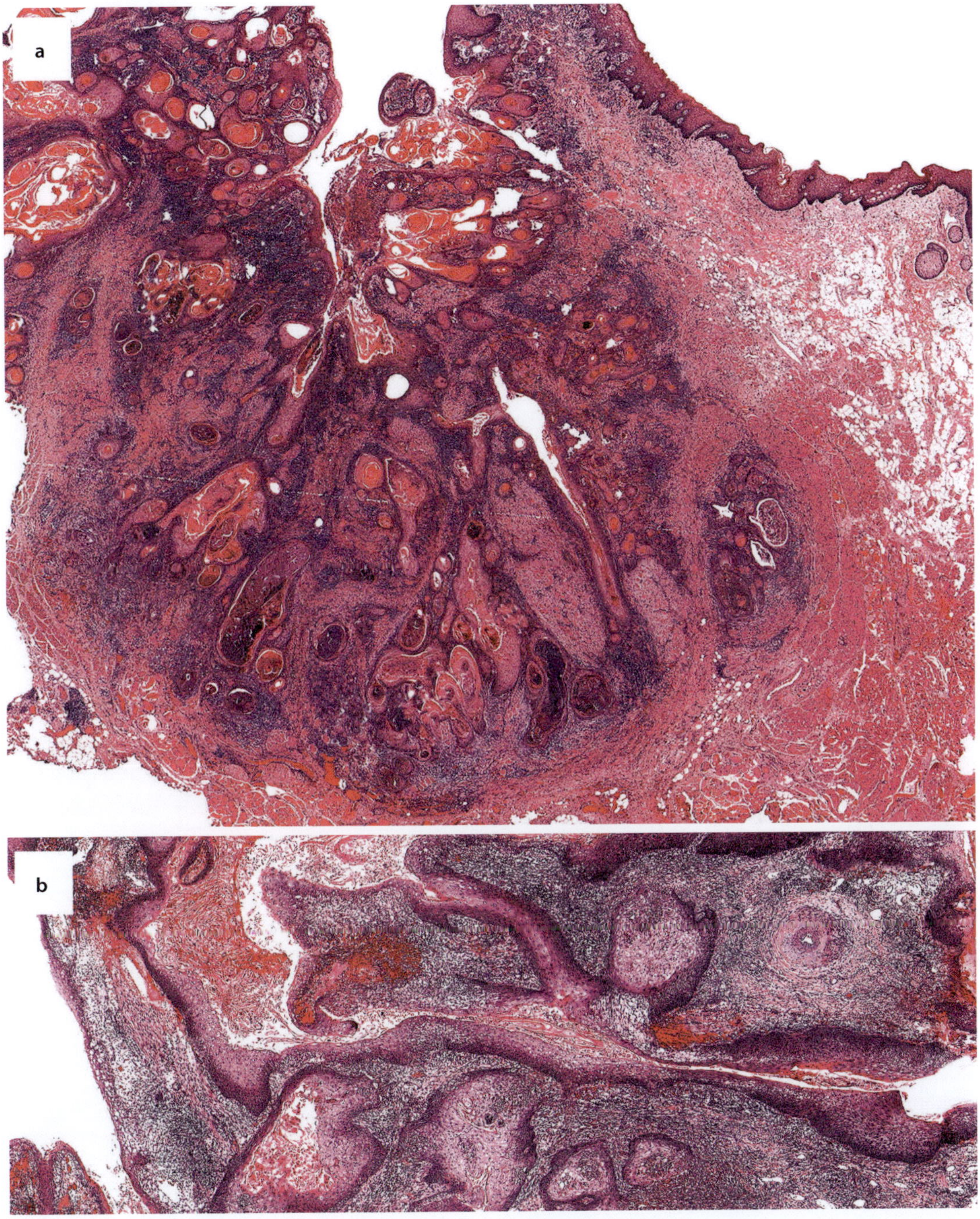

Fig. 3.37 **a, b** This buccal cuneiform carcinoma produced warrens-like burrows of keratinizing carcinoma. Cuneiform carcinoma has also been described as "inverted verrucous carcinoma"

HIV-Associated SCC

Squamous carcinoma of the head and neck is the third most common cancer non-AIDS defining malignancies for patients infected with human immunodeficiency virus (HIV). It is seen in excess among HIV-infected individuals, most commonly in the oropharynx and larynx [103, 104]. Histologically, multinucleated tumor giant cells are a distinct and common feature of HIV-associated SCC (◘ Fig. 3.38).

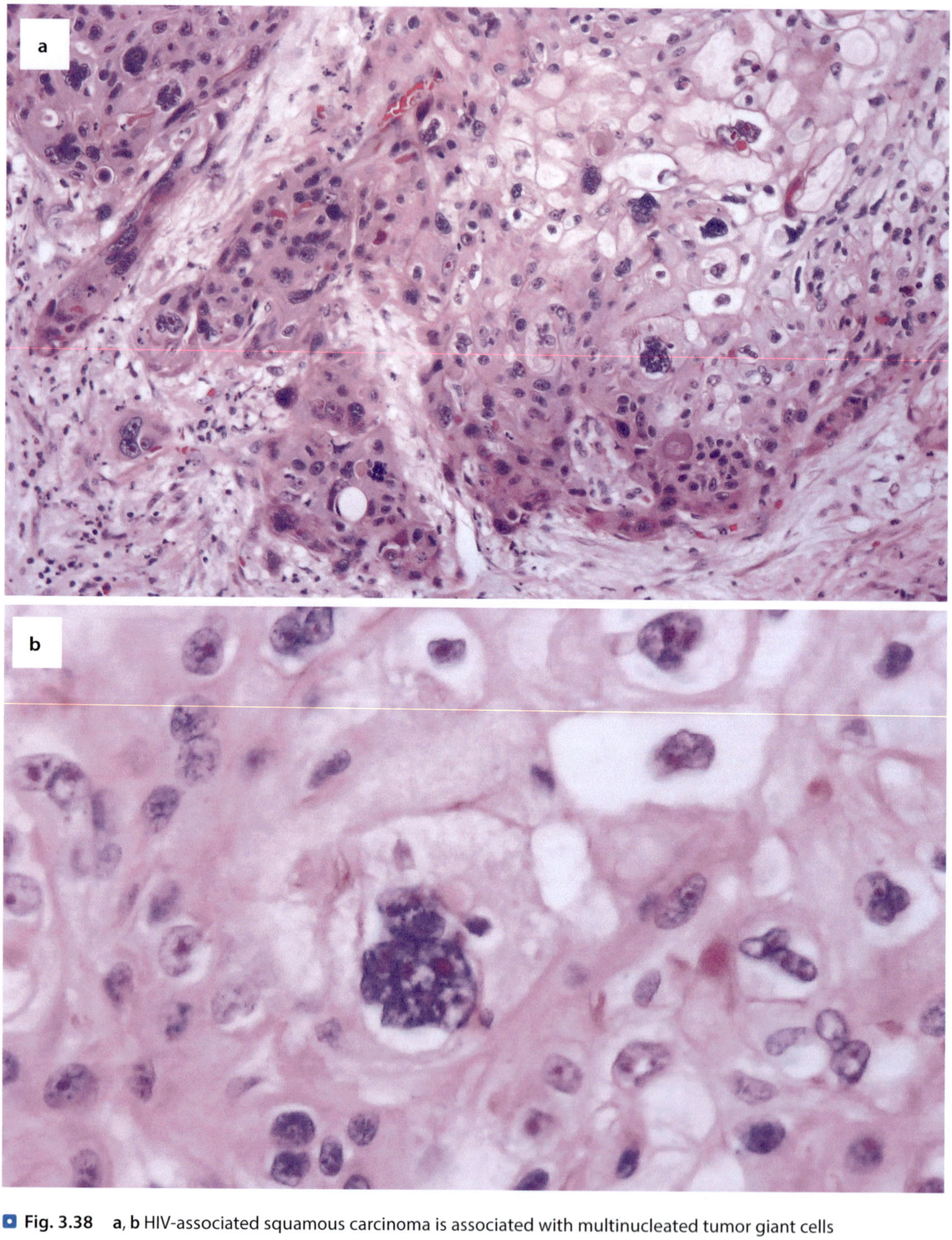

◘ **Fig. 3.38** **a, b** HIV-associated squamous carcinoma is associated with multinucleated tumor giant cells

Papillary Variant

This is a mixed group of tumors united by their exophytic papillary component. Laryngeal, oropharyngeal, and hypopharyngeal subsites are most common affected [105, 106]. ***The intraoral subsite distribution characteristicially involves the mandibular gingiva and buccal cavity*** [107–110]. Papillary variants of squamous carcinomas are described as pink, red, exophytic, pebbly, surface with filiform, finger-like projections. Importantly, they may be either entirely exophytic and noninvasive or may contain some invasive component.

Histologically, this tumor is defined by prominent fibrovascular cores. Cytologically, well-differentiated carcinomas with maturation and keratinization are more common than cytologically higher-grade carcinomas, which are easy to recognize as malignant on limited biopsies (◘ Figs. 3.39, 3.40, and 3.41). Well-differentiated papillary squamous carcinomas may be difficult to classify on initial biopsy, and may warrant the diagnosis of "squamoproliferative process". Not surprisingly, oropharyngeal papillary squamous carcinomas tend to harbor high-risk HPV and overexpress p16 [106]. The outcome for patients with oral cavity papillary squamous carcinoma appears to be good; locoregional and distant metastases are uncommon.

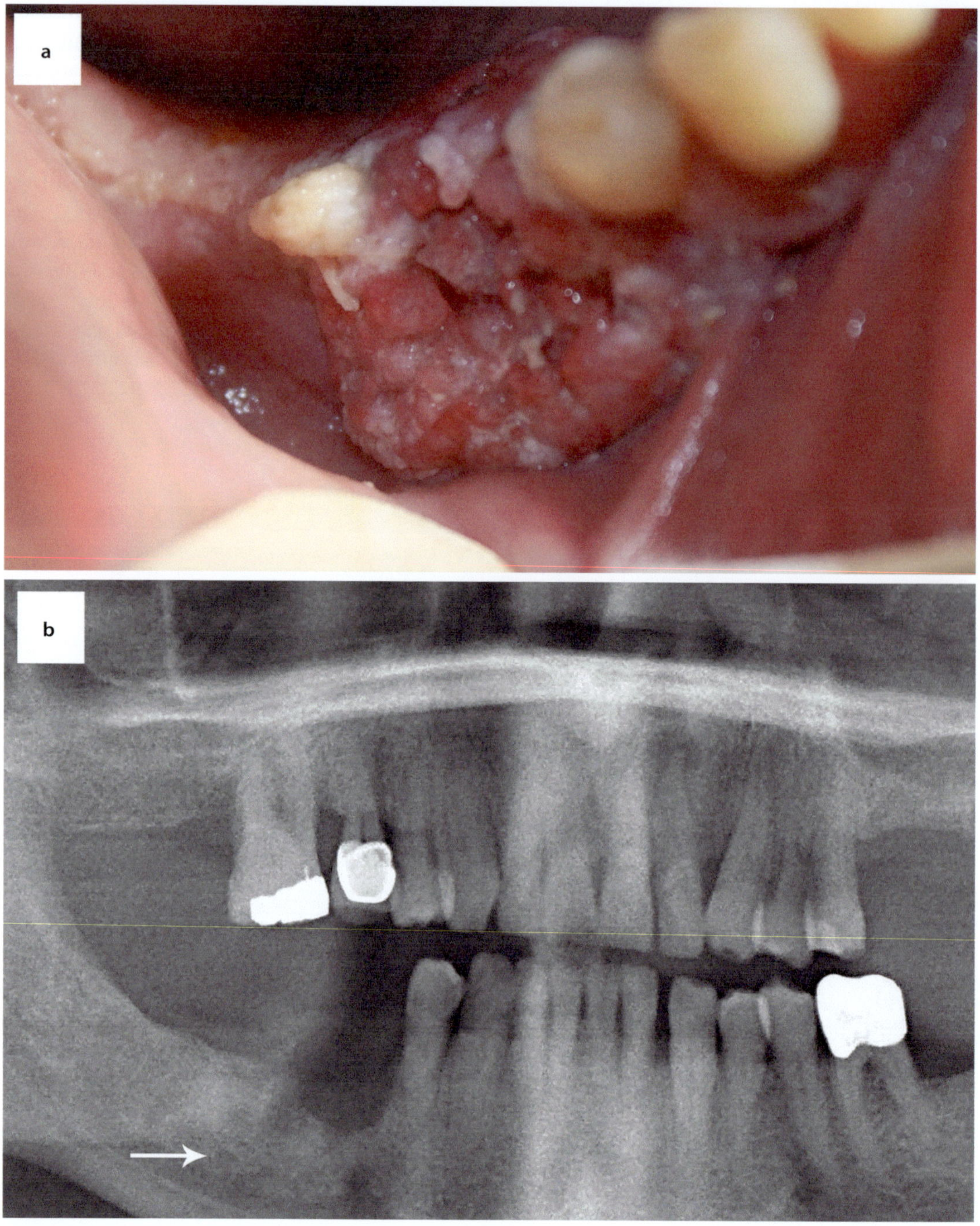

Fig. 3.39 **a** Papillary variant of squamous carcinoma. (Courtesy of Dr. Anthony Morland). **b** The plain film demonstrated boney erosion (*arrow*)

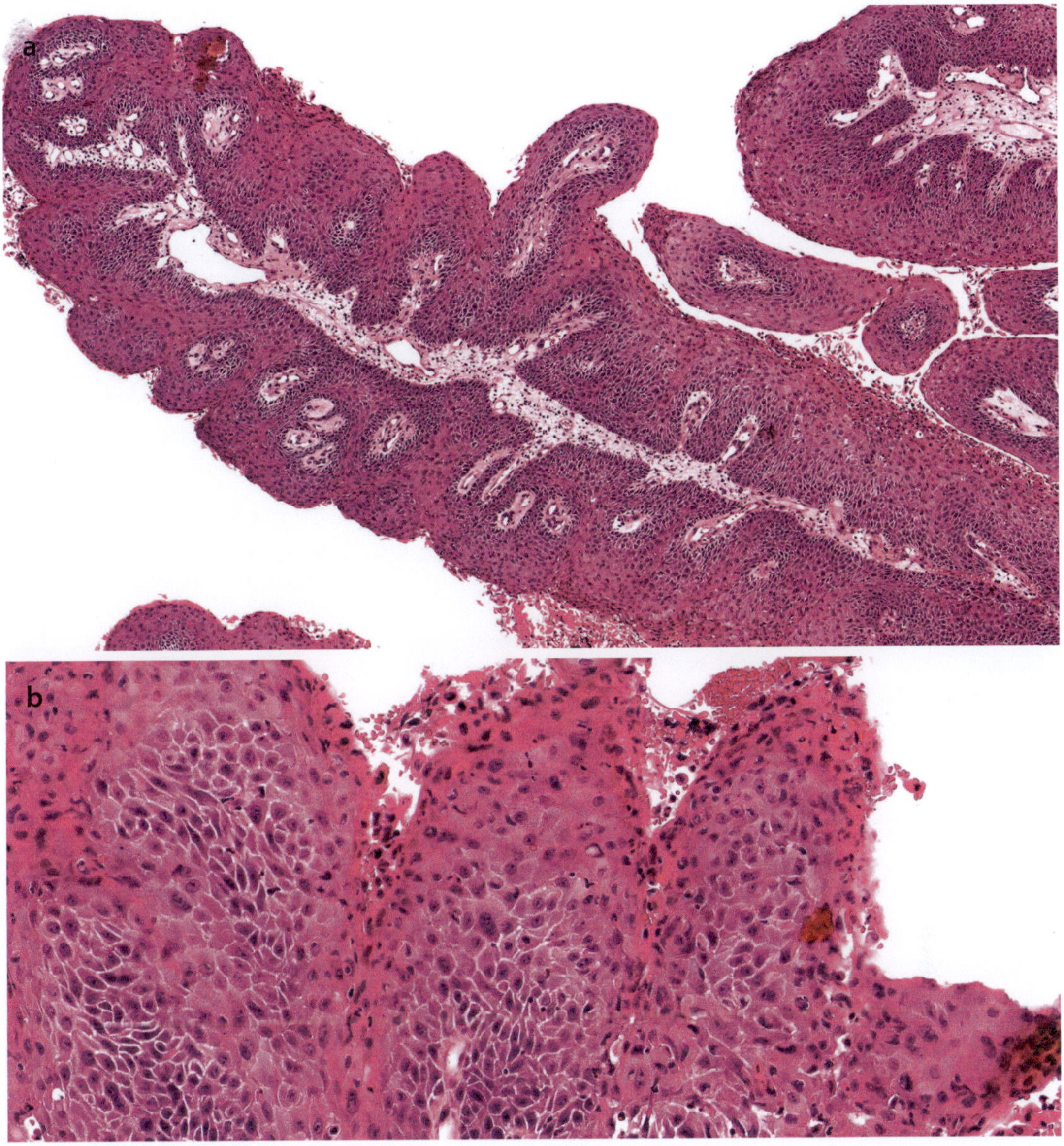

Fig. 3.40 **a, b** Papillary formation with discreet fibrovascular cores. This diagnosis can be straightforward in the face of cytologic pleomorphism

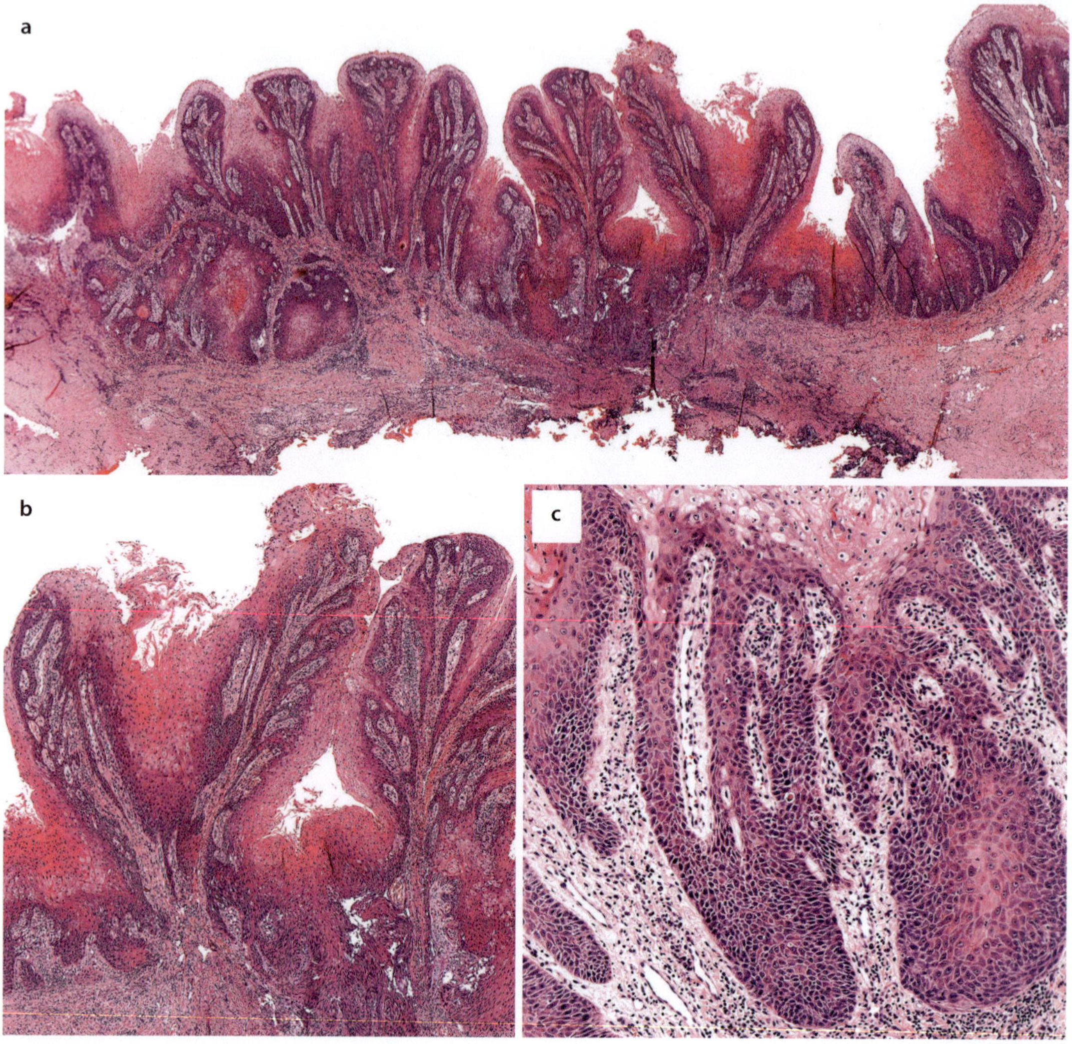

Fig. 3.41 a–c Papillary variant of squamous carcinoma. The diagnosis can require clinicopathologic correlation if pleomorphism is not striking, or absent

Pagetoid Spread

Although not a recognized variant, it is worthwhile to know that rare head and neck squamous carcinomas can be so discohesive as to also disperse along squamous mucosa and into minor salivary ducts and glands and are invariably associated with aggressive biology [111, 112] (◘ Fig. 3.42).

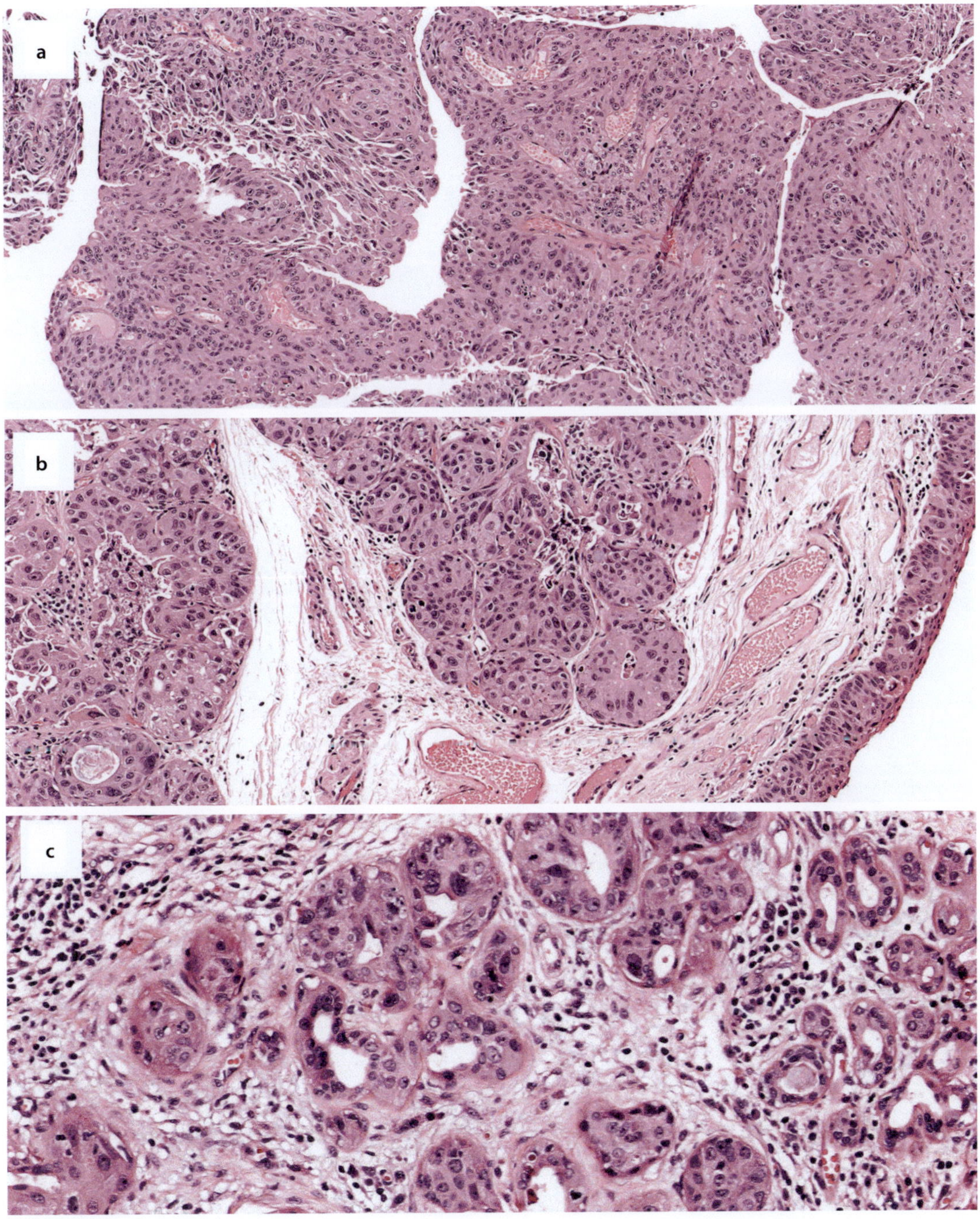

◘ **Fig. 3.42** **a–c** Pagetoid spread of mucosal squamous carcinoma into small minor salivary ducts

Pseudoangiosarcomatoid variant adenoid squamous carcinoma

This rare variant is kin to the acantholytic/adenoid variant, tumor discohesiveness leads to formation of pseudoglands and blood-filled channels that mimic angiosarcoma [113, 114] (Figs. 3.43 and 3.44). As with other rare variants, no conclusions about outcome can be drawn.

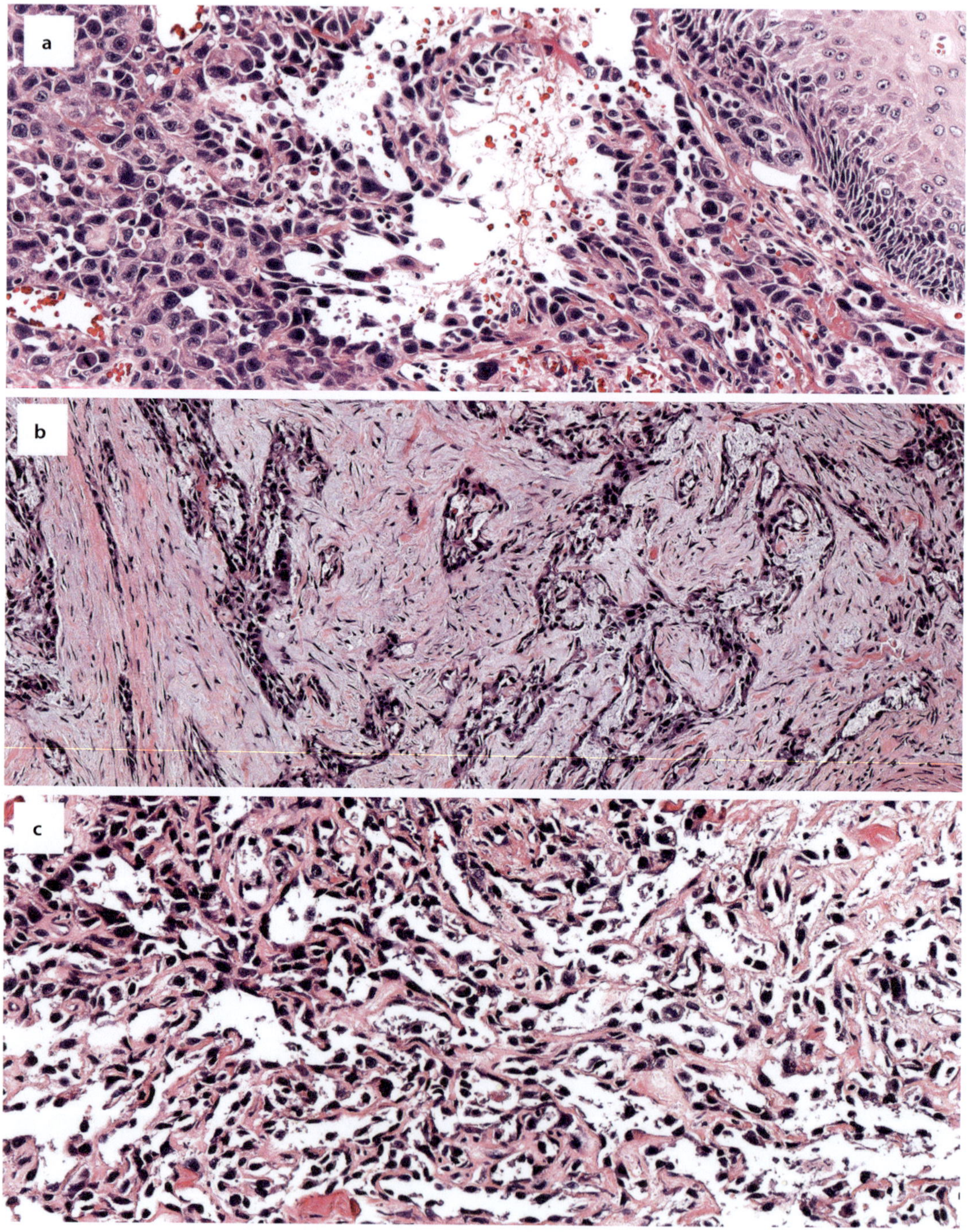

Fig. 3.43 **a–c** Pseudoangiosarcomatoid variant of squamous carcinoma – another variation on "cancer come apart". Here the inherent discohesion between cancer cells and extravasated erythrocytes mimic the serpiginous vascular spaces of angiosarcoma

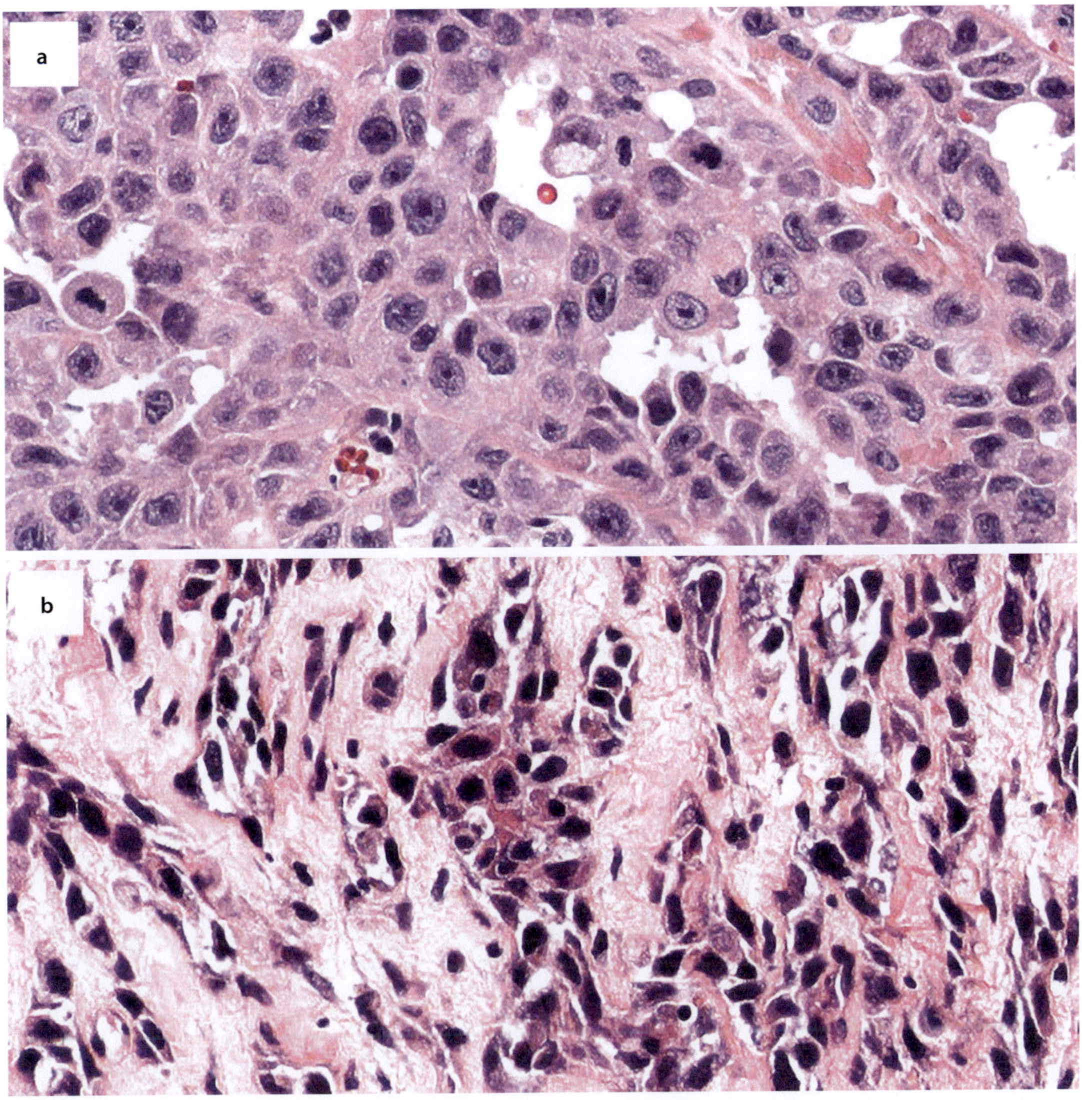

Fig. 3.44 **a** Pseudoangiosarcomatoid variant of squamous carcinoma mimicking epithelioid angiosarcoma. **b** Mimicking "hobnail" like tumor cells projecting into spaces

Spindle Cell Variant

Spindle cell squamous carcinoma (carcinosarcoma, pseudosarcoma, sarcomatoid carcinoma) refers to a variant with a prominent malignant spindle cell component. Demographically, it is seen predominantly in older individuals (sixth to seventh decade life) with a male predominance. Spindle cell carcinoma often grows as a polypoid tumor. The larynx is the most common site for this variant followed by the oral cavity, usually tongue, gingiva/alveolar ridge, retromolar trigone [115–118].

Histopathologically, the malignant spindle cells can have various appearances and grades. Often, the elongated tumor cells are epithelioid with abundant pink cytoplasm and therefore still recognizable as squamous carcinoma (Figs. 3.45 and 3.46). Other times, this variant may be indistinguishable from sarcoma, with hyperchromatic and very long nuclei, high nuclear/cytoplasmic ratio, forming a storiform fasicular pattern. Additional mesenchymal differentiation may be evident, such as osteoid-like matrix or chondroid matrix. Evidence of squamous differentiation may come in the following forms: focal islands of keratinizing SCC, either near mucosal surface or at the advancing edge,

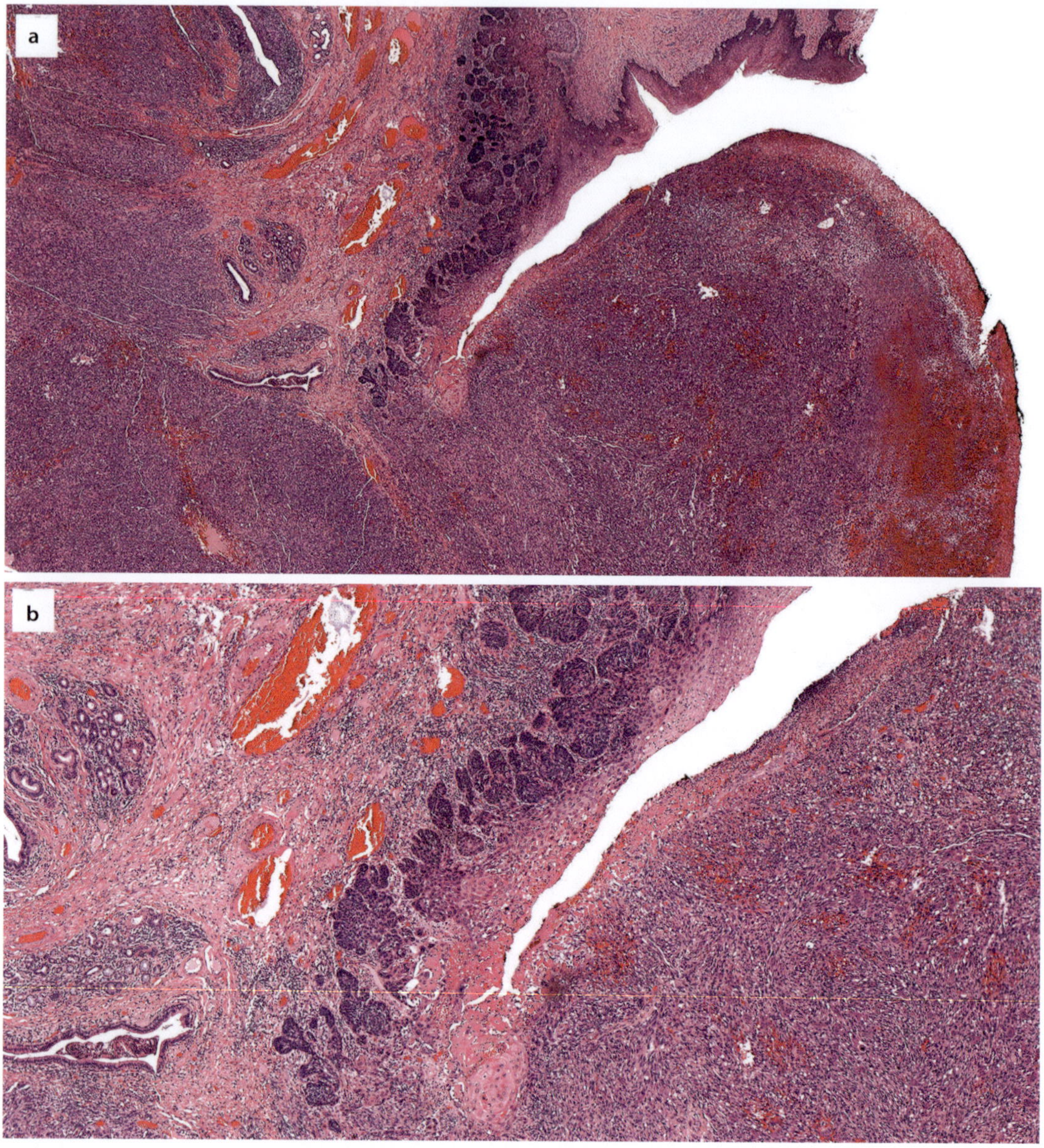

Fig. 3.45 **a** Spindle cell variant of squamous carcinoma. Here, we see a cellular, exophytic and polypoid neoplasm with an invasive component. **b** Squamous carcinoma-in-situ

mucosal *carcinoma-in-situ,* or keratin expression. The diagnosis of oral spindle cell variant is even justified in the absence of any of the above elements, as long as other malignancies (melanoma, true sarcomas) have been excluded. Grading based on cellularity, nuclear pleomorphism, mitotic activity, and necrosis.

Spindle cell variant represents "epithelial-mesenchymal transition writ large". Tumor cells often express vimentin, and may at times express smooth muscle actin. They are staged like conventional squamous carcinomas. Two recent studies bear mention, despite the SEER national database limitation regarding lack of pathology re-review. Spindle cell variants are more likely to present at Stage I compared with conventional squamous carcinomas, reflecting their polypoid tendency which is also protective against lymph node

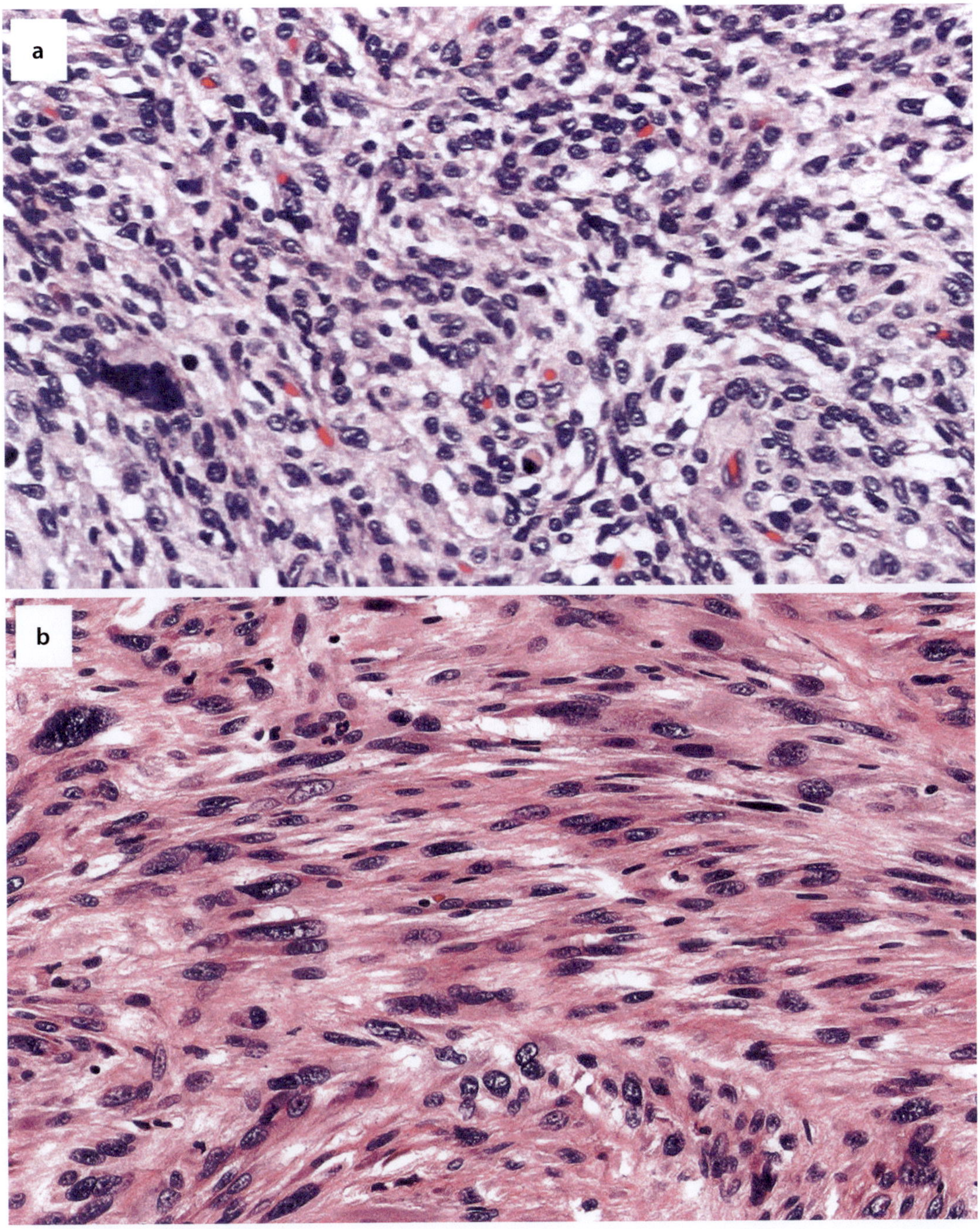

Fig. 3.46 **a** Spindle cell variant of squamous carcinoma. Epithelioid spindled tumor cells. **b** These tumor nuclei are elongated and more sarcoma-like

metastases. When approached according to subsite, both studies (using the same national data) demonstrated that oral cavity spindle cell variants was associated with significantly decreased disease-specific survival compared with conventional squamous carcinomas [119, 120].

Transitional Variant

This variant is mentioned here to emphasize two histological points: (1) Recognizing the polarity of ribbons (flattened maturing "up" side versus the "down" side which recapitulates the basal reserve layer) effectively excludes the possibility of adenocarcinoma, and confirms the squamoid nature of the carcinoma. (2) In the urinary bladder, this pattern is usually attributed to *in-situ* disease. In the head and neck, this pattern is usually associated with a non-aggressive pushing type pattern of invasion (Fig. 3.47).

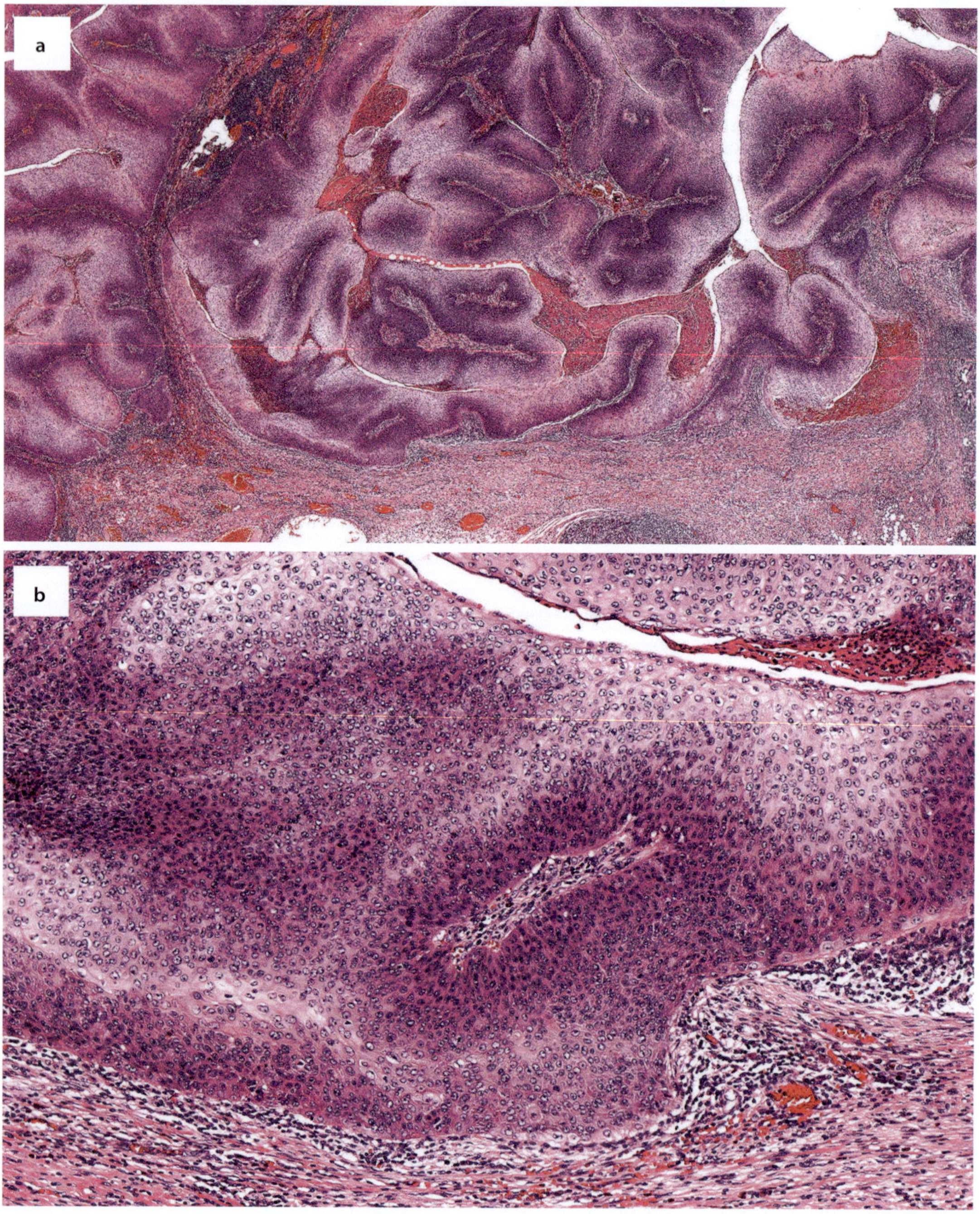

Fig. 3.47 **a, b** Transitional variant of squamous carcinoma forms smooth ribbons with polarized maturation ("down side and up side"). The transitional variant is associated with a non-aggressive pushing type pattern of invasion

Verrucous Carcinoma

Verrucous carcinoma is a slow-growing locally invasive malignancy ***with no metastatic potential.*** The oral cavity is the most common head and neck site, most often involving subsites of gums, buccal mucosa, oral commissure, and tongue [121, 122]. The larynx is the second most common head and neck site. There is a male predominance with male to female ratio of 3:2. The median age at diagnosis is the seventh decade. It is curious that while head and neck verrucous carcinoma represents a homogenous entity, it so rarely is associated with Human Papillomavirus, quite contrary to its genital counterpart [123].

Clinically, verrucous carcinoma presents as white, warty, cauliflower-like tumor. The inherent difficulties in establishing this diagnosis on initial biopsies alone are well-known and clinicopathologic correlation is often necessary. Superficial biopsies can be useless. The mucosa should be retracted and the biopsy forceps directed from the tumor periphery centripetally towards the deep tumor. Thus the diagnostic features of pushing fronds (see below) might be included in the biopsy.

Histopathologically, verrucous carcinoma is characteristically composed of cytologically bland keratinizing tumor cells with glassy cytoplasm, forming hyperkeratotic surface papillae and deep pushing fronds (◘ Figs. 3.48, 3.49, 3.50, 3.51, and 3.52). Invasion into underlying tissue is seen as pushing, finger-like pattern of invasion. The adjacent squamous mucosa usually reveals verrucoid hyperplasia. Usually mitoses are rare and cytologic atypia is absent. Hybrid squamous carcinoma/verrucous carcinoma merits consideration [124, 125]. Truly invasive squamous carcinoma should demonstrate discontinuity from the main tumor mass which may require deeper levels. If the squamous carcinoma component of a hybrid tumor is minimal, (≤2 mm), patient outcome is equally positive as with conventional verrucous carcinoma [125].

The differential diagnosis of verrucous carcinoma includes verrucous vulgaris and proliferative verrucoid hyperplasia. Verrucous vulgaris is a smaller lesion than verrucous carcinoma. The rete pegs of verrucous vulgaris are elongated and thin, pointing toward the lesion's center. Detached islands of infiltrating carcinoma SCC are not seen. Proliferative verrucoid hyperplasia demonstrates acanthosis, papillary hyperplasia, hyperkeratosis, wide, bulbous rete pegs and ***distinctive deep keratin clefts;*** the latter is absent from verrucous carcinoma. The pushing bulbous rete pegs of verrucoid hyperplasia are more superficial than verrucous carcinoma.

Verrucous carcinoma is primarily a surgical disease with great expected outcome and low rates of local recurrence after adequate resection. Primary radiation may be offered to poor surgical candidates, or to those patients wishing to preserve laryngeal function; however local control is poorer with primary radiation as compared to surgery. Cervical neck dissection is not indicated, even with palpable regional lymph nodes as these are invariably reactive.

Before we leave the topic of squamous carcinoma, look at ◘ Figs. 3.53, 3.54, 3.55, 3.56, 3.57, and 3.58 for squamous-related diagnostic pitfalls.

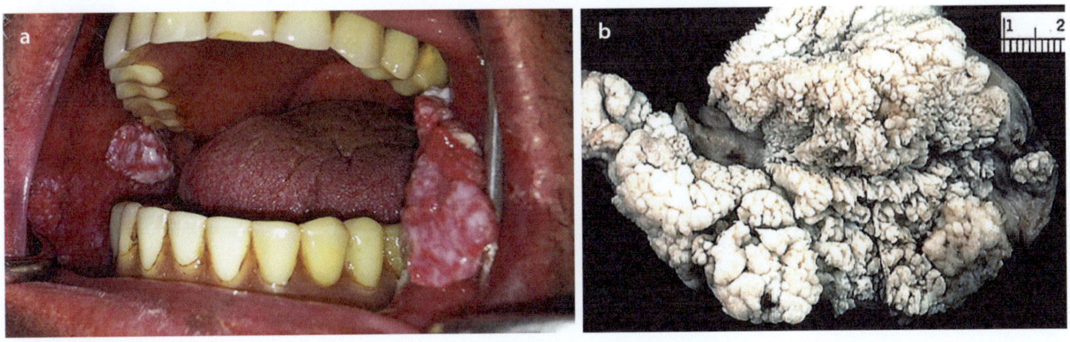

◘ **Fig. 3.48** **a** Bilateral buccal verrucous carcinomas. (Courtesy of Dr. Marilena Vered). **b** Cauliflower-like gross morphology

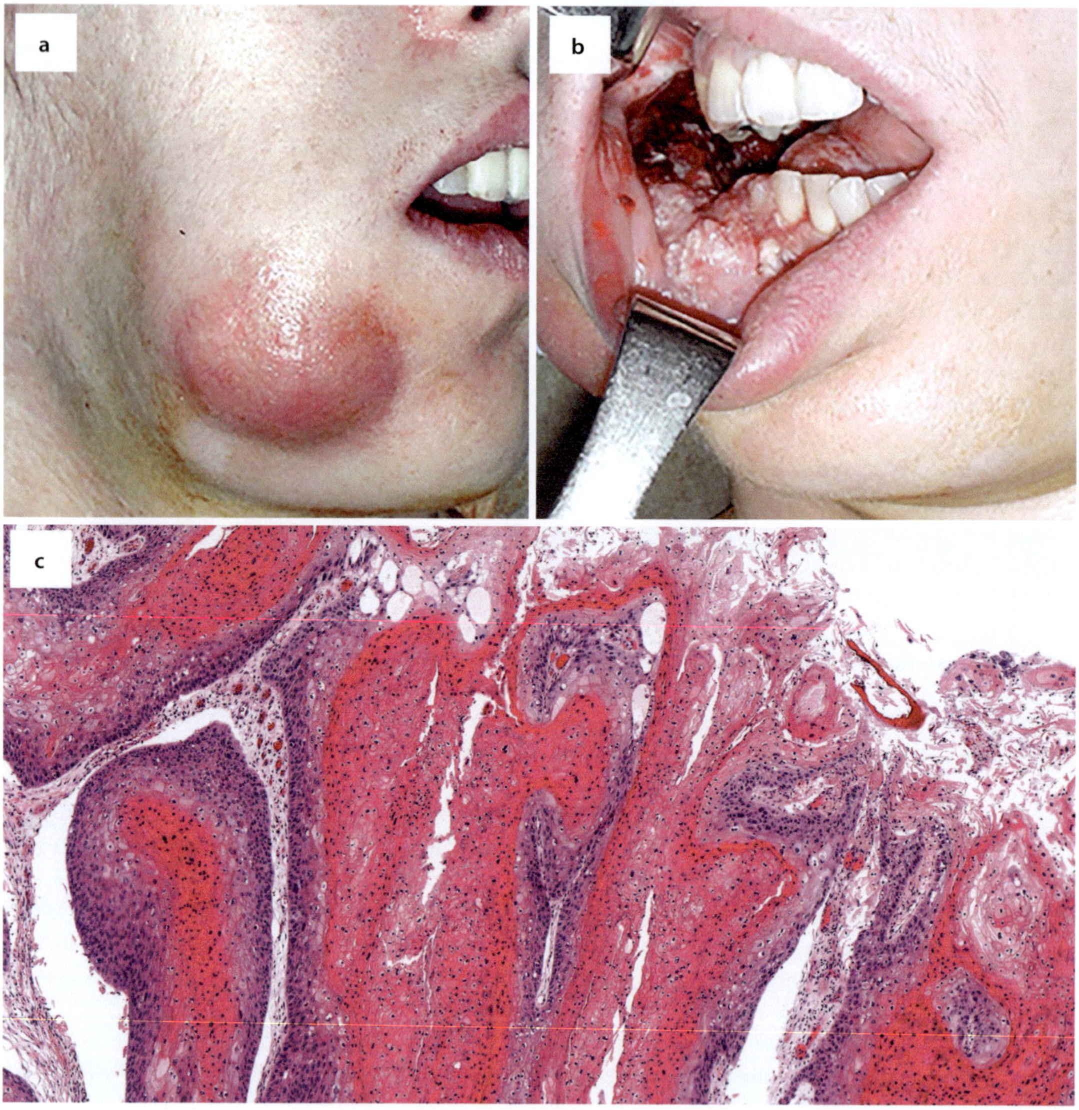

Fig. 3.49 **a**, **b** Another buccal verrucous carcinoma. (Courtesy of Dr. Eric Genden). **c** The superficial aspect of verrucous carcinoma is characterized by papillations with heaps of hyperkeratosis

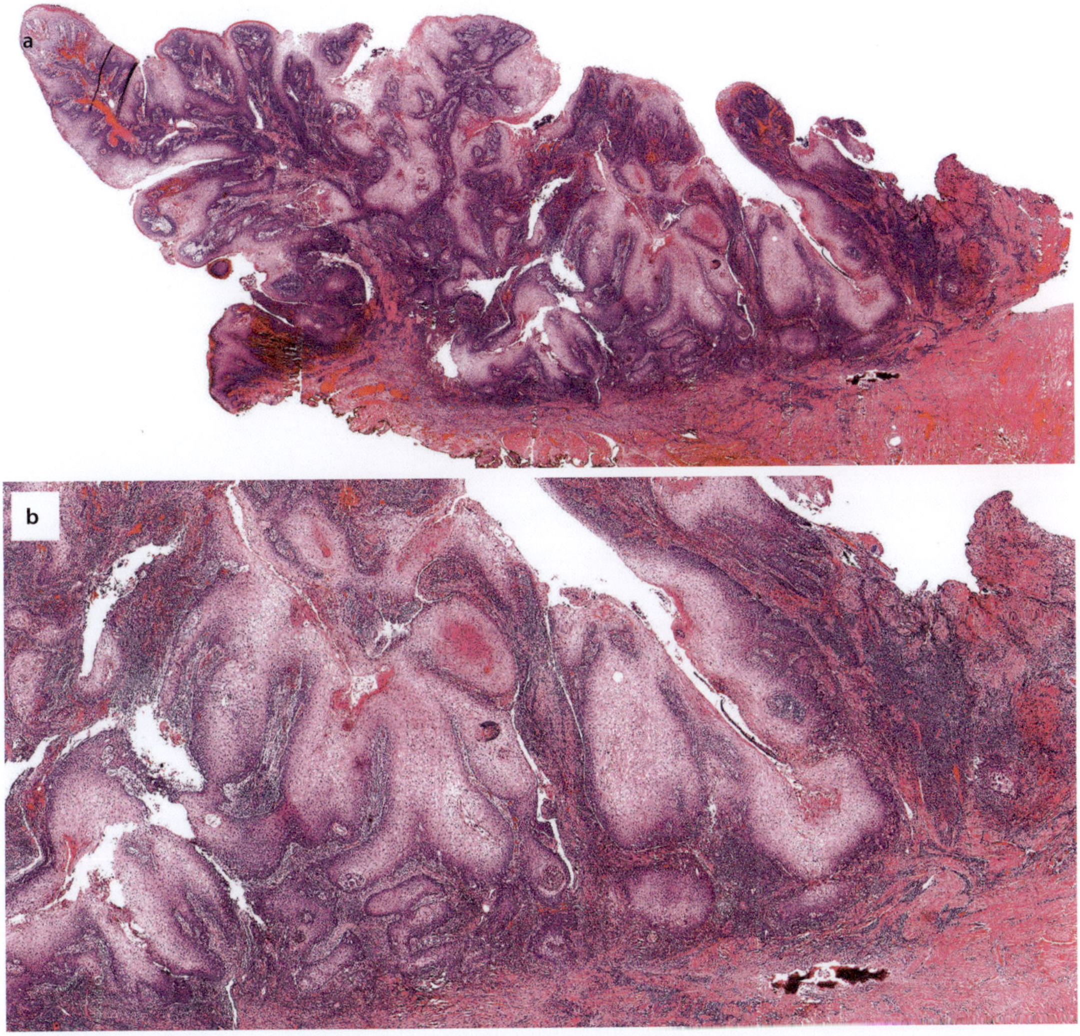

Fig. 3.50 **a**, **b** Verrucous carcinoma. The architectural silhouette, comprised of papillae and pushing rete pegs, is more complex than is seen with verrucoid hyperplasia (Fig. 3.16)

a

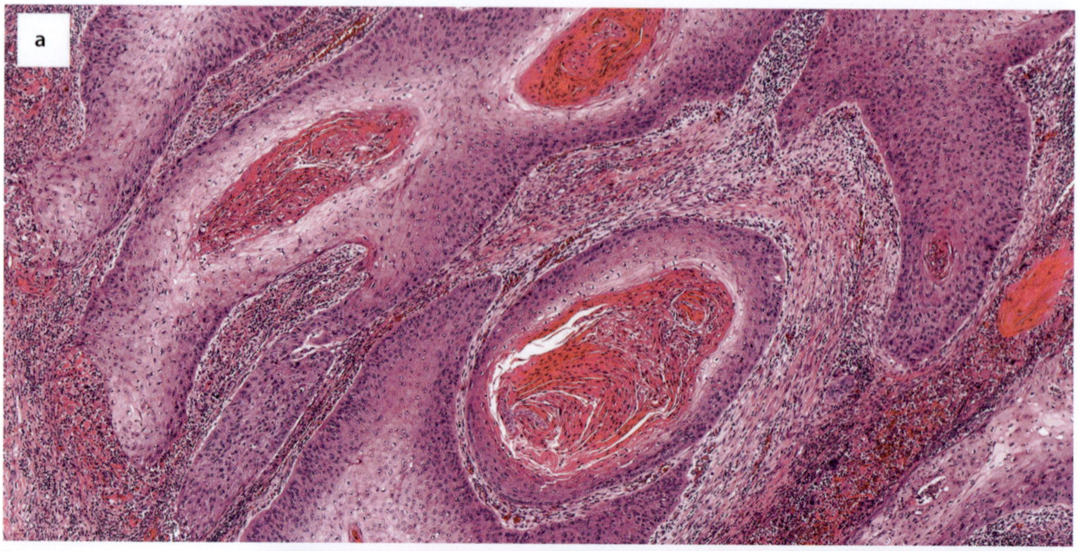

b

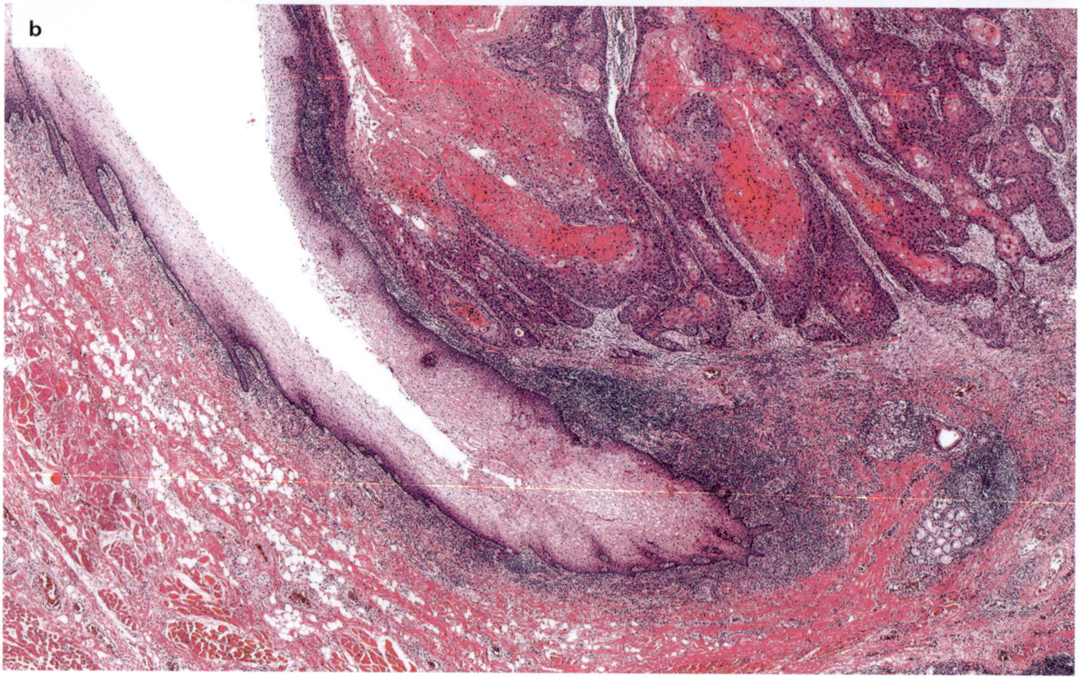

Fig. 3.51 **a** Verrucous carcinoma. **b** The lateral tumor border may reveal a characteristic "dip"

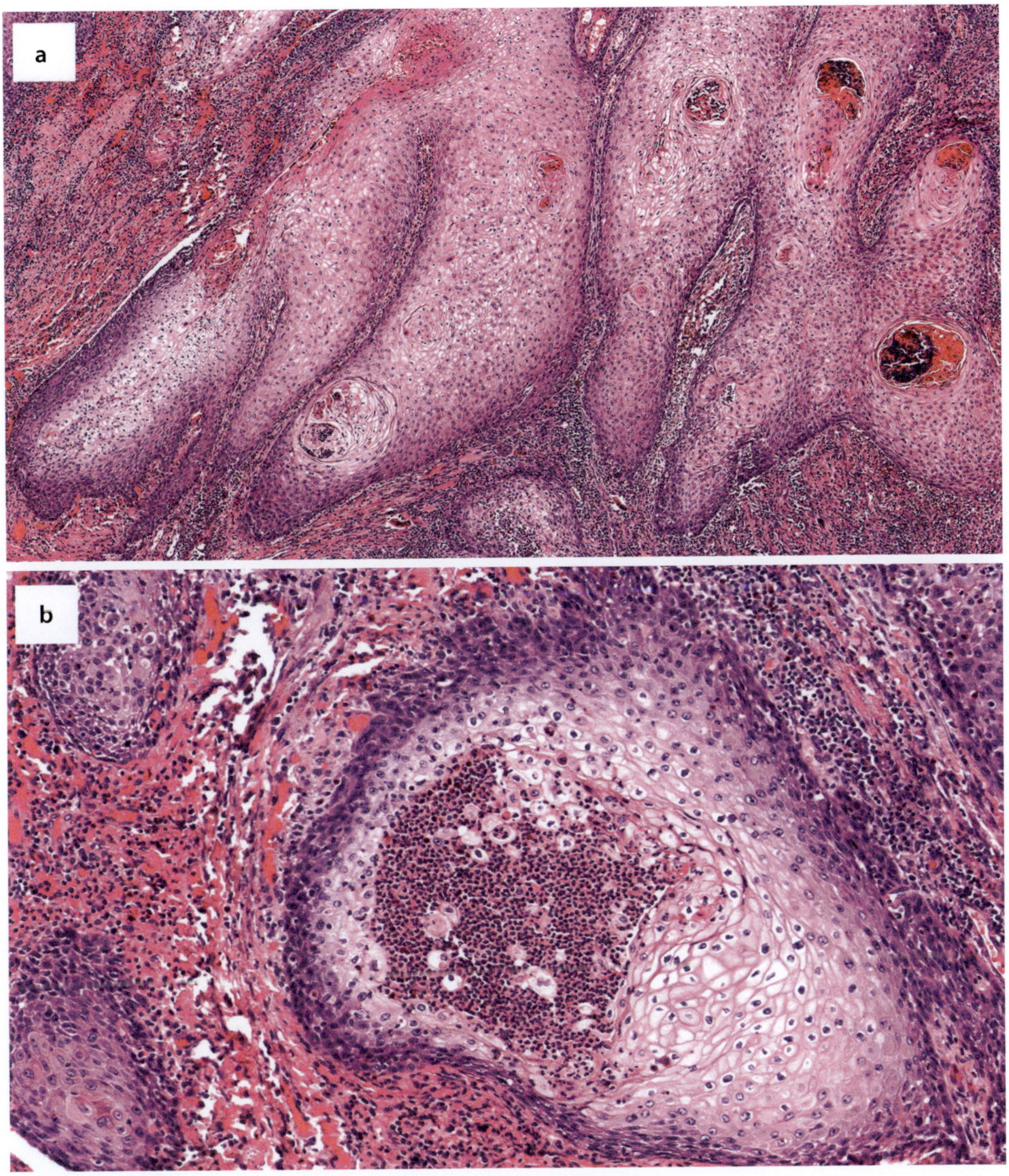

Fig. 3.52 **a**, **b** Verrucous carcinoma. Broad pushing advancing tumor front

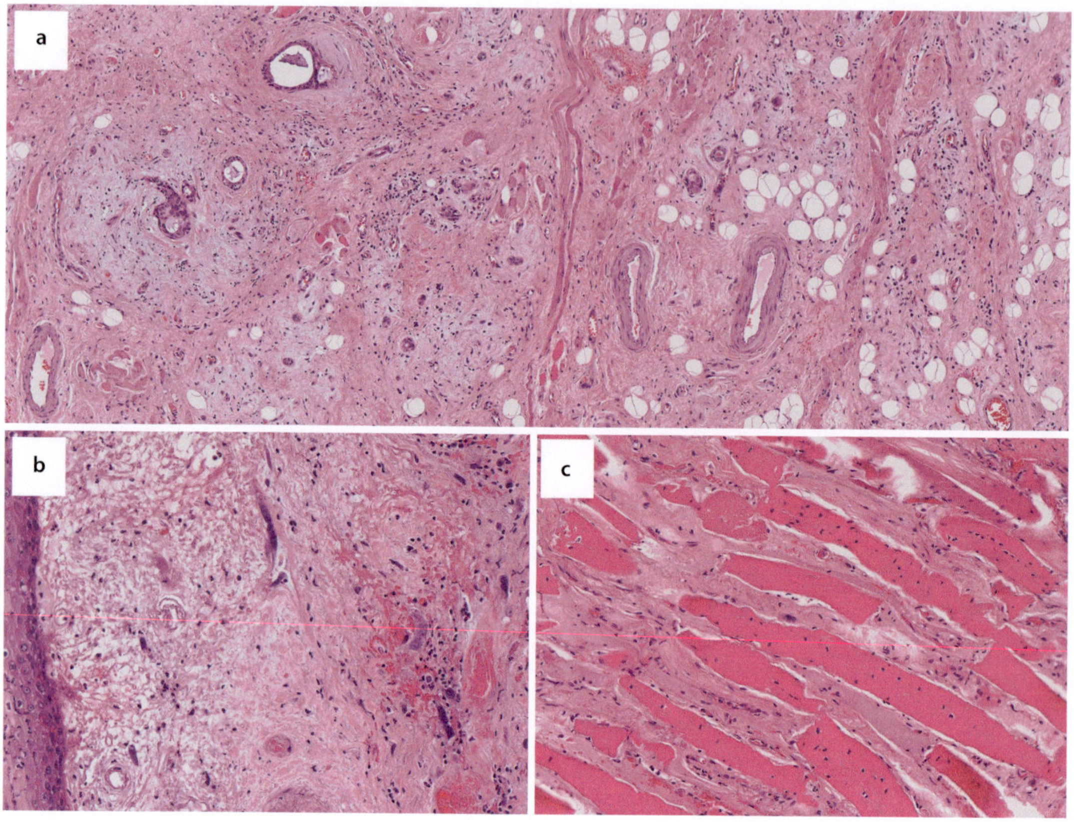

Fig. 3.53 Radiation changes to the upper airway include atrophic minor salivary acini **a**, radiation fibroblasts **b**, and atrophic skeletal muscle **c**

Fig. 3.54 There are many reasons pathologists commence with low-power examination, then move to high-power, not least of which is to avoid being startled by atypical cells taken out of context

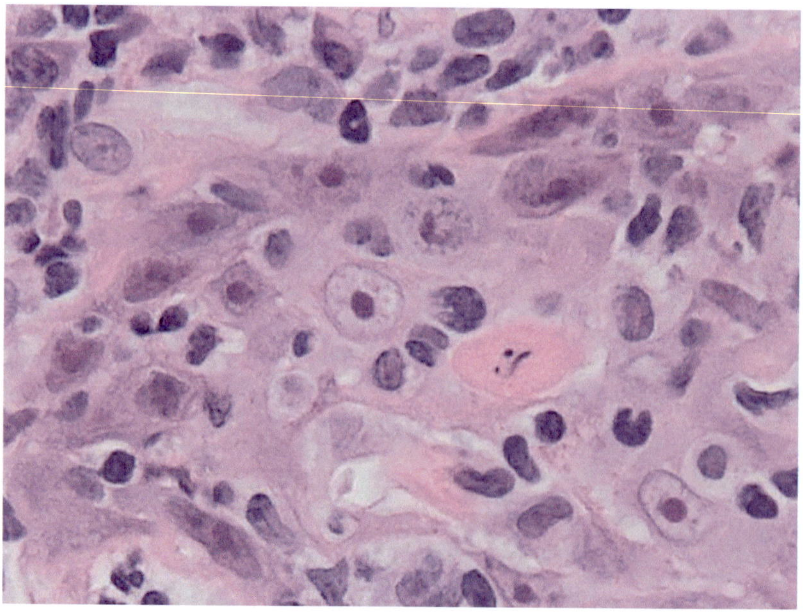

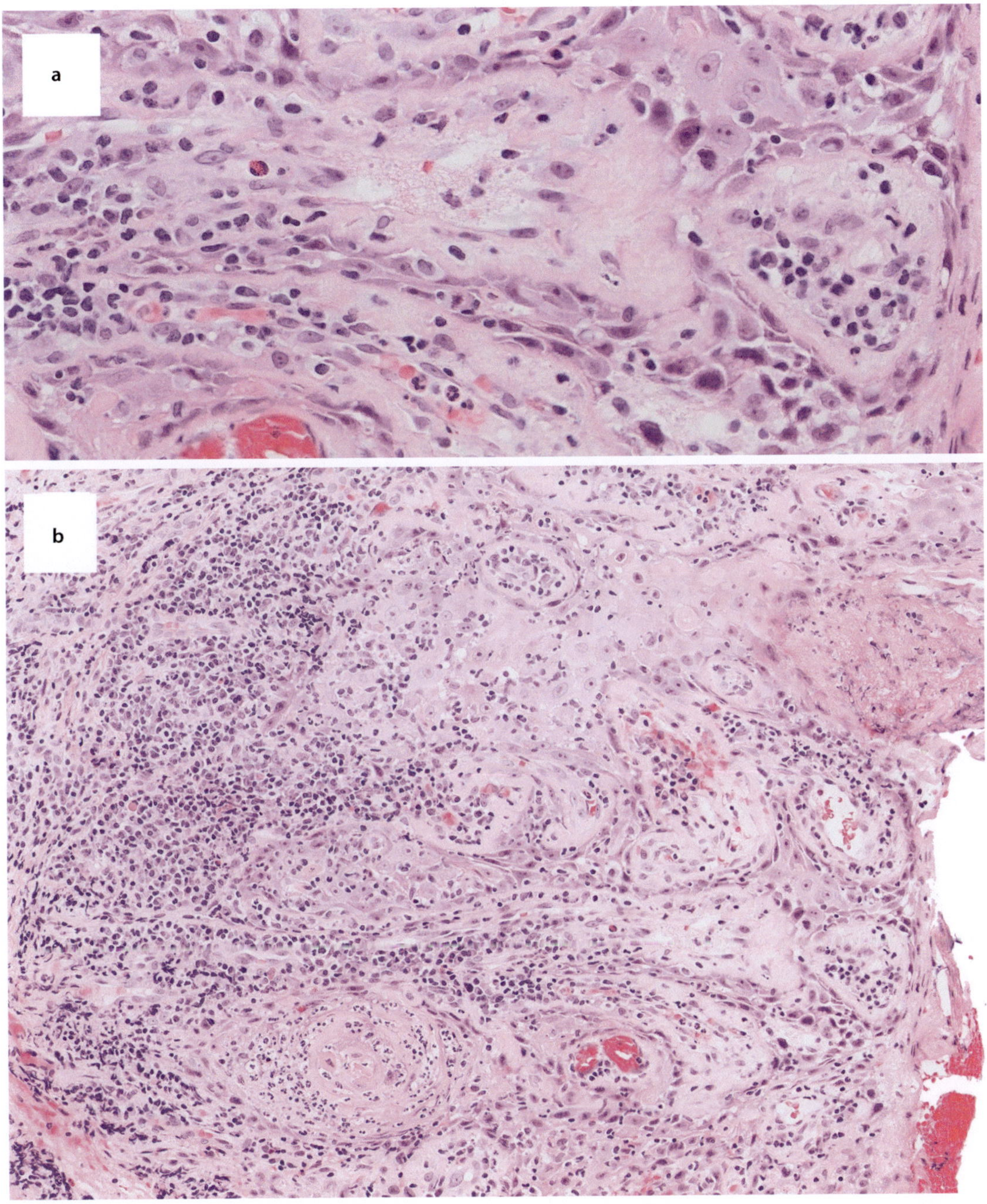

■ **Fig. 3.55** **a**, **b** The context for ■ Fig. 3.54 is that of a reactive regenerative process adjacent to mucosal ulceration

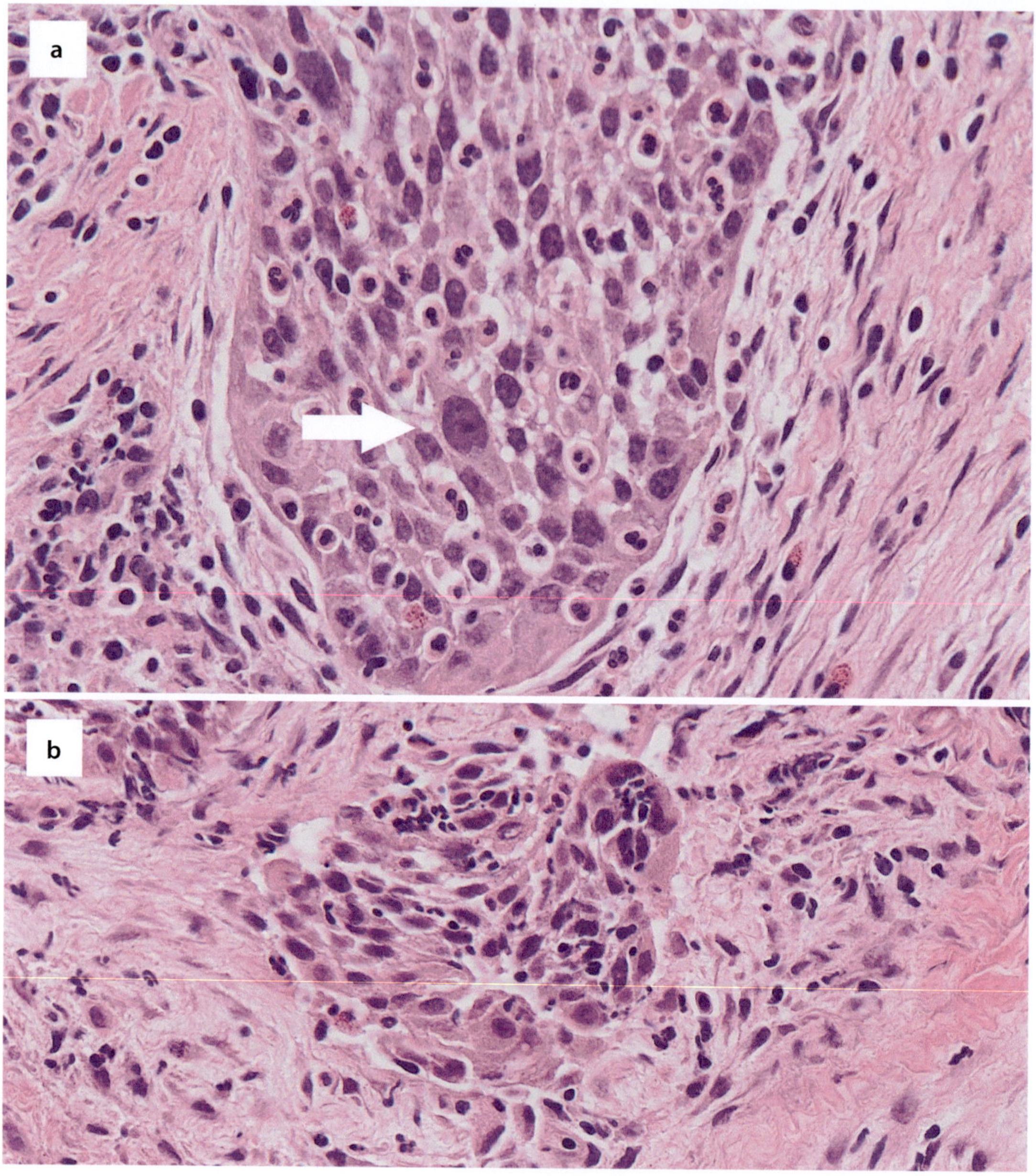

Fig. 3.56 **a**, **b** Another "look before you leap into a malignant diagnosis". Remember that large nucleoli in the context of fine chromatin (*arrow*), basophilic cytoplasm, and acute inflammation, suggest a reactive process

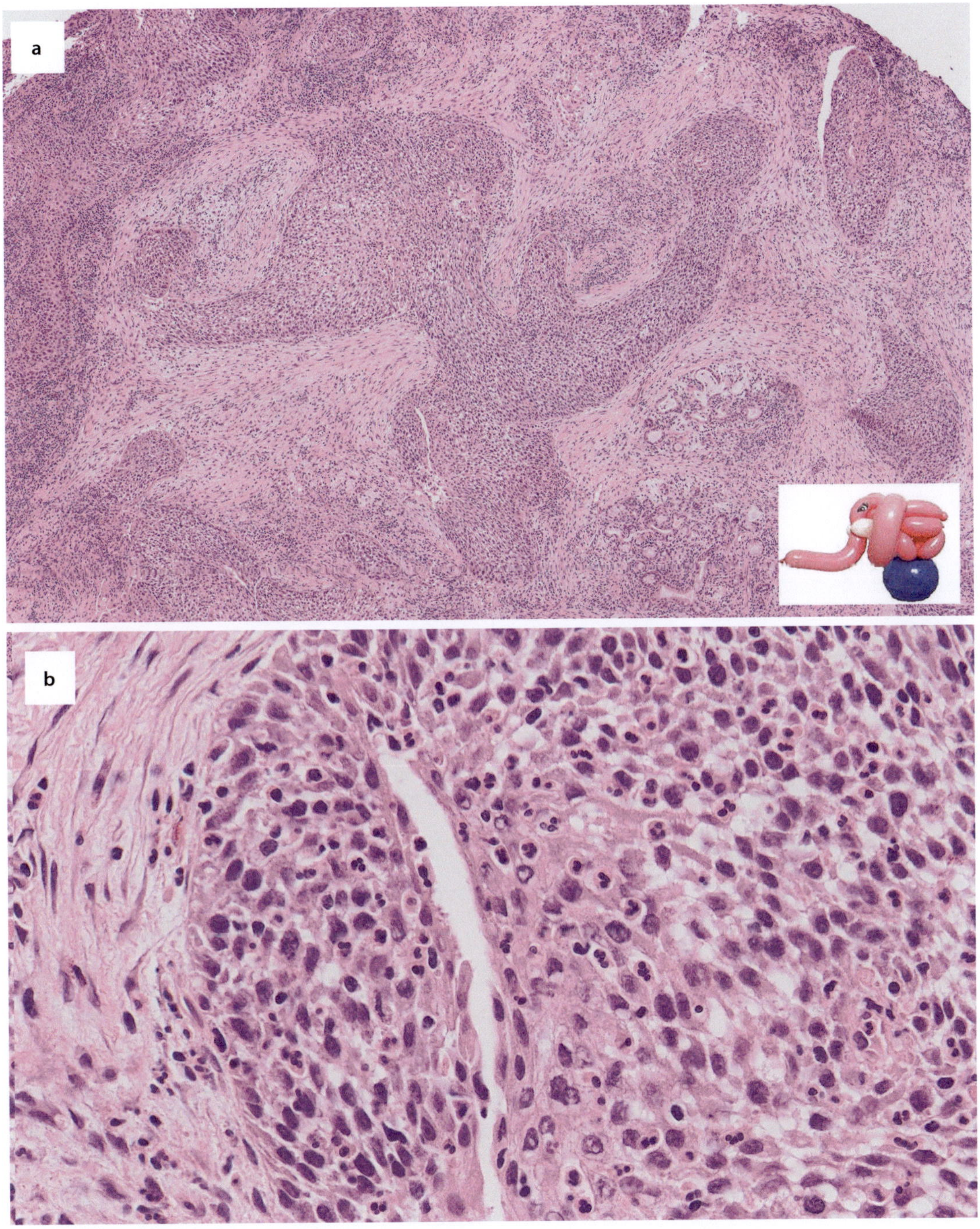

Fig. 3.57 Noticing the kinked tube appearance **a** and retained ductal lumena **b** steer you towards the correct diagnosis of sialometaplasia

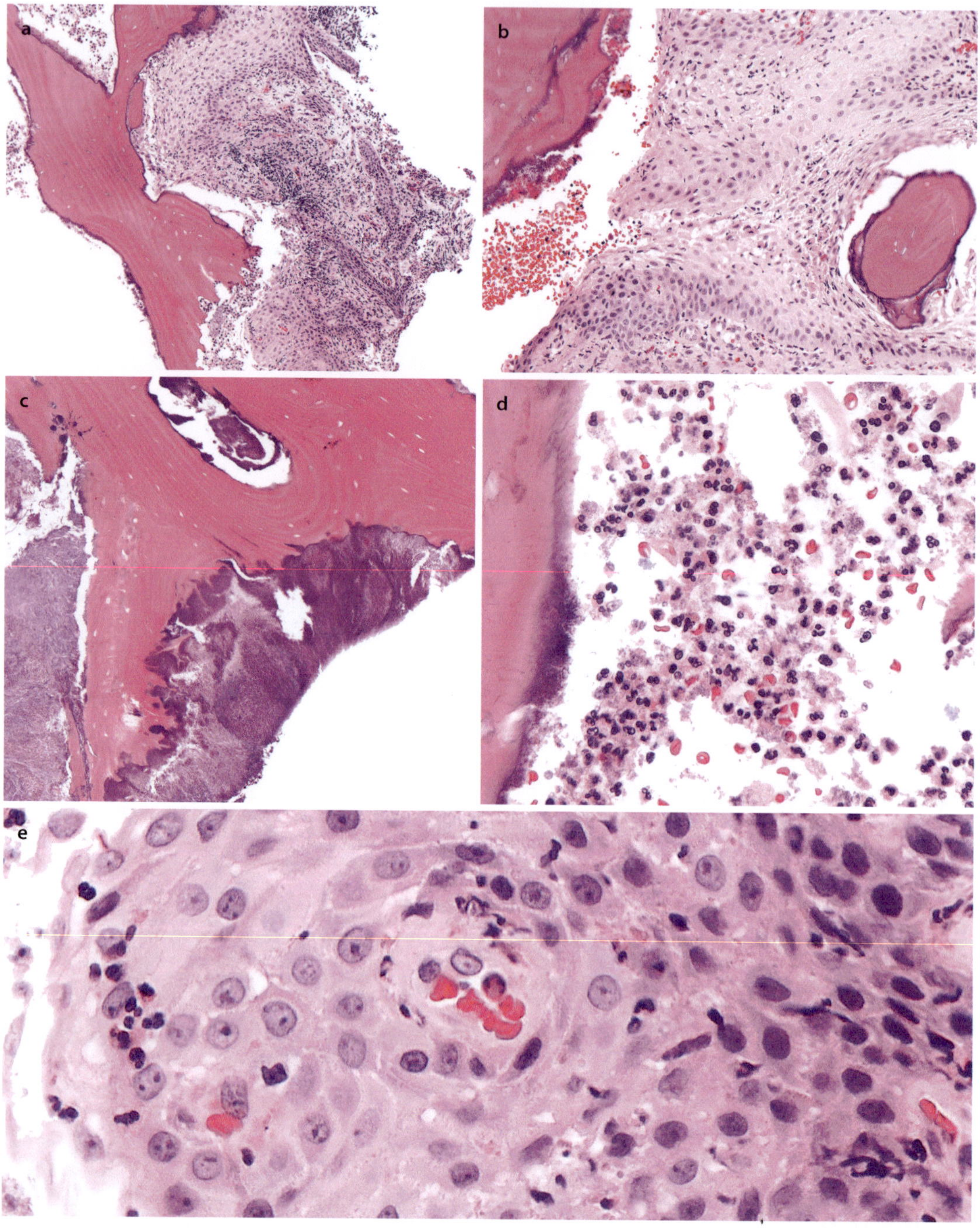

Fig. 3.58 **a–e** Another "look before you leap into a malignant diagnosis". Epithelialization of necrotic mandible leads to fistula formation. It might also lead to a misdiagnosis of squamous carcinoma. Again, go to low power to recognize the context of osteomyelitis and osteonecrosis

3.3 Kaposi's Sarcoma

Kaposi's sarcoma is vascular soft tissue neoplasm which is caused by KSHV (Kasposi's Sarcoma Herpesvirus or Human Herpesvirus 8 (HHV-8)) and classified into four forms: [126, 127]

1. **Classic or endemic Kaposi's sarcoma**, which occurs in elderly Mediterranean or Eastern European men who are not immunosuppressed and are HIV-negative. These patients present with macular/nodular lesions on the trunk and lower legs. Rarely, classic Kaposi's sarcoma can manifest as head and neck mucosal lesions [128].
2. **African Kaposi's sarcoma**, which is seen in HIV seronegative African men and boys. The less aggressive form of African Kaposi's sarcoma is similar in presentation and course to classic Kaposi's sarcoma. The more aggressive form of African Kaposi's sarcoma includes visceral and lymph node involvement in addition to dermal and mucosal lesions, manifests in pediatric HIV-negative patients, and is progressive and fatal.
3. **Iatrogenic Kaposi's sarcoma**, which develops in HIV seronegative immunosuppressed patients, most commonly in recipients of kidney other solid organs.
4. **Epidemic or HIV-associated Kaposi's sarcoma**, which remains the most common HIV-associated neoplasm; the risk for this is highest among male homosexuals compared to other HIV seropositive groups. Kapsosi's sarcoma is presented in this chapter as the oral cavity is the most extracutaneous site for HIV-associated Kaposi's sarcoma.

HIV-associated Kaposi's sarcoma commonly affects head and neck skin and upper airway mucosa. The most common extracutaneous sites are the oral cavity, gastrointestinal tract and lung. Oral Kaposi's sarcoma may be the first clinical manifestation of HIV infection [129]. The most commonly involved oral sites are hard palate and gingiva (◘ Fig. 3.59). Other potentially involved oral sites include tongue, floor of the mouth, and oropharyngeal sites such as tonsils, soft palate, and oropharynx. Early lesions present clinically as flat bluish plaques, older lesions form violaceious nodular, bulky submosal and ulcerating tumors. Oral Kaposi's sarcoma is usually asymptomatic, but can affect eating and speaking. The lesions progress to multifocal visceral involvement.

Histopathologically, the early macule or patch stage of Kaposi's sarcoma appears as a proliferation of thin-walled irregular vascular channels often lined by plump endothelium. These leaky vascular channels surround a pre-existing vessel (promontory sign), inflammation, extravasated erythrocytes, and hemosiderin deposition (◘ Fig. 3.60). The advanced nodular (placque, tumoral) stage demonstrates an infiltrate of long, plump, pleomorphic spindle tumor cells. Mitotic figures are abundant. Intracellular eosinophilic globules ('red bodies') can be seen; these bodies are smaller than erythrocytes and stain with phosphotungstic acid hematoxylin. Hemosiderin deposition and abundant erythrocytes can be seen within the slit-like spaces. The degree of "vascular space" formation correlates with tumor differentiation. **Well-differentiated Kaposi's sarcoma** is characterized by dilated ectatic vascular spaces, angiosarcomatous anastomotic spaces (blood filled mazes), and "glomeruloid" formations – loose "skein-like" clusters of capillaries resembling glomeruli. Poorly-differentiated Kaposi's sarcoma is characterized by a solid proliferation of tumor spindle cells +/− slit-like/cleft-like spaces which may be depleted of erythrocytes thus focally mimicking other soft tissue sarcomas. Immunohistochemstry reveals expression of HHV8, vimentin, CD31, and CD34.

Angiosarcoma should be considered in the differential diagnosis. Angiosarcoma forms incomplete, anastamosing channels, with protrusion of the malignant nuclei into lumina, whereas Kaposi's sarcoma forms "slit-like" spaces although angiosarcoma-like spaces may also be seen. Angiosarcoma will be negative for HHV-8.

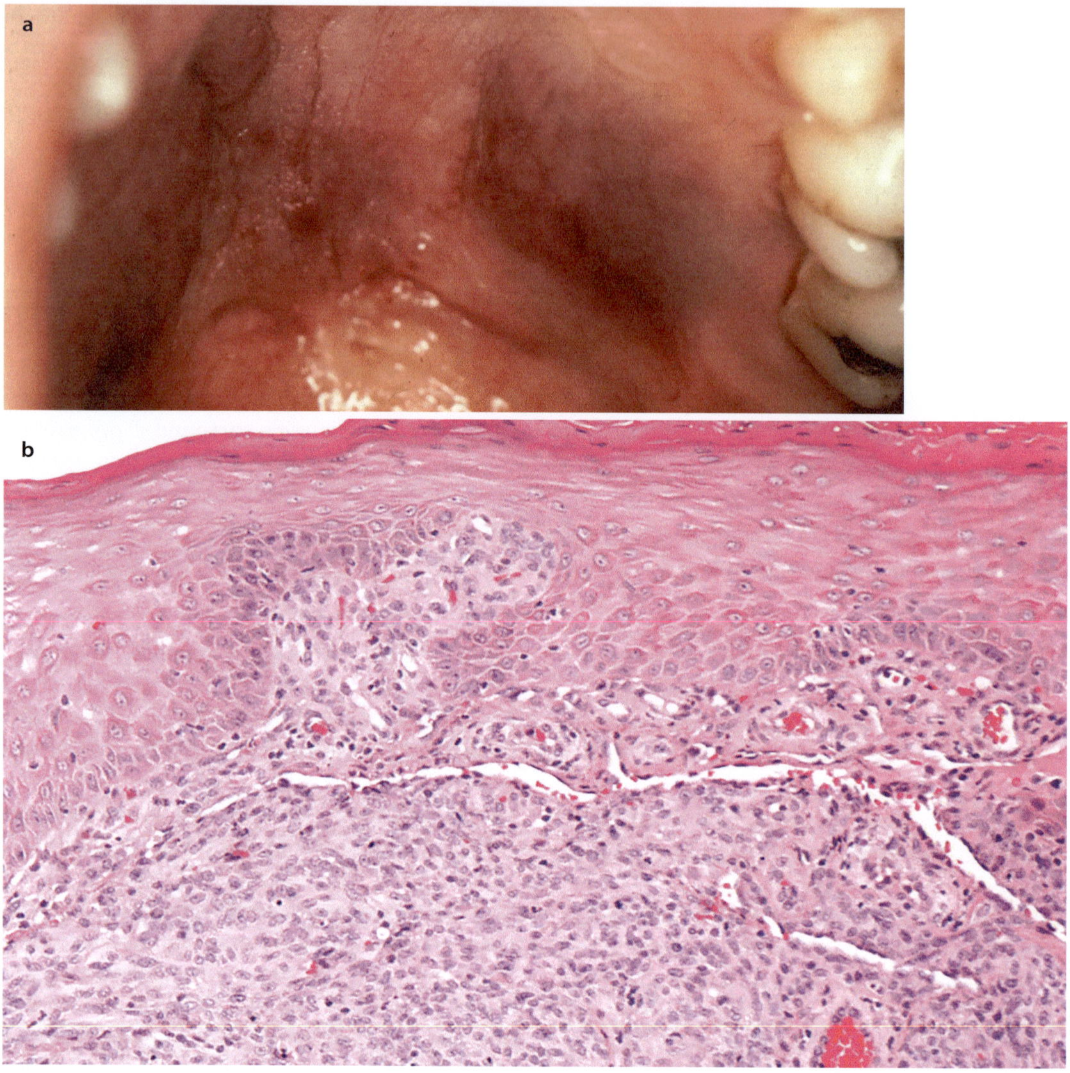

Fig. 3.59 **a** Kaposi's sarcoma: violaceous swelling of the left hard palate. **b** Submucosal spindle cell infiltrate with abundant vessels

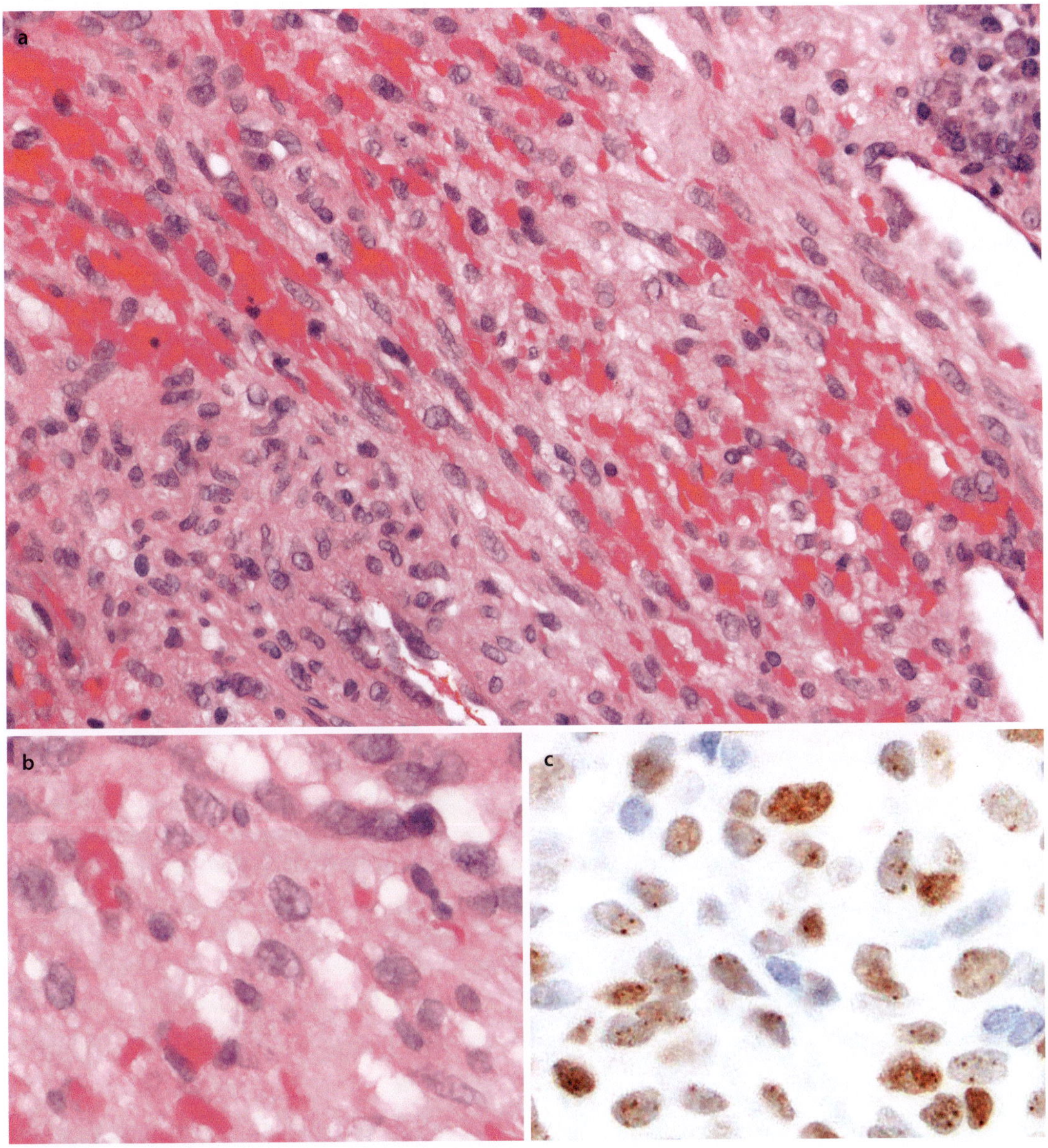

Fig. 3.60 **a** Kaposi's sarcoma: typical appearance of closely packed spindled tumor cells and extravasated erythrocytes. **b** Cytoplasmic vacuoles, some with erythrocytes. **c** IHC for HHV8

3.4 Oral Melanoma

Less than 1% of all melanomas develop within mucosal sites and 55% of mucosal melanomas involve the head and neck [130]. Approximately 67% of head and neck mucosal melanomas occur within the sinonasal tract; approximately 25% occur in the oral cavity [131–134]. Unusual case clustering suggests genetic predispositions among Japanese and Ugandans [132, 135]. Oral melanoma has been recently reported in a young woman with Li-Fraumeni syndrome (germline TP53 mutation) [136]. Primary oral melanomas occur over a very wide age range. In general, they develop more commonly in mucosal sites directly adjacent to bone (i.e. hard palate, gingiva, alveolar ridge) than soft tissues (i.e. tongue, lip, buccal mucosa). Palatal/maxillary tumors are more common than mandibular tumors. These tumors present as darkly pigmented, nodular, ulcerated masses. Melanin can rub off on a gauge pad and stain it black, which is a means of clinically confirming the suspicion of oral melanoma [133].

Histopathologically, mucosal lentiginous melanoma is the most commonly encountered primary oral melanoma [134]. Nests and single melanoma cells can be seen at the mucosal rete pegs extending laterally beyond the regions on confluent tumor growth. Confluent invasive oral melanoma is commonly composed of polytypic malignant cells such as spindled and epithelioid and oval cells [134]. Other melanoma cell types include plasmacytoid, pleomorphic, and clear cell. Growth patterns include nested/organoid, trabecular (◘ Fig. 3.61), fascicles, and pseudoalveolar. Beyond stage, histological predictors of poor outcome are high-mitotic rate ($\geq$25 mitoses/mm^2) and tumor ulceration [137]. Immunohistochemistry will reveal variable expression of S-100, Mart-1/melan-A, MITF, tyrosinase, Sox10 and HMB-45. A panel approach is necessary as not every single melanoma expresses S-100.

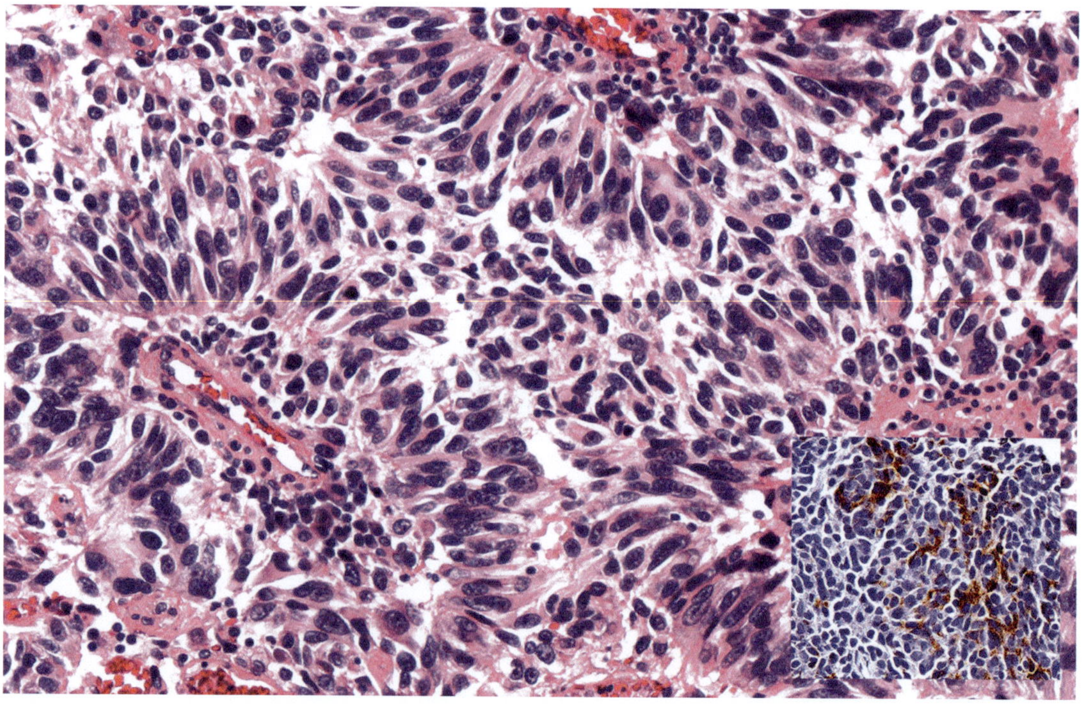

◘ **Fig. 3.61** Primary oral melanoma: "Cancers are bandits. They can do anything!" Sadao Otani (1892–1969) [139]. This primary melanoma, producing festoons, wants you to think it's a neuroendocrine carcinoma. Inset: IHC for HMB 45

▪ Staging

Approximately 60% of patients with oral melanoma present with positive lymph nodes [138]. To reflect the generally aggressive nature of mucosal melanomas, all tumors are broadly classified as **Stage III/IV.** Primary melanomas limited to the mucosa and soft tissues are **pT3**, regardless of tumor thickness or size. Advanced mucosal melanomas are classified as either T4a or T4b. Advanced **T4a** can involve deep soft tissue, cartilage, bone, or overlying skin. Very advanced **T4b** can involve brain, dura, skull base, lower cranial nerves (IX, X, XI, XII), masticator space, carotid artery, prevertebral space, or mediastinal structures. Regional lymph nodes are classified as either pNX: regional lymph nodes cannot be assessed, pN0: no lymph node metastases, or pN1: any regional lymph node metastases. **Stage III** is reserved for **pT3pN0** patients. Any other combination of TNM is grouped as Stage IV. **Stage IVA** is either **T4aN0M0** or **T3-T4a/N1 M0. Stage IVb** is **T4b/any N/M0. Stage IVC** is reserved for **M1**. The rate of distant metastases at presentation range from 10% to 50%, usually involving lungs, live, bones, and brain [138].

Primary wide resection with neck dissection, if feasible, is the therapeutic mainstay, with 1.0 to 1.5 cm of soft tissue and 2.0 cm of bone [138]. Adjuvant radiotherapy is also a standard approach and some studies have demonstrated significant improvement in local disease-free survival for patients receiving postoperative radiatherapy [140, 141]. Cisplatin, vinblastine, dacarbazine, and other chemotherapy agents have been used in either the primary or adjuvant setting. Ahn and colleagues demonstrated significantly improved survival with adjuvant chemotherapy on multivariate analysis [142]. Immunomodulatory therapies with immune checkpoint inhibitors show promising results for patients with metastatic melanoma, especially for combinations of drugs: ipilimumab is an FDA approved anti-cytotoxic T lymphocyte associated antigen-4 inhibitor; pembrolizumab is another FDA approved anti-cytotoxic T-cell inhibitor which inhibits PD-1 [143]. Phase III trials are underway investigating their efficacy in metastatic mucosal melanoma. Lastly, carbon-ion-based radiotherapy offers higher linear energy transfer and smaller linear scattering as compared to photon-based radiotherapy; preliminary outcomes have been reported using primary single modality therapy for mucosal melanomas [144].

3.5 Oral Myeloma

Multiple myeloma is a systemic disease caused by clonal proliferation of malignant plasma cells within the bone marrow. There is a male predisposition; patient age at presentation ranges from fifth to eighth decade of life. **Solitary plasmacytoma of bone** is very uncommon and can be a precursor to multiple myeloma. **Extramedullary plasmacytoma** represents a clonal plasma cell proliferation within the soft tissues. It is very common in patients with multiple myeloma, and mechanistically represents "stromal independent" plasmacytic proliferation [145]. Extramedullary plasmacytomas are also common in the setting of disease relapse for multiple myeloma patients [145]. ***Primary* extramedullary plasmacytomas** represents a rare presentation which is limited to the soft tissue, without contiguous bony involvement. **Eighty percent of *primary* extramedullary plasmacytomas occur in the head and neck soft tissues, most commonly nasopharynx and sinonasal tract.**

Systemic manifestations of multiple myeloma include increased blood viscosity secondary to immune globulin production, impaired renal function, amyloid deposition, coagulopathy, multiple lytic bony lesions, back pain due to vertebral lesions, anemia, and fatigue. Light chains of immunoglobulins are detected as proteinuria. The skull is involved by lytic lesions in 46.7% of myeloma patients, the mandible is involved in 15.6% of the same [146]. Boney radiolucent lesions are described as" moth-eaten", "punched out" without sclerotic rimming (◘ Fig. 3.62) [147–151].

Histopathologically, plasmacytic proliferations can range from well- to poorly-differentiated. The better differentiated the neoplasm, the more recognizable it is as plasmacytic. Normal plasma cells may be admixed with atypical binucleate cells, and more overtly pleomorphic plasma cells with atypical mitotic figures (◘ Fig. 3.63). The "clock-

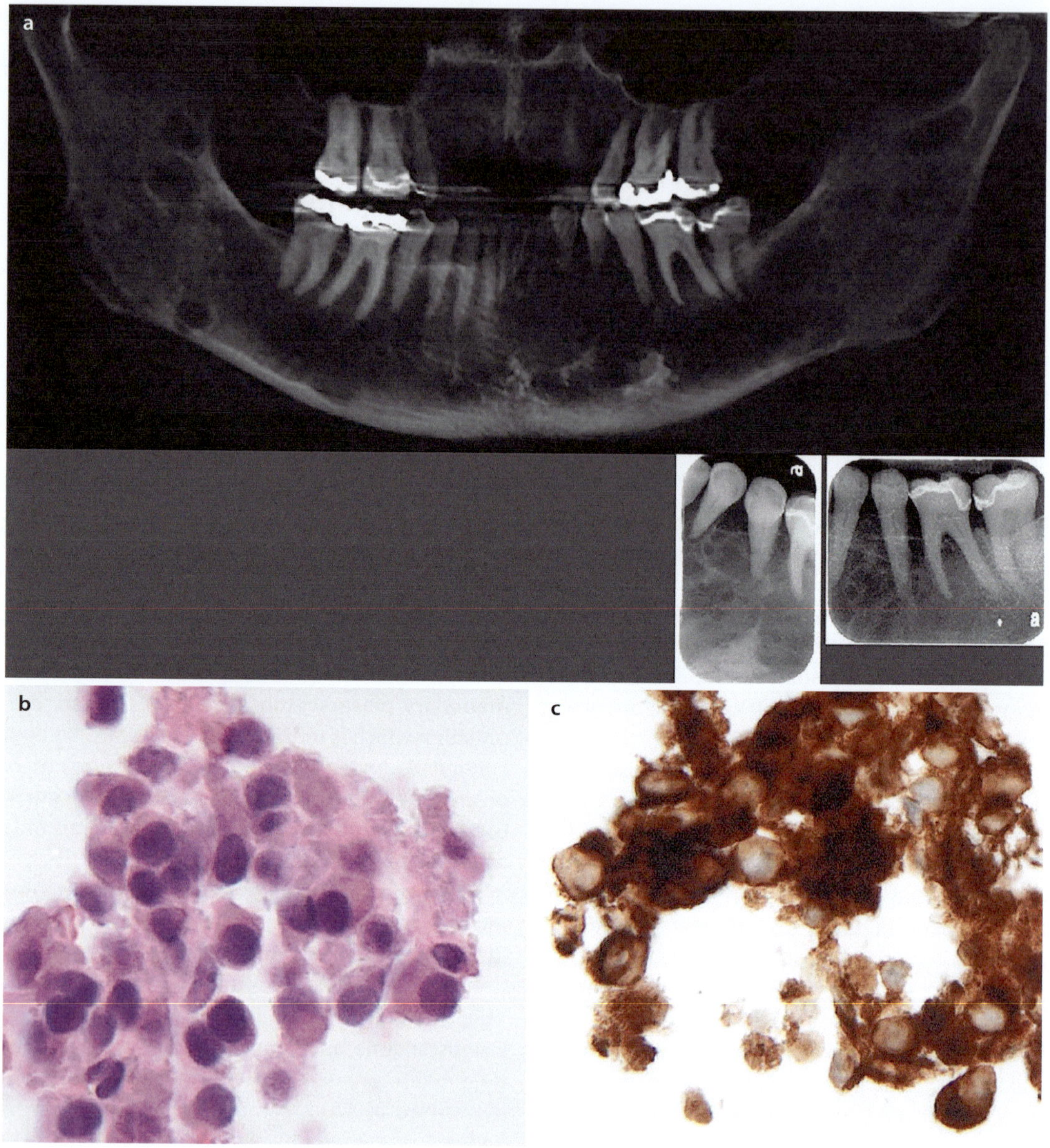

■ **Fig. 3.62** **a** Jaw myeloma: typical diffuse, multifocal, osteolytic lesions radiographically diagnostic for myeloma. **b** These plasma cells are atypical in that you can see variation in nuclear size and shape. **c** IHC for CD138

face" chromatin pattern may still be preserved. Alternatively, a pleomorphic, poorly-differentiated plasmacytic tumor may offer up hints as to its plasmacytic origins by the eosinophilic perinuclear "hof" (■ Fig. 3.64). Immunohistochemistry for CD 138/CD38/CD79a and kappa and lambda light chains can be used to establish the diagnosis. Expression of CD19 and CD20 are often lost.

Although myeloma cannot be considered a curable disease, advances in genetic risk stratification and therapeutics, have revolutionized treatment approaches and significantly improved patient survival [152, 153]. Thalidomides, next-generation immunomodulators such as lenalidomide, and proteaosome inhibitors such as bortezomib, impact multiple pathways associated with plasma cell proliferation, survival, migration, and drug resistance; they also inhibit processes of tumor-supporting stromal cells such as bone marrow angiogenesis, which are directly involved in

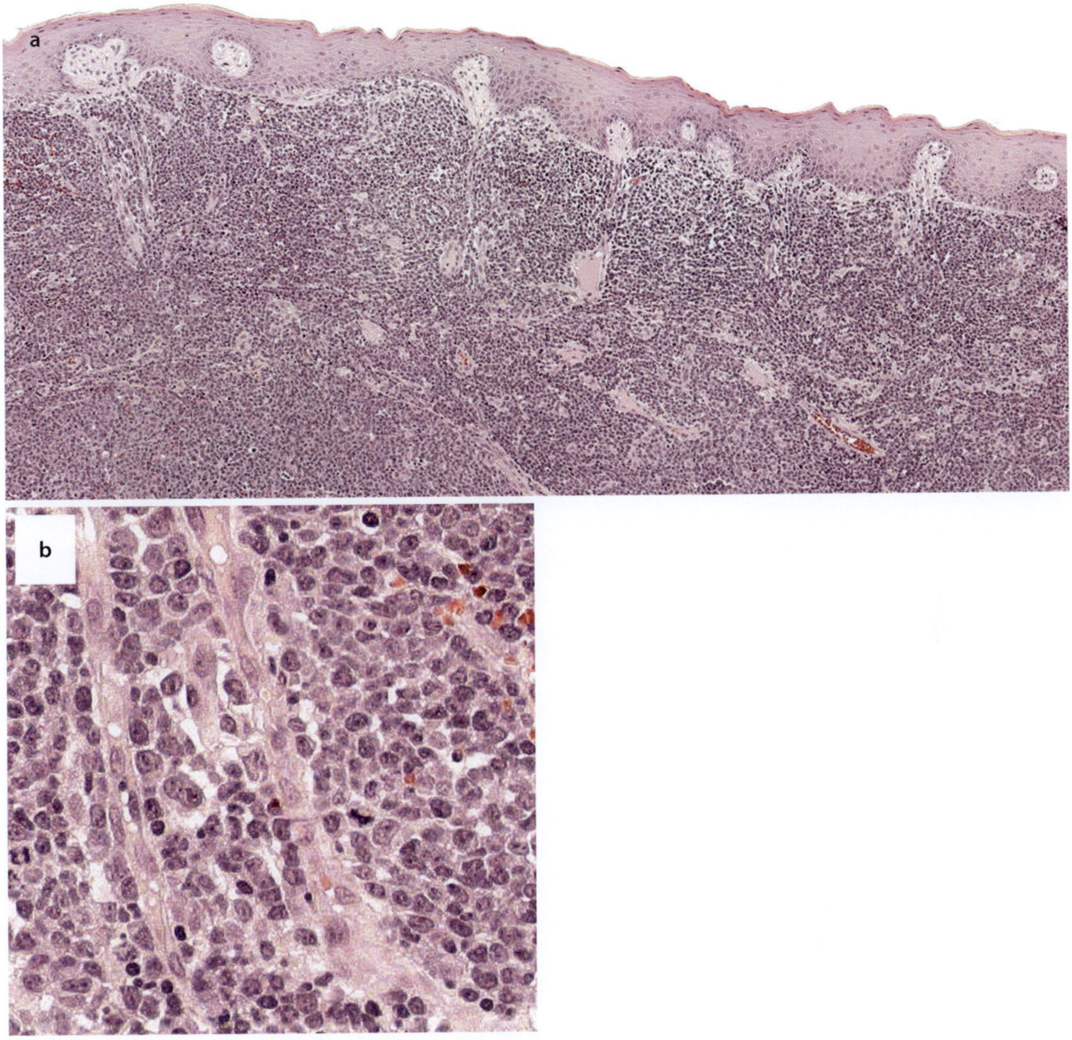

■ **Fig. 3.63** **a** Palatal plasmacytoma. **b** Higher power: Atypical plasma cells, atypical mitotic figure (*arrow*)

lytic bone lesions. Myeloma treatment varies by Durie Salmon stage (■ Table 3.5) and risk stratification. Genetic profiling and epigenetic analyses can identify high-risk groups and become the rationale for tailoring therapies. Patients with asymptomatic Stage I disease may not be treated; bone loss can be managed with bisphosphonates (BONJ). An associated side effect is bisphosphonates osteoradionecrosis of the jaws (■ Fig. 3.65) [154, 155]. This may present with oral mucosal fenestration and exposed necrotic bone. Patients may have pain, loose teeth, pathological mandibular fracture, sinus tract/fistula formation, soft tissue abscess, in the absence of exposed bone.

Stage II disease, or light chain amyloidosis can be treated with combination thalidomides and steroids, or vincristine, doxorubicin, and steroids. Autologous stem cell transplant after high-dose chemotherapy can significantly prolong disease-free survival, although it is not curative. Radiation may be used to treat vertebral lesions causing impending spinal cord compression. At initial presentation, 14% of patients can be stratified as “ultra-high-risk” based on 17p deletion and chromosome 1 abnormalities. They are expected to have a median survival of <2 years, and are offered novel treatment strategies [153].

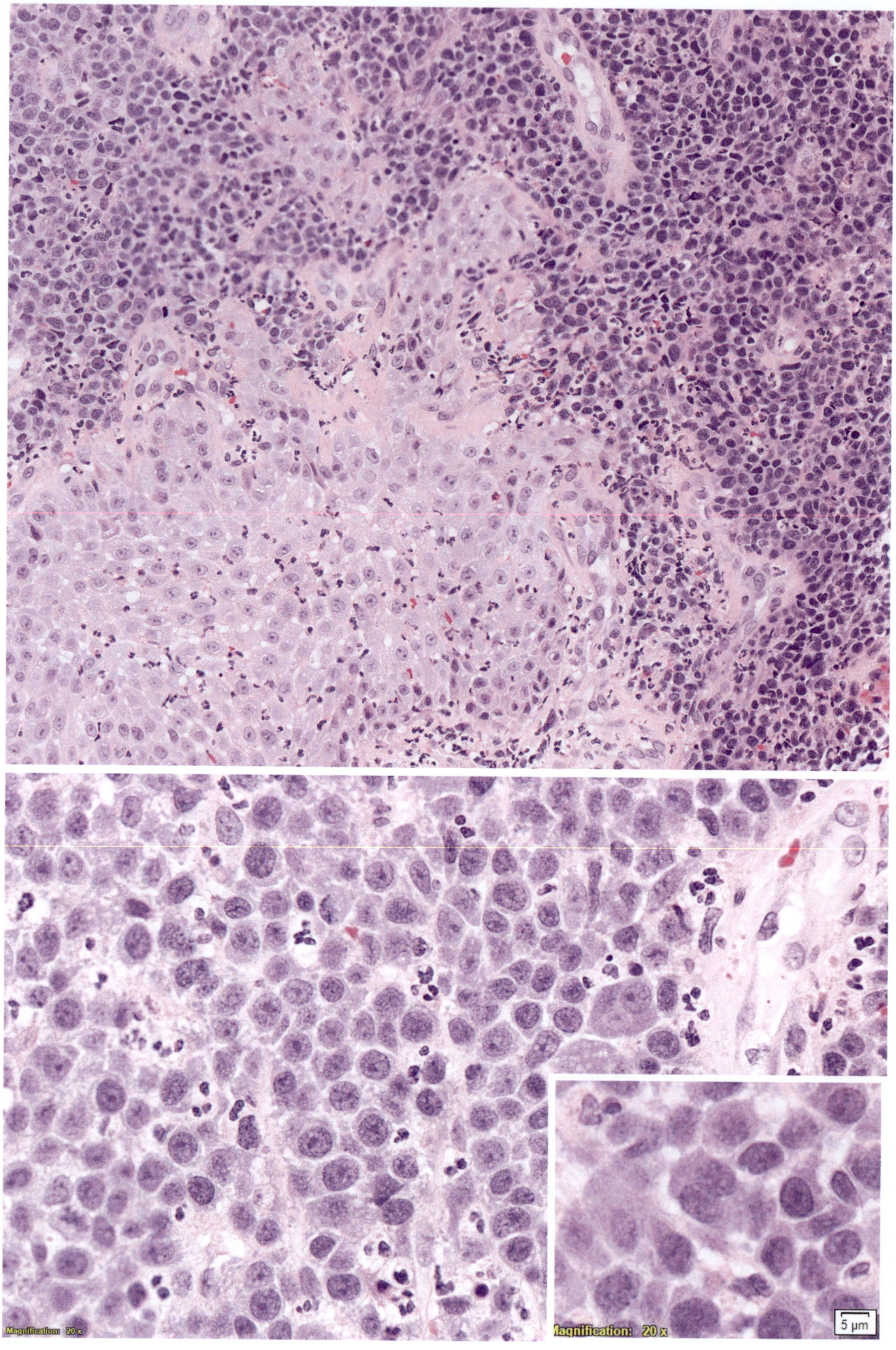
Magnification: 20 x
Magnification: 20 x
5 µm

Table 3.5 Durie Salmon Staging System

	Monoclonal immuno-globulins blood/urine	Serum Ca	Bone damage	Serum Hg
Stage 1	Relatively small amount	Normal (<12 mg/dl)	Normal or 1 area of damage	Slightly < normal, but >10 g/dl
Stage 2	More than Stage 1		2 areas of damage	Between 8.5 and 10 g/dl
Stage 3	Large amount monoclonal immunoglobulins in blood or urine	>12 mg/dl	≥3 areas of bone destruction	<8.5 g/dl

Fig. 3.64 **Top** Gingival biopsy from a woman previously in remission for myeloma. **Bottom** Plasma cells are "sticky" mimicking a carcinoma-like pattern. Looks at the perinuclear hofs, which are expected in plasmacytic tumors. Inset: This binucleated malignant plasma cell is another valuable diagnostic hint

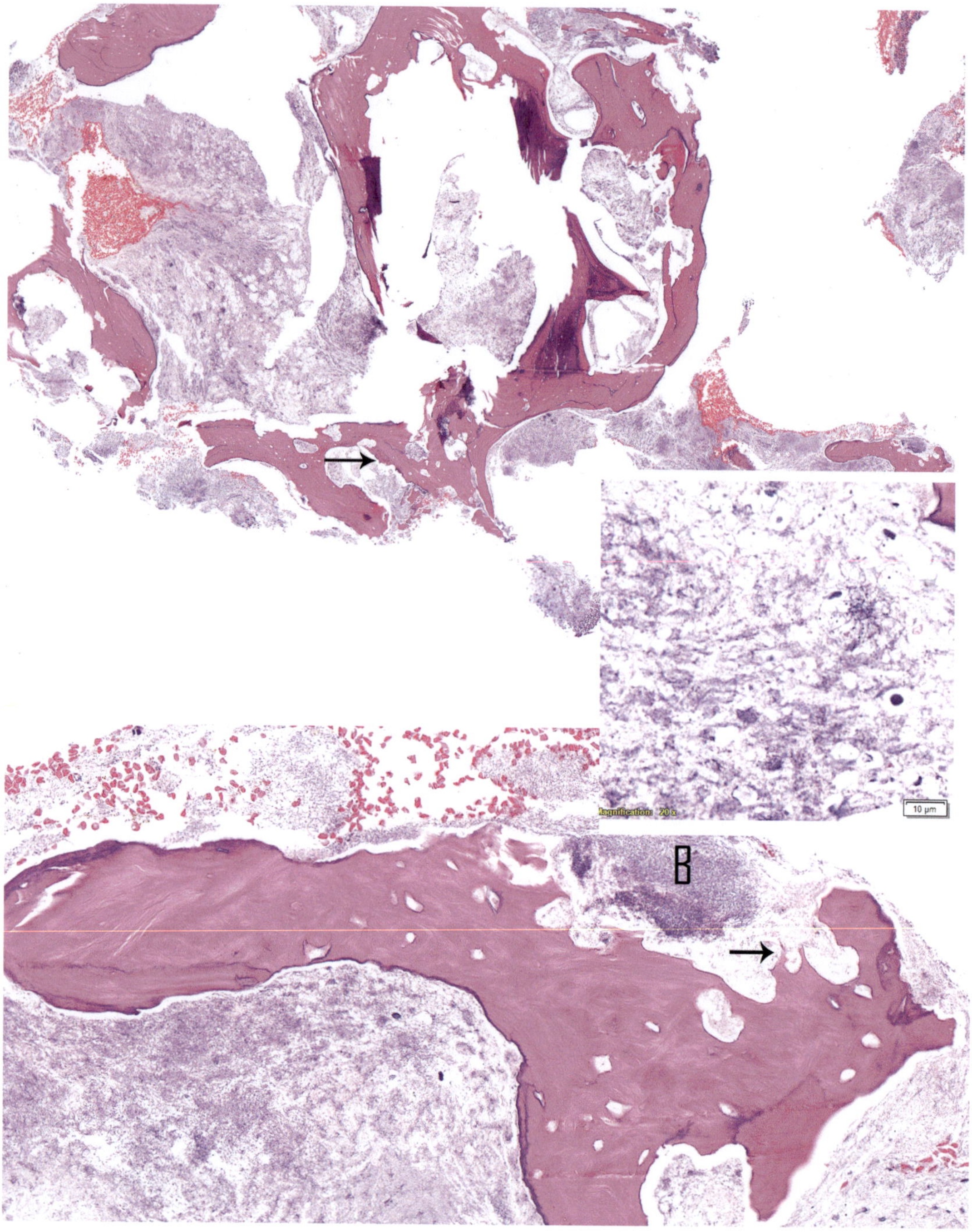

Fig. 3.65 Bisphosphonates osteoradionecrosis: **Top** The typical appearance is that of dead bone and florid bacterial proliferation with little or no acute inflammation. **Bottom** In addition to empty lacunae, look for irregular jagged bony contours (*arrows*) imparting a "moth-eaten" appearance. The amphophilic regions (**B and inset**) represent mixed bacterial colonies

3.6 Oral Basal Cell Carcinoma

The **Nevoid Basal Cell Carcinoma syndrome (Gorlin-Goltz Syndrome)** represents a rare genetic disorder with an autosomal dominant pattern of inheritance, high penetrance, and variable expressivity. These patients are predisposed to developing basal cell carcinomas, a variety of benign tumors, and congenital skeletal malformations. The clinical diagnosis is established by either two major criteria, or one major and two minor criteria (◘ Table 3.6). The underlying genetic disorder is caused by heterozygous germline mutation of the **patched1 (*PTCH1*)** tumor suppressor gene on chromosome 9. One third to half of syndromic patients have spontaneous *de-novo* germline mutations, while the remainder patients demonstrate familial inheretance [156]. PTCH1 is a membrane receptor/repressor for smoothened (SMO). Binding of a hedgehog ligand, most commonly sonic hedgehog (SHH) to PTCH1 activates SMO which leads to downstream effects on proliferation, migration, differentiation, and developmental patterning. *PTCH1* mutation leads to constitutive activation of the hedgehog pathway; *PTCH2* or *SUFU* (SUppressor of FUsed homolog) mutations are alternative germline mutations [157]. *PTCH-1* mutation alone is insufficient to promote carcinogenesis, and a second hit, such as solar radiation, is necessary to promote basal cell carcinoma.

The most common features of the Nevoid Basal Cell Carcinoma syndrome are maxillary odontogenic keratocysts/keratocytic odontogenic tumors (◘ Fig. 3.66) and multiple basal cell carcinomas [158, 159]. The most common site for all keratocystic odontogenic tumors is the posterior body and ramus of the mandible; keratocytic odontogenic tumors of the posterior maxilla are often syndromic. Basal cell carcinoma of the oral mucosa (◘ Fig. 3.67), and within syndromic keratocytic odontogenic tumors are rare events [160, 161].

◘ **Table 3.6** Diagnostic criteria for Gorlin-Goltz Syndrome

Major criteria	Minor criteria
Basal cell carcinoma (BCC) before 20 years of age, or >2 BCC after age 20	Radiographic abnormalities such as wedge-shaped vertebrae, bridging sella turcica
Jaw keratocytic odontogenic tumor before the age of 20.	Other skeletal abnormalities such as short fourth metacarpal, polydactyly, syndactyly, Sprengel's deformity (congenital high scapula)
≥3 palmar or plantar pitting	Macrocephaly
Lamellar calcifications falx cerebri	Cleft lip or palate, frontal bossing, (◘ Fig. 3.68)
Bifib, fused, or splayed ribs	Ovarian or cardiac fibroma
First degree relative with syndrome	Stabismus, hypertelorism, congenital cataracts, glaucoma, coloboma
	Lymphomesenteric cysts
	Medulloblastoma

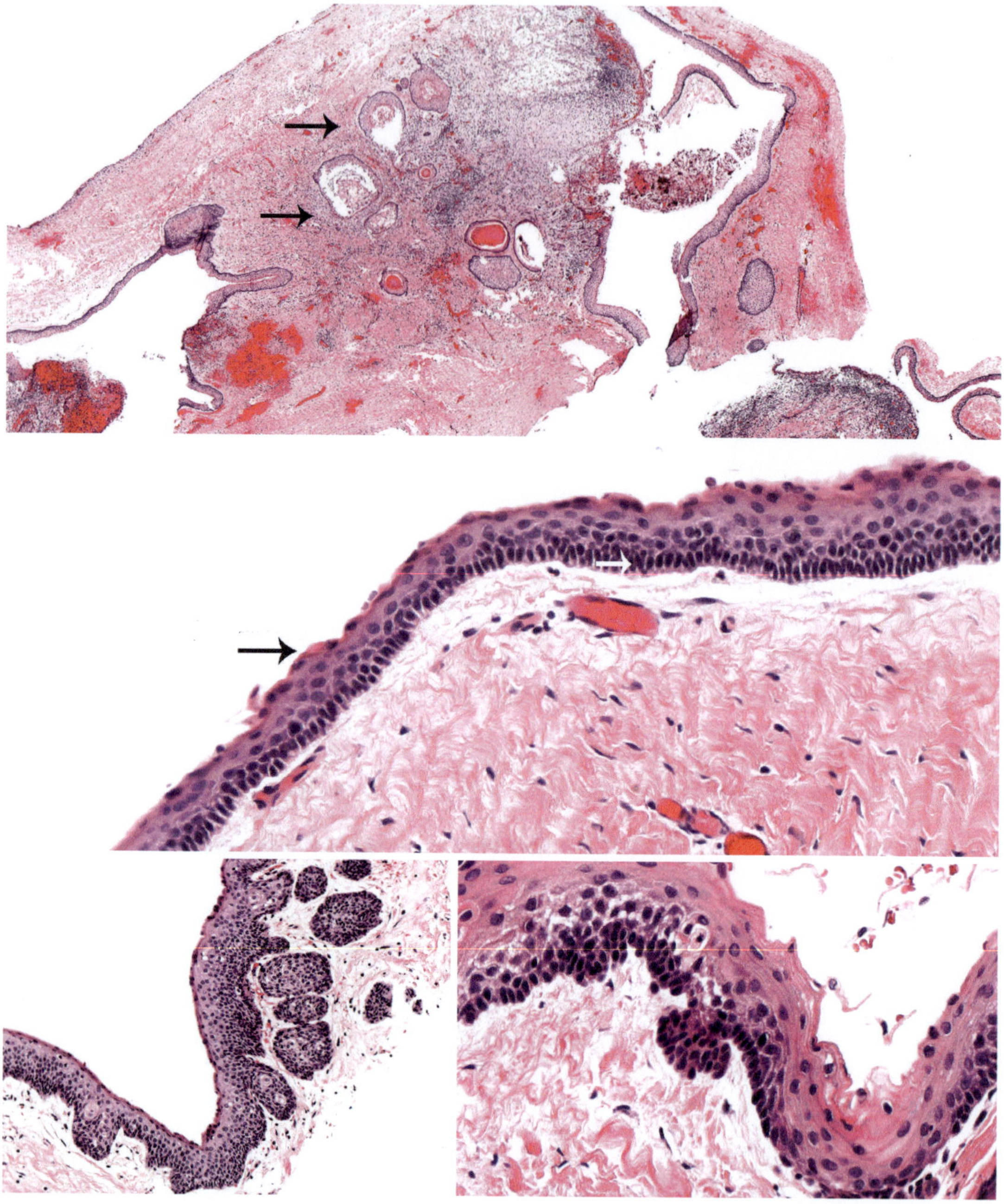

Fig. 3.66 Keratocystic Odontogenic Tumors: **Top** The multiple keratin-filled cysts hint at daughter-cysts. This finding is rare, and not specific for syndromic keratocystic odontogenic tumors. **Middle** Corrugated parakeratosis (*black arrow*) and nuclear palisading (*white arrow*). **Bottom** Basaloid daughter budding may be seen in syndromic and nonsyndromic, recurrent keratocystic odontogenic tumors

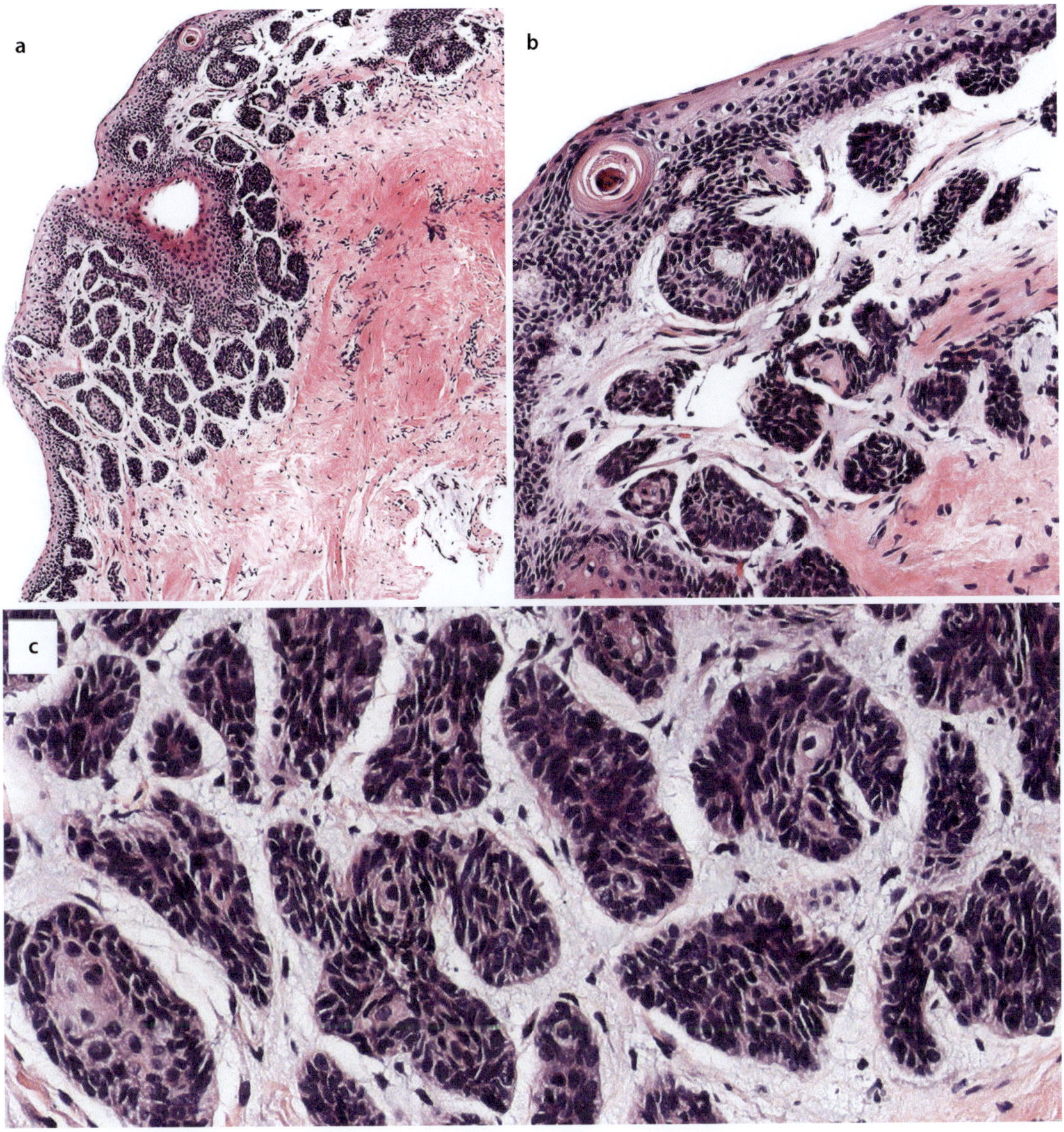

Fig. 3.67 Intraoral basal cell carcinoma in a patient with Gorlin's Syndrome. **a**, **b** The tumor forms a main nodular mass, with multifocal mucosal basaloid budding directly from the basal reserved layer. **c**. Islands of BCC with prominent peripheral palisading

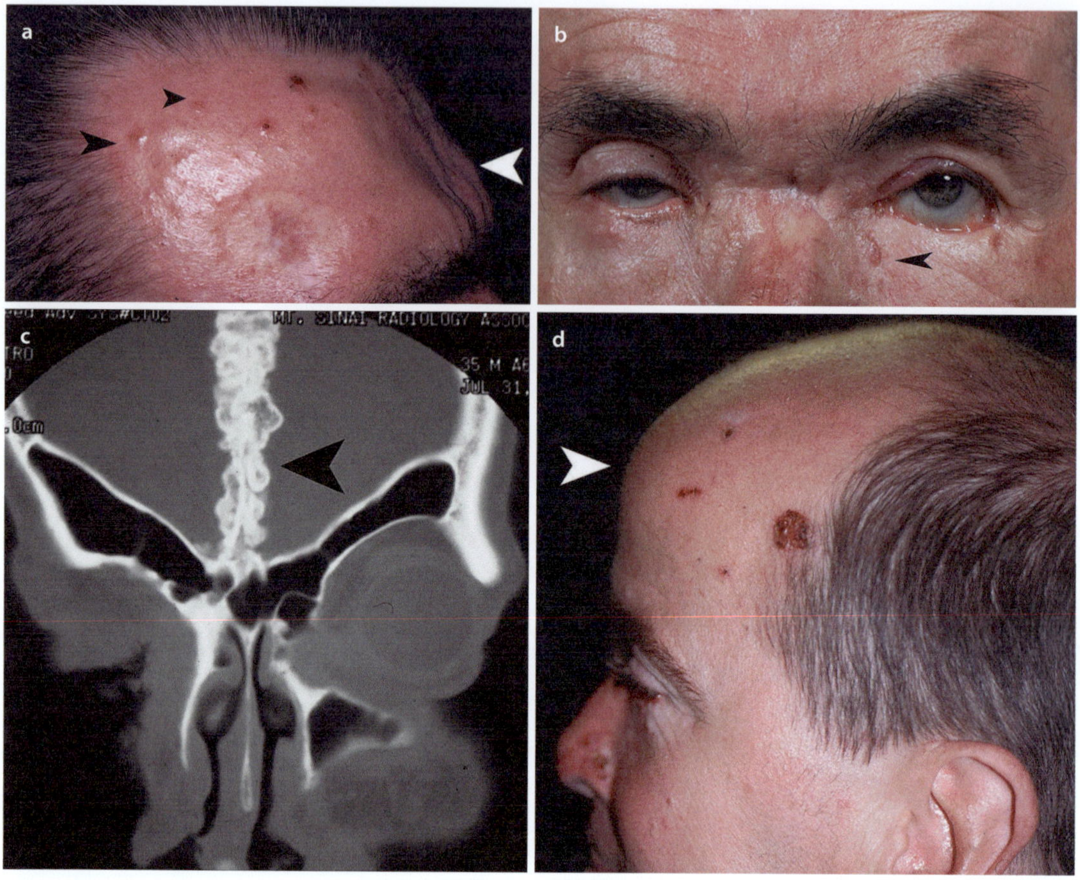

Fig. 3.68 Gorlin's syndrome – Frontal bossing refers to an unusually prominent forehead sometimes associated with a heavy brow ridge (white arrows in upper left and bottom right panels). Multiple basal cell carcinomas appear as pearly papules (black arrows, upper left and upper right panels). The depressed scars bespeak prior resections for basal cell carcinomas. Calcified falx cerebri (black arrow, bottom left panel). (Courtesy of Dr. William Lawson)

Self Study

1. Look at the three illustrations (Figures 3.69, 3.70, and 3.71). Which one correctly measures depth of invasion?

Figure 3.69 – The "plumb line" (top, green line) measures 1.6 mm

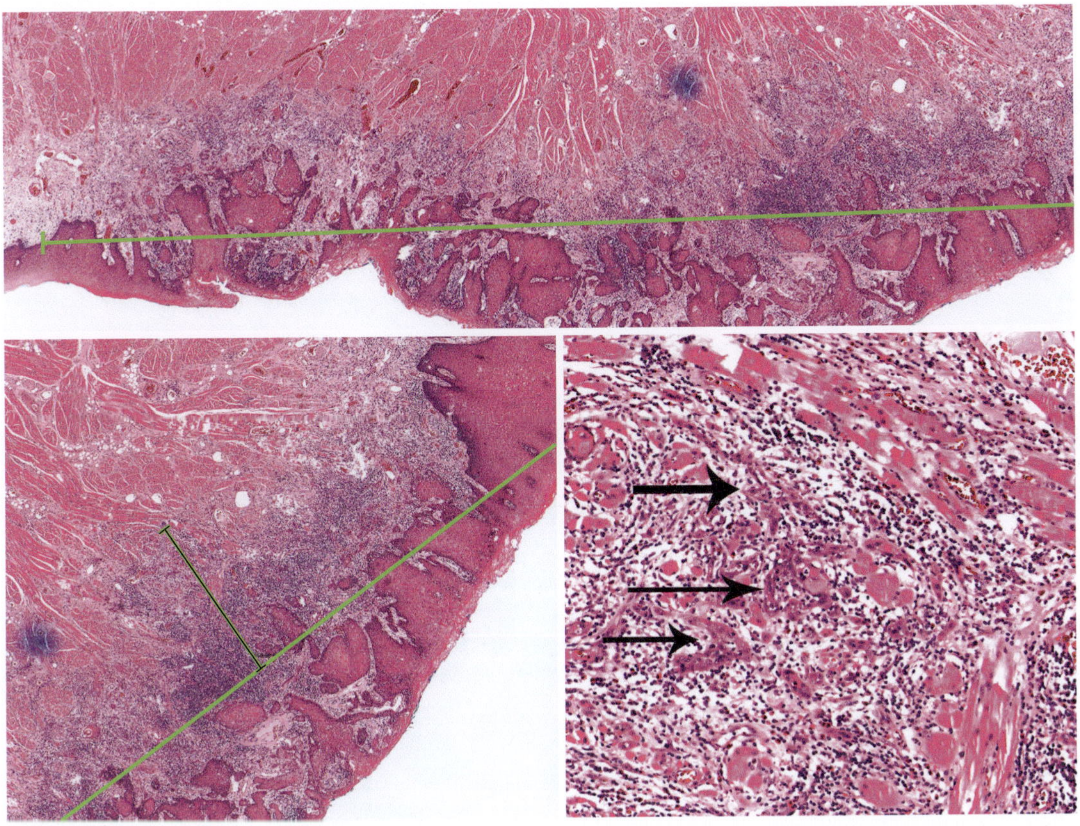

Fig. 3.69 Self study #1

Figure 3.70 – The plumb line (green line) measures 2.9 mm

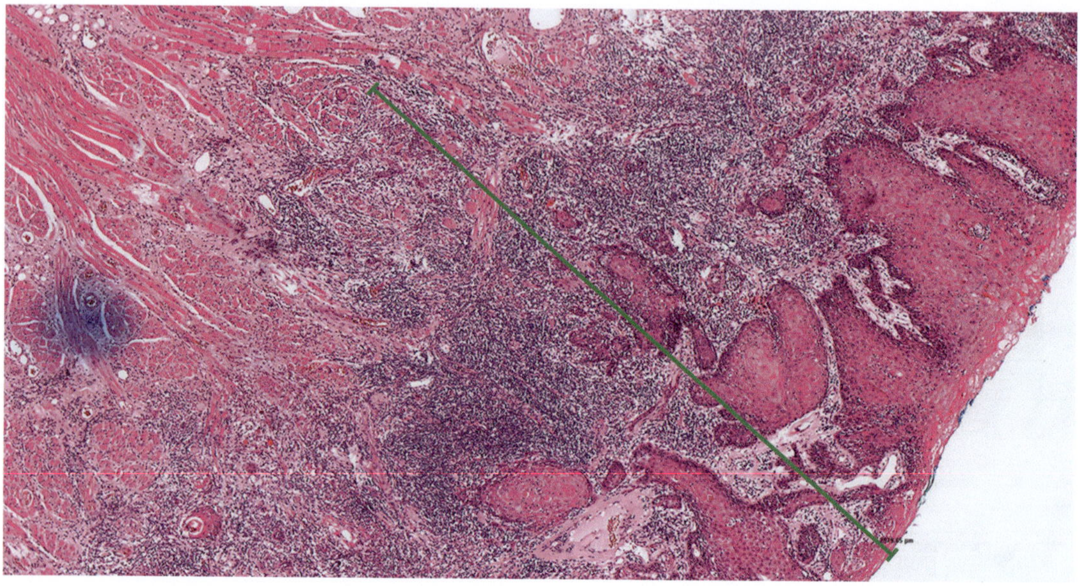

Fig. 3.70 Self study #1

■ Figure 3.71 – The plumb line measures 2.6 mm

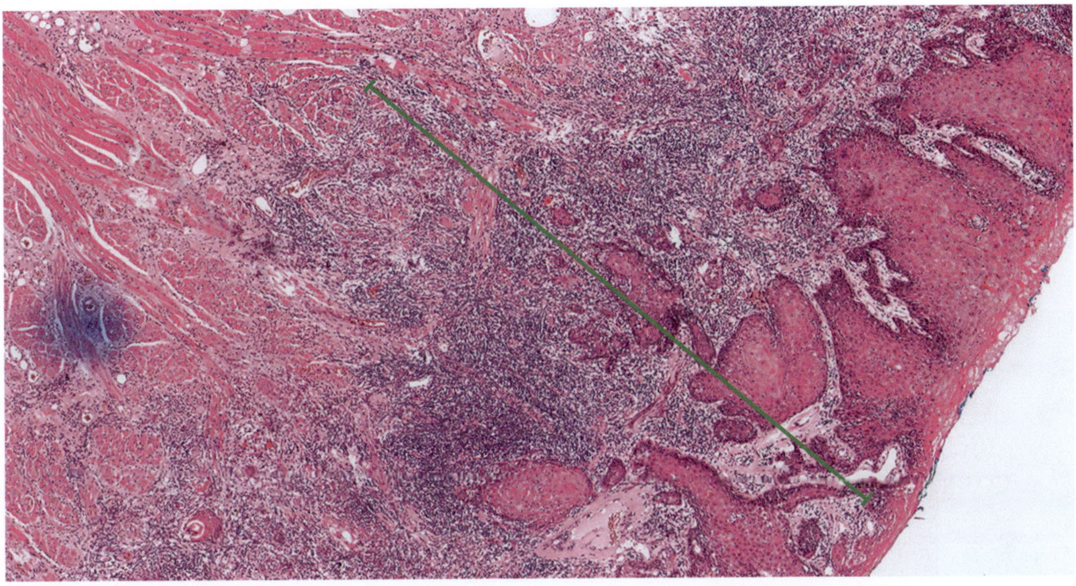

■ **Fig. 3.71** Self study #1

2. Study ◘ Figs. 3.72, 3.73 and 3.74, which represent the same tumor. The inset for ◘ Fig. 3.72 confirms the nature of the satellite. The plumb line in ◘ Fig. 3.73 measures 5.9 mm. The distance measured in ◘ Fig. 3.74 is 1.5 mm. What is the pT stage and WPOI (worst pattern of invasion)?

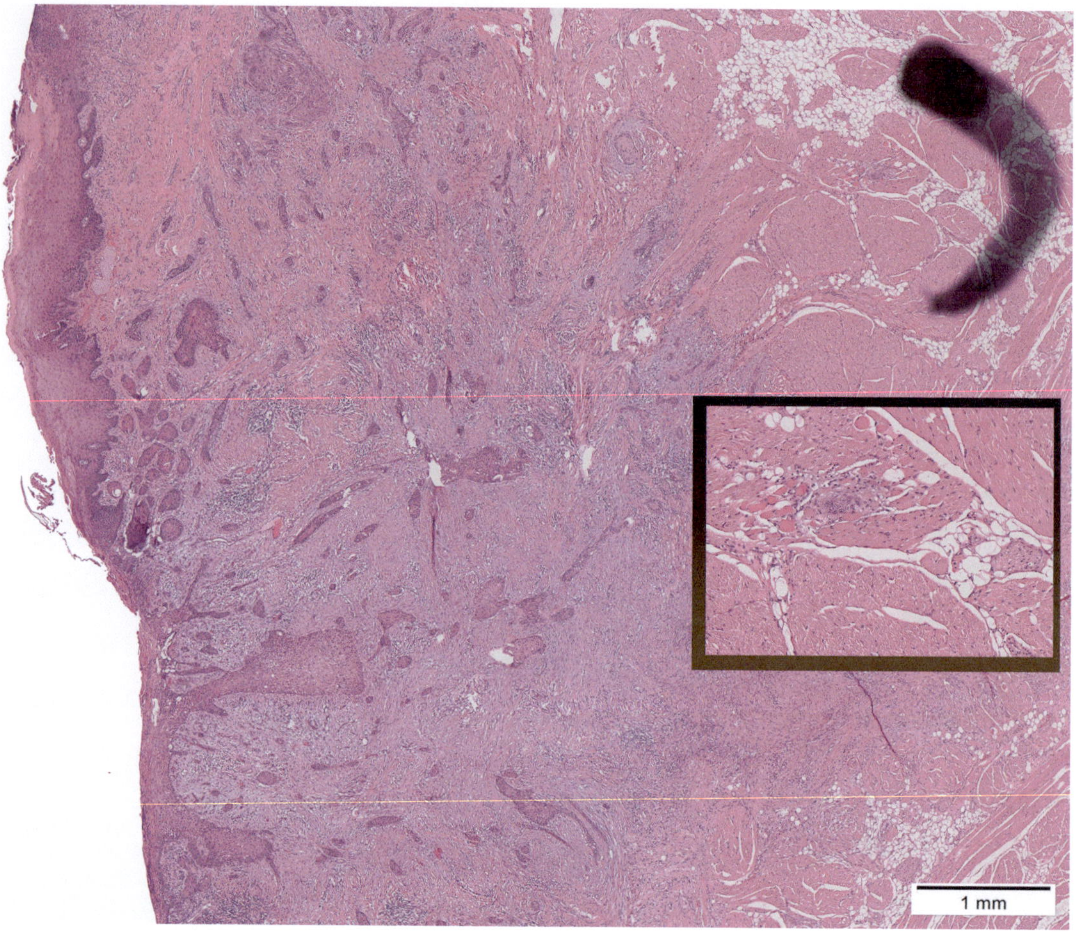

◘ **Fig. 3.72** Self study #2

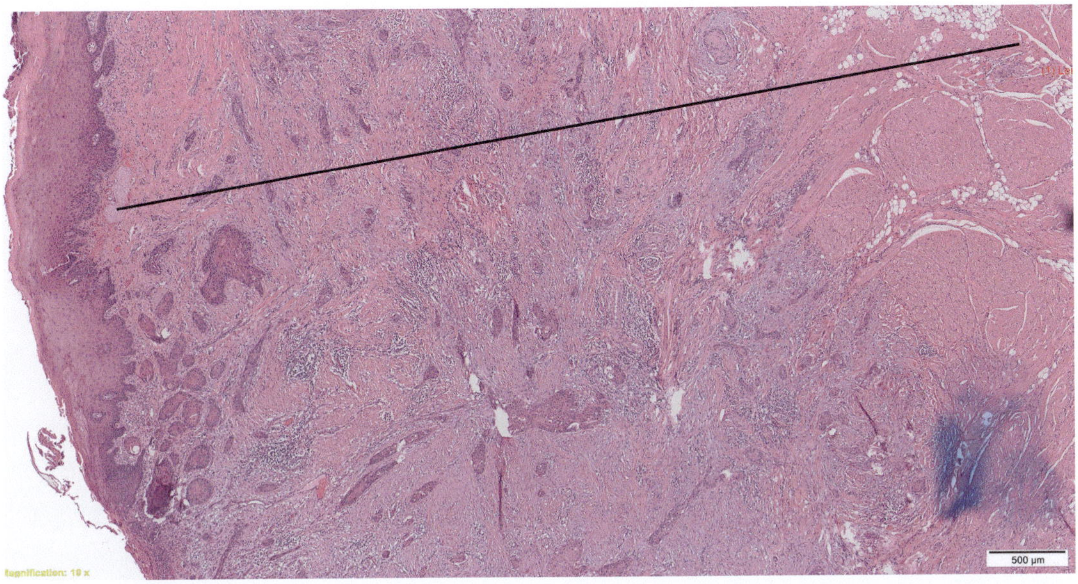

Fig. 3.73 Self study #2

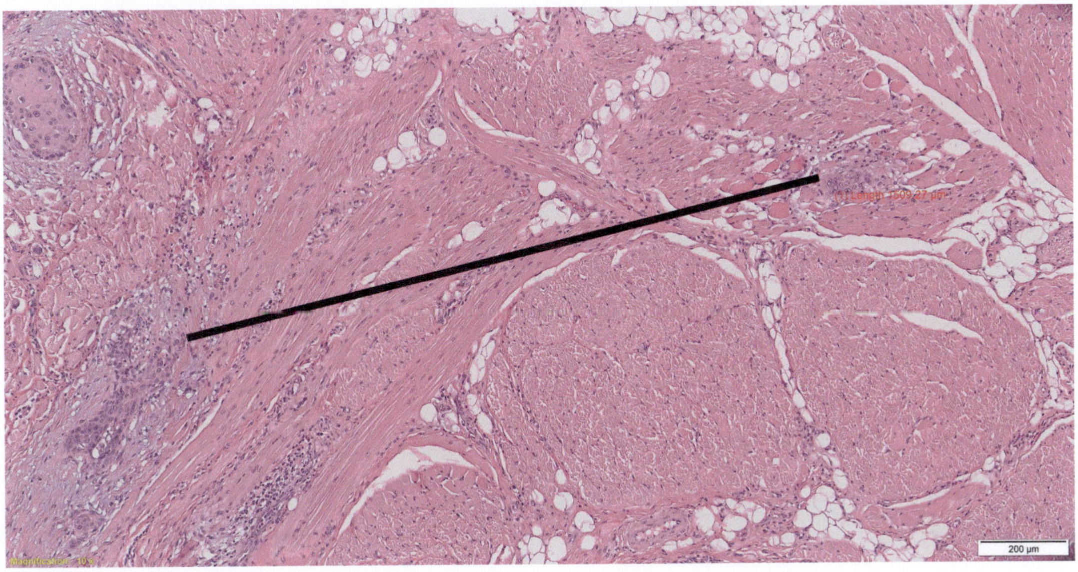

Fig. 3.74 Self study #2

3. Study ◻ Figs. 3.75 and 3.76. Notice the placement of the horizon for ◻ Fig. 3.75. The plumb line (red) measures 1.9 mm. The green line in ◻ Fig. 3.76 measures 0.2 mm. What is the pT stage and WPOI?

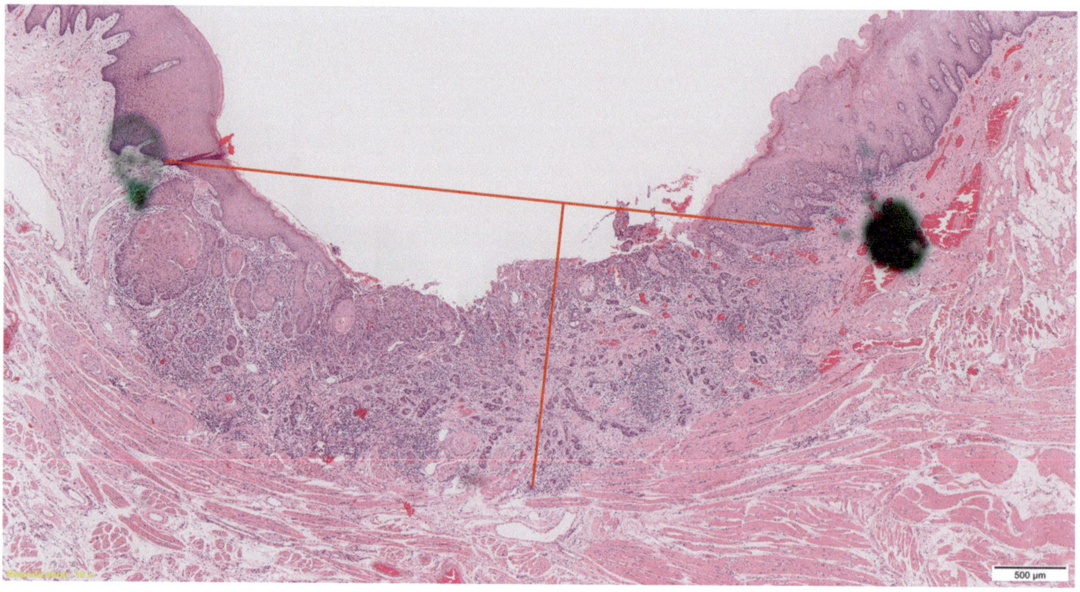

◻ **Fig. 3.75** Self study #3

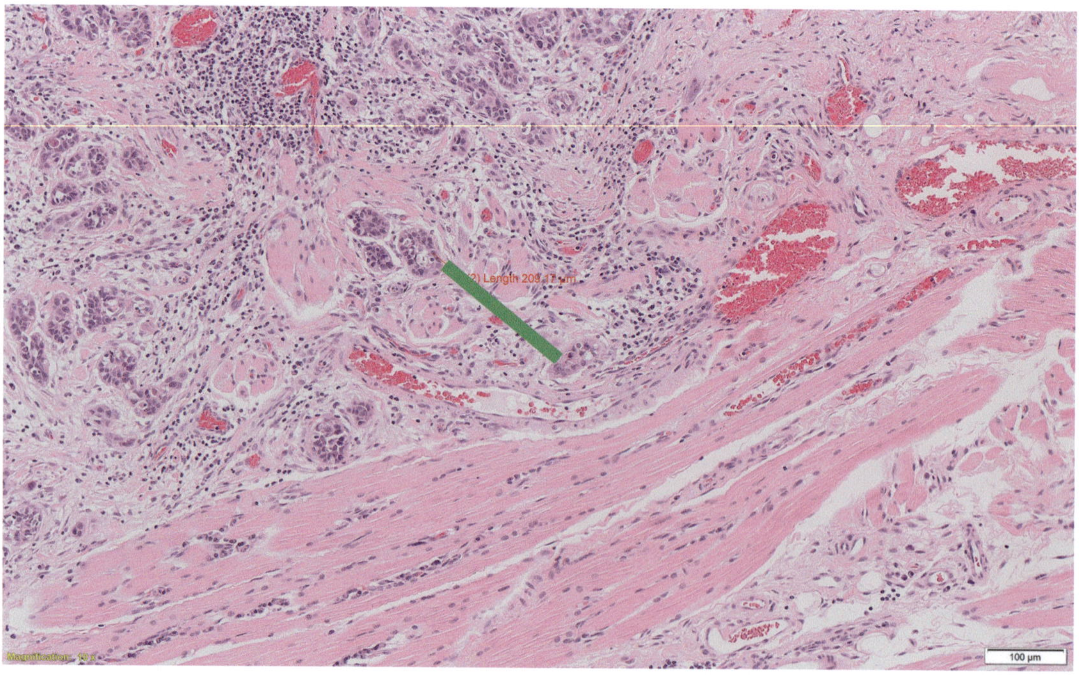

◻ **Fig. 3.76** Self study #3

4. Study ▫ Fig. 3.77 (plumb line (green) 5.4 mm) and ▫ Fig. 3.78 (plumb line (green) 5.2 mm). ▫ Figures 3.79 and 3.80 survey the advancing edge and illustrate the WPOI. What is the pT stage and WPOI?

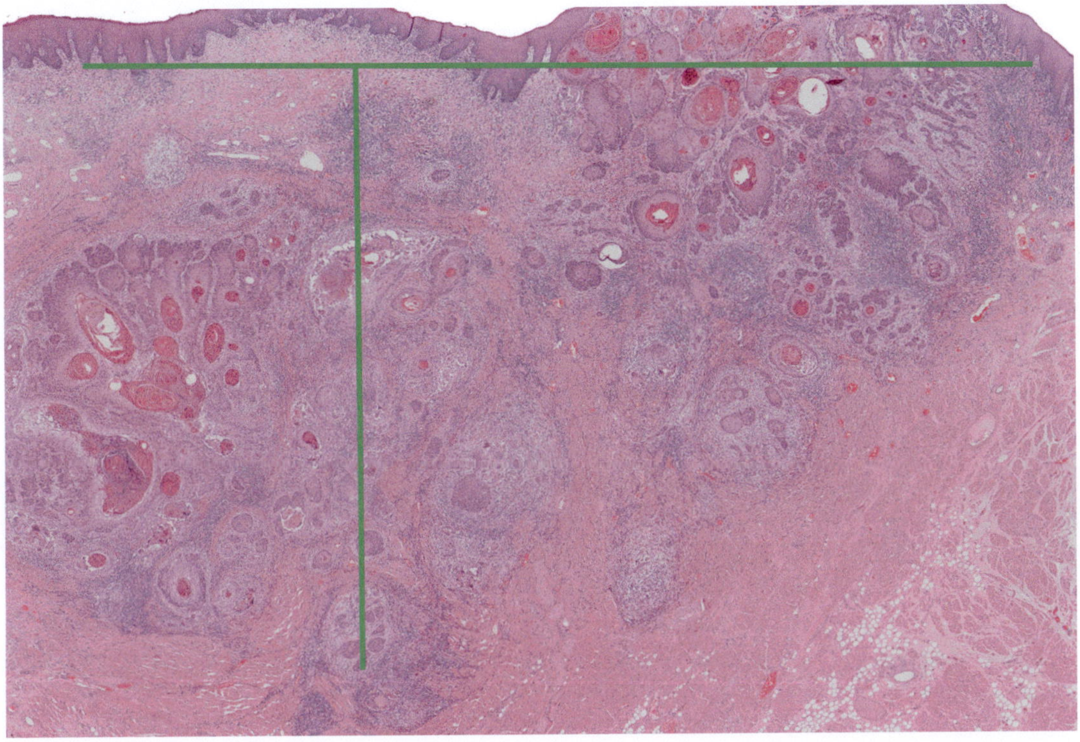

▫ **Fig. 3.77** Self study #4 DOI

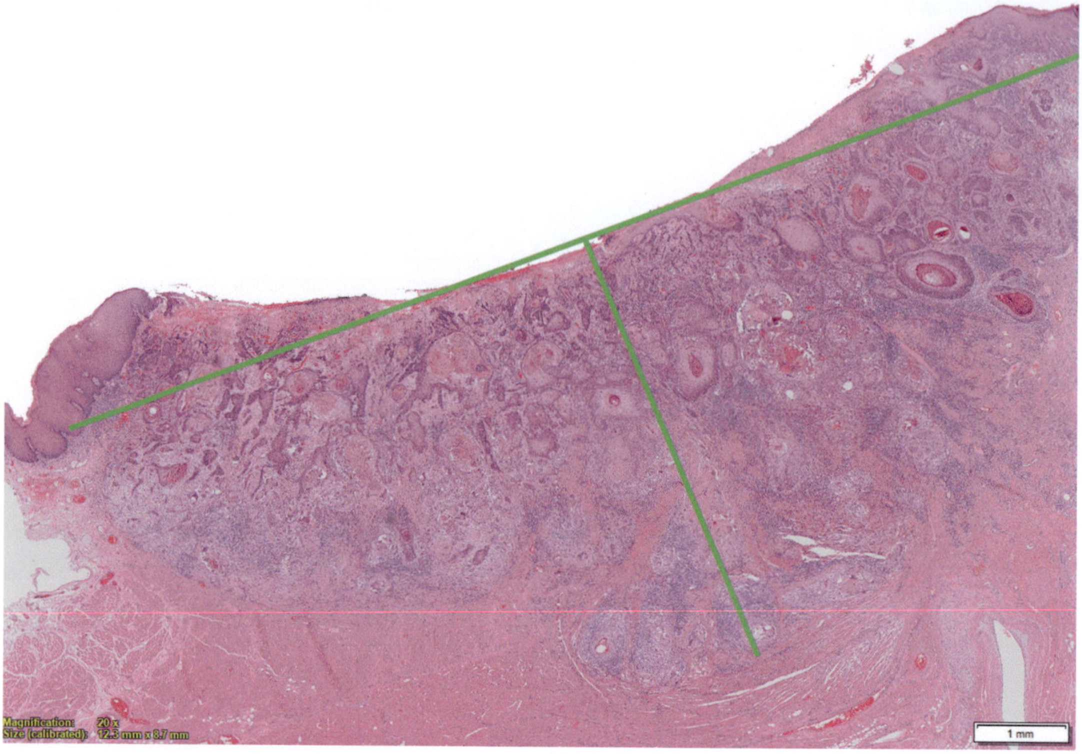

Fig. 3.78 Self study #4 DOI

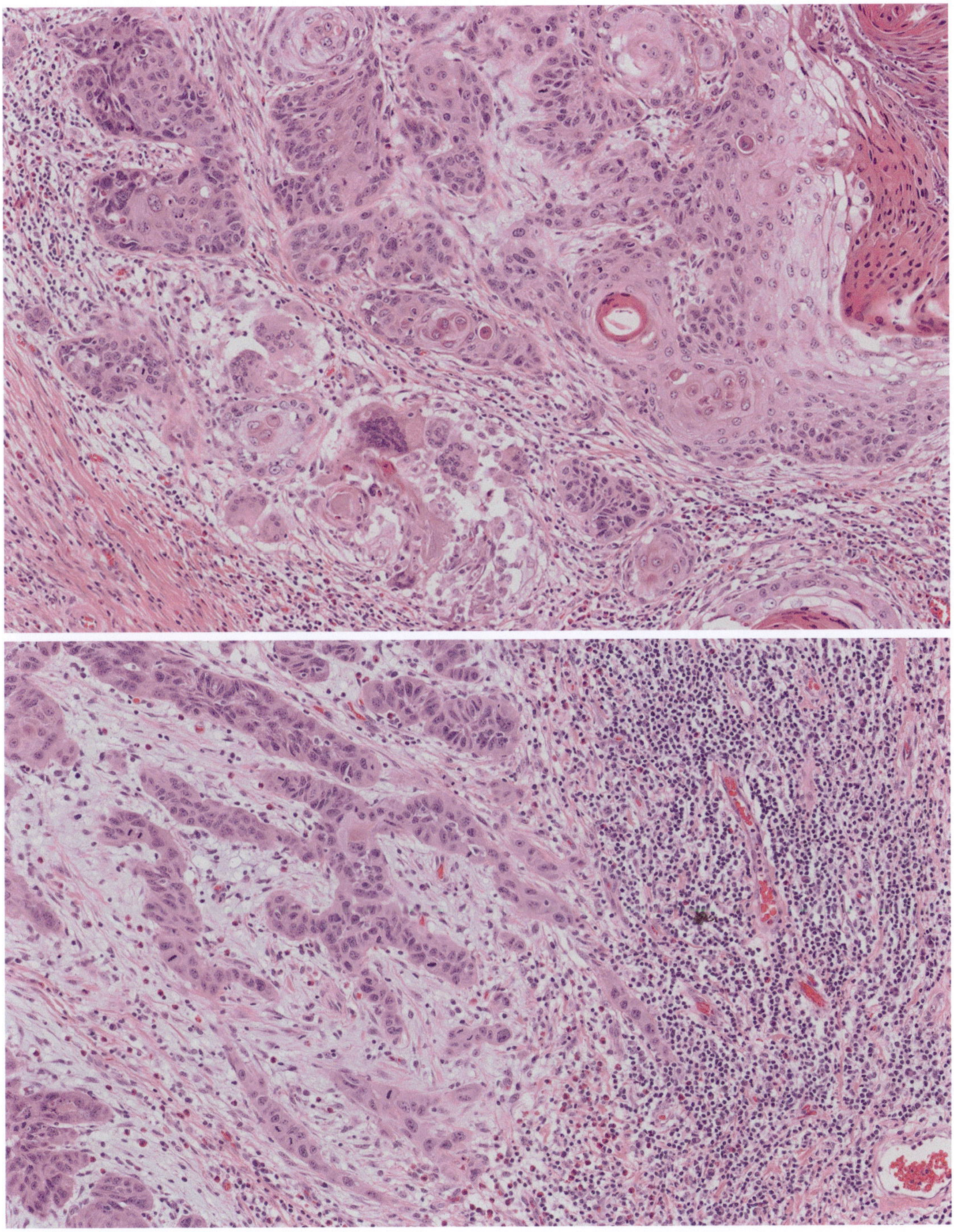

Fig. 3.79 Self study #4 WPOI

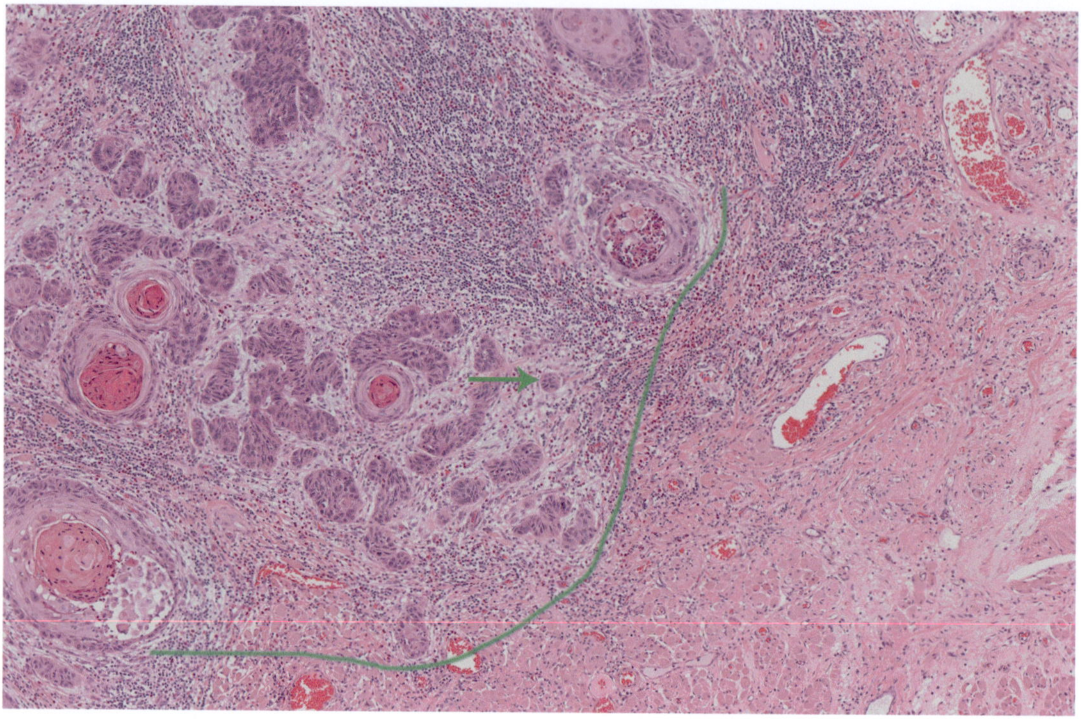

Fig. 3.80 Self study #4 WPOI

5. Let's practice some more WPOI, shall we?
   What is WPOI for ◘ Fig. 3.81?

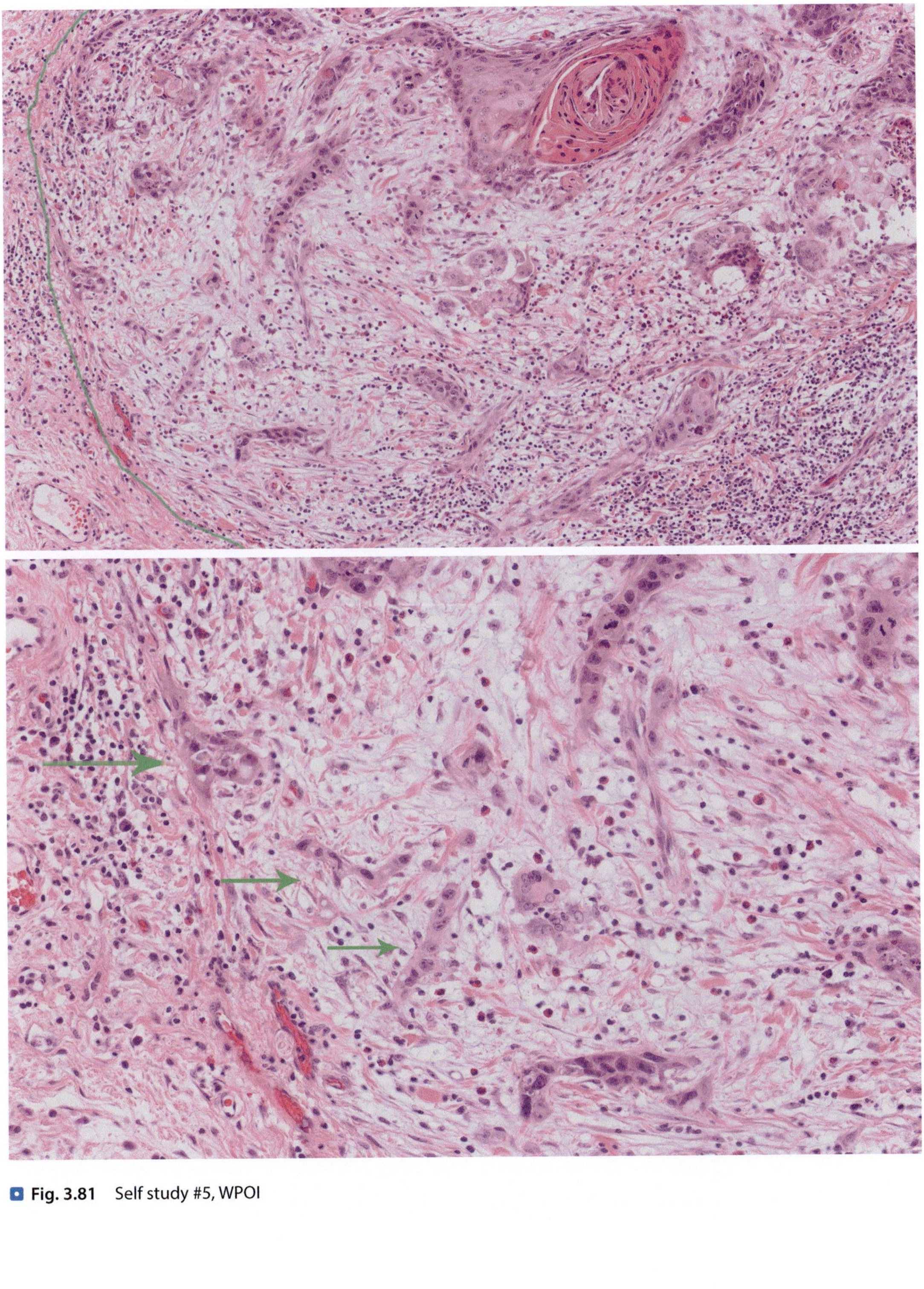

◘ **Fig. 3.81** Self study #5, WPOI

6. What is WPOI for Fig. 3.82?

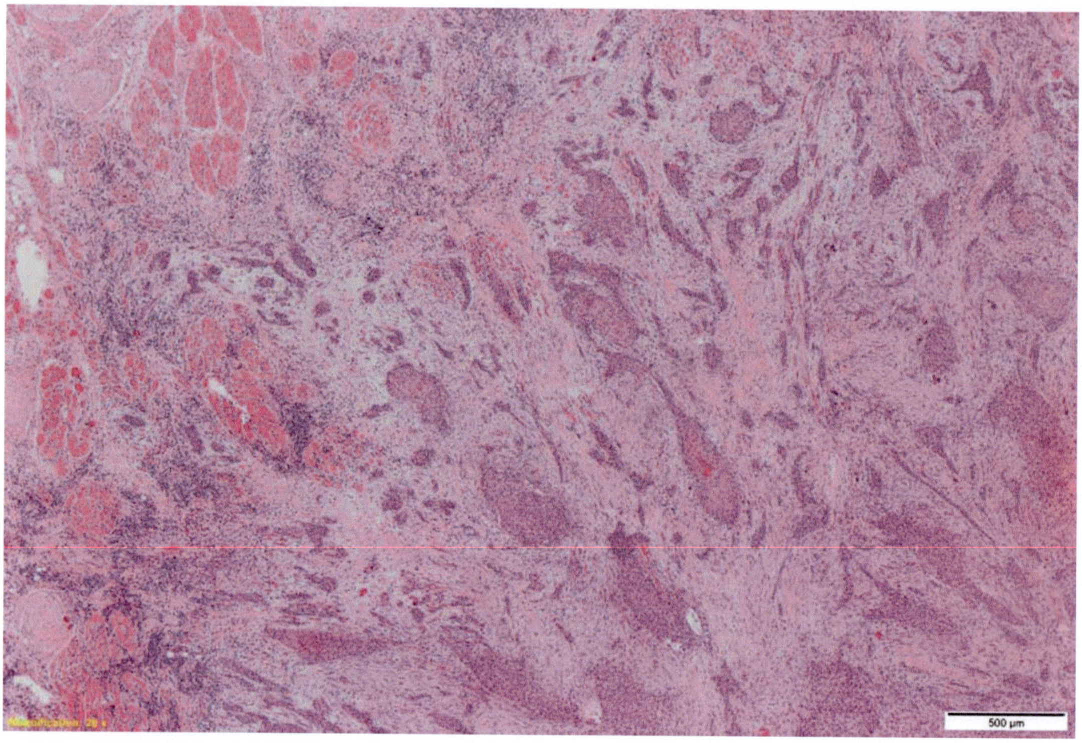

Fig. 3.82 Self study #6, WPOI

7. Last one: What is WPOI for ◘ Figs. 3.83 and 3.84 (same tumor)?

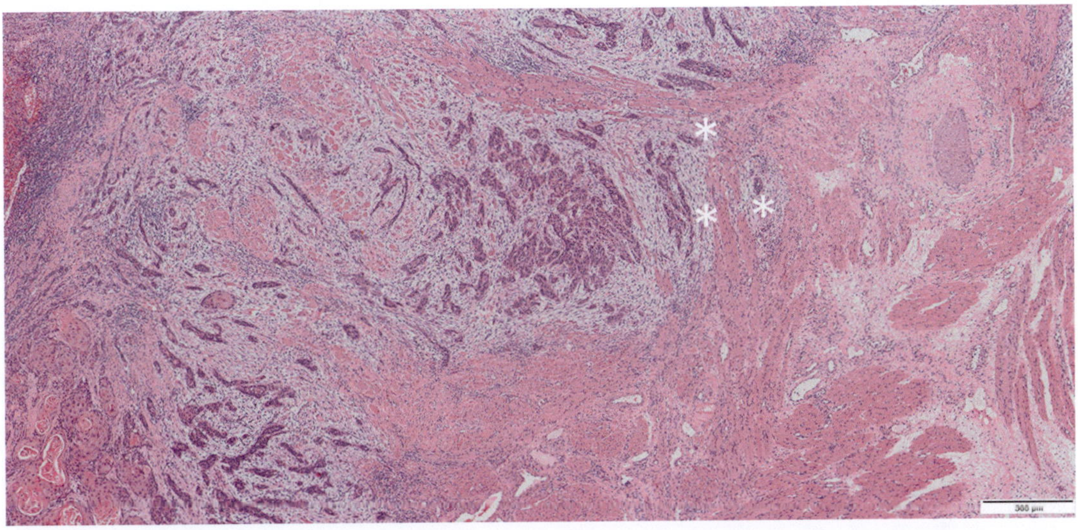

◘ **Fig. 3.83** Self study #7, WPOI

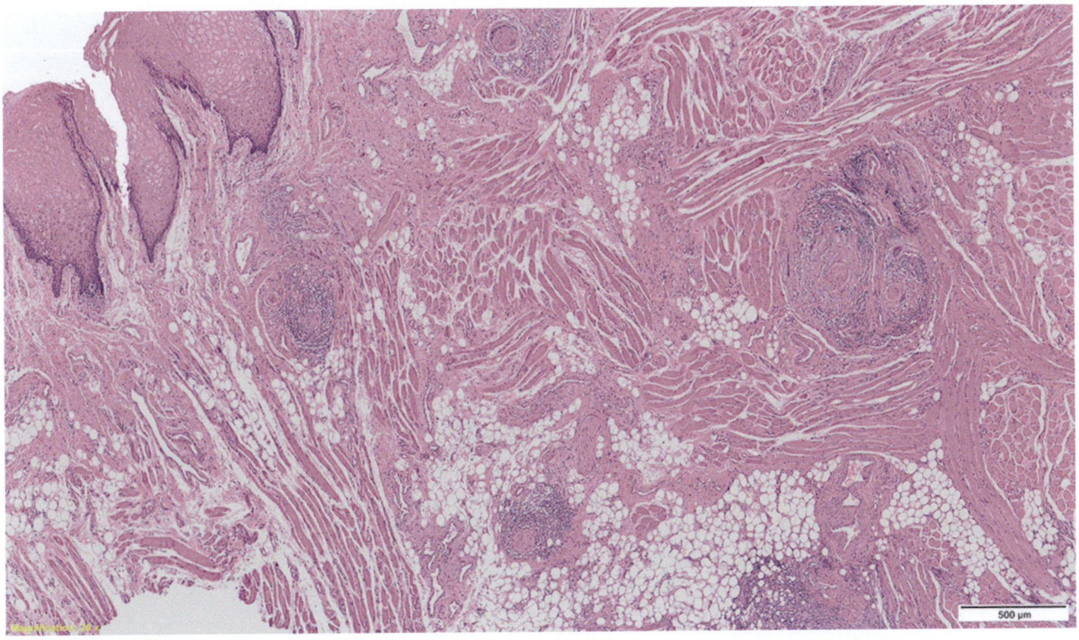

◘ **Fig. 3.84** Self study #7, WPOI

8. ▣ Figure 3.85 represents an excisional biopsy. Which of the following statements is/are true?
   A. This has a predilection for elderly woman and is usually multifocal
   B. This is caused by HPV 16/18
   C. This is caused by cigarette and alcohol exposure.
   D. All statements are true.
   E. No statements are true.

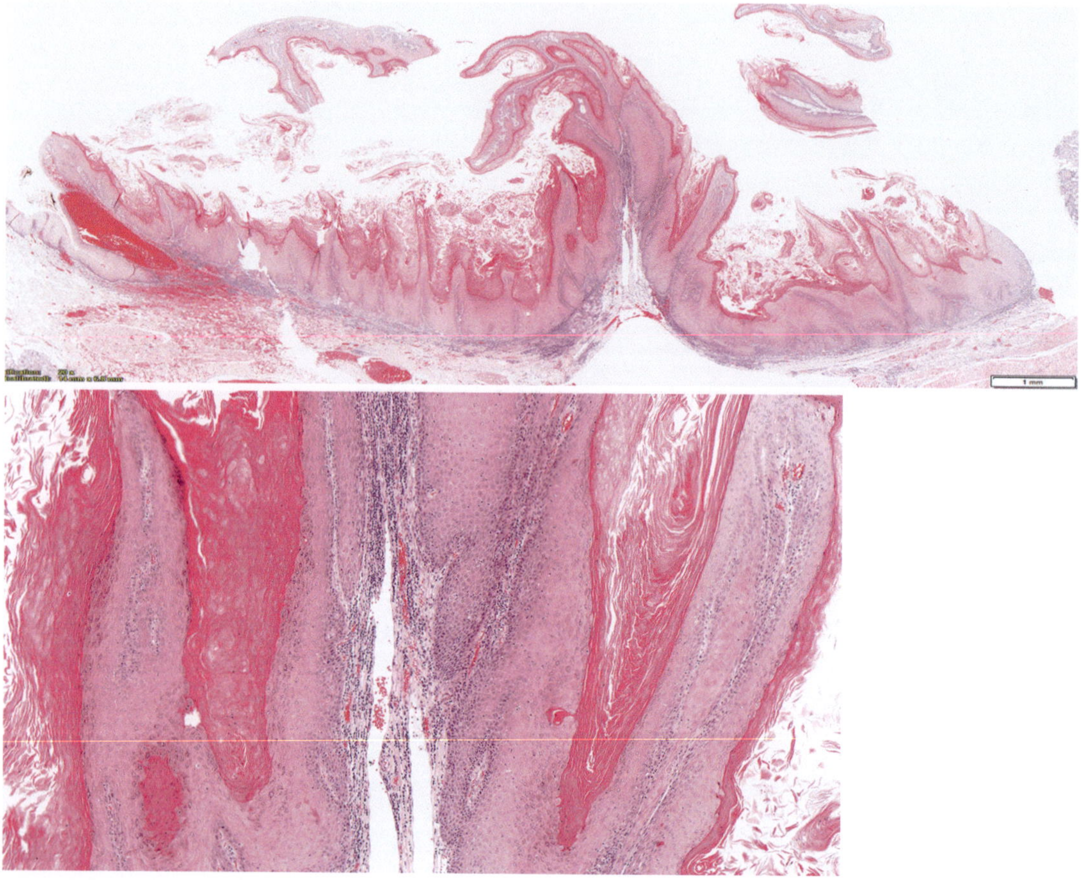

▣ **Fig. 3.85** Self study #8

9. ◘ Figures 3.86 and 3.87 are from the same patient. What is the stage and WPOI?

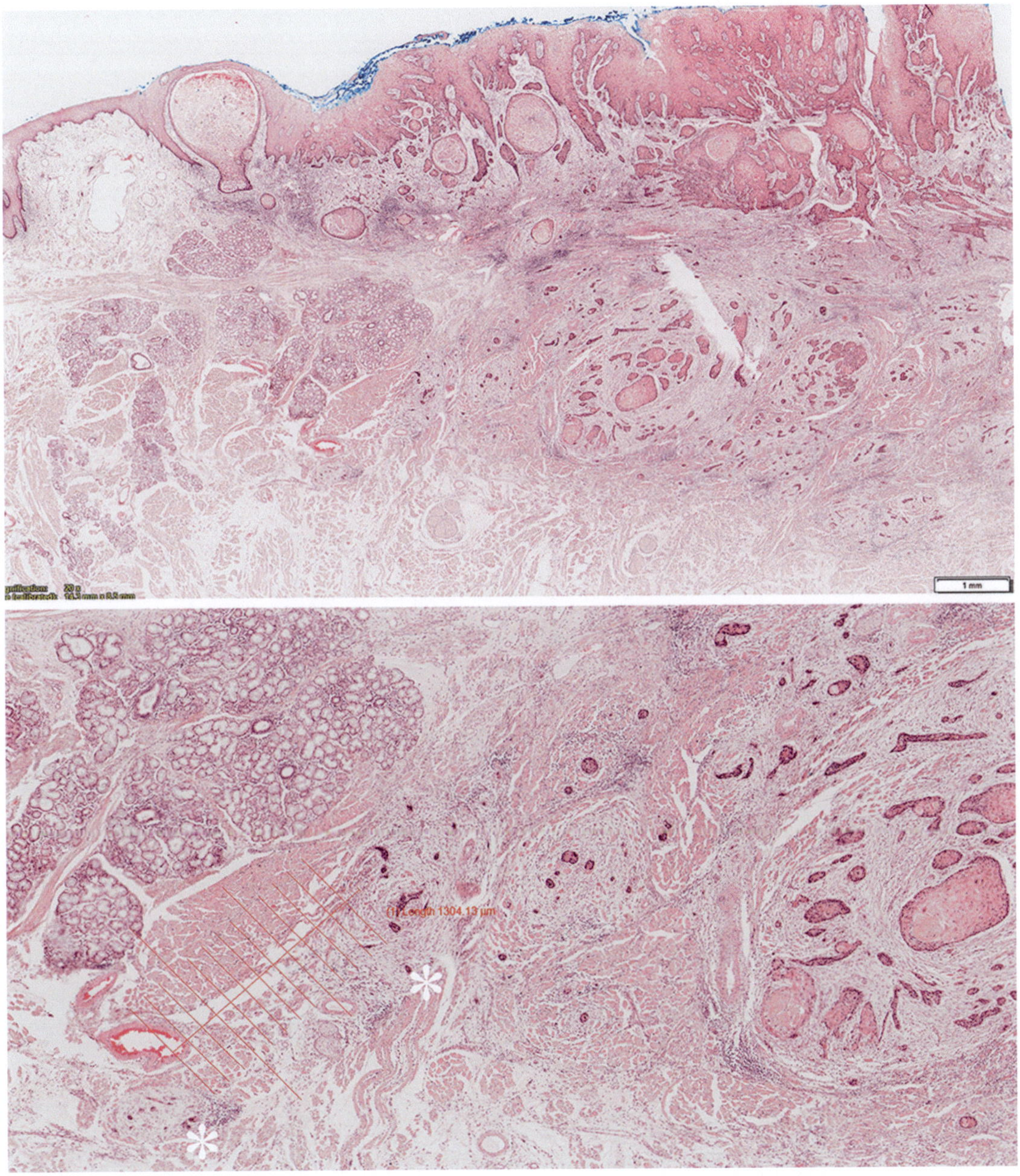

◘ **Fig. 3.86** Self study # 9

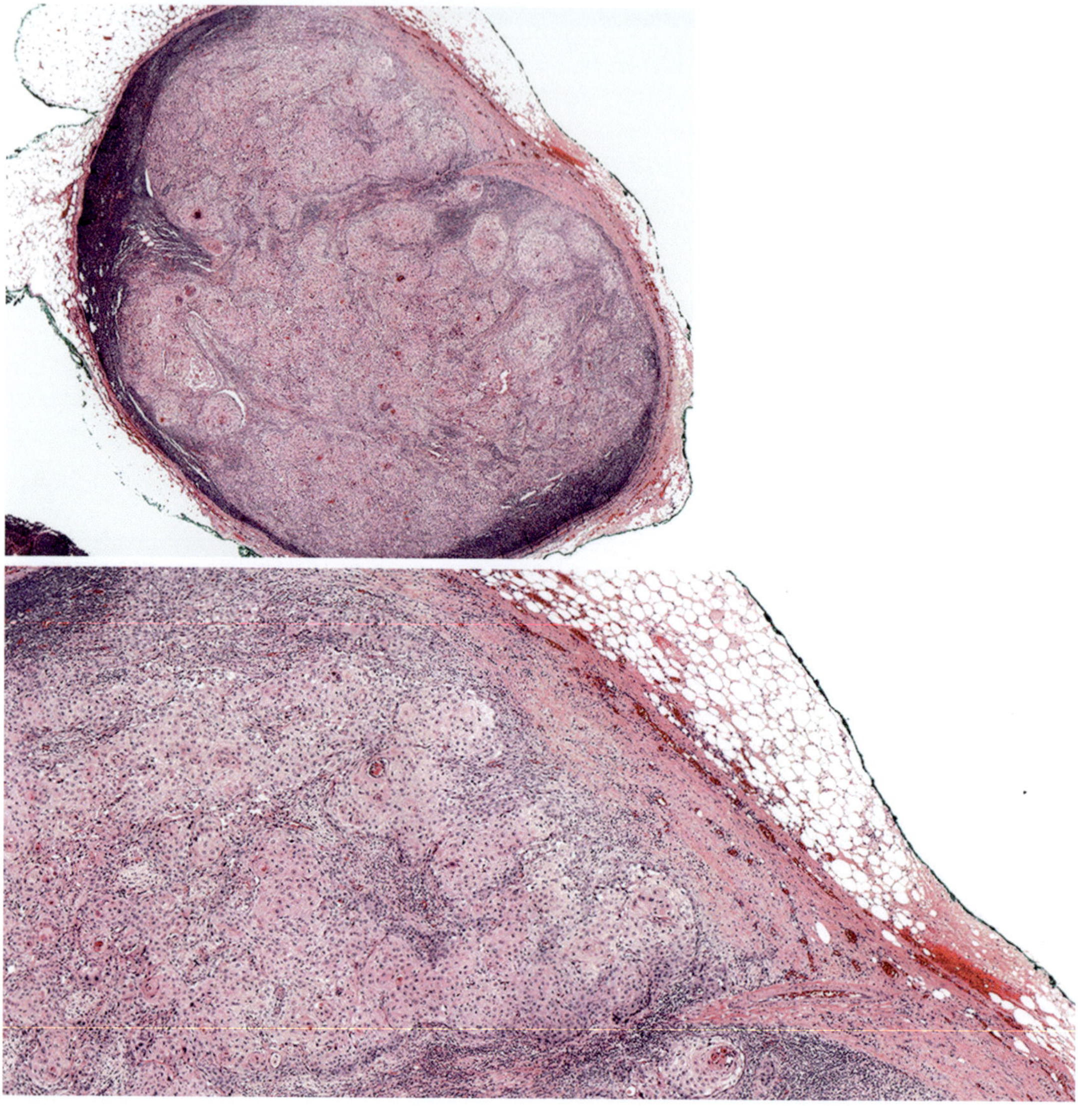

Fig. 3.87 Self study # 9

10. Study Fig. 3.88. Where is this from?
What is your diagnosis?

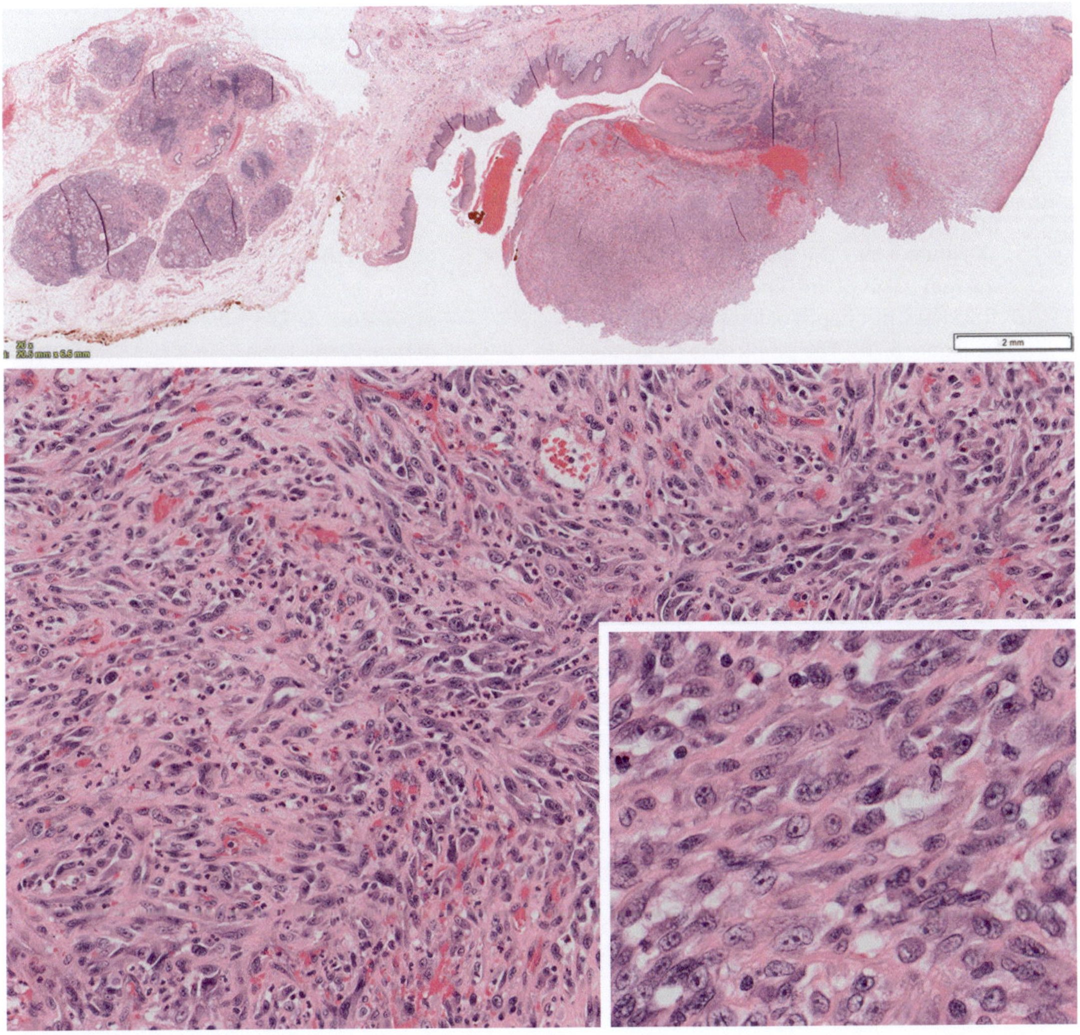

Fig. 3.88 Self study # 10

Answers

1. Which of the three illustrations is correct for determining depth of invasion (DOI)?
   Figure 3.68 – The "plumb line" measures 1.6 mm – **Correct.** The top image gives you the "long view" as to the nearest normal basal reserve layer. A "plumb line" is dropped from this horizon **(Bottom left**). The **Bottom right** panel confirms that this region represents cancer satellites.
   Figure 3.69 – The plumb line measures 2.9 mm – This plumb line measures tumor thickness, not depth of invasion.
   Figure 3.70 – The plumb line measures 2.6 mm – This plumb line does not start from the nearest normal mucosal basal reserve layer.
2. Study Figs. 3.71, 3.72, and 3.73, which represents the same tumor. The inset for Fig. 3.71 confirms the nature of the satellite. What is the pT stage and WPOI (worst pattern of invasion)?
   Answer: pT2 – DOI = **5.9 mm.** Notice how you can appreciate tumor dispersion on low-power. This is an example of **WPOI-5,** as tumor dispersion **is ≥ 1 mm.**
3. Study Figs. 3.74 and 3.75. Notice the placement of the horizon for Fig. 3.74. This is a depressed ulcerated tumor. The plumb line measures 1.9 mm. Notice how on low-power, the tumor islands are "convincingly" separate. This "contextual" determination is based in part on the shapes of the satellites. "Feathery" contours suggest that islands may all interconnect on deeper sections, whereas smooth rounded contours support the opposite conclusion. The green line in Fig. 3.75 measures 0.2 mm. What is the pT stage and WPOI (worst pattern of invasion)? **Answer: pT1 – depth of invasion is 1.9 mm. WPOI-4, as there are convincingly separate tumor satellite, which are *not* dispersed.**
4. Study Fig. 3.76 (plumb line 5.4 mm) and Fig. 3.77 (plumb line 5.2 mm). What is the pT stage and WPOI?
   Figs. 3.78, 3.79, 3.80, and 3.81 survey the advancing edge and illustrate the WPOI. **Answer:** Both figures illustrate **pT2.** Remember (in the words of Andy Huvos, may her rest in peace) "Ace beats King". If DOI ≤ 5 mm in one region, but >5 mm in another, then **pT2.** Now we survey the advancing edge to look for WPOI. The gestalt of Figs. 3.76 and 3.77 **is "nondispersed"** and therefore **not WPOI-5.** The purpose of fine tuning higher power survey is to confirm this impression and avoid missing the possibility of few scattered dispersed satellites. Remember that WPOI-5 usually occurs in the context of generalized tumor dispersion. But the exceptions prove the rule. Figure 3.78 **top** demonstrates large islands (> 15 nuclei/ island). Figure 3.78 **bottom** is a nice example of **"not convincingly detached".** These small tumor strands have feathery contours, and are too close to adjacent cancer islands to be considered "convincingly detached". Therefore, both regions represent WPOI-3.
   Figure 3.79 introduces **"the perimeter rule".** In your mind's eye (that plane where pathology is writ large), draw out a perimeter at the very advancing edge (green line). Small, convincingly detached tumor islands ***not*** at the advancing edge (green arrow) don't count! Therefore, this region also represent WPOI-3.
   Figure 3.80 **top** demonstrates another perimeter (green line). Figure 3.80 **bottom** demonstrates small tumor strands. While they also demonstrate a feathery contour, they are far enough away from neighboring islands as to be convincingly detached. Therefore, this region represents **WPOI-4** (small and convincingly detached islands). Now, from a collapsed and more practical point of view, it suffices to say, ***not WPOI-5!***
5. What is WPOI for Fig. 3.81?
   Answer: WPOI-4, not WPOI-5. At this advancing edge you get a real sense of convincingly detached small islands with some dispersion. The more intervening normal tissue seen, the more dispersion present. Use the size bar on the lower right is 500 um or 0.5 mm to assess distance between the outermost islands at the advancing edge with the next closest islands. Eyeballing the closest

distance between the two furthest satellites (**asterisks**) is <1.0 mm, therefore **WPOI-4, not WPOI-5.**

6. What is WPOI for ◘ Fig. 3.82?
   Answer: WPOI-4, not WPOI-5. Same discussion as for question 5.
7. Last one: What is WPOI for ◘ Fig. 3.83?
   Answer: WPOI-5. This low-power view gives you a sense of scale. Use the size bar on the lower right is 500 um or 0.5 mm to assess distances. Now look at ◘ Fig. 3.89, which is a tumor silhouette or "mugshot" of "ground truth" produced from annotating high resolution images to serve the dual purposes of graphic based analyses and machine learning (see below). The blue denotes mucosal surface. The black islands denote cancer satellites. As the scale is identical to ◘ Fig. 3.83, it is easy to appreciate that these dispersed satellites are >1 mm from their closest neighbors, hence **WPOI-5!**

Why 1 mm? Even the most robust pathologist-driven classifications schemas are based on arbitrary, albeit intuitive, classes. To define "dispersed" I needed to pick a number. So I picked "1.0 mm". At the same moment that I "picked a number", I was also keenly aware of the need to examine all possible distances as a continuous variable. In fact, Scott Doyle, PhD, (State University of New York at Buffalo) and I are engaged in finding this optimized predictive cut-point through graphic-based analyses of these tumor "mugshots".

Why machine learning? Machine learning or deep learning, is a method of "teaching the computer" to recognize cancer, faces (as in Facebook), letters on a page, or scenes from a car window ("driverless cars") through exposing the computer to many many known examples ("ground truth"). **Having the computer correctly recognize cancer allows for high-through analyses.** ◘ Figure 3.90, **top** and **middle left panels** represent ***computer renderings*** derived from ***top and middle right panels,*** which are original regions of interest. Blue = carcinoma, red = stroma, yellow = lymphocytes. The **top** and **middle middle panels** represent intermediary ground truth hand annotations of carcinoma. The "machine" is also "fed" examples of inflammatory cells and normal stroma.

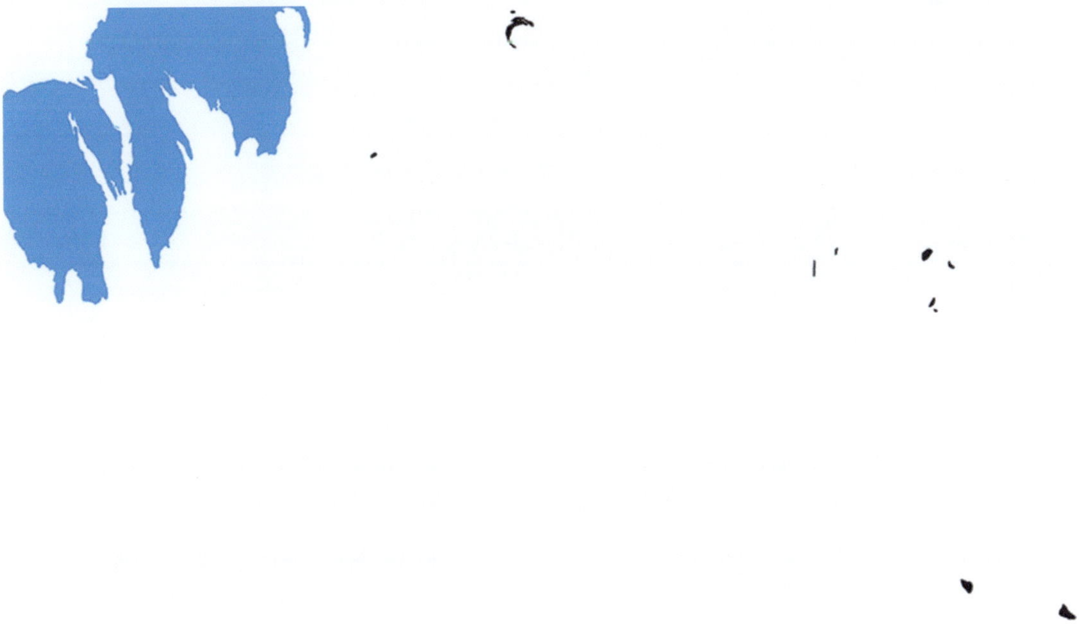

◘ **Fig. 3.89** Answer for self study #7

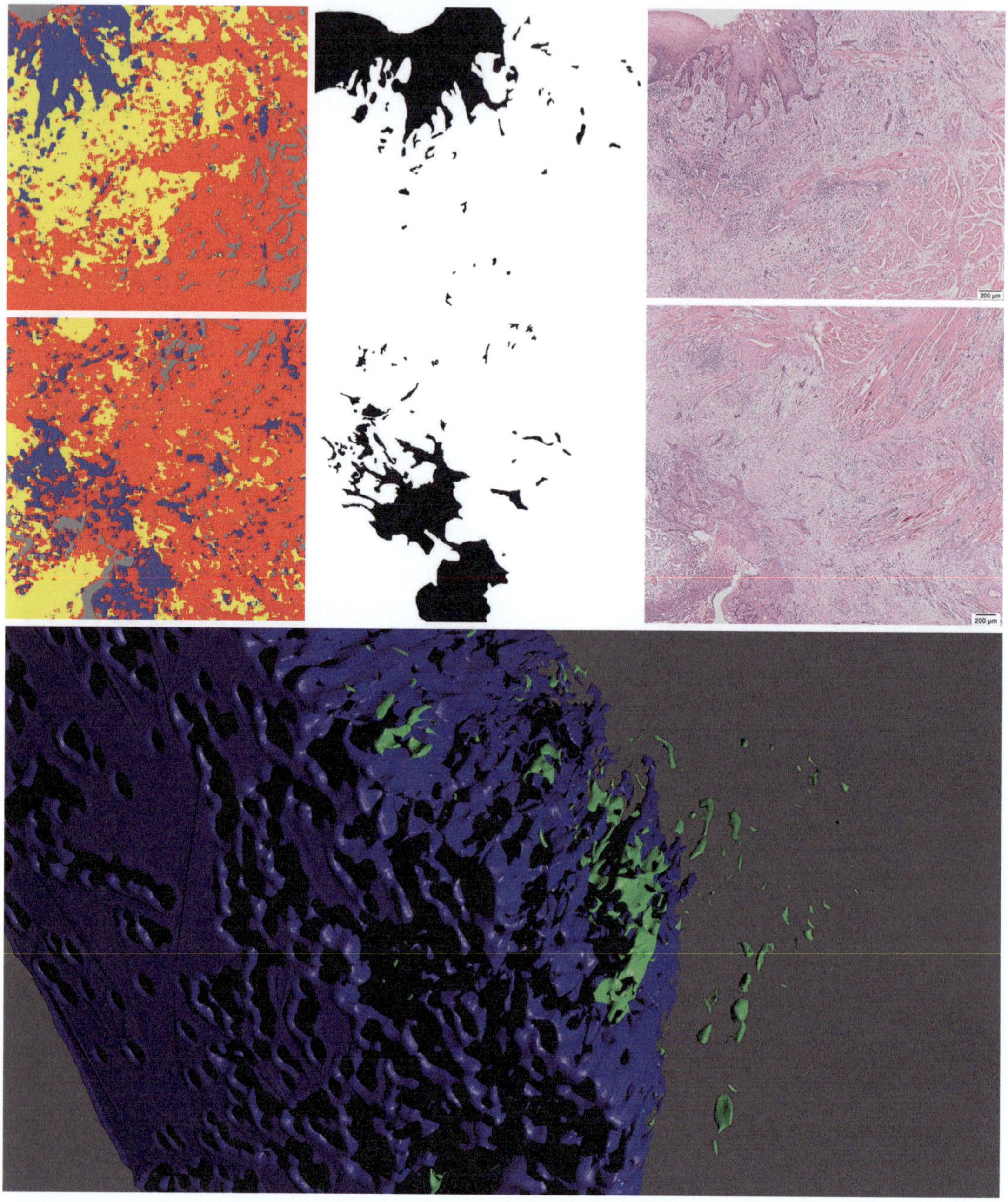

■ **Fig. 3.90** Self study #7, WPOI

The bottom panel represents a machine-generated three-dimensional model of a **WPOI-5 carcinoma.** This was generated by running this classifier (machine learning algorhythm) on 90 consecutive digitalized slides from a WPOI-5 carcinoma. The computer is programed to code all cancer green, but the largest body of cancer blue. Thus the designation of "main tumor" and "satellites" is machine generated.

8. ■ Figure 3.86 represents an excisional biopsy. Which of the following statements is/are true?
   A. This has a predilection for elderly woman and is usually multifocal. **CORRECT.** You are looking at a low-power image (top) of a papillary

squamoproliferative process. This low-power view deliberately demonstrates intact basement membrane. A suggestion of a "pushing border" is seen on the right hand side. The lower panel confirms the lack of pleomorphism. The material allowed me to conclude I could dispense with the usual disclaimer of, "invasive squamous carcinoma cannot be ruled out." I chose to classify this as proliferative verrucoid hyperplasia. This entity is known for its predilection for elderly woman, and multifocality.

B. This is caused by HPV 16/18. The cause of proliferative verrucoid hyperplasia is unknown.
C. This is caused by cigarette and alcohol exposure. The cause of proliferative verrucoid hyperplasia is unknown.
D. All statements are true. False.
E. No statements are true. False.

9. ◘ Figures 3.87 and 3.88 are from the same patient. What is the stage and WPOI?
Stage III, pT2N1, no ENE, WPOI-5
Use the 1.0 mm scale bar in the bottom of the **top panel** for ◘ Fig. 3.87**.** Establish the horizon then drop a plumb line. The DOI is 6.7, therefor **pT2**. Notice the faint red ruler on the left hand side of the **bottom** of ◘ Fig. 3.87**?** The shortest distance between the outmost group of satellites and the next closest group is >1 mm (1.3 mm). **Therefore WPOI-5.** In looking for the shortest distance between two satellites or group of satellites, imagine you are crossing a river stepping over stones. You want to find the closest next stone to step on. ◘ Figure 3.88 represents the only positive lymph node. The lower panel represents a reaction at the level of the lymph node capsule. This sort of reaction, and even stretching of the capsule by metastatic carcinoma, does not represent extranodal extension (ENE). Therefore, this is pN1, no ENE.

10. Study ◘ Fig. 3.89. Where is this from? What is your diagnosis?
This is a **spindle cell variant of squamous carcinoma** from the **floor of mouth**. Let's first address the "where". Look at the large lobules of minor salivary tissue with their large ducts on the left side of the upper panel. The minor salivary tissue is embedded in loose fibroconnective tissue. No skeletal muscle is seen. This only happens in the floor of mouth. As for the "what", notice the exophytic polypoid nature of this tumor. This is typical, although not specific, for spindle cell variant of squamous carcinoma. ***Remember that spindle cell variant of squamous carcinoma is much more likely encountered than a true sarcoma***. Always consider the possibility that the patient may have had a prior sarcoma, and this might represent metastases. The lower panel reveals a high-grade spindle cell malignancy with a storiform ("rush mat") pattern. The inset shows a higher power view of these tumor cells. These spindle cells are more epithelioid, have more pink cytoplasm, than would a true sarcoma. The open chromatin pattern and prominent amphophilic nucleolus are also typical of a squamous carcinoma, compared with a true sarcoma. The diagnosis of spindle carcinoma can be confirmed if (1) adjacent squamous carcinoma-in-situ is present. (2) squamous differentiation with keratinization is observed, (3) IHC expression of keratins, p63, or p40. In the absence of these three conditions, you can still make this diagnosis with confidence, as long you have considered the possibility of metastases (◘ Fig. 3.90).

References

1. Reibel J, Tilakaratnew WM, Gale N, Westra WH, Hille J, Williams MD, Hunt JL, Vigneswaran N, Lingen M, Fatani HA, Muller S, Odell EW, Sloan P, Zain RB. Oral potentially malignant disorders and oral epithelial dysplasia. In: El-Naggar AK, JKC C, Grandis JR, Takata T, Slootweg PJ, editors. WHO classification of head and neck tumors. 4th ed. Lyon: IARC. 2015; p. 112–5.
2. Gopinath D, Thannikunnath BV, Neermunda SF. Prevalence of carcinomatous foci in oral leukoplakia: a clinicopathologic study of 546 Indian samples. J Clin Diagn Res. 2016;10(8):ZC78–83.

3. Bradley G, Odell EW, Raphael S, Ho J, Le LW, Benchimol S, Kamel-Reid S. Abnormal DNA content in oral epithelial dysplasia is associated with increased risk of progression to carcinoma. Br J Cancer. 2010;103:1432–42.
4. Liu W, Wang YF, Zhou HW, Shi P, Zhou ZT, Tang GY. Malignant transformation of oral leukoplakia: a retrospective cohort study of 218 Chinese patients. BMC Cancer. 2010;10:685. Published online 2010 Dec 16. https://doi.org/10.1186/1471-2407-10-685.
5. Liu W, Shi LJ, Wu L, Feng JQ, Yang X, Li J, Zhou ZT, Zhang CP. Oral cancer development in patients with leukoplakia – clinicopathological factors affecting outcome. PLoS One. 2012;7(4):e34773. https://doi.org/10.1371/journal.pone.0034773.
6. Dost F, Lê Cao K, Ford PJ, Ades C, Farah CS. Malignant transformation of oral epithelial dysplasia: a real-world evaluation of histopathologic grading. Oral Surg Oral Med Oral Pathol Oral Radiol. 2014;117:343–52.
7. Mehanna HM, Rattay T, Smith J, McConkey CC. Treatment and follow-up of oral dysplasia – a systematic review and meta-analysis. Head Neck. 2009;31:1600–9.
8. Warnakulasuriya S, Ariyawardana A. Malignant transformation of oral leukoplakia: a systematic review of observational studies. J Oral Pathol Med. 2016;45:155–66.
9. Wang YY, Tail YH, Wang WC, Chen CY, Kao YH, Chen YK, Chen CH. Malignant transformation in 5071 southern Taiwanese patients with potentially malignant oral mucosal disorders. BMC Oral Health. 2014. https://doi.org/10.1186/1472-6831-14-99.
10. Abadie WM, Partington EJ, Fowler CB, Schmalbach CE. Optimal management of proliferative verrucous leukoplakia: a systematic review of the literature. Otolaryngol Head Neck Surg. 2015;153:504–11.
11. Akrish S, Ben-Izhak O, Sabo E, Rachmiel A. Oral squamous cell carcinoma associated with proliferative verrucous leukoplakia compared with conventional squamous cell carcinoma–a clinical, histologic and immunohistochemical study. Oral Surg Oral Med Oral Pathol Oral Radiol. 2015;119:318–25.
12. Gillenwater AM, Vigneswaran N, Fatani H, Saintigny P, El-Naggar AK. Proliferative verrucous leukoplakia (PVL): a review of an elusive pathologic entity! Adv Anat Pathol. 2013;20:416–23.
13. Gillenwater AM, Vigneswaran N, Fatani H, Saintigny P, El-Naggar AK. Proliferative verrucous leukoplakia: recognition and differentiation from conventional leukoplakia and mimics. Head Neck. 2014;36:1662–8.
14. Arakeri G, Patil SG, Aljabab AS, Lin KC, Merkx MA, Gao S, Brennan PA. Oral submucous fibrosis: an update on pathophysiology of malignant transformation. J Oral Pathol Med. 2017. https://doi.org/10.1111/jop.12582.
15. Arakeri G, Boraks G, Patil SG, Aljabab AS, Merkx MA, Carrozzo M, Brennan PA. Current protocols in the management of oral submucous fibrosis: an update. J Oral Pathol Med. 2017. https://doi.org/10.1111/jop.12583.
16. Niaz K, Maqbool F, Khan F, Bahadar H, Ismail Hassan F, Abdollahi M. Smokeless tobacco (paan and gutkha) consumption and its prevalence contributing toward oral cancer. Epidemiol Health. 2017. https://doi.org/10.4178/epih.e2017009.
17. Yang PY, Chen YT, Wang YH, Su NY, Yu HC, Chang YC. Malignant transformation of oral submucous fibrosis in Taiwan: a nationwide population-based retrospective cohort study. J Oral Pathol Med. 2017. https://doi.org/10.1111/jop.12570.
18. Shirsat PM, Desai RS, Bansal S, Prasad P. Oral epithelial dysplasia in oral submucous fibrosis: a challenge. Oral Oncol. 2016;54:e19. https://doi.org/10.1016/j.oraloncology.2015.11.005. Epub 2015 Nov 19
19. Pandya S, Chaudhary AK, Singh M, Singh M, Ravi Mehrotra R. Correlation of histopathological diagnosis with habits and clinical findings in oral submucous fibrosis. Head Neck Oncol. Published online. 2009. https://doi.org/10.1186/1758-3284-1-10.
20. Haniffa AM, Saitoh M, Abiko Y, Takeshima M, Nishimura M, Yamazaki M, Nagayasu H, Sugiura C, Muthumala M, Kaku T, Chiba I, Shibata T. Expression pattern of p63 in oral epithelial lesions and submucous fibrosis associated with betel-quid chewing in Sri Lanka. Med Mol Morphol. 2007;40(4):203–7.
21. Gadbail AR, Chaudhary M, Gawande M, Hande A, Sarode S, Tekade SA, Korde S, Zade P, Bhowate R, Borle R, Patil S. Oral squamous cell carcinoma in the background of oral submucous fibrosis is a distinct clinicopathological entity with better prognosis. J Oral Pathol Med. 2017. https://doi.org/10.1111/jop.12553.
22. Sujatha D, Hebbar PB, Pai A. Prevalence and correlation of oral lesions among tobacco smokers, tobacco chewers, areca nut and alcohol users. Asian Pac J Cancer Prev. 2012;13:1633–7.
23. Greer RO Jr. Oral manifestations of smokeless tobacco use. Otolaryngol Clin N Am. 2011;44:31–56.
24. Mehta FS, Jalnawalla PN, Daftary DK, Gupta PC, Pindborg JJ. Reverse smoking in Andhra Pradesh, India: variability of clinical and histologic appearances of palatal changes. Int J Oral Surg. 1977;6:75–83.
25. Mehta FS, Sahiar BE, Daftary DK, Gupta PC, Pindborg JJ. A correlative histocytological study of carcinoma and epithelial atypia of the palate among Indian reverse smokers. Br J Cancer. 1972;26:230–3.
26. Pindborg JJ, Mehta FS, Gupta PC, Daftary DK, Smith CJ. Reverse smoking in Andhra Pradesh, India: a study of palatal lesions among 10,169 villagers. Br J Cancer. 1971;25:10–20.
27. Pednekar MS, Gupta PC, Yeole BB, Hébert JR. Association of tobacco habits, including bidi smoking, with overall and site-specific cancer incidence: results from the Mumbai cohort study. Cancer Causes Control. 2011;22:859–68.
28. Hongal BP, Kulkarni VV, Deshmukh RS, Joshi PS, Karande PP, Shroff AS. Prevalence of fungal hyphae in potentially malignant lesions and conditions—does its occurrence play a role in epithelial dysplasia? J Oral Maxillofac Pathol. 2015;19:10–7.
29. McCullough M, Jaber M, Barrett AW, Bain L, Speight PM, Porter SR. Oral yeast carriage correlates with presence of oral epithelial dysplasia. Oral Oncol. 2002;38:391–3.
30. de Sousa LVNF, Santos VL, Monteiro AS, Dias-Souza MV, Marques SG, Faria ES, Assunção EAO, Santos SG, Zonis JM, Alvarenga DG, Holanda RA, de Sousa JG, Santos KV, Stoianoff MAR. Isolation and identification of Candida species in patients with orogastric cancer: susceptibility to antifungal drugs, attributes of virulence in vitro and immune response phenotype. BMC

Infect Dis. 2016;16:86. Published online 2016 Feb 23. https://doi.org/10.1186/s12879-016-1431.
31. Bakri MM, Hussaini HM, Holmes AR, Cannon RD, Rich AM. Revisiting the association between candidal infection and carcinoma, particularly oral squamous cell carcinoma. J Oral Microbiol. 2010. https://doi.org/10.3402/jom.v2i0.5780.
32. Czerninski R, Zeituni S, Maly A, Basile J. Clinical characteristics of lichen and dysplasia vs lichen planus cases and dysplasia cases. Oral Dis. 2015;21:478–82.
33. Patil S, Rao RS, Sanketh DS, Warnakulasuriya S. Lichenoid dysplasia revisited – evidence from a review of Indian archives. J Oral Pathol Med. 2015;44:507–14.
34. Fitzpatrick SG, Hirsch SA, Gordon SC. The malignant transformation of oral lichen planus and oral lichenoid lesions: a systematic review. J Am Dent Assoc. 2014; 145:45–56.
35. Liu W, Shen ZY, Wang LJ, Hu YH, Shen XM, Zhou ZT, Li J. Malignant potential of oral and labial chronic discoid lupus erythematosus: a clinicopathological study of 87 cases. Histopathology. 2011;59:292–8.
36. Fernandes MS, Girisha BS, Viswanathan N, Sripathi H, Noronha TM. Discoid lupus erythematosus with squamous cell carcinoma: a case report and review of the literature in Indian patients. Lupus. 2015;24:1562–6.
37. Jadotte YT, Schwartz RA. Solar cheilosis: an ominous precursor: part I. Diagnostic insights. J Am Acad Dermatol. 2012;66:173–84.
38. Cavalcante AS, Anbinder AL, Carvalho YR. Actinic cheilitis: clinical and histological features. J Oral Maxillofac Surg. 2008;66:498–503.
39. Speight PM, Abram TJ, Floriano PN, James R, Vick J, Thornhill MH, McDevitt JT. Inter-observer agreement in dysplasia grading: towards an enhanced gold standard for clinical pathology trials. Oral Surg Oral Med Oral Pathol Oral Radiol. 120(4):474–482.e2.
40. Bouquot JE, Speight PM, Farthing PM. Epithelial dysplasia of the oral mucosa—Diagnostic problems and prognostic features. Curr Diagn Pathol. 2006;12:11–21.
41. http://globocan.iarc.fr/Pages/fact_sheets_population.aspx
42. Simard EP, Torre LA, Jemal A. International trends in head and neck cancer incidence rates: differences by country, sex and anatomic site. Oral Oncol. 2014;50:387–403.
43. Tataru D, Mak V, Simo R, Davies EA, Gallagher JE. Trends in the epidemiology of head and neck cancer in London. Clin Otolaryngol. 2017;42:104–14.
44. Shridhar K, Rajaraman P, Koyande S, Parikh PM, Chaturvedi P, Dhillon PK, Dikshit RP. Trends in mouth cancer incidence in Mumbai, India (1995–2009): an age-period-cohort analysis. Cancer Epidemiol. 2016;42:66–71.
45. Shield KD, Ferlay J, Jemal A, Sankaranarayanan R, Chaturvedi AK, Bray F, Soerjomataram I. The global incidence of lip, oral cavity, and pharyngeal cancers by subsite in 2012. CA Cancer J Clin. 2017;67:51–64.
46. Siddiqi K, Shah S, Abbas SM, Vidyasagaran A, Jawad M, Dogar O, Sheikh A. Global burden of disease due to smokeless tobacco consumption in adults: analysis of data from 113 countries. BMC Med. 2015;13: 194–216.
47. Mishra A, Meherotra R. Head and neck cancer: global burden and regional trends in India. Asian Pac J Cancer Prev. 2014;15:537–50.
48. Gupta B, Johnson NW, Kumar N. Global epidemiology of head and neck cancers: a continuing challenge. Oncology. 2016;91:13–23.
49. Smith EM, Rubenstein LM, Haugen TH, Pawlita M, Turek LP. Complex etiology underlies risk and survival in head and neck cancer human papillomavirus, tobacco, and alcohol: a case for multifactor disease. J Oncol. 2012;2012:571862. Published online 2012 Jan 23. https://doi.org/10.1155/2012/571862.
50. Zhang Y, Wang R, Miao L, Zhu L, Jiang H, Yuan H. Different levels in alcohol and tobacco consumption in head and neck cancer patients from 1957 to 2013. PLoS One. 2015;10(4):e0124045.
51. Radoï L, Menvielle G, Cyr D, Lapôtre-Ledoux B, Stücker I, Luce D. ICARE study group Population attributable risks of oral cavity cancer to behavioral and medical risk factors in France: results of a large population-based case–control study, the ICARE study. BMC Cancer. 2015;15:827. Published online 2015 Oct 31. https://doi.org/10.1186/s12885-015-1841-5.
52. Isayeva T, Xu J, Ragin C, Dai Q, Cooper T, Carroll W, Dayan D, Vered M, Wenig B, Rosenthal E, Grizzle W, Anderson J, Willey CD, Yang ES, Brandwein-Gensler M. The protective effect of p16(INK4a) in oral cavity carcinomas: p16(Ink4A) dampens tumor invasion-integrated analysis of expression and kinomics pathways. Mod Pathol. 2015;28:631–53.
53. Alamgir MM, Jamal Q, Mirza T. Conventional clinical and prognostic variables in 150 oral squamous cell carcinoma cases from the indigenous population of Karachi. Pak J Med Sci. 2016;32(3):672–6. https://doi.org/10.12669/pjms.323.9905.
54. Gupta B, Johnson NW. Systematic review and meta-analysis of association of smokeless tobacco and of betel quid without tobacco with incidence of oral cancer in South Asia and the Pacific. PLoS One. 2014;9(11):e113385. Published online 2014 Nov 20. https://doi.org/10.1371/journal.pone.0113385.
55. Maxwell JH, Thompson LD, Brandwein-Gensler MS, Weiss BG, Canis M, Purgina B, Prabhu AV, Lai C, Shuai Y, Carroll WR, Morlandt A, Duvvuri U, Kim S, Johnson JT, Ferris RL, Seethala R, Chiosea SI. Early oral tongue squamous cell carcinoma:sampling of margins from tumor bed and worse local control. JAMA Otolaryngol Head Neck Surg. 2015;141:1104–10.
56. Buchakjian MR, Tasche KK, Robinson RA, Pagedar NA, Sperry SM. Association of main specimen and tumor bed margin status with local recurrence and survival in oral cancer surgery. JAMA Otolaryngol Head Neck Surg. 2016;142:1191–8.
57. Liao CT, Chang JT, Wang HM, Ng SH, Hsueh C, Lee LY, Lin CH, Chen IH, Huang SF, Cheng AJ, Yen TC. Analysis of risk factors of predictive local tumor control in oral cavity cancer. Ann Surg Oncol. 2008;15(3):915–22.
58. Tasche KK, Buchakjian MR, Pagedar NA, Sperry SM. Definition of "close margin" in oral cancer surgery and association of margin distance with local recurrence rate. JAMA Otolaryngol Head Neck Surg. 2017. https://doi.org/10.1001/jamaoto.2017.0548.

59. Zanoni DK, Migliacci JC, Xu B, Katabi N, Montero PH, Ganly I, Shah JP, Wong RJ, Ghossein RA, Patel SG. A proposal to redefine close surgical margins in squamous cell carcinoma of the oral tongue. JAMA Otolaryngol Head Neck Surg. 2017. https://doi.org/10.1001/jamaoto.2016.4238.
60. Ebrahimi A, Gil Z, Amit M, Yen TC, Liao CT, Chaturvedi P, Agarwal JP, Kowalski LP, Kreppel M, Cernea CR, Brandao J, Bachar G, Bolzoni Villaret A, Fliss D, Fridman E, Robbins KT, Shah JP, Patel SG, Clark JR. Primary tumor staging for oral cancer and a proposed modification incorporating depth of invasion: an international multicenter retrospective study. JAMA Otolaryngol Head Neck Surg. 2014;140:1138–48.
61. Prabhu RS, Hanasoge S, Magliocca KR, Moeller BJ, Milas ZL, Hall WA, El-Deiry M, Wadsworth JT, Higgins KA, Beitler JJ. Extent of pathologic extracapsular extension and outcomes in patients with nonoropharyngeal head and neck cancer treated with initial surgical resection. Cancer. 2014;120:1499–506.
62. Wreesmann VB, Katabi N, Palmer FL, Montero PH, Migliacci JC, Gönen M, Carlson D, Ganly I, Shah JP, Ghossein R, Patel SG. Influence of extracapsular nodal spread extent on prognosis of oral squamous cell carcinoma. Head Neck. 2016;38(Suppl 1):E1192–9. https://doi.org/10.1002/hed.24190.
63. Subramaniam N, Balasubramanian D, Murthy S, Limbachiya S, Thankappan K, Iyer S. Adverse pathologic features in early oral squamous cell carcinoma and the role of postoperative radiotherapy-a review. Oral Surg Oral Med Oral Pathol Oral Radiol. 2017;pii: S2212–4403(17):30104–9. https://doi.org/10.1016/j.oooo.2017.03.002.
64. Chatzistefanou I, Lubek J, Markou K, Ord RA. The role of perineural invasion in treatment decisions for oral cancer patients: A review of the literature. J Craniomaxillofac Surg. 2017;pii: S1010–5182(17):30082–3. https://doi.org/10.1016/j.jcms.2017.02.022.
65. Barry CP, Wong D, Clark JR, Shaw RJ, Gupta R, Magennis P, Triantafyllou A, Gao K, Brown JS. Postoperative radiotherapy for patients with oral squamous cell carcinoma with intermediate risk of recurrence: A case match study. Head Neck. 2017. https://doi.org/10.1002/hed.24780. [Epub ahead of print] PubMed.
66. Brandwein-Gensler M, Teixeira M, Lewis C, et al. Oral squamous cell carcinoma: histological risk assessment, but not margin status, is strongly predictive of local disease-free and overall survival. Am J Surg Pathol. 2005;29:167–78.
67. Brandwein-Gensler M, Smith RV, Wang B, Penner C, Thielken A, Broughel D, Schiff B, Owen RP, Smith J, Sarta C, Hebert T, Nason R, Ramer M, Delacure M, Hirsch D, Myssiorek D, Heller K, Prystowsky M, Schlecht N, Negassa A. Validation of the histological risk model in a new patient cohort with primary head and neck squamous cell carcinoma. Am J Surg Pathol. 2010;34:676–88.
68. Li Y, Bai S, Carroll W, Dayan D, Dort JC, Heller K, Jour G, Lau H, Penner C, Prystowsky M, Rosenthal E, Schlecht NF, Smith RV, Urken M, Vered M, Wang B, Wenig B, Negassa A, Brandwein-Gensler M. Validation of the risk model: high-risk classification and tumor pattern of invasion predict outcome for patients with low-stage oral squamous cell carcinoma. Head Neck Pathol. 2013;7:211–23.
69. Jakobsson PÅ, Eneroth CM, Killander D, et al. Histologic classification and grading of malignancy in carcinoma of the larynx. Acta Radiol Ther Phys Biol. 1973;12:1–8.
70. Bryne M. Is the invasive front of an oral carcinoma the most important area for prognostication? Oral Dis. 1998;4:70–7.
71. Bryne M, Koppang HS, Lilleng R, et al. New malignancy grading is a better prognostic indicator than Broders' grading in oral squamous cell carcinomas. J Oral Pathol Med. 1989;18:432–7.
72. Miller ME, Palla B, Chen Q, Elashoff DA, Abemayor E, St John MA, Lai CK. A novel classification system for perineural invasion in noncutaneous head and neck squamous cell carcinoma: histologic subcategories and patient outcomes. Am J Otolaryngol. 2012;33:212–5.
73. Arora A, Husain N, Bansal A, Neyaz A, Jaiswal R, Jain K, Chaturvedi A, Anand N, Malhotra K, Shukla S. Development of a new outcome prediction model in early-stage squamous cell carcinoma of the oral cavity based on histopathologic parameters with multivariate analysis: the Aditi-Nuzhat lymph-node prediction score (ANLPS) system. Am J Surg Pathol. 2017. https://doi.org/10.1097/PAS.0000000000000843.
74. Hori Y, Kubota A, Yokose T, Furukawa M, Matsushita T, Takita M, Mitsunaga S, Mizoguchi N, Nonaka T, Nakayama Y, Oridate N. Predictive significance of tumor depth and budding for late lymph node metastases in patients with clinical N0 early oral tongue carcinoma. Head Neck Pathol. 2017. https://doi.org/10.1007/s12105-017-0814-1.
75. Attramadal CG, Kumar S, Boysen ME, Dhakal HP, Nesland JM, Bryne M. Tumor budding, EMT and cancer stem cells in T1-2/N0 oral squamous cell carcinomas. Anticancer Res. 2015;35:6111–20.
76. Numico G, Silvestris N, Grazioso RE. Advances in EGFR-directed therapy in head and neck cancer. Front Biosci (Schol Ed). 2011;3:454–66.
77. Koch DT, Pickhard A, Gebel L, Buchberger AMS, Bas M, Mogler C, Reiter R, Piontek G, Wirth M. Epidermal growth factor receptor variant III in head and neck squamous cell carcinoma is not relevant for targeted therapy and irradiation. Oncotarget. 2017;8(20):32668–82. https://doi.org/10.18632/oncotarget.15949.
78. Alterio D, Marvaso G, Maffini F, Gandini S, Chiocca S, Ferrari A, Preda L, Rocca MC, Lepanto D, Fodor C, Volpe S, Dicuonzo S, Laudati A, Giugliano G, Ansarin M, Jereczek-Fossa BA. Role of EGFR as prognostic factor in head and neck cancer patients treated with surgery and postoperative radiotherapy: proposal of a new approach behind the EGFR overexpression. Med Oncol. 2017;34(6):107. https://doi.org/10.1007/s12032-017-0965-7.
79. Boeckx C, Weyn C, Vanden Bempt I, Deschoolmeester V, Wouters A, Specenier P, Van Laer C, Van den Weyngaert D, Kockx M, Vermorken JB, Peeters M, Pauwels P, Lardon F, Baay M. Mutation analysis of genes in the EGFR pathway in head and neck cancer patients: implications for anti-EGFR treatment response. BMC Res Notes. 2014;7:337. https://doi.org/10.1186/1756-0500-7-337.

80. de Boer E, Warram JM, Tucker MD, Hartman YE, Moore LS, de Jong JS, Chung TK, Korb ML, Zinn KR, van Dam GM, Rosenthal EL, Brandwein-Gensler MS. *In Vivo* fluorescence immunohistochemistry: localization of fluorescently labeled cetuximab in squamous cell carcinomas. Sci Rep. 2015;5:101692015.
81. Even AJ, Hamming-Vrieze O, van Elmpt W, Winnepenninckx VJ, Heukelom J, Tesselaar ME, Vogel WV, Hoeben A, Zegers CM, Vugts DJ, van Dongen GA, Bartelink H, Mottaghy FM, Hoebers F, Lambin P. Quantitative assessment of Zirconium-89 labeled cetuximab using PET/CT imaging in patients with advanced head and neck cancer: a theragnostic approach. Oncotarget. 2017;8(3):3870–80.
82. Bauman JE, Duvvuri U, Gooding WE, Rath TJ, Gross ND, Song J, Jimeno A, Yarbrough WG, Johnson FM, Wang L, Chiosea S, Sen M, Kass J, Johnson JT, Ferris RL, Kim S, Hirsch FR, Ellison K, Flaherty JT, Mills GB, Grandis JR. Randomized,placebo-controlled window trial of EGFR, Src, or combined blockade in head and neck cancer. JCI Insight. 2017;2(6):e90449. https://doi.org/10.1172/jci.insight.90449.
83. Mann JE, Hoesli R, Michmerhuizen NL, Devenport SN, Ludwig ML, Vandenberg TR, Matovina C, Jawad N, Mierzwa M, Shuman AG, Spector ME, Brenner JC. Surveilling the potential for precision medicine-driven PD-1/PD-L1-targeted therapy in HNSCC. J Cancer. 2017;8:332–44.
84. Kogashiwa Y, Yasuda M, Sakurai H, Nakahira M, Sano Y, Gonda K, Ikeda T, Inoue H, Kuba K, Oba S, Ishikawa J, Enoki Y, Matsumura S, Minami K, Ebihara Y, Sugasawa M. PD-L1 expression confers better prognosis in locally advanced oral squamous cell carcinoma. Anticancer Res. 2017;37:1417–24.
85. Sajin M, Hodorogea Prisăcaru A, Luchian MC, Pătraşcu OM, Dumitru A, Costache D, Dumitrescu D, Vrînceanu D, Voinea LM, Simionescu O, Costache M. Acantholytic squamous cell carcinoma: pathological study of nine cases with review of literature. Romanian J Morphol Embryol. 2014;55:279–83.
86. Mardi K, Singh N. Acantholytic squamous cell carcinoma of the oral cavity: a rare entity. J Oral Maxillofac Pathol. 2014;18:S128–30.
87. Gu X, Jiang R, Fowler MR. Acantholytic squamous cell carcinoma in upper aerodigestive tract: histopathology, immunohistochemical profile and epithelial mesenchymal transition phenotype change. Head Neck Pathol. 2012;6:438–44.
88. Lee RJ, Lin T, Lee SA, Lee KK, Christensen RE. Importance of tumor extent in adenosquamous carcinoma of the head and neck: a retrospective cohort study. Oral Surg Oral Med Oral Pathol Oral Radiol. 2017;pii: S2212–4403(17):30106–2. https://doi.org/10.1016/j.oooo.2017.03.004.
89. Sravya T, Rao GV, Kumar MP, Sudheerkanth K. Oral adenosquamous carcinoma: report of a rare entity with a special insight on its histochemistry. J Oral Maxillofac Pathol. 2016;20:548.
90. Satomi T, Kohno M, Hasagawa O, Enomoto A, Abukawa H, Chikazu D, Yoshida M, Matsubayashi J, Nagao T. Adenosquamous carcinoma of the tongue: clinicopathologic study and review of the literature. Odontology. 2017;105:127–35.
91. Kass JI, Lee SC, Abberbock S, Seethala RR, Duvvuri U. Adenosquamous carcinoma of the head and neck: molecular analysis using CRTC-MAML FISH and survival comparison with paired conventional squamous cell carcinoma. Laryngoscope. 2015;125:E371–6.
92. Masand RP, El-Mofty SK, Ma XJ, Luo Y, Flanagan JJ, Lewis JS. Adenosquamous carcinoma of the head and neck: relationship to human papillomavirus and review of the literature. Head Neck Pathol. 2011;5:108–16.
93. Heera R, Ayswarya T, Padmakumar SK, Ismayil P. Basaloid squamous cell carcinoma of oral cavity: report of two cases. J Oral Maxillofac Pathol. 2016;20:545.
94. Patel PN, Mutalik VS, Rehani S, Radhakrishnan R. Basaloid squamous cell carcinoma of oral cavity with incongruent clinical course. BMJ Case Rep. 2013;2013. pii:bcr2013200441. https://doi.org/10.1136/bcr-2013-200441.
95. Fritsch VA, Gerry DR, Lentsch EJ. Basaloid squamous cell carcinoma of the oral cavity: an analysis of 92 cases. Laryngoscope. 2014;124:1573–8.
96. Khoury ZH, Bugshan A, Lubek JE, Papadimitriou JC, Basile JR, Younis RH. Glycogen-rich clear cell squamous cell carcinoma originating in the oral cavity. Head Neck Pathol. 2017. https://doi.org/10.1007/s12105-017-0812-3.
97. Kaliamoorthy S, Sethuraman V, Ramalingam SM, Arunkumar S. A rare case of clear cell variant of oral squamous cell carcinoma. J Nat Sci Biol Med. 2015;6:245–7.
98. Nainani P, Singh HP, Paliwal A, Nagpal N. A rare case report of clear cell variant of oral squamous cell carcinoma. J Clin Diagn Res. 2014;8:QD07–9.
99. Frazier JJ, Sacks H, Freedman PD. Primary glycogen-rich clear cell squamous cell carcinoma of the mandibular gingiva. Oral Surg Oral Med Oral Pathol Oral Radiol. 2012;114:e47–51.
100. Datar UV, Kale A, Mane D. Oral carcinoma cuniculatum: a new entity in the clinicopathological spectrum of oral squamous cell carcinoma. J Clin Diagn Res. 2017;11:ZD37–9.
101. Thavaraj S, Cobb A, Kalavrezos N, Beale T, Walker DM, Jay A. Carcinoma cuniculatum arising in the tongue. Head Neck Pathol. 2013;6:130–4.
102. Goh GH, Venkateswaran K, Leow PC, Loh KS, Thamboo TP, Petersson F. Carcinoma cuniculatum of the esophagus and tongue: report of two cases, including TP53 mutational analysis. Head Neck Pathol. 2014;8:261–8.
103. D'Souza G, Carey TE, William WN, Nguyen ML, Ko EC, Riddell J, Pai SI, Gupta V, Walline HM, Lee JJ, Wolf WT, Shin DM, Grandis JR, Ferris RL. Epidemiology of head and neck squamous cell cancer among HIV-infected patients. J Acquir Immune Defic Syndr. 2014;65:603–10.
104. Beachler DC, Abraham AG, Silverberg MJ, Jing Y, Fakhry C, Gill MJ, Kitahata MM, Klein MB, Burchell AN, Korthuis PT, Moore RD, D'Souza G. Incidence and risk factors of HPV-related and HPV-unrelated head and neck squamous cell carcinoma in HIV-infected individuals. Oral Oncol. 2017;50:1169–76.
105. Mehrad M, Carpenter DH, Chernock RD, Wang H, Ma XJ, Luo Y, Luo J, Lewis JS, El-Mofty SK. Papillary squamous cell carcinoma of the head and neck: clinicopathologic and molecular features with special reference to human papillomavirus. Am J Surg Pathol. 2013;37:1349–56.

106. Jo VY, Mills SE, Stoler MH, Stelow EB. Papillary squamous cell carcinoma of the head and neck: frequent association with human papillomavirus infection and invasive carcinoma. Am J Surg Pathol. 2009;33:1720–4.
107. Fitzpatrick SG, Neuman AN, Cohen DM, Bhattacharyya I. Papillary variant of squamous cell carcinoma arising on the gingiva: 61 cases reported from within a larger series of gingival squamous cell carcinoma. Head Neck Pathol. 2013;7:320–6.
108. Terada T. Papillary squamous cell carcinoma of the mandibular gingiva. Int J Clin Exp Pathol. 2012;5:707–9.
109. Terada T. Papillary squamous cell carcinoma of the oral cavity with acantholytic and pseudovascular features. Int J Clin Exp Pathol. 2011;4:794–6.
110. Ding Y, Ma L, Shi L, Feng J, Liu W, Zhou Z. Papillary squamous cell carcinoma of the oral mucosa: a clinicopathologic and immunohistochemical study of 12 cases and literature review. Ann Diagn Pathol. 2013;17:18–21.
111. Sarioglu S, Dogan E, Sahin Y, Uzun E, Bekis R, Ada E, Sagot O, Akman F. Undifferentiated laryngeal carcinoma with pagetoid spread. Head Neck Pathol. 2016;10:252–5.
112. Tan T, Jennings T, Carlson JA. Dedifferentiated salivary hybrid carcinoma of the maxillary sinus with pagetoid spread to the overlying lining mucosa. Head Neck Pathol. 2015;9:293–9.
113. Vidyavathi K, Prasad C, Kumar HM, Deo R. Pseudovascular adenoid squamous cell carcinoma of oral cavity: a mimicker of angiosarcoma. J Oral Maxillofac Pathol. 2012;16:288–90.
114. Zidar N, Gale N, Zupevc A, Dovsak D. Pseudovascular adenoid squamous-cell carcinoma of the oral cavity–a report of two cases. J Clin Pathol. 2006;59:1206–8.
115. Bavle RM, Govinda G, Venkataramanaiah PG, Muniswamappa S, Venugopal R. Fallacious carcinoma- spindle cell variant of squamous cell carcinoma. J Clin Diagn Res. 2016. https://doi.org/10.7860/JCDR/2016/16400.8099.
116. Reyes M, Pennacchiotti G, Valdes F, Montes R, Veloso M, Matamala MA, Zanolli L, Rojas-Alcayaga G. Sarcomatoid (spindle cell) carcinoma of tongue: a report of two cases. Case Rep Dent. 2015. https://doi.org/10.1155/2015/780856.
117. Romañach MJ, Azevedo RS, Carlos R, de Almeida OP, Pires FR. Clinicopathological and immunohistochemical features of oral spindle cell carcinoma. J Oral Pathol Med. 2010;39:335–41.
118. Watson RF, Chernock RD, Wang X, Liu W, Ma XJ, Luo Y, Wang H, El-Mofty SK, Lewis JS Jr. Spindle cell carcinomas of the head and neck rarely harbor transcriptionally-active human papillomavirus. Head Neck Pathol. 2013;7:250–7.
119. Bice TC, Tran V, Merkley MA, Newlands SD, van der Sloot PG, Wu S, Miller MC. Disease-specific survival with spindle cell carcinoma of the head and neck. Otolaryngol Head Neck Surg. 2015;153:973–80.
120. Gerry D, Fritsch VA, Lentsch EJ. Spindle cell carcinoma of the upper aerodigestive tract: an analysis of 341 cases with comparison to conventional squamous cell carcinoma. Ann Otol Rhinol Laryngol. 2014;123:576–83.
121. Terada T. Verrucous carcinoma of the oral cavity: a histopathologic study of 10 Japanese cases. J Maxillofac Oral Surg. 2011;10:148–51.
122. Candau-Alvarez A, Dean-Ferrer A, Alamillos-Granados FJ, Heredero-Jung S, García-García B, Ruiz-Masera JJ, Arévalo-Arévalo R, Zafra-Camacho F, Valenzuela-Salas B. Verrucous carcinoma of the oral mucosa: An epidemiological and follow-up study of patients treated with surgery in 5 last years. Med Oral Patol Oral Cir Bucal. 2014;19:e506–11.
123. Odar K, Kocjan BJ, Hošnjak L, Gale N, Poljak M, Zidar N. Verrucous carcinoma of the head and neck – not a human papillomavirus-related tumour? J Cell Mol Med. 2014;18:635–45.
124. Terada T. Squamous cell carcinoma arising within verrucous carcinoma of the oral cavity: a case report. Int J Clin Exp Pathol. 2012;5:363–6.
125. Patel KR, Chernock RD, Sinha P, Müller S, El-Mofty SK, Lewis JS. Verrucous carcinoma with dysplasia or minimal invasion: a variant of verrucous carcinoma with extremely favorable prognosis. Head Neck Pathol. 2015;9:65–73.
126. Wakeham K, Johnston WT, Nalwoga A, Webb EL, Mayanja BN, Miley W, Elliott AM, Whitby D, Newton R. Trends in Kaposi's sarcoma-associated Herpesvirus antibodies prior to the development of HIV-associated Kaposi's sarcoma: a nested case-control study. Int J Cancer. 2015;136:2822–30.
127. Douglas JL, Gustin JK, Moses AV, Dezube BJ, Pantanowitz L. Kaposi sarcoma pathogenesis: a triad of viral infection, oncogenesis and chronic inflammation. Transl Biomed. 2010;1:72.
128. Crosetti E, Succo G. Non-human immunodeficiency virus-related Kaposi's sarcoma of the oropharynx: a case report and review of the literature. J Med Case Rep. 2013;7:293. Published online 2013 Dec 31. https://doi.org/10.1186/1752-1947-7-293.
129. Kennedy-LeJeune E, Cataldo VD. Kaposi's sarcoma of the oral cavity. N Engl J Med. 2017;376:1268.
130. Carvajal RD, Spencer SA, Lydiatt W. Mucosal melanoma: a clinically and biologically unique disease entity. J Natl Compr Cancer Netw. 2012;10:345–56.
131. Rapini RP, Golitz LE, Greer RO Jr, Krekorian EA, Poulson T. Primary malignant melanoma of the oral cavity: a review of 177 cases. Cancer. 1985;55:1543–51.
132. Takagi M, Ishikawa G, Mori W. Primary malignant melanoma of the oral cavity in Japan: with special reference to mucosal melanosis. Cancer. 1974;34:358–70.
133. Aguas SC, Quarracino MC, Lence AN, Lanfranchi-Tizeira HE. Primary melanoma of the oral cavity: ten cases and review of 177 cases from the literature. Med Oral Patol Oral Cir Bucal. 2009;14:E265–E71.
134. Smith MH, Bhattacharyya I, Cohen DM, Islam NM, Fitzpatrick SG, Montague LJ, Damm DD, Fowler CB. Melanoma of the oral cavity: an analysis of 46 new cases with emphasis on clinical and histopathologic characteristics. Head Neck Pathol. 2016;10:298–305.
135. Broomhall C, Lewis MG. Malignant melanoma of the oral cavity in Ugandan Africans. Br J Surg. 1967;54:581–4.

136. Klein JD, Kupferman ME. Li-Fraumeni syndrome presenting as mucosal melanoma: case report and treatment considerations. Head Neck. 2017;39:E20–2.
137. Liu YS, Yang CH, Sun YF, Geng B, Yuan KF. Multivariate analysis of the prognostic factors in 230 surgically treated oral mucosal malignant melanomas. Shanghai Kou Qiamg Yi Xue. 2005;14:466–71.
138. Chatzistefanou I, Kolokythas A, Vahtsevanos K, Antoniades K. Primary mucosal melanoma of the oral cavity: current therapy and future directions. Oral Surg Oral Med Oral Pathol Oral Radiol. 2016;122:17–27.
139. Perloff JK. Remembering Sadao Otani. Am J Cardiol. 2013;111:1537–8.
140. Temam S, Mamelle G, Marandas P, Wibault P, Avril MF, Janot F, Julieron M, Schwaab G, Luboinski B. Postoperative radiotherapy for primary mucosal melanoma of the head and neck. Cancer. 2005;103:313–9.
141. Meleti M, Leemans CR, de Bree R, Vescovi P, Sesenna E, van der Waal I. Head and neck mucosal melanoma: experience with 42 patients, with emphasis on the role of postoperative radiotherapy. Head Neck. 2008;30:1543–51.
142. Ahn HJ, Na II, Park YH, Cho SY, Lee BC, Lee GH, Koh JS, Lee YS, Shim YS, Kim YK, Kang HJ, Ryoo BY, Yang SH. Role of adjuvant chemotherapy in malignant mucosal melanoma of the head and neck. Oral Oncol. 2010;46:607–11.
143. Margolin K. The promise of molecularly targeted and immunotherapy for advanced melanoma. Curr Treat Options in Oncol. 2016 Sep;17(9):48. https://doi.org/10.1007/s11864-016-0421-5.
144. Koto M, Demizu Y, Saitoh JI, Suefuji H, Tsuji H, Okimoto T, Ohno T, Shioyama Y, Takagi R, Nemoto K, Nakano T, Kamada T, Japan Carbon-Ion Radiation Oncology Study Group. Multicenter study of carbon-ion radiation therapy for mucosal melanoma of the head and neck: subanalysis of the Japan Carbon-Ion Radiation Oncology Study Group (J-CROS) study (1402 HN). Int J Radiat Oncol Biol Phys. 2017;97:1054–60.
145. Bladé J, Fernández de Larrea C, Rosiñol L, Cibeira MT, Jiménez R, Powles R. Soft-tissue plasmacytomas in multiple myeloma: incidence, mechanisms of extramedullary spread, and treatment approach. J Clin Oncol. 2011;29:3805–12.
146. Witt C, Borges AC, Klein K, Neumann HJ. Radiographic manifestations of multiple myeloma in the mandible: a retrospective study of 77 patients. J Oral Maxillofac Surg. 1997;55:450–3.
147. Sreeja C, Vijayabanu B, Vijayalakshmi D, Devi M, Ramakrishnan K, Dhivya K. Multiple myeloma involving mandible: In an elderly female. J Pharm Bioallied Sci. 2015;7:S763–5.
148. Kasamatsu A, Kimura Y, Tsujimura H, Kanazawa H, Koide N, Miyamoto I, Endo-Sakamoto Y, Shiiba M, Tanzawa H, Uzawa K. Maxillary swelling as the first evidence of multiple myeloma. Case Rep Dent. 2015;2015:439536. https://doi.org/10.1155/2015/439536.
149. Goetze E, Walter C, Kämmerer PW. Osseous plasma cell neoplasm of the mandible for initial diagnosis of multiple myeloma: case report and literature review. J Maxillofac Oral Surg. 2015;14:469–74.
150. Ramaiah KK, Joshi V, Thayi SR, Sathyanarayana P, Patil P, Ahmed Z. Multiple myeloma presenting with a maxillary lesion as the first sign. Imaging Sci Dent. 2015;45:55–60.
151. Wei H, Pinting L, Enyi T, Zhiyong W. Initial finding of mandible mass in multiple myeloma. J Craniofac Surg. 2012;23:e599–600.
152. Vallet S, Podar K. New insights, recent advances, and current challenges in the biological treatment of multiple myeloma. Expert Opin Biol Ther. 2013;13:S35–53.
153. Highsmith KN, Chen SE, Horowitz S. Carfilzomib and pomalidomide: recent advances in the treatment of multiple myeloma. Pharmacotherapy. 2014;34:927–40.
154. Campisi G, Fedele S, Fusco V, Pizzo G, Di Fede O, Bedogni A. Epidemiology, clinical manifestations, risk reduction and treatment strategies of jaw osteonecrosis in cancer patients exposed to antiresorptive agents. Future Oncol. 2014;10:257–75.
155. Vescovi P, Nammour S. Bisphosphonate-Related Osteonecrosis of the Jaw (BRONJ) therapy. A critical review. Minerva Stomatol. 2010;59:181–203–204–13.
156. Lazaridou MN, Katopodi T, Dimitrakopoulos I. Gorlin-Goltz syndrome: a 25-year follow-up of a familial case. Oral Maxillofac Surg. 2015;19:79–84.
157. Onodera S, Saito A, Hasegawa D, Morita N, Watanabe K, Nomura T, Shibahara T, Ohba S, Yamaguchi A, Azuma T. Multi-layered mutation in hedgehog-related genes in Gorlin syndrome may affect the phenotype. PLoS One. 2017;12(9):e0184702. https://doi.org/10.1371/journal.pone.0184702.
158. Bresler SC, Padwa BL, Granter SR. Nevoid basal cell carcinoma syndrome (Gorlin syndrome). Head Neck Pathol. 2016;10:119–24.
159. de Santana ST, Vajgel A, Martins-Filho PR, de Albuquerque Maranhao Filho AW, De Holanda Vasconcellos RJ, Frota R, Filho JR. Nevoid Basal cell carcinoma syndrome: A long-term study in a family. Craniomaxillofac Trauma Reconstr. 2016;9:94–104.
160. Koutlas IG, Koch CA, Vickers RA, Brouwers FM, Vortmeyer AO. An unusual ostensible example of intraoral basal cell carcinoma. J Cutan Pathol. 2009;36:464–70.
161. Lazaridou MN, Dimitrakopoulos I, Tilaveridis I, Iliopoulos C, Heva A. Basal cell carcinoma arising in association with a maxillary keratocyst in a patient with Gorlin-Goltz syndrome. Report of a case. Oral Maxillofac Surg. 2012;16:127–31.
162. Ridge JA, Lydiatt WM, Patel SG, Glastonbury CM, Brandwein-Gensler M, Ghossein RA, Shah JP. Lip and oral cavity. In: Amin MB et al., editors. AJCC cancer stagin manual. 8th ed. 2016; p. 79–101.

Oropharynx, Hypopharynx, and Parapharyngeal Space: Anatomy, Histology, Benign and Malignant Neoplasia

M. S. Brandwein-Weber, *Textbook of Head and Neck Pathology*,
https://doi.org/10.1007/978-3-319-76106-0_4

Key Points

- Each pathology department has a policy for exempting tissue from submission to pathology. The published literature support the idea that bilateral tonsillectomy specimens for obstructive sleep apnea or chronic tonsillitis may undergo gross examination only.
- Parapharyngeal space tumors present as intraoral soft palate bulge. Expect to encounter pleomorphic adenomas and Schwannomas in this setting.
- Many a low-grade liposarcoma of the hypopharynx has been initially diagnosed as something else. However, polypoid hollow-organ lipomatous tumors all warrant the same conservative surgical approach. Well-differentiated liposarcomas can manifest their unique potential in the form of multiple local recurrences, which still can be treated conservative re-excision.
- p16 overexpression is a surrogate biomarker for high-risk Human Papillomavirus (HR-HPV) only in the ***limited context*** of oropharyngeal cancers. p16 overexpression may be observed in other malignancies, even non-epithelial malignancies, with no relationship to HR-HPV.
- *In-situ* hybridization for HR-HPV is recommended in the setting of metastatic carcinoma from unknown tumor primary.
- The four histologic features that suggest HPV-mediated cancer are: (1) nonkeratinizing morphology, (2) multinucleated tumor giant cells, (3) "inside out" maturation, (4) cystic metastases.

4.1 Anatomy and Histology

The anterior anatomic boundaries of the oropharynx are the border of the soft palate, the anterior tonsillar pillars, and the lingual circumvallate papillae. The level of the soft palate separates the oropharynx from the nasopharynx (◘ Figs. 4.1, 4.2, and 4.3). The level of the tip of the epiglottis separates the oropharynx from the hypopharynx (laryngopharynx). ◘ Table 4.1 details the anatomic structures contained within these two anatomic compartments.

The parapharyngeal space is a fibrofatty potential space which becomes clinically manifest when involved by inflammation (parapharyngeal abscess) or tumor. It is shaped like an inverted pyramid; its base reaches superiorly to the skull base and its apex points to the greater cornu of the hyoid bone. The anterior margin is the deep cervical fascia which surrounds the medial pterygoid muscle. The posterior margin is the prevertebral layer of the deep cervical fascia. The medial margin is the pretracheal layer of the deep cervical fascia. The lateral margin is the fascia that invests the deep cervical fascia which covers the deep parotid lobe. The parapharyngeal space can be divided into pre-styloid and post-styloid compartments by the fascia which extends from the styloid process to the tensor veli palatini. The contents of the pre-styloid compartment include the deep lobe of the parotid gland and minor salivary glands, lymph nodes, and parapharyngeal fat. These tissues can then give rise to salivary tumors, lymphomas, and lipomas. The post-styloid compartment contains the carotid artery, jugular vein, cranial nerves IX–XII, lymph nodes, cervical sympathetic chain, and glomus tissue. The contents of the post-styloid compartment can give rise to paragangliomas, nerve sheath tumors, ganglioneuromas, lymphomas, and connective tissue tumors.

The extreme paradigm shift when contrasting the pathobiologies of squamous carcinomas from the oral cavity and from the oropharynx can be understood by comparing the normal histology and function of these two anatomic sites. The "*raison d'etre*" of the oropharynx is maintainence of local immunity by the mucosal associated lymphoid tissue (MALT) of Waldeyer's ring. The epithelial crypts of Waldeyer's ring are lined by specialized **reticulated epithelium**, which is thinner than stratified squamous epithelium and characterized by abundant intraepithelial lymphocytes and mononuclear cells. Additionally, the basement membrane in this region is composed of fine, discontinuous fibers, thus enabling

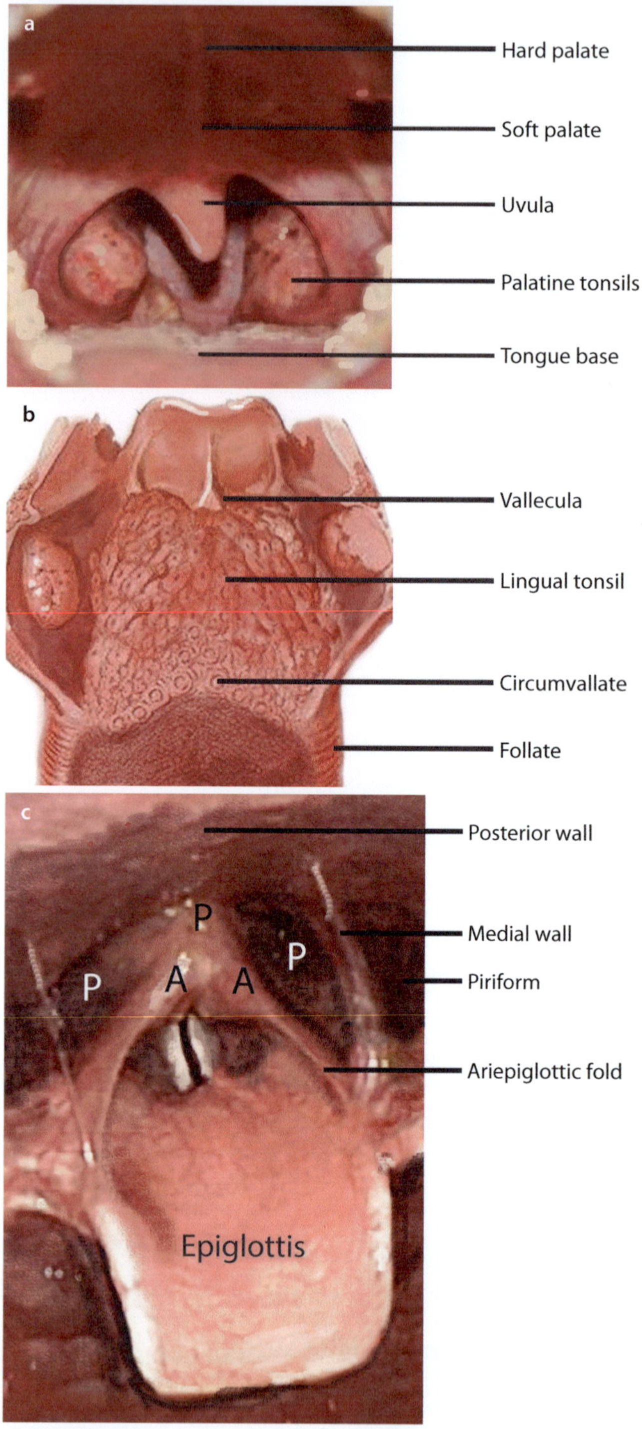

Fig. 4.1 **a**, **b** The anterior border of the oropharynx commences at the anterior tonsillar pillar (*white arrow*). The soft palate represents the superior border. The oropharynx is comprised of the base of tongue, anterior and posterior tonsillar pillars, palatine (pharyngeal) tonsils, glossotonsillar sulci (*black arrow*), vallecular, and lateral and posterior pharyngeal walls. **c** The hypopharynx represents the postcricoid region, which terminates in the esophagus. The two piriform sinuses act as gutters leading to the esophagus. **P**: postcricoid region, **A**: arytenoids. The lateral aspect of the postcricoid region forms the medial wall of the piriform

lymphocyte trafficking [1–3] (Fig. 4.4). By analogy to the uterine cervical squamocolumnar transition zone, the basal and parabasal cells of the reticulated epithelium are more accessible to HPV infection. Conversely, it is known that *intact* keratinizing stratified squamous epithelium is protected from HPV infection, requiring some level of microtrauma for access to

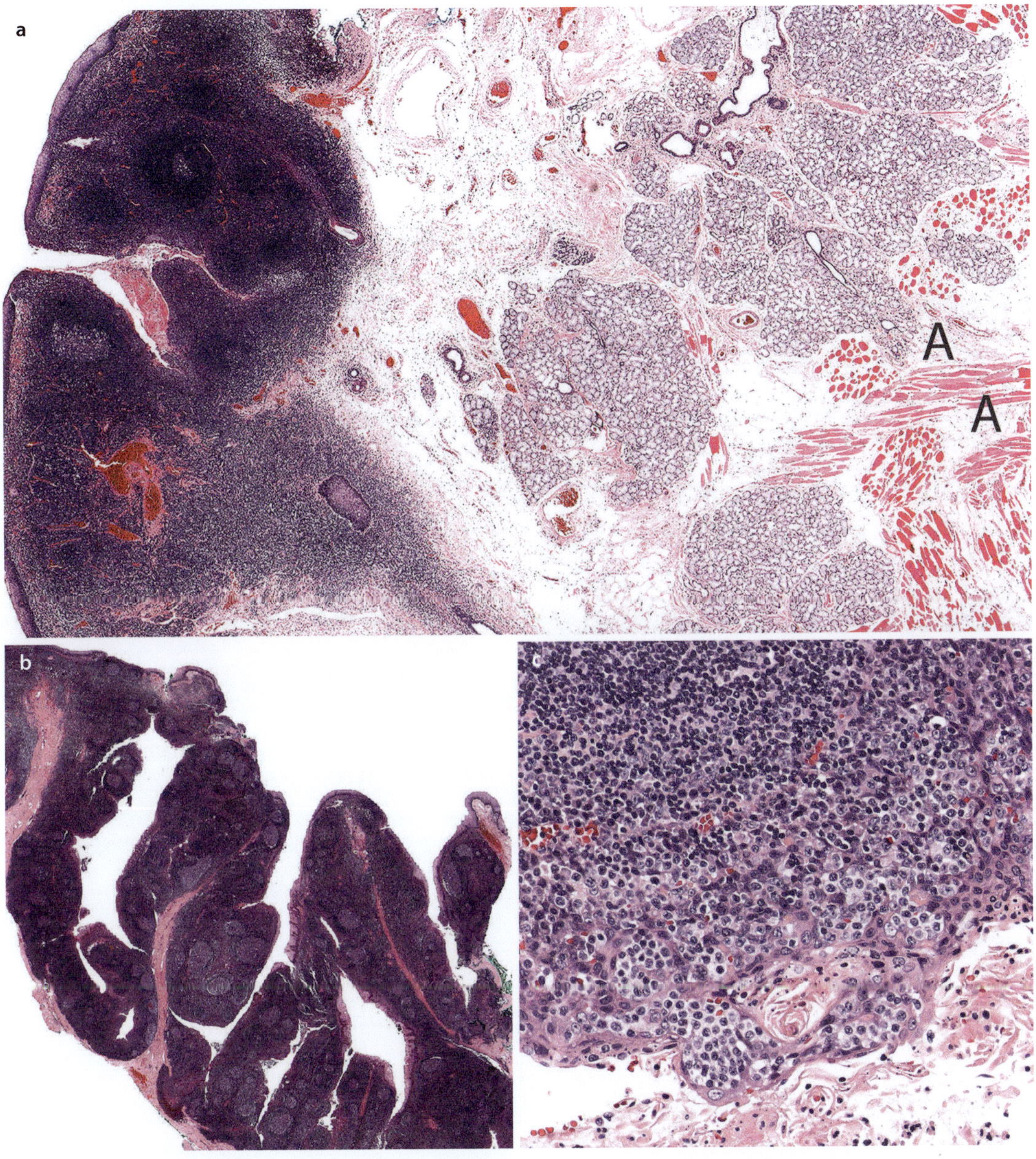

Fig. 4.2 **a** The tongue base is directly posterior to the circumvallate papillae and contain a variable amount of lingual tonsillar tissue. Note the windows of adipose tissue **a** which are more abundant in the posterior tongue and tongue base. **b** The palatine tonsils (faucial tonsils) have more extensive epithelial crypts than the other tonsillar tissues. The reticulated epithelium of this crypts have incomplete basement membranes, which allow for lymphocyte trafficking

basal/parabasal cells, where HPV is maintained [4, 5]. It is also known that the cycle of HPV from early to productive infection is entwined with the state of differentiation of squamous epithelium; ***virion production requires keratinizing epithelium*** [6].

4.2 Tonsillectomy Specimens

It is quite timely to revisit the issue of cost-effectiveness of histological examination of tonsillectomy specimens. The clinical indications for routine bilateral tonsillectomy are multiple

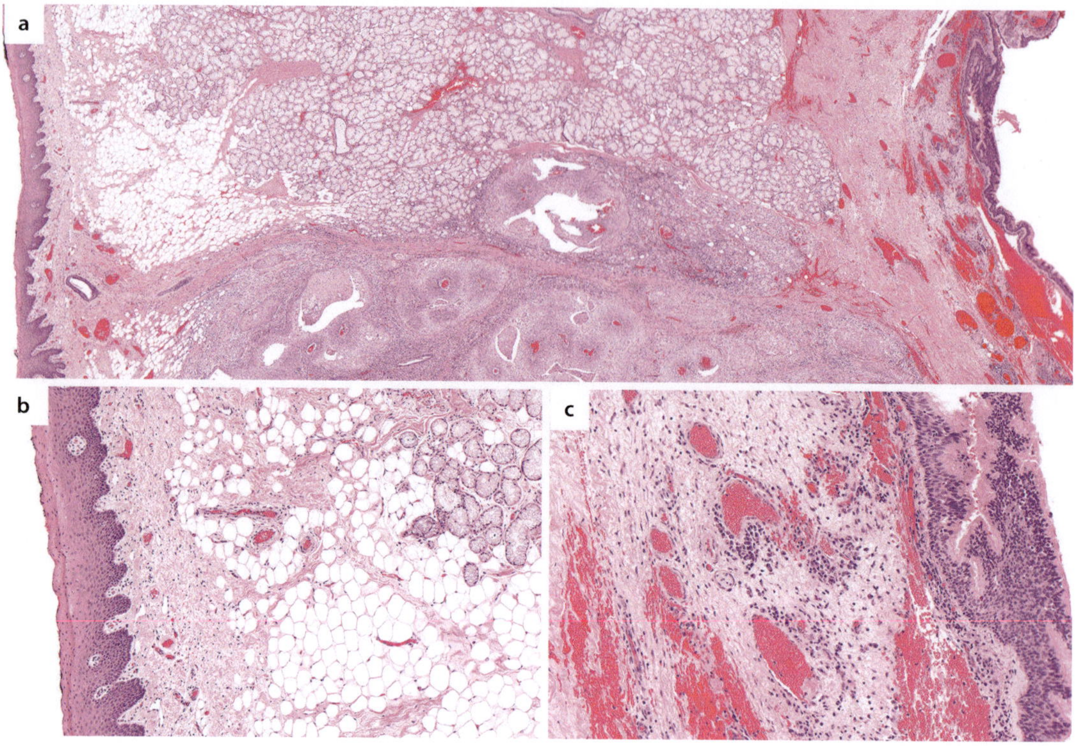

Fig. 4.3 **a** The soft palate is also within the oropharynx. This soft palate is resected for carcinoma. **b** The oral aspect of the soft palate is lined by stratified squamous epithelium. **c** The nasopharyngeal surface is lined by stratified ciliated respiratory mucosa

Table 4.1 Anatomic definitions

Oropharynx	Borders: Superior surface soft palate to superior hypoid bone/valleculla
	Inferior, anterior soft palate, and uvula
	Base of tongue, lingual tonsils
	Anterior and posterior tonsillar pillars
	Palatine (pharyngeal) tonsils
	Vallecula
	Glossotonsillar sulci
	Lateral and posterior pharyngeal walls
Hypopharynx	Borders: Superior hypoid bone/vallecullae to Inferior cricoid/esophagus
	Piriform sinuses
	Lateral and posterior hypopharyngeal walls
	Posterior cricoid region: including arytenoids and aryepiglottic folds
Parapharyngeal space	Glossopharyngeal nerve (IX)
	Vagus nerve (X)
	Internal carotid artery
	Internal jugular vein
	Accessory nerve (XI)
	Hypoglossal (XII)
	Sympathetic trunk and superior cervical ganglion
	Ascending pharyngeal artery
	Deep cervical lymph nodes

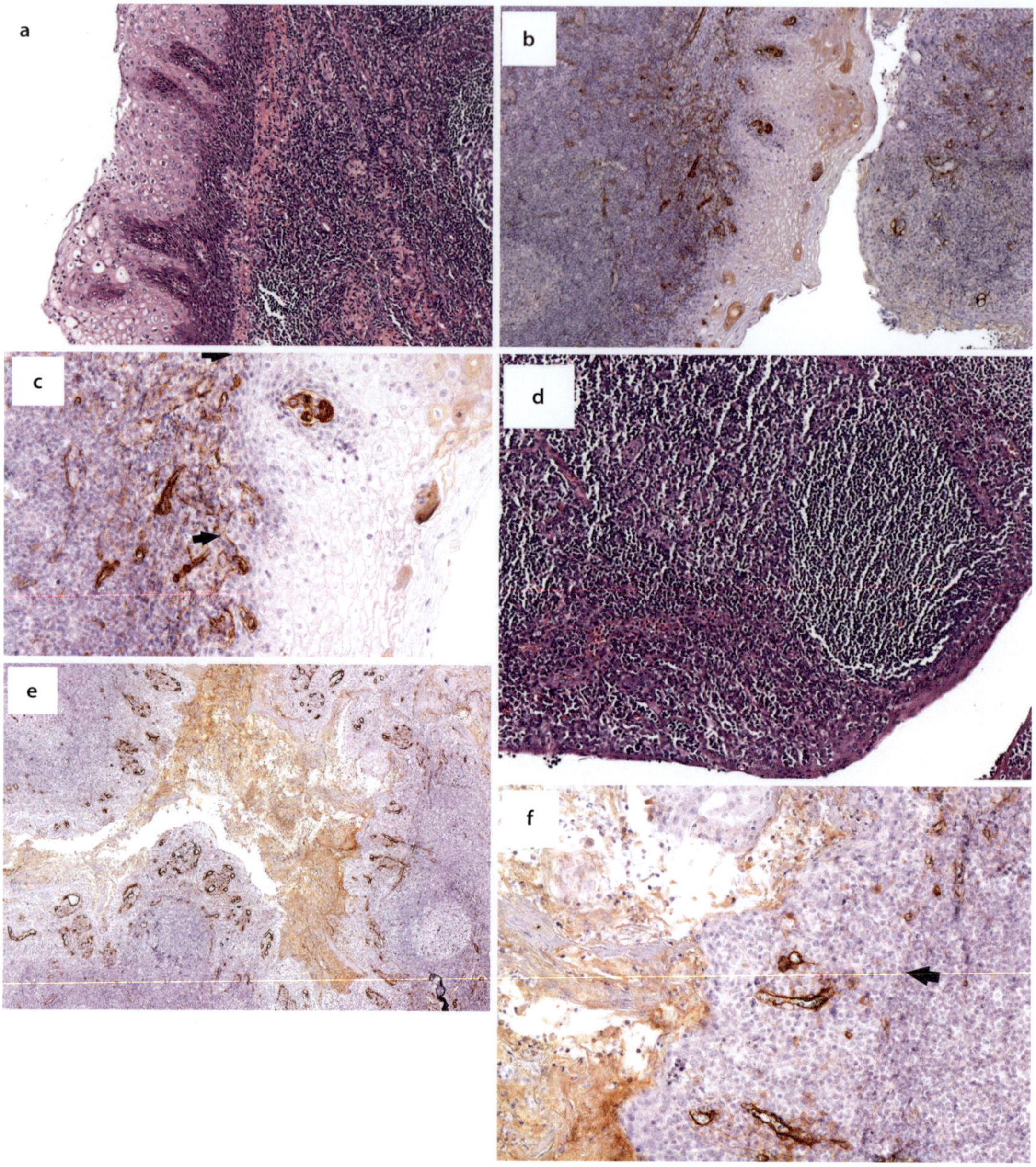

Fig. 4.4 **a–c** Stratified squamous epithelium of the tonsil versus reticulated epithelium **d–f** The stratified squamous epithelium demonstrates distinct boundary between epithelium and lymphoid tissue and linear collagen IV at basement membrane zone (**b**, **c**, *black arrow*). Reticulated epithelium is characterized by abundant migrating intraepithelial lymphocytes and a more subtle epithelial/lymphocyte boundary. Discontinuity of the supporting basement membrane fibers enables lymphocyte trafficking. The basement membrane zone here lacks collagen IV deposition (**e**, **f**, *black arrow*). Perivascular collagen is seen at both sites

episodes of tonsillitis, history of peritonsillar abscess, and obstructive sleep apnea. The concern with foregoing histological analysis would naturally be missing unexpected occult malignancies. *Recent systematic literature reviews support that conclusion that histological examination is unnecessary for routine bilateral tonsillectomies performed for the above indications, in both pediatric and adult populations* [7, 8]. Clinical setting requiring histological examination of tonsillectomies include: immunosuppression, organ transplantation, enlarged cervical lymph nodes, documentation or suspicion of malignancy, and unilateral tonsillar enlargement. Not surprisingly, 94% of patients with HPV-mediated oropharyngeal carcinomas have positive cervical lymph nodes, supporting the idea that HPV-mediated tonsillar cancer is highly unlikely to be an incidental finding in a routine adult tonsillectomy with normal gross appearence [9]. In one clinical review, a 45 year old male undergoing uvulopalatoplasty for obstructive sleep apnea was found to have an incidental HPV-mediated tonsillar carcinoma [7]. Unfortunately, the gross characteristics for this patient's specimens was not discussed. It would be hard to believe that the tonsils in this case appeared entirely normal on palpation and examination. Residents and pathology assistants are not absolved from careful gross inspection, palpation, serially sectioning, and examination of these specimens.

4.3 Lingual Thyroid

Lingual thyroid refers the persistence of thyroid tissue in the region of the foramen cecum (◘ Fig. 4.5). Thyroid embryogenesis commences around day 24 as a thickening in the floor of the primitive pharynx. The thyroid diverticulum migrates caudally reaching its final location inferior to the hyoid bone, anterior to the trachea, by week 7. Failure of the thyroid anlage to migrate results in lingual thyroid ectopy, which is only ***rarely*** associated with orthotopic thyroid [10, 11]. Persistent thyroglossal duct is caused by failure of this migratory track to regress. Cystic dilation of this thyroglossal duct manifests as a midline neck cyst; orthotopic thyroid is very common in the setting of a thyroglossal duct cyst. Concurrent lingual and thyroglossal ectopia and absent orthotopic thyroid are rare [12, 13]. Lingual ectopic thyroid may be asymptomatic, or may cause dysphonia, dysphagia, or dyspnea [14]. The development of papillary thyroid carcinoma within lingual thyroid is extraordinarily rare [15]. Corrective surgery is called a Sistrunk procedure, which includes dissection back to the hyoid bone. The bony segment should be documented during gross examination, but need not submitted for evaluation. The cyst wall is composed of simple respiratory mucosa. Thyroid tissue may or may not be identified in the specimen; IHC for thyroglobulin is unnecessary.

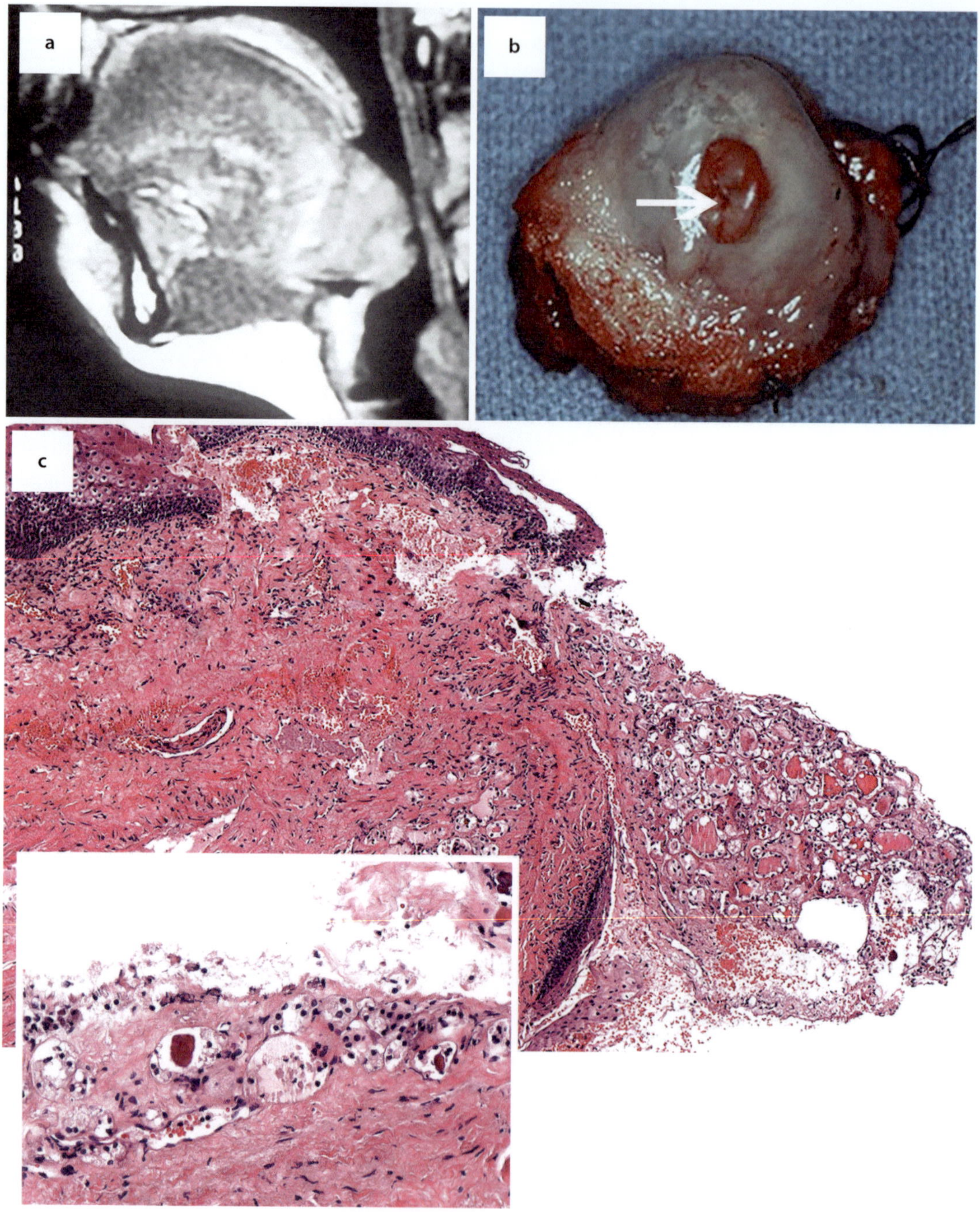

Fig. 4.5 **a** Undescended thyroid tissue may cause a symptomatic mass. Notice how this mass touches the epiglottis. **b** Tongue base resection with a submucosal mass with an area of ulceration and neovascularization (*arrow*). **c** and **inset**: Normal thyroid tissue in a tongue base excision for "mass". (Courtesy of Dr. S Wei)

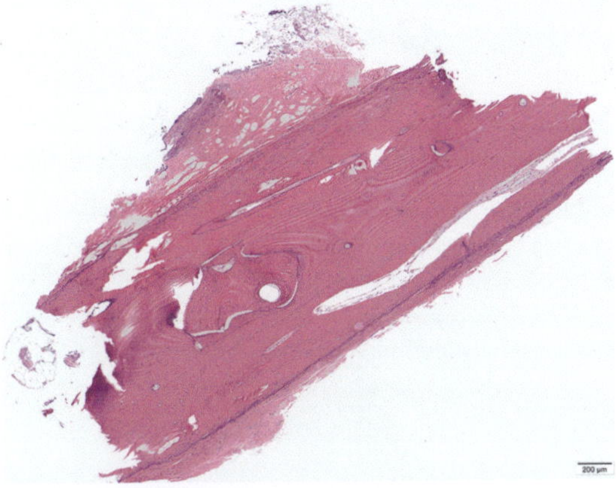

Fig. 4.6 Eagle's syndrome – This specimen might not look like anything specific to you, but look again! Resection of the hyoid bone, as seen in a Sistrunk procedure, shows sharp saw cuts. It does not have the slightly irregular contours of an ossified ligament. There is no other normal bony structures to consider with this tube-like appearance

4.4 Eagle's Syndrome

Eagle's syndrome represents a rare condition characterized by sharp pain throat while swallowing. It is caused by ossification of the stylohyoid ligament or elongation of the styloid process. This ossified ligament or elongated styloid process can be seen on a plain radiograph. Excision is curative. The specimen consists of an elongated tube of mature bone (Fig. 4.6).

4.5 Lymphangioma of Tonsil

A lymphangioma represents a benign proliferation of lymphatic channels, which can be classified as either: simple, cavernous, or cystic, based on the characteristics of the formed lymphatic spaces. The majority (90%) of lymphangiomas occur in the head and neck, usually skin and subcutaneous tissues. Cystic hygroma represents, as the name implies, a lymphangioma of the neck which forms massive cystic spaces. Lymphangiomas of other, nonsubcutaneous head and neck sites are very uncommon. Tonsillar lymphangiomas have been reported under other names such as tonsillar lymphangiomatous polyp, angiofibroma, fibrolipoma, hamartomatous tonsillar polyp, and lymphangiectatic fibrous polyp. Tonsillar lymphangiomas present as polypoid or pedunculated lesions [16–20]. They are commonly asymptomatic, but occasionally may become large enough to cause upper airway symptoms. Excisional biopsy is necessary to establish the diagnosis. Excision is curative [16].

Histologically, these pedunculated lesions have intact overlying squamous epithelium; the stroma contains abundant dilated simple lymphatic spaces. Lymphatic valves may be observed within these spaces. Lymphoid aggregates (lymphocytic epitheliotropsm) can be seen either within stroma and/or lymphatic spaces. Occasionally the lymphocytic epitheliotropsm may be quite robust, almost obliterating the diagnostic abundant dilated simple lymphatic spaces [20]. Immunohistochemistry confirms D2–40 expression, as well as FVIII, CD31 and CD34. The intervening stroma is collagenized and may contain adipose tissue.

4.6 Squamous Papilloma

Squamous (exophytic) papillomas are routinely encountered in the soft palate and tonsillar pillae [21]. Clinically, these lesions have frond-like white projections, which histologically represent stratified squamous epithelium covering fibrovascular cores.

4.7 Lymphoid Papillary Hyperplasia

This rare entity can clinically appear as numerous papillary projections, similar to squamous papilloma. However, these projections are histologically composed of excess lymphoid germinal centers covered by reticulated epithelium [22, 23].

4.8 Inlet Patch

Inlet patch refers to islands of heterotopic gastric mucosa in the cervical esophagus which can be observed in 1.4%–14% of patients undergoing upper gastrointestinal endoscopy [24–28]. Endoscopically, this appears as a salmon colored mucosal patch, which may be asymptomatic. Histologically, columnar gastric epithelium is present with either gastric body or gastric cardia glands, +/− intestinal metaplasia (Fig. 4.7).

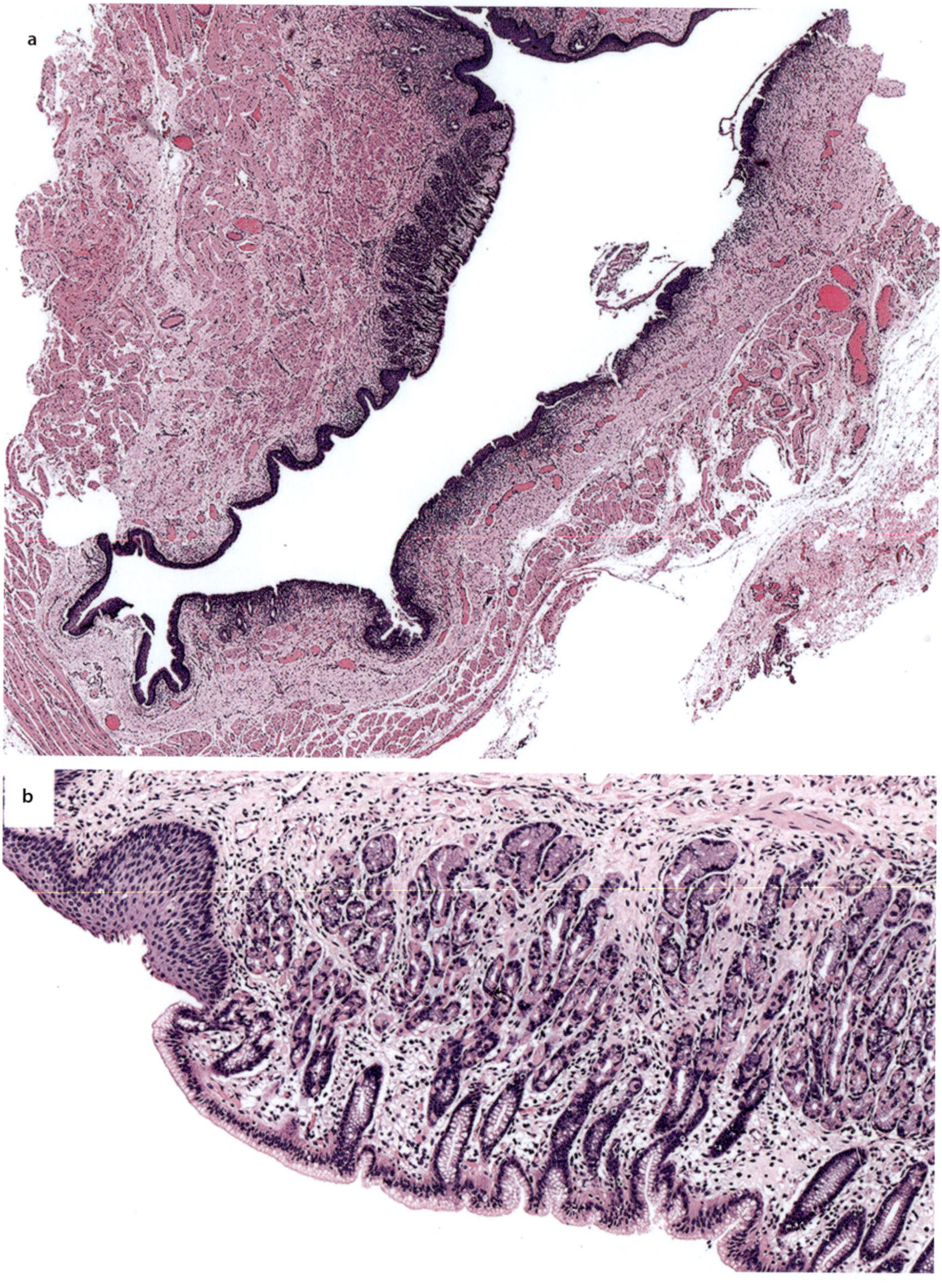

Fig. 4.7 Inlet patch: **a** Low power, **b** High power. Heterotopic gastric mucosa may be present in the superior esophagus discovered incidentally during a gastric pull-up reconstruction

4.9 Lymphoepithelial Cyst

A lymphoepithelial cyst in the tonsillar region results from obstruction of a tonsillar crypt, and has no association with persistence of branchial clefts [29, 30]. Histologically, it is composed of cystically dilated reticular epithelium (tonsillar crypt) surrounded by tonsillar lymphoid tissue (◘ Fig. 4.8).

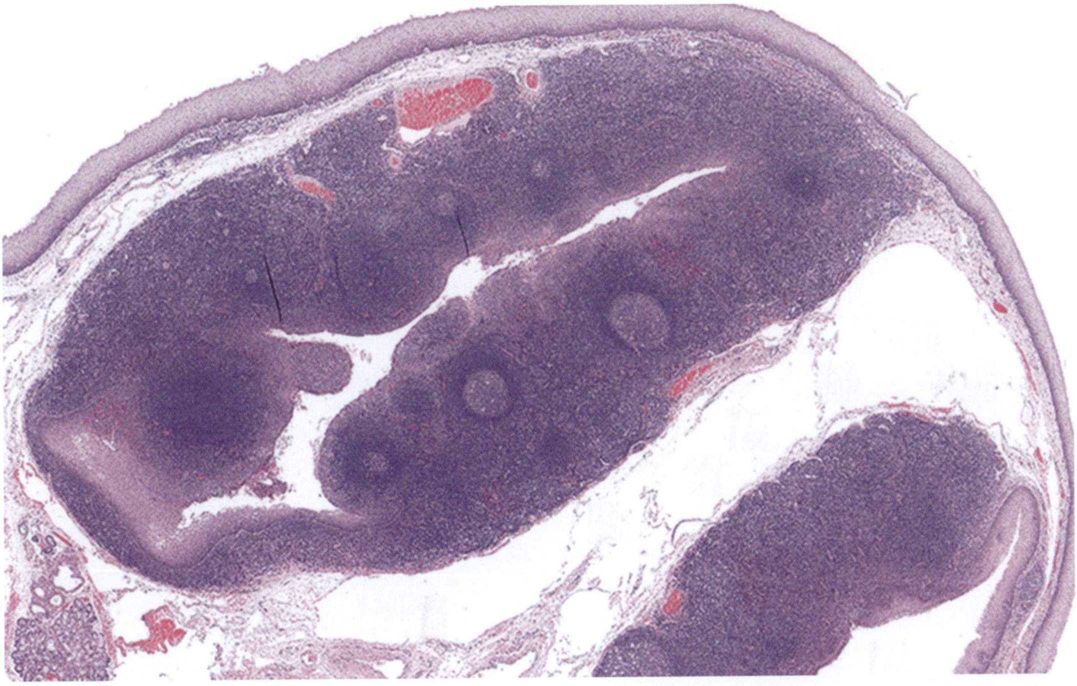

◘ **Fig. 4.8** Lymphoepithelial cyst of lingual tonsil

4.10 Mucinosis

Focal mucinosis is rare cause for a submucosal oropharyngeal lesion (◘ Fig. 4.9). Histopathologically, one sees a submucosal localized, lightly basophilic deposition of loose mucinous material, containing scattered stellate fibroblasts and capillaries. No inflammation should be seen. Mucicarmine stain will be negative or weakly positive. Alcian blue stain should be positive, and staining is abolished with hyaluronidase treatment. The stellate fibroblasts are S100 negative.

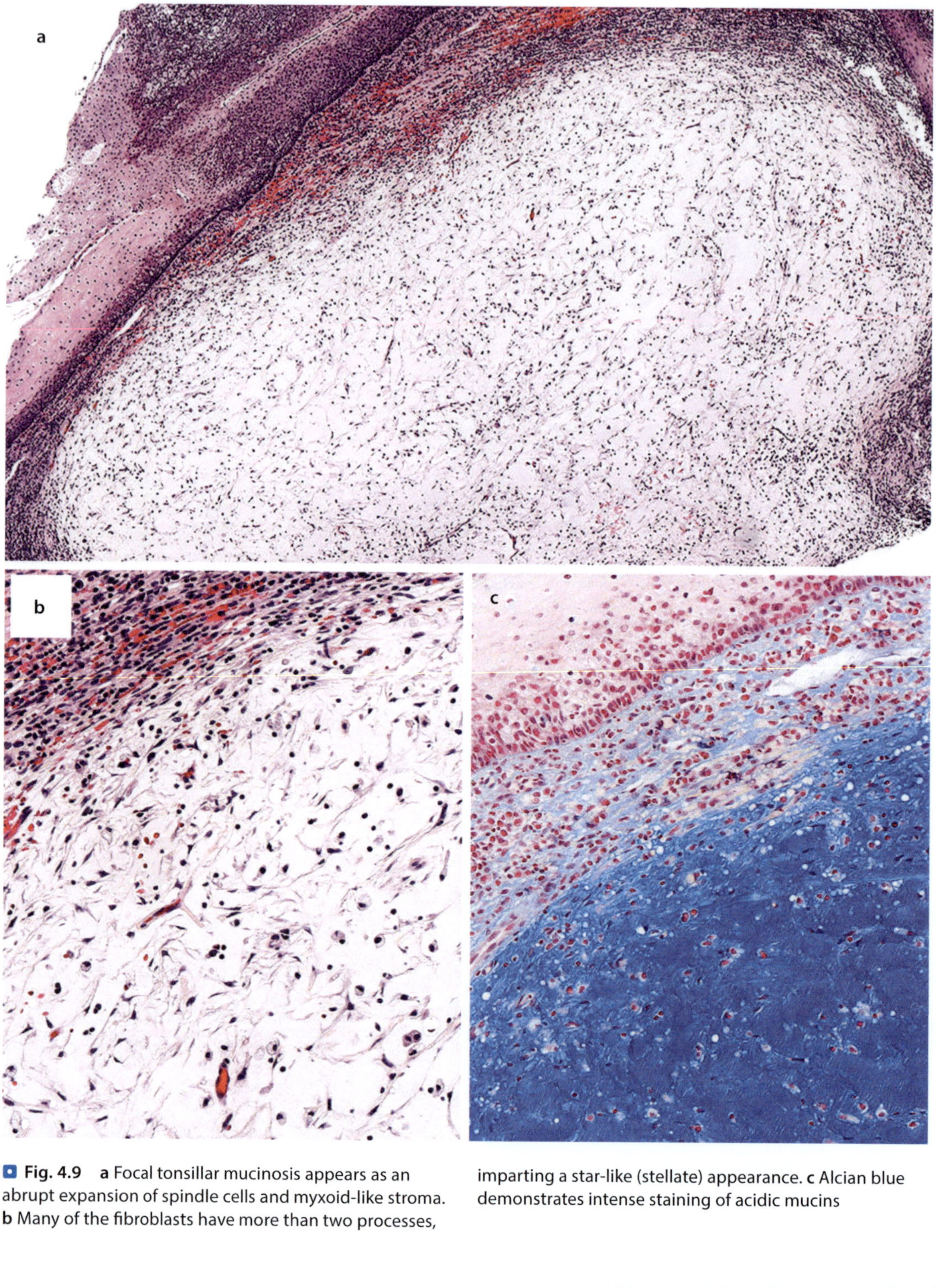

◘ **Fig. 4.9** **a** Focal tonsillar mucinosis appears as an abrupt expansion of spindle cells and myxoid-like stroma. **b** Many of the fibroblasts have more than two processes, imparting a star-like (stellate) appearance. **c** Alcian blue demonstrates intense staining of acidic mucins

4.11 Myxoma

Myxomas represent rare benign, expansile soft tissue tumors histologically composed of bland stellate fibroblasts. Myxomas of the pharynx are extraordinarily rare [31–33].This is an exclusionary diagnosis, after consideration of other myxoid neoplasia: myxoid liposarcoma, extraskeletal myxoid chondrosarcoma, myxoid change in other sarcomas, chordoma, peripheral nerve sheath tumor. Hisotlogically, myxomas are circumscribed, paucicellular, bland, and lack diagnostic elements of other neoplasia. They are vimentin + / CD34 + / S100-negative. Of note, oropharyngeal myxomas may be seen as part of the Carney complex, which is defined by skin pigmentary abnormalities, myxomas, most commonly cardiac, endocrine tumors or overactivity, and schwannomas [34].

4.12 Choristoma

By definition, a choristoma is the abnormal present of benign tissue at an aberrant location. Lingual thyroid (above) can also be considered a choristoma with a clear embryologic etiology. Oropharyngeal cartilaginous choristoma are very rare and have been described in the tongue base (foramen cecum) and tonsil [35–37]. Lingual chondroid choristomas within the anterior tongue have also been described [38]. Histologically, chondroid choristomas appear just as one would expect, well-circumscribed, smooth nodules of mature cartilage with blue matrix, and bland chondrocytes within lacunae. Chondroid choristomas, as chondromas, lack a lobulated pushing border, increased cellularity, and cellular pleomorphism of a Grade I chondrosarcoma.

4.13 Parapharyngeal Space Tumors

Tumors of the parapharyngeal space may become quite large before causing symptoms. Patients may note an intraoral soft palate bulge (◘ Fig. 4.10) or may complain of hoarseness, pain on swallowing, difficulty swallowing, impaired hearing or tinnitus. Some parapharyngeal masses may be totally asymptomatic, and come to attention as incidental radiographic findings.

The parapharyngeal space can be divided into pre-styloid and post-styloid compartments by the fascia which extends from the styloid process to the tensor veli palatini. The pre-styloid compartment

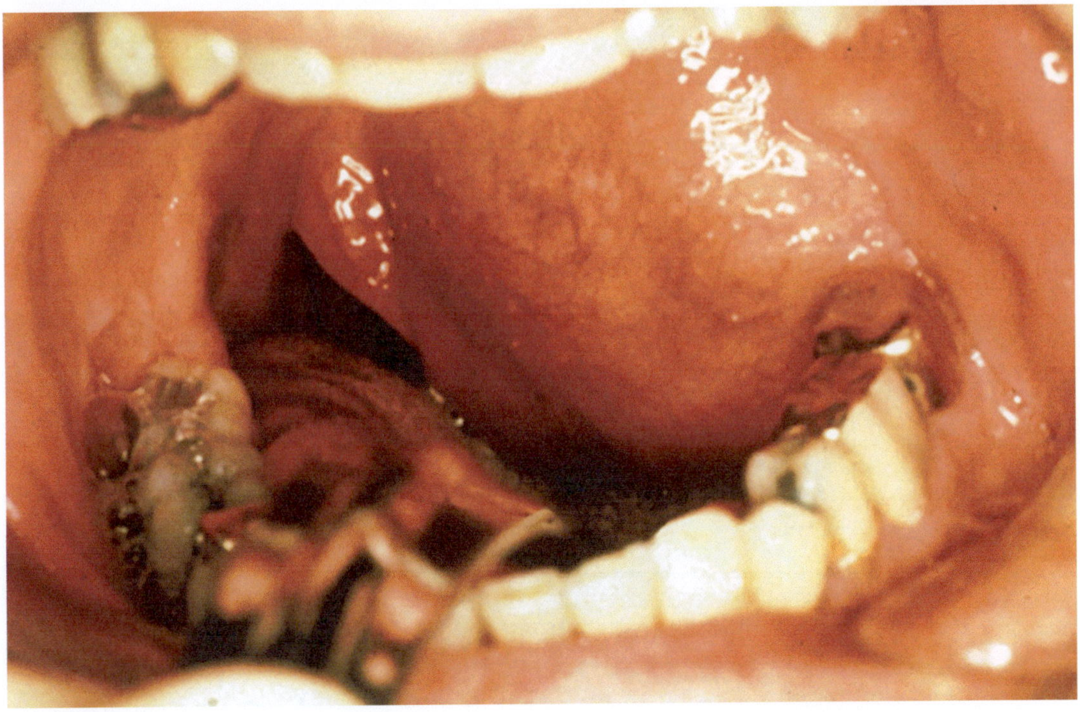

◘ **Fig. 4.10** The two most common parapharyngeal space tumors are benign mixed tumor arising from the deep parotid lobe, and vagal Schwannoma. A parapharyngeal space mass displaces the soft palate. (Courtesy of Dr. Richard V Smith)

includes the deep lobe of the parotid and minor salivary glands, lymph nodes, and parapharyngeal fat. These tissues can then give rise to salivary tumors, lymphomas, and lipomas. The post-styloid compartment contains the carotid artery, jugular vein, cranial nerves IX–XII, lymph nodes, cervical sympathetic chain, and glomus tissue. The contents of the post-styloid compartment can give rise to paragangliomas, nerve sheath tumors, ganglioneuromas, lymphomas, and connective tissue tumors. About 80% of parapharyngeal tumors will be benign [39–45]. The most common diagnoses are pleomorphic adenoma (Figs. 4.11 and 4.12), paraganglioma, and Schwannoma (Figs. 4.13 and

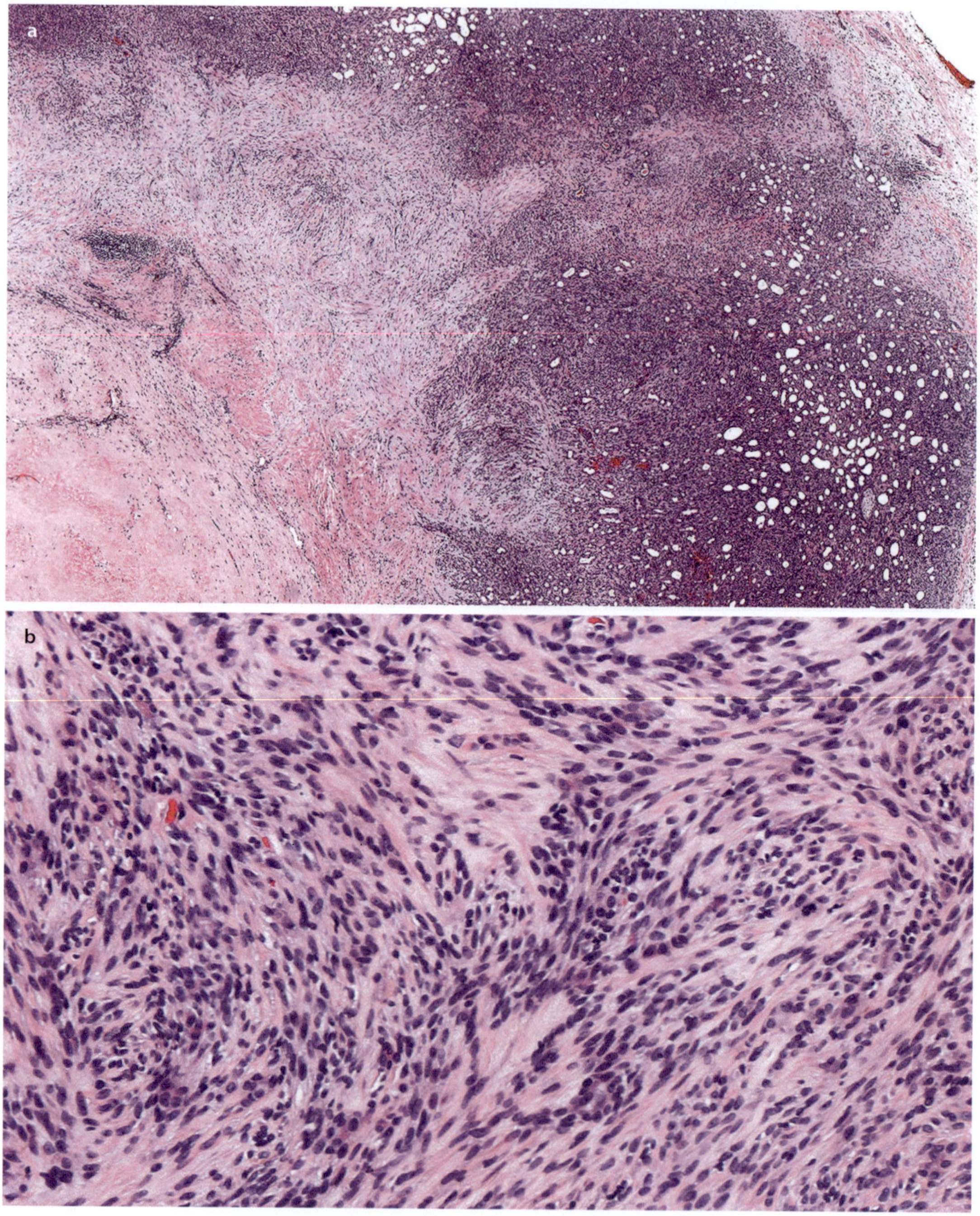

Fig. 4.11 **a** Benign mixed tumor of the deep parotid lobe revealing hyalinization and dense cellularity. **b** "Palisading" refers to these spindle cells lining up to form a striped pattern. Here this is reminiscent of a peripheral nerve sheath tumor

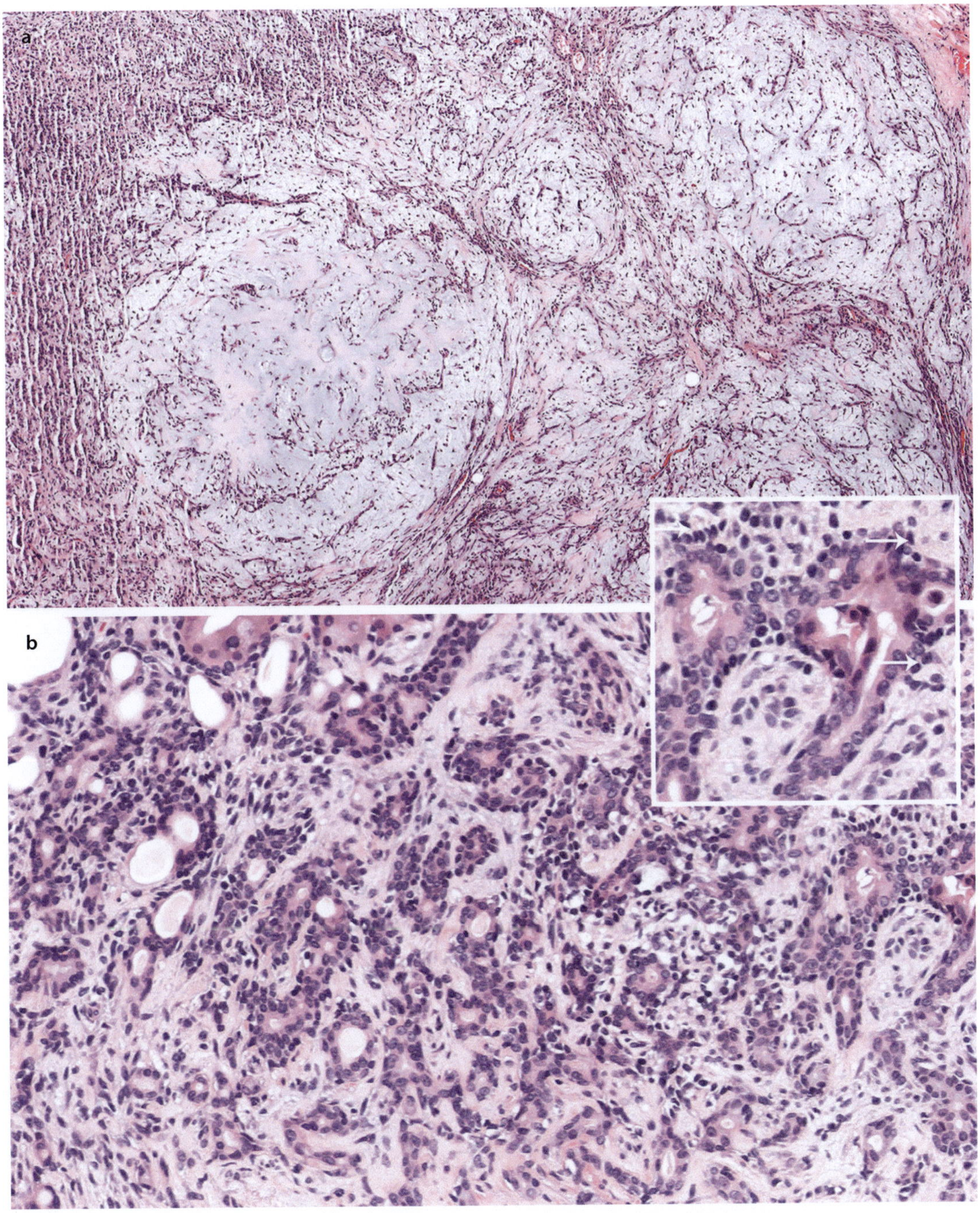

Fig. 4.12 **a** Chondroid matrix typical for benign mixed tumor. **b** Bilayered ductal structures with the "swarm of bees" appearance, emblematic of benign mixed tumor. **Inset:** The white arrows point out myoepithelial cells oriented perpendicularly to the duct. The "swarm of bees" refers to the overall haphazard pattern of myoepithelial cells as they "dissociate" from the ductal structures to form matrix material. Another way to appreciate this is to look at the border between ductal elements and matrix. This transition zone is sharply demarcated in basal cell adenoma or canalicular adenoma. This transition is zone is "fuzzy" in benign mixed tumors, because of the "swarming" myoepithelial cells

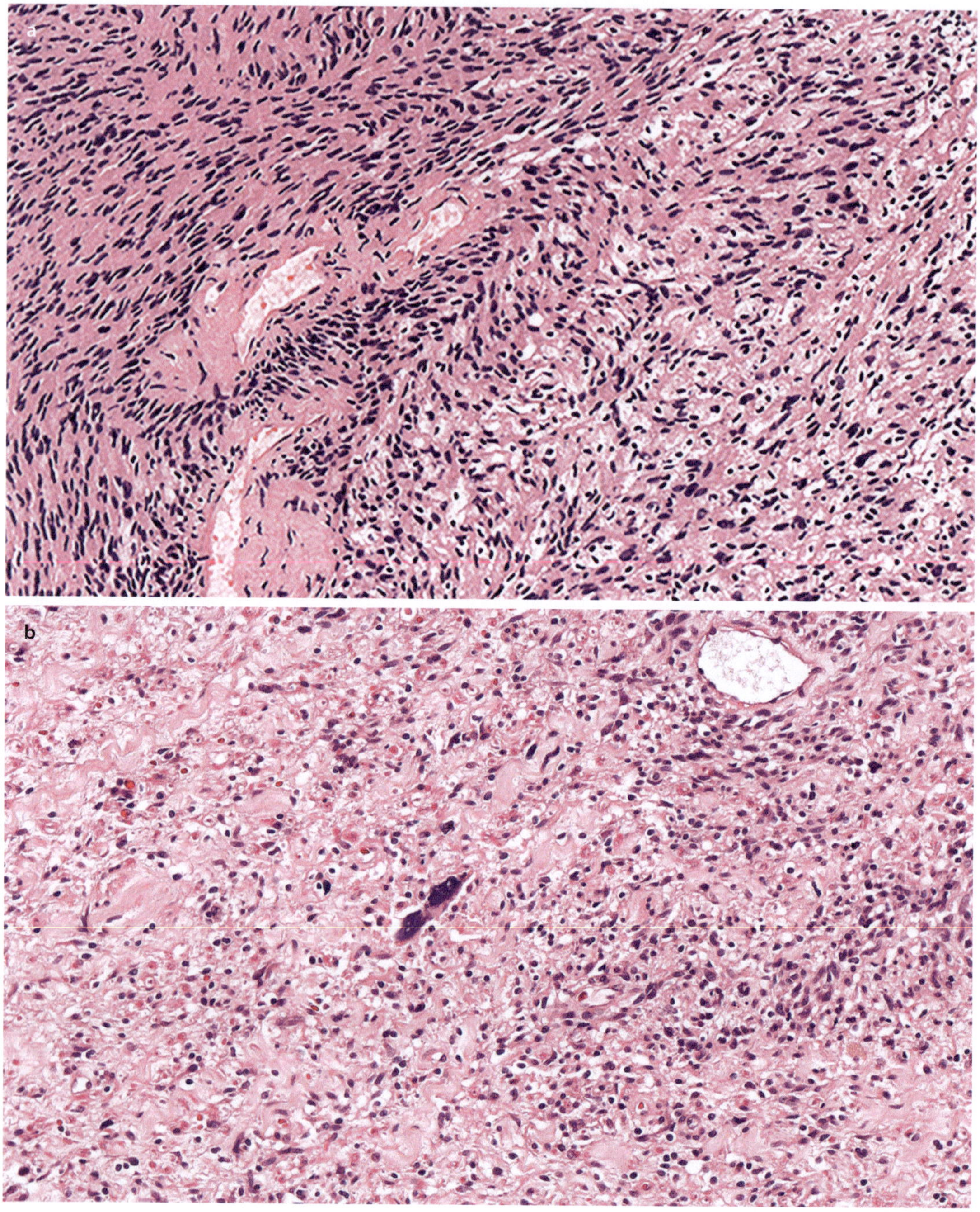

Fig. 4.13 **a** Parapharyngeal Schwannoma: The Antoni A region in the upper left shows a dense infiltrate of palisading spindle cells and hyaline matrix. Note the perivascular hyalinization. The Antoni B region in the lower right is less cellular. **b** Atypical degenerative cells can be seen ("ancient Schwannoma")

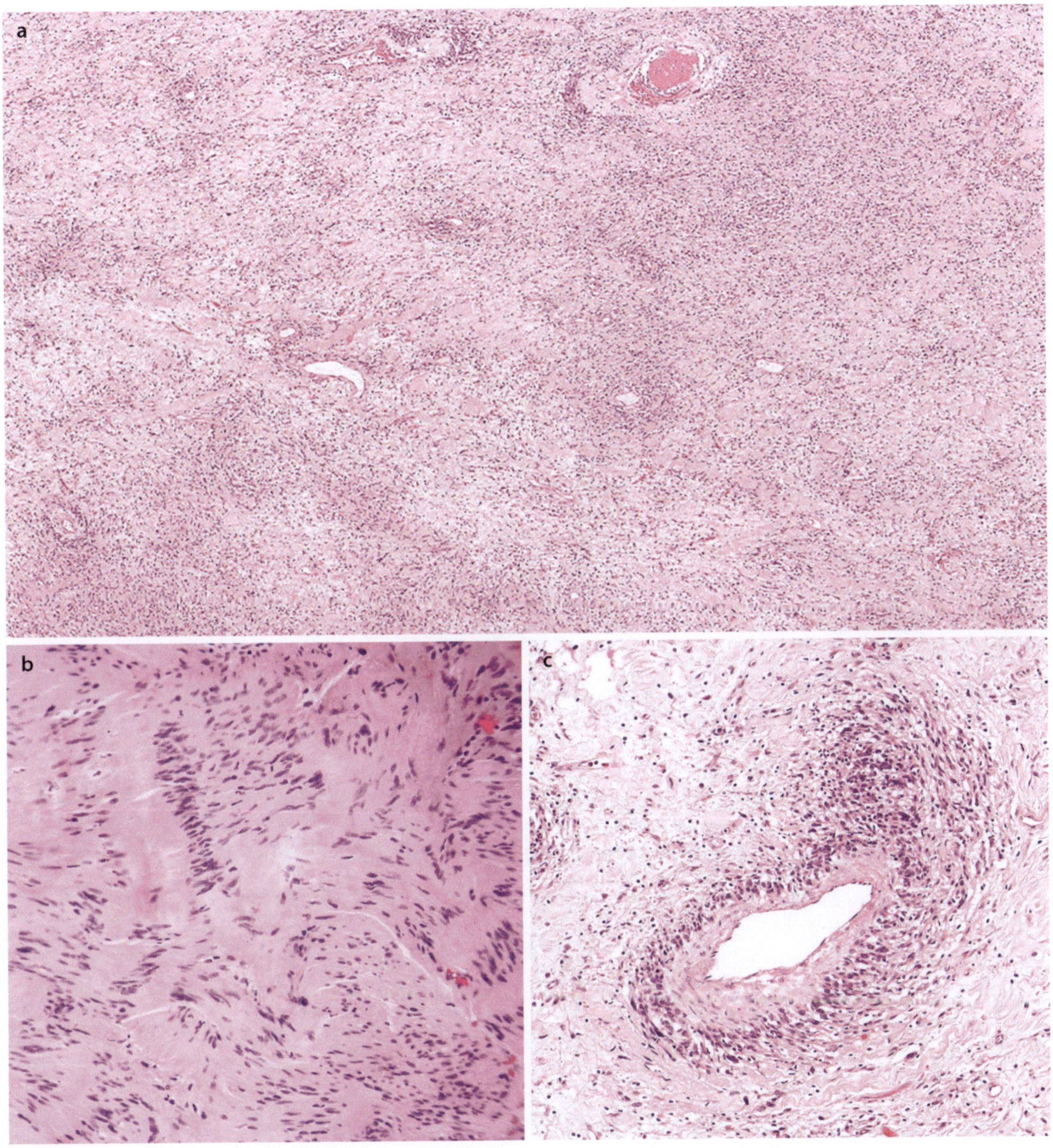

Fig. 4.14 **a** Another low-power view demonstrating the alternating Antoni A and Antoni B patterns. **b** Verrucay bodies represent groups of palisading nuclei lined up to form a striped pattern. **c** Another vessel with perivascular hyalinization

4.14). Malignant parapharyngeal tumors include adenoid cystic carcinoma, mucoepideroid carcinoma, lymphomas, and sarcomas.

4.14 Myofibroma

Myofibromas are uncommon benign tumors of myofibroblastic origin which can occur in both children and adults [46–51]. A recent report of oral and oropharyngeal myofibromas included 245 patients with median and mean ages of 19 and 30 years, respectively. Oral cavity tumors are more common than pharyngeal myofibromas; the most common sites are mandibular alveolar tissue, intraosseous mandible, buccal mucosa, tongue, labial mucosa and palate. The rates of multiple lesions and local recurrences (single or multiple) were less than 4%, each.

Histologically, myofibromas are characterized by well-circumscribed, unencapsulated tumors composed of short fascicles and whorls of plump

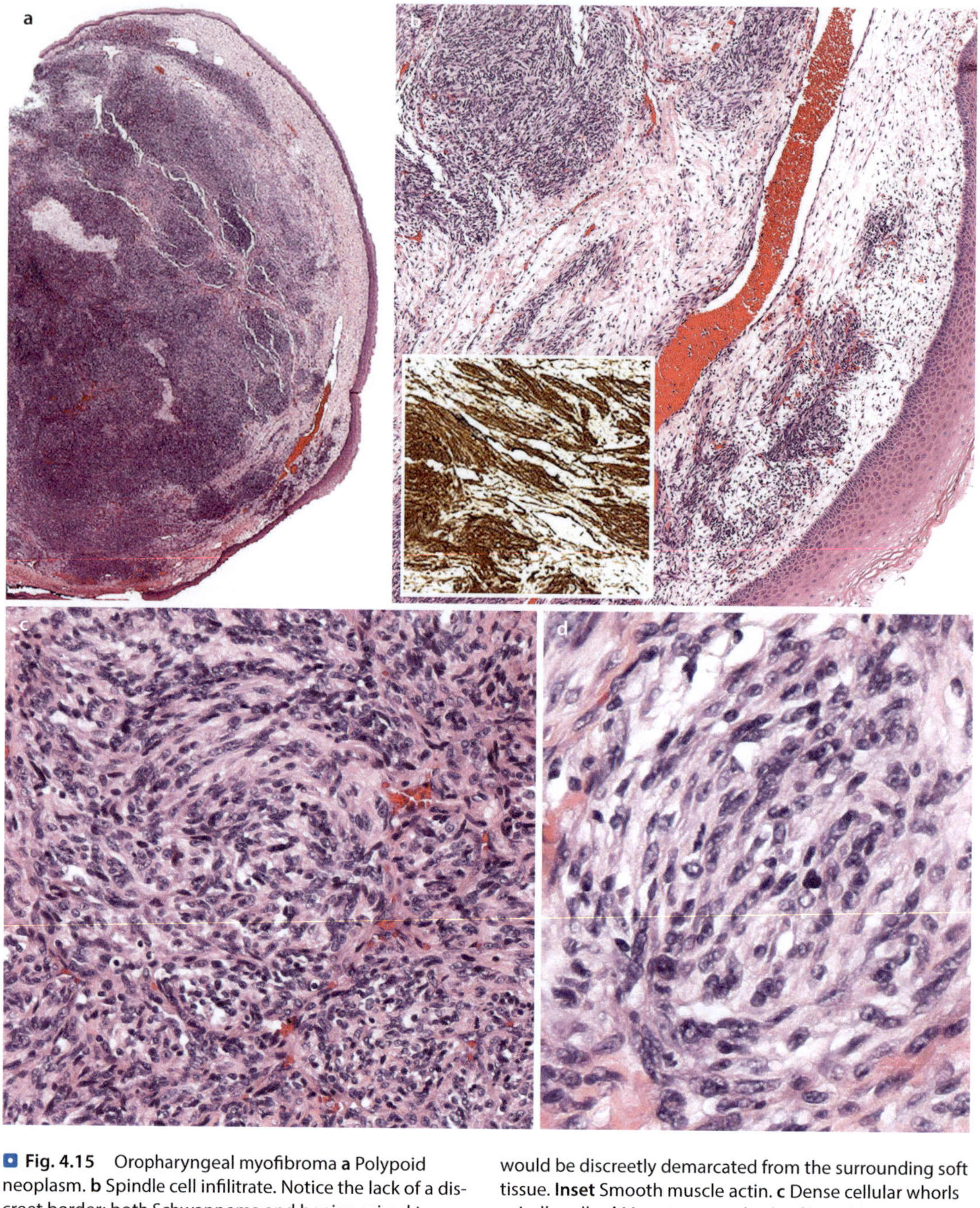

Fig. 4.15 Oropharyngeal myofibroma **a** Polypoid neoplasm. **b** Spindle cell infilitrate. Notice the lack of a discreet border; both Schwannoma and benign mixed tumor would be discreetly demarcated from the surrounding soft tissue. **Inset** Smooth muscle actin. **c** Dense cellular whorls spindle cells. **d** Monotonous whorls of long bland nuclei

spindle cells (Fig. 4.15). An architectural "zonal" pattern has been described which alternates less cellular regions with eosinophilic pink collagen and more cellular regions where tumor cells have less cytoplasm, thus appearing more blue. An abrupt transition between zones is characteristic. Typically, myofibroblasts have long tapered nuclei and may demonstrate perinuclear vacuoles. Tumor matrix may be "collagen" pink, with possible "pseudochondroid" blue regions. Vessels can be prominent and staghorn-like. Giant cells can be present. The mitotic rate is usually low. Myofibromas may also demonstrate aggressive features that are linked to recurrence, such as necrosis, perineural invasion, and vascular invasion. The immunohistochemical profile is alpha smooth muscle actin + / muscle specific actin + / calponin +.

4.15 Rhabdomyoma

Rhabdomyomas represent benign tumors of skeletal muscle origin [52–56]. Cardiac rhabdomyomas are the more commonly encountered type, associated with pediatric presentation and the tuberous sclerosis complex, an autosomal dominant disorder caused by mutations in either *TSC1* or *TSC2* tumor suppressor genes. The tuberous sclerosis complex is characterized by central nervous system tumors such as giant cell astrocytoma, cortical dysplasias, subependymal nodules, renal angiomyolipomas, pulmonary lymphangioleiomyomatosis, intracardiac rhabdomyomas, facial angiofibromas, periungual fibromas, hypomelanotic macules, and retinal astrocytic hamartomas.

Extracardiac rhabdomyomas are further subclassified as either **adult-type, fetal-type, or genital-type.** The most common site for extracardiac rhabdomyomas is the head and neck, specifically pharynx, parapharyngeal space, and larynx. Approximately 7% of adult rhabdomyomas are multifocal [54]. Of note, adult rhabdomyomas are associated with a significant likelihood of recurrence. A recurrence rate of 36% was compiled from a literature review (8/22 patients, parapharyngeal rhabdomyomas, adequate clinical follow-up) [56]. There is no potential for malignant transformation.

Histologically, adult rhabdomyomas are composed of closely packed, mixed large round to polygonal cells with abundant pink cytoplasm plus vacuolated polygonal cells (◘ Fig. 4.16). Cytoplasmic cross-striations can be observed. The "fetal" part of "**fetal rhabdomyomas**" refers to histological **immaturity** of tumor skeletal muscle cells; fetal rhabdomyomas can present at any age. Tumor rhabdomyoblasts range from primitive-appearing oval to spindled cells, immature ("fetal") skeletal muscle cells in a myxoid matrix, to mature skeletal muscle differentiation with little to no myxoid matrix. Genital rhabdomyomas lack vacuolated cells, and demonstrate more rhabdomyoblastic maturation than fetal rhabdomyomas.

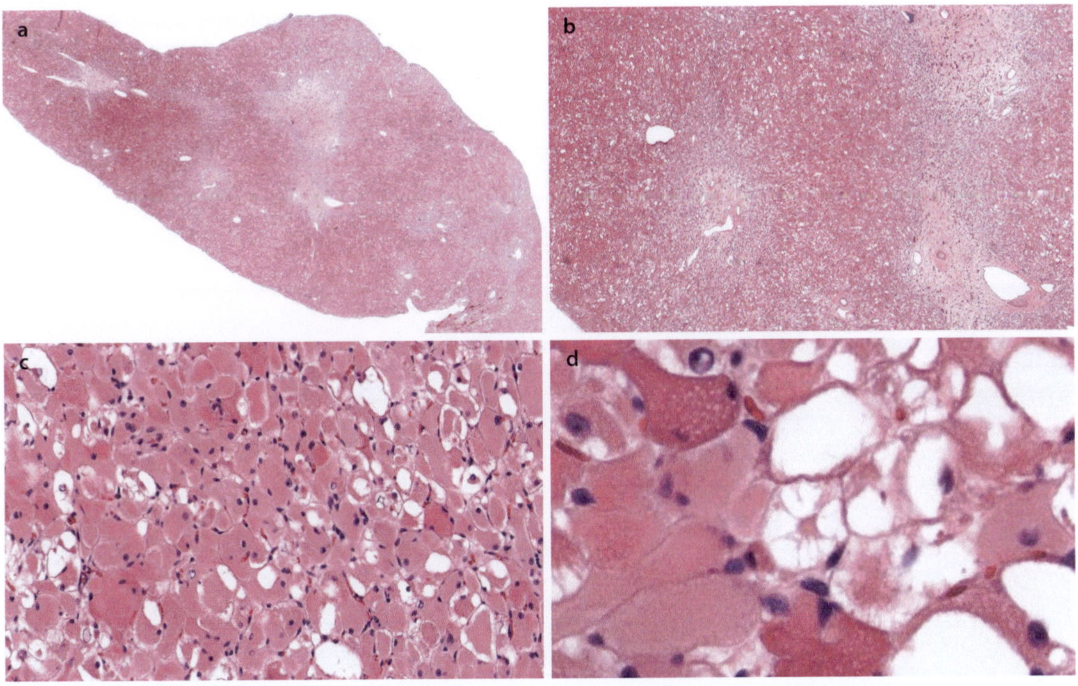

◘ **Fig. 4.16** Oropharyngeal adult rhabdomyoma **a** This polypoid vascular tumor resembles liver on low-power. **b** Solid proliferation of densely packed tumor cells with dense, deeply eosinophilic cytoplasm. **c, d** Retraction of cytoplasm from the cell membranes produces a star-like appearance. The rhabdomyocyte nuclei are condensed and peripheral

4.16 Lipomas and Liposarcomas

One should conceptualize ***lipoma-like*** oropharyngeal adipose tumors as existing on a spectrum. On one end, sit soft tissue lipomatous tumors composed of entirely of mature adipose tissue with well-defined capsules that are easily diagnosed as lipomas or their variants [57–59] (◘ Figs. 4.17 and 4.18). At the other end of the spectrum, sit polypoid lipomatous tumors which protrude into hollow lumena (◘ Fig. 4.19). Some polypoid tumors are entirely composed of mature lipocytes, thus can still be classified as lipomas or their variants [60]. Others contain a variable component of immature spindle cells. Some of these have been reported in the literature as **pleomorphic lipomas, spindle cell lipomas, atypical lipomas, or giant fibro-inflammatory polyps.** The waters become murky when some of these lesions recur after conservative excision. Some of these tumors really warrant the pathological classification of "well-differentiated liposarcomas". MDM2/CDK4 amplification has been demonstrated in these tumors [61]. ***However, the same initial surgical approach is warranted for all polypoid hollow-organ lipomatous tumors; the distinction between lipoma and well-differentiated liposarcoma may not be crucial for the purposes of initial resection.*** Conservative excision with preservation of function is recommended. Well-differentiated liposarcomas can manifest their unique potential in the form of multiple local recurrences [61, 62]. The literature bears out that recurrences can be treated by conservative re-excision. No adverse outcomes (metastases, grade progression, disease-specific mortality) have been reported for patients that have been conservatively managed. A recurrent "fibrolipoma" should raise the suspicion of a sclerosing liposarcoma. On the other hand, no harm has been done in the initial misclassified of a recurrent low-grade liposarcoma. In fact, harm has been avoided by the conservative nature of the excision.

Higher grade liposarcomas of the head and neck pose no diagnostic challenge as they are obviously malignant. In a study of 36 cases of superficial pleomorphic liposarcomas, seven occurred in the head and neck, however anatomic subsite was not mentioned [63]. In a series of 30 liposarcomas specifically involving the head and neck, 20 were classified as either pleomorphic liposarcoma, round cell liposarcoma, or myxoid liposarcoma; they developed in subsites such as scalp, neck or parotid, upper aerodigestive tract, skull base, and orbit [64]. The prognosis for higher-grade liposarcomas is related to tumor grade, stage, and resectibility. Myxoid liposarcomas can be considered as intermediate-grade sarcomas, which may be associated with local recurrence but not metastasis or disease-specific mortality [64, 65]. The round cell and pleomorphic variant of liposarcoma behave as high-grade sarcomas, and cause disease-specific mortality.

Histopathologically, lipomas are composed of abundant mature benign adipose tissue which is

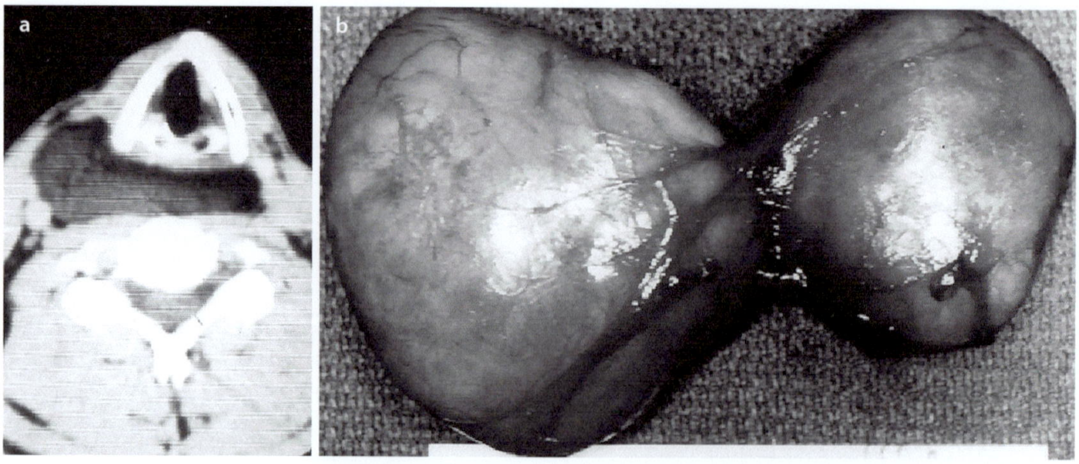

◘ **Fig. 4.17** **a** MRI scan of a retropharyngeal lipoma. **b** Encapsulated dumbbell-shaped tumor. This was composed entirely of mature adipose tissue. (Courtesy of Dr. Hugh Biller)

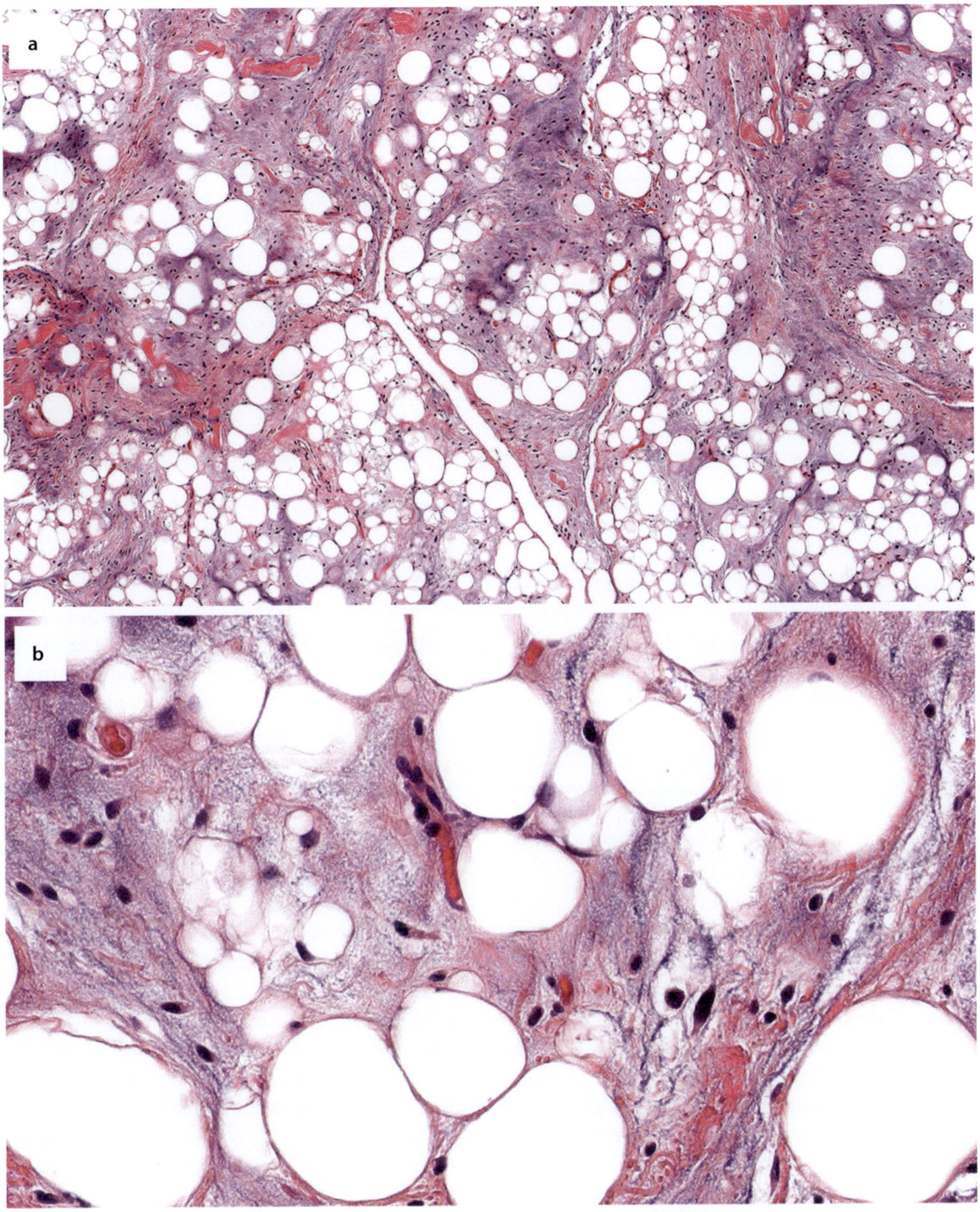

Fig. 4.18 Spindle cell lipoma **a**, **b** Mature adipose tissue intermixed with bland fibroblastic proliferation elaborating a basophilic myxoid matrix

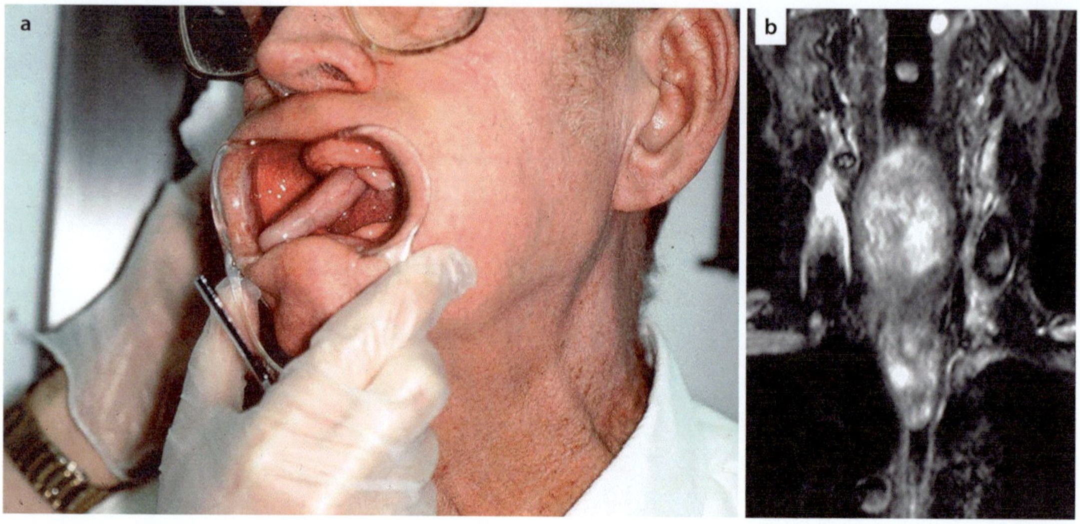

Fig. 4.19 **a** Regurgitated polypoid well-differentiated liposarcoma in a Caucasian male. (Courtesy of Dr. J Mark Reed, Jackson, MS). **b** MRI of an endolaryngeal lipoma-sarcoma. Top: Polypoid well-differentiated liposarcoma in the laryngeal submucosa. Bottom: Variable sized adipose lobules with cellular fibrous septae. Segmented look.

traversed by collagenous fibrous septae. Wisps of smooth connective tissue capsule can be appreciated at the periphery. Lipoma variants include: **spindle cell lipoma**, which is admixed with bland fibroblastic spindle cells. If the spindle cell component consists of dense mature fibroblasts, the designation of **fibrolipoma** can be made. **Pleomorphic lipoma** is characterized by variable-sized fat cells, spindle cells and bizarre, pleomorphic, multinucleated giant cells. Floret-like cells and ropy collagen can be seen. Pleomorphic lipomas are usually superficially located and well circumscribed. Spindle cell/pleomorphic lipomas are well-circumscribed and lack MDM2 amplification.

Angiolipoma appears as encapsulated with mature adipose tissue, coursed by fibrous septae with abundant branching capillaries and thick-walled vessels concentrated mostly at the tumor periphery. Intravascular hyaline fibrin thrombi are present. An **intramuscular lipoma** represents a lipoma with interspersed skeletal muscle cells. Remember that not all lipomas will demonstrate abundant adipose differentiation [66, 67]. "**Low-fat**" or "**fat-free**" **lipomas** have little or no interposed adipocytes. These well-circumscribed tumors are composed of ropey collagen, possible myxoid change, and atypical fibroblasts, and floret-like cells. Diffuse CD34 expression is seen.

The designation of **well-differentiated lipoma-like liposarcoma/atypical lipomatous neoplasm** may be used in tumors which contain ropy collagen, myxoid background, ***lipoblasts,*** and ***atypical lipoblasts*** (Figs. 4.20 and 4.21). Lipoblasts may be focal; they reveal characteristic "chicken claw" shaped nuclei, indented by cytoplasmic fat globules. Chromatin is dense and pyknotic, with enlarged nucleoli. ***Atypical lipoblasts have large, irregular nuclei and smudged chromatin.*** Florette cells can be seen in both benign and malignant lipomatous tumors, they demonstrate multiple nuclei in a wreath-like pattern. Sclerosing liposarcoma demonstrates abundant collagenous, bland fibroblastic background in addition to the requisite lipoblasts. This is the most common form to affect the hypopharynx and form polypoid growths.

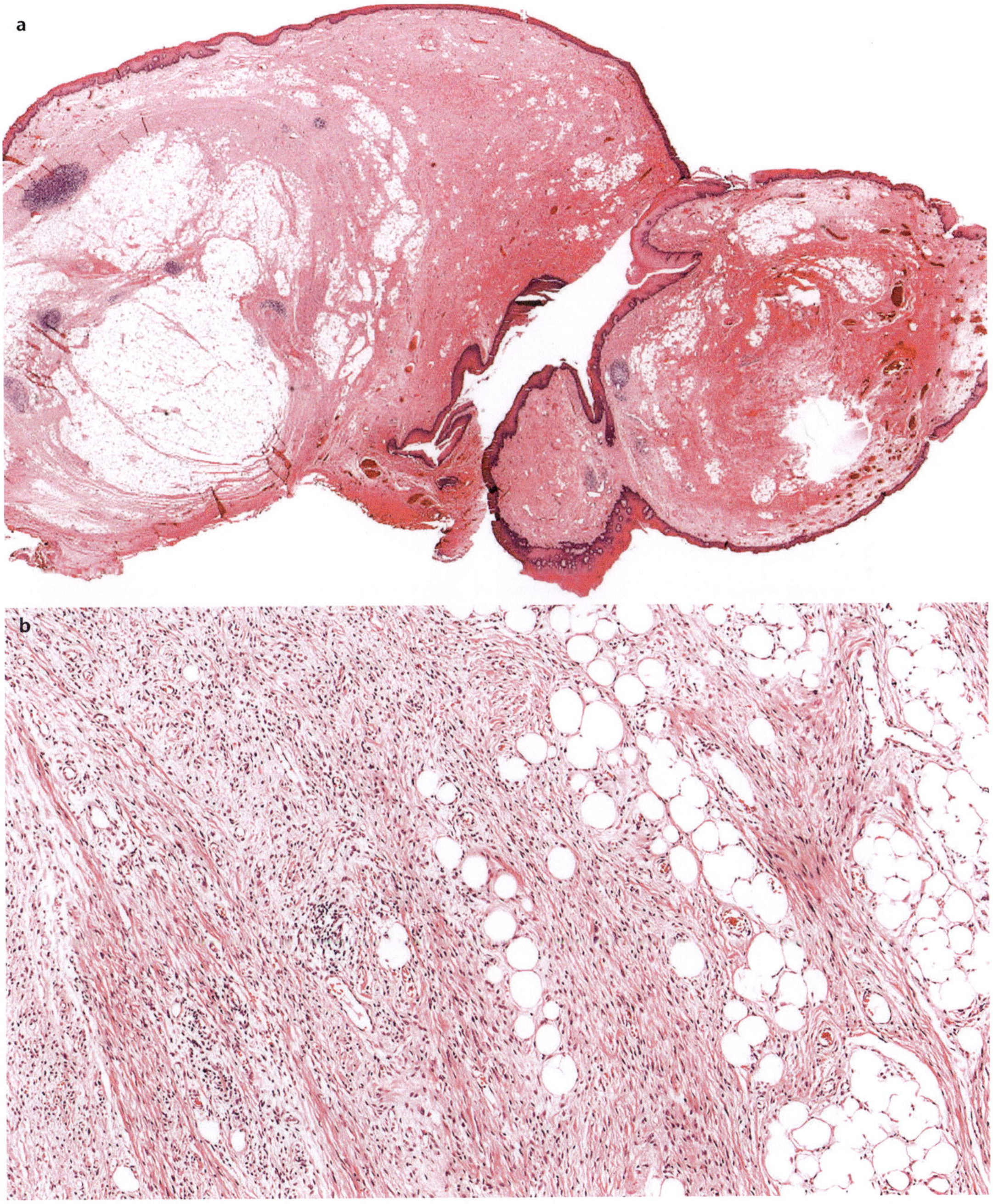

Fig. 4.20 **a** Polypoid hypopharyngeal well-differentiated liposarcoma. **b** Low-power view of bland fibroblastic and lipomatous components

Immunohistochemistry for MDM2 can reveal protein over-expression for the majority of tumor nuclei. **FISH for *MDM2* is sensitive and specific for demonstrating amplification, which is diagnostic for well-differentiated lipoma-like liposarcoma/atypical lipomatous tumor and distinguishes it from pleomorphic/spindle cell lipoma** (Fig. 4.22).

Myxoid liposarcoma is an intermediate-grade sarcoma which contains loose, myxoid stroma and a "chicken-wire" meshwork of arborizing

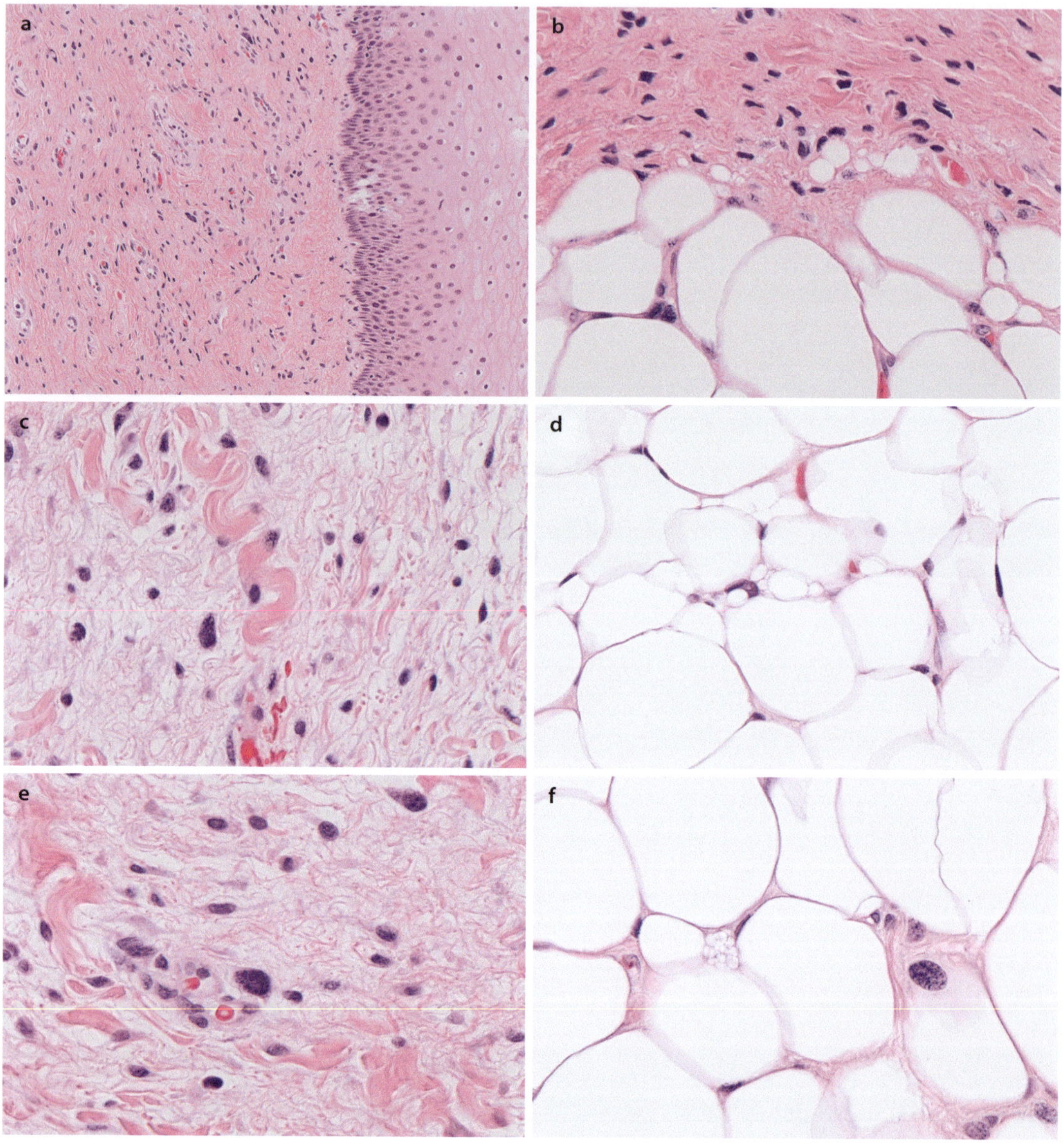

Fig. 4.21 **a** The lesional infiltrate extends up to the overlying squamous mucosa. **b** Interface between fibroblastic and lipomatous elements. **c, e** Atypical fibroblasts with large, pleomorphic nuclei and dark, smudgy chromatin and occasional intranuclear holes. **d, f** Rare lipoblasts and atypical lipocytes

vessels. Lipoblasts can be seen as univacuolated signet ring cells and multivaculolated cells tumor cells with atypical nuclei. Lipoblasts may be scarce and congregated at the periphery of the expanding tumor lobules.

Pleomorphic liposarcoma and round cell liposarcoma are high-grade sarcomas. A pleomorphic liposarcomas is composed of crowded malignant spindle cells and bizarre, highly pleomorphic forms; the lipoblastic component (lipoblasts and signet ring cells) may be minimal. Round cell liposarcoma refers to a sarcoma composed of closely packed signet ring type lipoblasts and little intervening myxoid or adipose stroma.

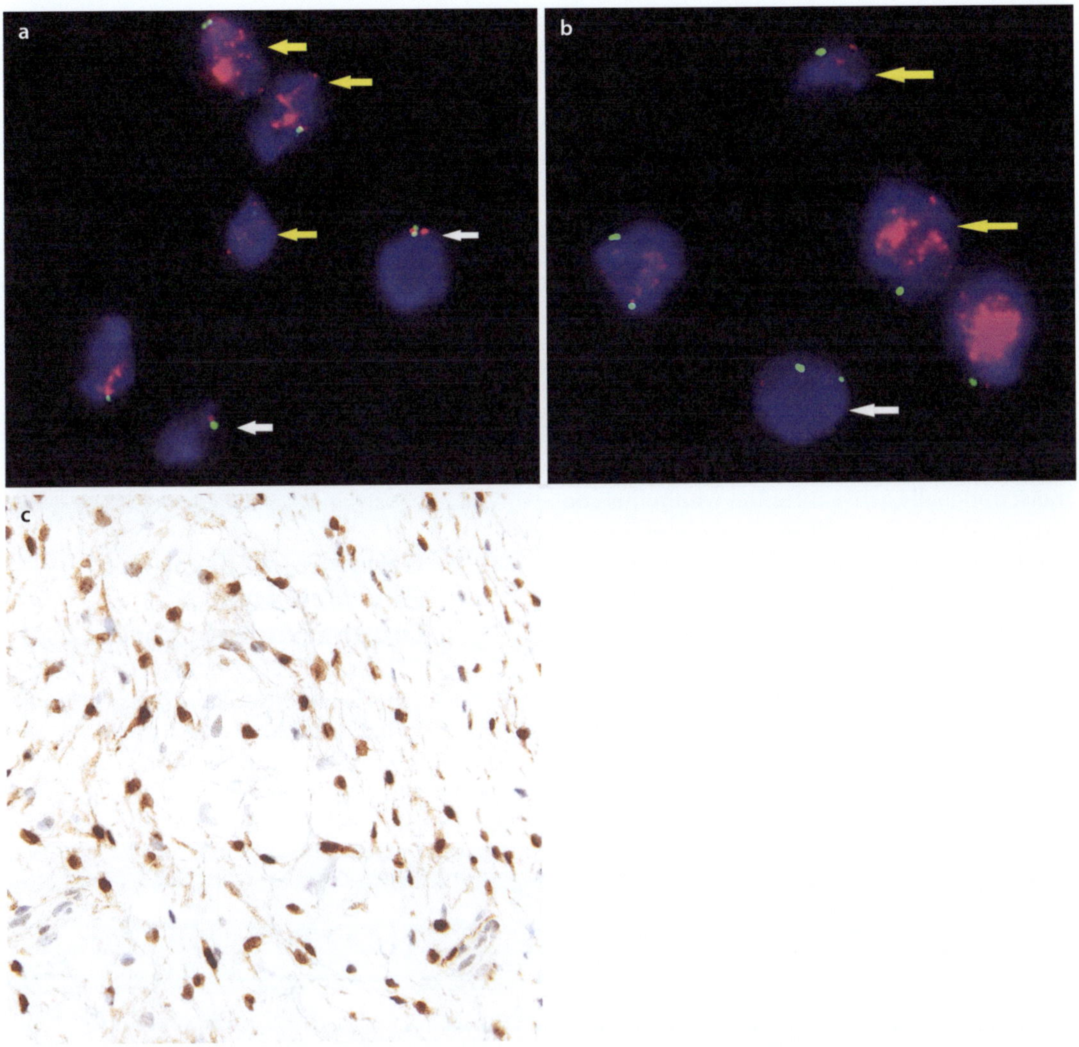

Fig. 4.22 **a, b** *MDM2*/CEP12 FISH assay in hypopharyngeal liposarcomas The white arrows are examples of normal complement of signals (*MDM2*-red signals and CEP12-green signals). Yellow arrows are examples of increased FISH signals, corresponding to *MDM2* gene amplification. **c** MDM2 nuclear expression

4.17 HPV-mediated Squamous Carcinoma

The onset of the high-risk Human Papillomavirus (HR-HPV) mediated oropharyngeal carcinogenesis could be observed in the midcentury, as the SEER data demonstrated a four-fold increase in the incidence of tonsillar carcinoma in women during the period of 1945–1994 [68]. This was indirect evidence of the increasing impact of HR-HPV. It is well-established that transcriptionally active HPV promotes cancer in >50% of oropharyngeal SCC, and 70–80% of the subset of patients with tonsillar SCC, predominantly HPV16; HPV18 is associated with 5–10% of virally mediated oropharyngeal cancers [69–82]. Other causative HR-HPV types are HPV31, HPV33, HPV35, HPV51, HPV56, HPV58, and HPV59. The proclivity for HPV-mediated cancers to develop in Waldeyer's ring reflects the fact that the basal reserve cells of the reticulated epithelium are normally exposed and thus vulnerable to HR-HPV infection.

Typically, HPV-mediated oropharyngeal cancers develop in patients who are significantly younger, with greater number of sexual partners, greater oral sex exposure, and have never smoked or drank. On the other hand, cigarette and alcohol exposure may overlap in this group. It is alsowellestablished that the vast majority of HPV-mediated oropharyngeal carcinoma patients have positive lymph nodes yet improved outcome as compared to HPV-negative oropharyngeal cancer. The tendency for early metastases was discussed early in this chapter in the context of the specialized reticulated epithelium of Waldeyer's ring. The basement membrane here is composed of fine, discontinuous fibers, thus enabling lymphocyte trafficking. "True" carcinoma-*in-situ* cannot exist in the setting of a discontinuous basement membrane [83, 84].

The overexpression of tumor suppressor protein p16 became synonymous with high-risk HPV mediated oropharyngeal cancers as it was demonstrated to be an excellent surrogate biomarker for transcriptionally active infection within this context. It's also been established as a biomarker of improved outcome. One of the early supporting studies was the DAHANCA trial, which included 331 patients with oropharyngeal and supraglottic cancers. This trial demonstrated that a hypoxic cell radiosensitizer improved local disease free survival for p16 negative patients, but had no impact on p16+ who demonstrated significantly better local disease-free survivals [85].

Immunohistochemical assessment of p16 overexpression is relatively straightforward, as it tends to be an "all or nothing" phenomena. Tumor nuclear p16 expression is requisite, cytoplasmic p16 may or may not be present. The optimal cutpoint for p16 overexpression correlating with the presence of HR-HPV in oropharyngeal cancers is ≥75% staining of tumor nuclei [86]. A subset oropharyngeal cancers will harbor HR-HPV, yet p16 is silenced. A number of studies have validated the finding that outcomes for HPV/p16 discordant oropharyngeal cancer patients stratify according to p16 status; survival curves for HPV+/p16 silenced patients are similar to patients with HPV−/p16-negative oropharyngeal tumors [87–90].

4.17.1 Genomic Landscapes of HPV-Mediated Oropharyngeal Cancers

High-risk HPV promotes carcinogenesis through E6 and E7 viral oncoprotein-mediated functional disabling of the p53 and Rb tumor suppressor proteins (◘ Fig. 4.23). The p53 tumor suppressor

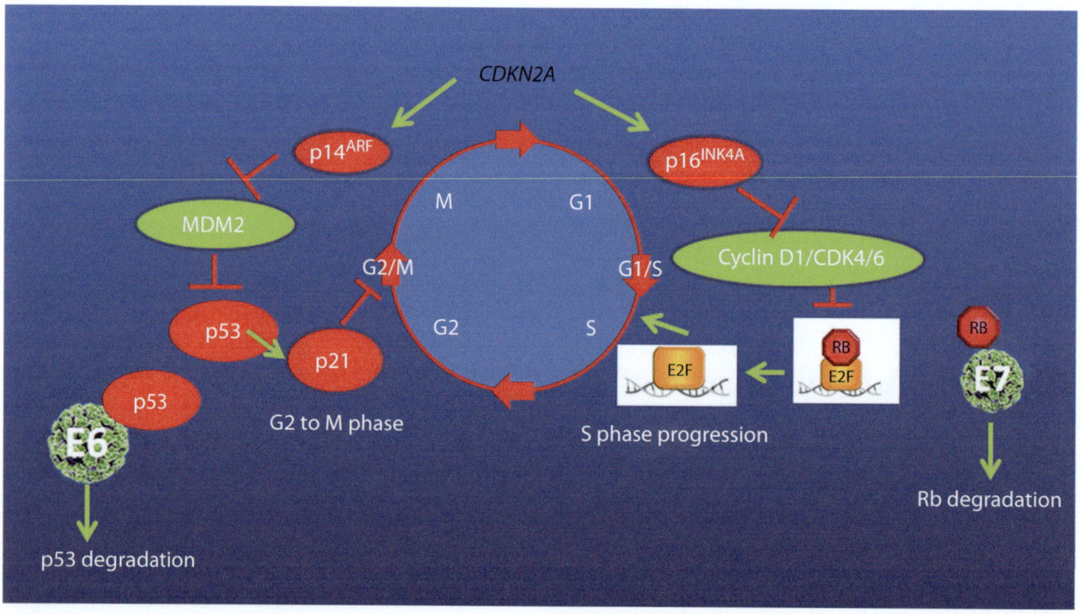

◘ **Fig. 4.23** HR-HPV oncoproteins disrupt cell cycle regulation: *CDKN2A* encodes tumor suppressor proteins $p14^{ARF}$ and $p16^{INK4A}$. $p14^{ARF}$ suppresses MMDM2, which disinhibits p53 activation of p21, which halts G2 to M phase progression. HR-HPV E6 protein functionally deactivates p53 by binding and targeting it for degradation; p53-mediated G2/M checkpoint regulation through p21 is lost. $p16^{INK4A}$ suppresses the cyclin D1/CDK4/6 complex, which normally deactivates Rb tumor suppressor protein, and drives G1/S4 progression through transcription factor E2F. HR-HPV E7 protein functionally deactivates Rb by binding4 and targeting it for degradation; E2F is now derepressed to drive G1/S progression

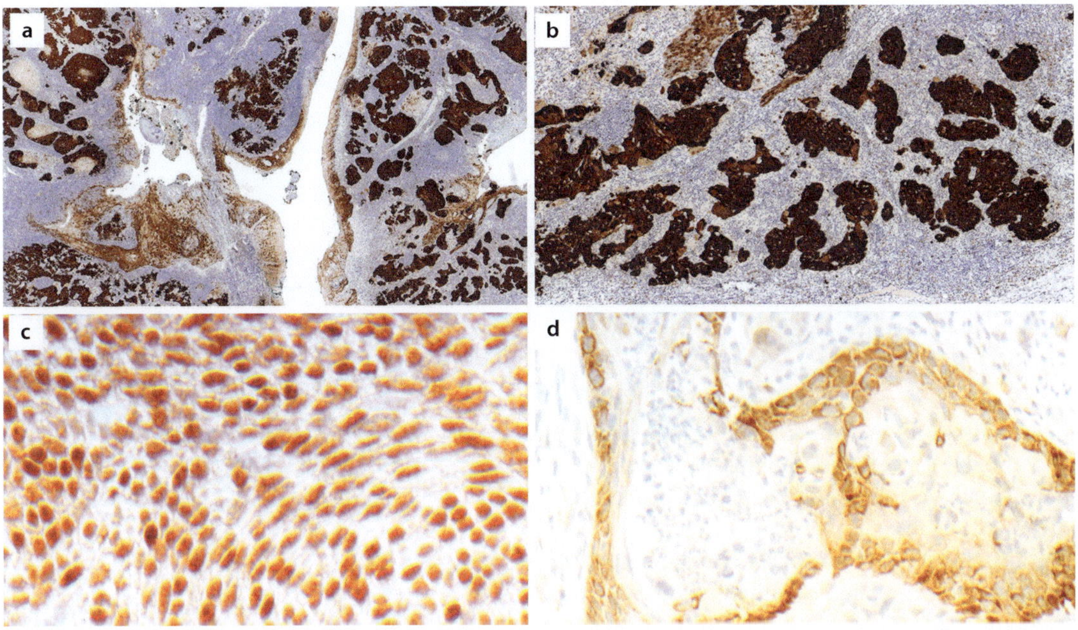

Fig. 4.24 **a**, **b** Diffuse, robust p16 overexpression is typical of an HR-HPV-mediated tonsillar carcinoma. **c** A rarer pattern of strong p16 overexpression limited to nuclei. **d** Nonspecific cytoplasmic p16 expression is usually associated with limited staining distribution. Carcinomas with this staining pattern are considered not overexpressers

protein normally regulates cell cycle progression from G2 to M phase and also regulates response to DNA damage. High-risk HPV E6 proteins binds p53 and induces ubiquitin-dependent proteolysis. Normally, $p16^{INK4a}$ binds and inactivates cyclin-kinase complex, while hypophosphorylated Rb, the activated tumor suppressor protein, binds transcription activator E2F, thus intact $p16^{INK4a}$ and Rb function as the gatekeepers to S phase progression. Activated cyclin D kinase inactivates Rb, which promotes S phase progression. In HPV-mediated carcinogenesis high-risk HPV E7 viral oncoproteins bind Rb, and induce ubiquitin-dependent proteolysis, thus driving S phase progression. 16^{INK4a} is overexpressed due to loss of feedback inhibition in the oncogenic stress that follows Rb inactivation (Fig. 4.24).

> It is infinitely fascinating to have a front-row seat in the theater of new diseases. I witnessed the unfolding and elucidation of AIDS from its very beginning, prior to the appreciation of its infectious nature from the front row vision as a resident in the autopsy suite. Witnessing the emerging entity of HPV-mediated oropharyngeal cancers, its impact on pathologic diagnostics and staging, and revolutionary changes surgical approaches (TORS) and treatment paradigms has been another privilege which should remind us all of the importance of pathologic observation.

HPV-mediated oropharyngeal cancers have a distinct mutational landscape and generally harbor half the mutational load as compared with HPV-negative tobacco and alcohol mediated head and neck cancers. HPV-mediated oropharyngeal cancers typically ***lack*** deletion mutations in tumor suppressor genes *TP53, CDKN2A, PIK3CA, TERT* and *NOTCH,* or increased copy number events for *EGFR, CCND1,* and *FGFR1,* these are common events in HPV-negative, tobacco and alcohol-mediated head and neck cancers [91–96]. By contrast, **activating mutations of *E2F*** can be seen in HPV-mediated cancers, further driving the S phase progression impact of E7-mediated Rb degradation [94]. Activating mutations of *PIK3CA* are also unique to HPV-mediated oropharyngeal cancer, which drive the *AKT*/m*TOR* pathway that normally controls cell survival, proliferation, adhesion, and motility [94]. *DDX3x* mutations were found exclusive to HPV-mediated tumors, *DDX3x* encodes ATP-dependent RNA helicase involved in RNA processing [93]. HPV-mediated cancers can also harbor mutations in *CYLD*, which is common to HPV-mediated cervical cancers, and involved in cellular differentiation, and NFκB signaling [93]. Inactivating *TRAF3* mutation is also unique to HPV mediated cancers, blocking apoptosis [93].

Of interest, two distinct genomic profiles have been discerned in HPV-mediated cancers: HPV-positive classical type, which have some degree of keratinization and demonstrate significant enrichment of polyamine degradation pathway, E2F3 amplification, and increased proliferation, and the HPV-mediated inflamed mesenchymal type which is associated with better outcome, demonstrates nonkeratinizing phenotype, less proliferation, **prominent CD8+ lymphocyte infiltration**, and expression of vimentin and metalloproteases [95]. Additionally, high-risk HPV E6 is responsible for epigenetic silencing through hypermethylation of genes involved in cell cycle regulation (*CDKN2A, CCNA1*), JAK-STAT pathway (*JAK3, STAT5A*), and cadherin (*CDH8, CDH15, PCDH8–10*) [97].

HR-HPV preferentially infects the basal reserve cells, persisting at a level of 20–50 episomal copies per cell. HPV integrates into host genome at the expense of *E1* and *E2* genes, which control viral replication. The majority of HPV16-mediated oropharyngeal tumors retain viral episomes, but some episomes are re-established *after* integration, as HPV-human hybrid sequences are detected in some episomes [98]. Viral integration occurs over known chromosomal fragile spots similar to those observed in HPV-mediated cervical cancers; integration can be the result of, or further promote chromosomal instability [99–101].

4.17.2 New Staging Criteria

Observations that patients with p16 overexpressing oropharyngeal carcinomas have improved outcomes despite presenting as "high-stage" begs for new prognostic schema that can discriminate outcome for this uniform patient group. The 8th AJCC staging criteria for p16 overexpressing oropharyngeal cancers is based on an exploratory analysis of 704 patients with p16 overexpressing oropharyngeal cancers treated by primary surgery +/− adjuvant therapy, with curative intent [9].

Table 4.2 HPV mediated (p16+) oropharyngeal cancer

T category	**T0**	No primary identified
	T1	≤2 cm
	T2	>2 cm but ≤4 cm
	T3	>4 cm or extension to lingual epiglottis
	T4	Invades larynx, extrinsic muscle of tongue, medial pterygoid, hard palate, or mandible of beyond
N category	**Nx**	Cannot be assessed
	No	Negative lymph nodes
	N1	Metastases in 1–4 lymph nodes
	N2	Metastases in 5 or more lymph nodes
M category	**M0**	None
	M1	Distant metastases

If T is...	And N...	And M...	Then Stage...
T0, T1, T2	N0, N1	M0	I
T0, T1, T2	N2	M0	II
T3, T4	N0, N1	M0	II
T3, T4	N2	M0	III
Any T	Any N	M1	IV

Only 6% were N_0. Not surprisingly, the 7th AJCC staging criteria failed to adequately discriminate outcome groups specifically for N staging. Conjunction consolidation demonstrated that the cutpoint of ≤4 versus ≥5 positive lymph nodes has the greatest discrimination of outcome survival curves. The new staging criteria for p16 over-expressing oropharyngeal carcinomas are presented in Table 4.2. Note that there is no "*Tis*" or carcinoma-*in-situ*" category, which refers back to the fact that the discontinuous basement membrane of Waldeyer's ring abrogates that possibility. Also, note that extranodal extension in positive lymph nodes does not impact staging; however it is used in some clinical trials for risk stratification. Carcinomas of the oropharynx that are p16-negative, and all hypopharyngeal carcinomas are staged according to Table 4.3.

Table 4.3 p16 negative oropharyngeal cancers

T category	Tx	Cannot be assessed
	Tis	Carcinoma-*in-situ*
	T1	≤ 2 cm
	T2	> 2 cm, ≤ 4 cm
	T3	> 4 cm, or lingual epiglottis
	T4a	Invades larynx, extrinsic tongue, medial pterygoid, hard palate, or mandible
	T4b	Lateral pterygoid, pterygoid plates, lateral nasopharynx, skull base, encases carotid artery
All Hypopharyngeal Cancers		
T category	Tx	Cannot be assessed
	Tis	Carcinoma-*in-situ*
	T1	One subsite and/or ≤2 cm
	T2	More than one subsite, or adjacent site, or >2 cm, ≤ 4 cm, without fixation of hemilarynx
	T3	> 4 cm, or fixation hemilarynx, or extension to esophagus
	T4a	Invades thyroid/cricoid cartilage, hyoid bone, thyroid gland, central compartment soft tissue
	T4b	Prevertebral fascia, encases carotid artery, mediastinal involvement
N category	Nx	Cannot be assessed
	N0	No metastases
	N1	One positive lymph node ≤3 cm, no ENE
	N2a	One positive lymph node ≤3 cm with ENE+, or one positive lymph node >3 cm, ≤ 6 cm, no ENE
	N2b	Multiple lymph nodes ≤6 cm, no ENE
	N2c	Bilateral or contralateral lymph nodes ≤6 cm, no ENE
	N3a	One positive lymph node >6 cm no ENE
	N3b	One positive lymph node >3 cm with ENE+, or multiple lymph nodes, either ipsilateral, contralateral, bilateral with ENE+
M category	M0	None
	M1	Distant metastases

If T is…	And N…	And M…	Then Stage…
Tis	N0	M0	0
T1	N0	M0	I
T2	N0	M0	II
T3	N0	M0	III
T1/T2/T3	N1	M0	III
T4a	N0, N1	M0	IVA
T1/T2/T3/T4a	N2	M0	IVA
Any T	N3	M0	IVB
T4b	Any N	M0	IVB
Any T	Any N	M1	IVC

The rationale for designating p16 overexpression as the gatekeeper to this staging schema is that p16 immunohistochemistry is widely available, robust, and easy to interpret. *In-situ* hybridization for HR-HPV is not necessary in clinical practice; it is only recommended in the setting of metastatic carcinoma from unknown tumor primary. Lastly, it cannot be overemphasized that that p16 overexpression is a surrogate biomarker for HR-HPV only in the limited context of oropharyngeal cancers. p16 overexpression may be observed in other malignancies, even non-epithelial malignancies, with no relationship to HR-HPV.

4.17.3 New Treatment Strategies

The improved outcome for HPV-mediated oropharyngeal cancers has become the basis for developing new treatment strategies. The standard 70GY dose with concurrent chemotherapy is associated with significant toxicities such as severe mucositis and dysphagia, necessitating gastrostomy tubes, and long-term chronic dysphagia and xerostomia. The long-term quality of life issues associated with dysphagia and feeding tube dependence are far from negligible. The goal of new treatment strategies is to decrease the risk of treatment toxicity yet not compromise disease-free survival [102]. Cetuximab, a monoclonal antibody targeting the EGFR extracellular ligand binding domain is approved for the treatment of locally advanced head and neck squamous cell carcinoma, as it was demonstrated to improve overall survival at three years for patients receiving radiotherapy in combination with cetuximab as compared to radiotherapy alone, 55% versus 45%, respectively, without increased toxicities as would be expected with multimodality therapies [103]. Subgroup analysis indirectly pointed to the greatest benefits seen among patients with the demographics of HPV-mediated oropharyngeal cancers (young age, positive lymph nodes, low T stage).

Multiple ongoing clinical trials explore the impact of replacing cisplatin with cetuximab for p16 overexpressing oropharyngeal carcinomas (RTOG 1016, NCT01302834, NCT01874171, NCT01855451), the results of which will ultimately confirm or refute the idea that cetuximab plus 70 Gy is beneficial in decreasing treatment related toxicities without negatively impacting outcome. There are ongoing Phase 2 clinical trials evaluating the impact of lower intensity-modulated radiation therapy (IMRT) dosing. NCT01530997 delivered ***60 Gy*** IMRT over 6 weeks with concurrent weekly cisplatin for HPV+ patients. The rate of complete pathologic response was 86%; the rates of grade 3 toxicities compare favorably to historical controls with a gastrostomy tube rate of 39% and long-term feeding tube dependence rate of 0%.

ECOG 1308 (NCT01084083), a Phase 2 trial, examines radiation de-intensification based on response to induction chemotherapy in patients with resectable stage III-IV T3e4b N0e3 HPV-associated oropharyngeal carcinoma. Patients receive 3 cycles of induction chemotherapy with cisplatin, paclitaxel, and cetuximab. Patients with clinical ***complete response*** at the primary site receive ***54 Gy*** over 5 1/2 weeks with concurrent cetuximab. Patients with a ***partial response*** or stable disease at the primary site receive ***69.3 Gy*** over 6 1/2 weeks with concurrent cetuximab. Complete clinical response was seen in 87% of patients. Progression-free survival rates at one year ranged from 87% for patients with partial response or stable disease receiving 69.3 Gy plus cetuximab, to 97% for patients with complete response receiving 54 Gy radiotherapy and only 1% of patients exhibiting grade 4 toxicity and the rate of grade 3 toxicity was low [104]. The lower IMRT doses significantly decreased the likelihood of late toxicities of dysphagia (100% versus 35%) supporting the idea that **doses < 55 Gy are less likely to impair swallowing** [105].

Prior to the revolution of robotic surgery, tonsillar cancers were resected via open mandibulotomy to gain surgical access, resulting in severe functional and cosmetic deformities. Transoral approaches include transoral robotic surgery (TORS), which uses miniaturized instruments, robotic control, and magnification, allowing for adequate access and resection of small pharyngeal tumors through the open mouth. Better surgical access increases surgical success and can potentially decrease the need for adjuvant radiotherapy. ECOG 3311 (NCT01898494) explores TORS plus de-intensified adjuvant radiotherapy or chemoradiotherapy in patients with cT1/T2 cN0/N1 HPV-mediated oropharyngeal cancer. ***Low-risk*** patients (***margin-negative resection, pN0/N1 disease, no extranodal extension***) receive no adjuvant therapy. ***Intermediate-risk*** patients (***margins < 1 mm, extranodal extension, or 2–4 positive lymph nodes***) receive either 50 Gy or 60 Gy. ***High-risk*** patients ***(>1 mm extranodal extension, positive margins, or 5 or greater positive lymph nodes***) receive 66 Gy and weekly cisplatin. Results of this trial will support or refute the idea that minimally invasive surgical techniques plus reduced intensity adjuvant therapy is less toxic than current standard of care management. NCT02215265 also calls for risk-based stratification after TORS with the pathologic features of lymphovascular invasion and perineural invasion added to risk stratification.

Histologically, HPV-mediated oropharyngeal carcinomas are typically nonkeratinizing [106, 107] (◘ Figs. 4.25 and 4.26). That is to say, frank keratinization is generally not observed at low-power. On the other hand, at high-power, one can see cellular maturation and cytoplasmic keratinization. A transitional type ribbon-like morphology can be observed which recapitulates squamous mucosa: one side has basal reserve-like cells while the cells at the opposite side of the ribbon reveal maturation in the form of flattening and keratinization (◘ Figs. 4.27 and 4.28). Cytologically, tumor cells are "basaloid" in that they contain little cytoplasm and have a high nuclear/cytoplasmic ratio. By comparison, tumor cells from the usual keratinizing squamous carcinoma are polygonal with abundant pink "glassy" cytoplasmic keratin, discernable cell membranes, and intercellular bridges. One should resist the temptation to label these nonkeratinizing tumors "poorly" differentiated" [108]. Actually, there is usually not much pleomorphism between tumor nuclei. In a biopsy setting, how might one correctly recognize focal carcinoma, without the aid of immunohistochemistry? How would this be distinguished from tangential sectioning through tonsillar epithelial crypts?" Two features help with this distinction: the size of the nuclei, and the relative lack of lymphocyte percolation. Compare the next tonsillar epithelial crypt you come across with the next HPV-mediated oropharyngeal carcinoma. The majority of tumor cells will be at least 4 times, or larger than surrounding lymphocytes. The majority of benign epithelial cells are smaller than this cut-off. Normal reticulated epithelium demonstrates heavy lymphocyte trafficking, much greater than the tumor infiltrating lymphocytes seen in HPV-mediated oropharyngeal carcinoma.

Three additional features also suggest HPV-mediated cancer: "Inside out" maturation (◘ Fig. 4.29), multinucleated tumor cells (◘ Fig. 4.30), and cystic metastases (◘ Fig. 4.31). Usual squamous carcinoma typically reveals tumor islands in with peripheral proliferation and central maturation. Keratin pearls are generally seen in the center of tumor islands. In many HPV-mediated oropharyngeal carcinomas one sees this maturation pattern reversed. The centers of these islands can be cellular, filled with proliferating tumor cells, while the flattened maturing cells rim the island periphery. Multinucleated and anaplastic tumor cells can be commonly observed in HPV-mediated oropharyngeal carcinoma. Multinucleated tumor cells are defined as any high-power field containing three or more tumor cells with multiple nuclei; tumor anaplasia is defined as any high-power field with three or more tumor cells with nuclei ≥5 lymphocytes wide (~25 μm) [109]. Tumor anaplasia can be observed in usual, non-HPV-mediated cancers. However, multinucleated tumor cells are suggestive of HPV-mediation. Interestingly, both findings of multinucleated cells and anaplastic cells correlated with poorer disease-specific outcomes on multivariate analysis [109]. Validation of this finding is important in the context of determining which patients might not be suitable for treatment de-intensification paradigms [110].

Typically, HPV-mediated oropharyngeal cancers form cystic metastases with paradoxical "tumor normalization". This refers to the phenomenon of malignancy mimicking benignity. The fact that segments of cystic metastases can mimic benign squamous epithelium probably accounts for "malignant branchial cleft cysts" of dubious repute. Cilia may be observed at the luminal aspect of cystic metastases and may become the basis of another benign mimicker [111, 112].

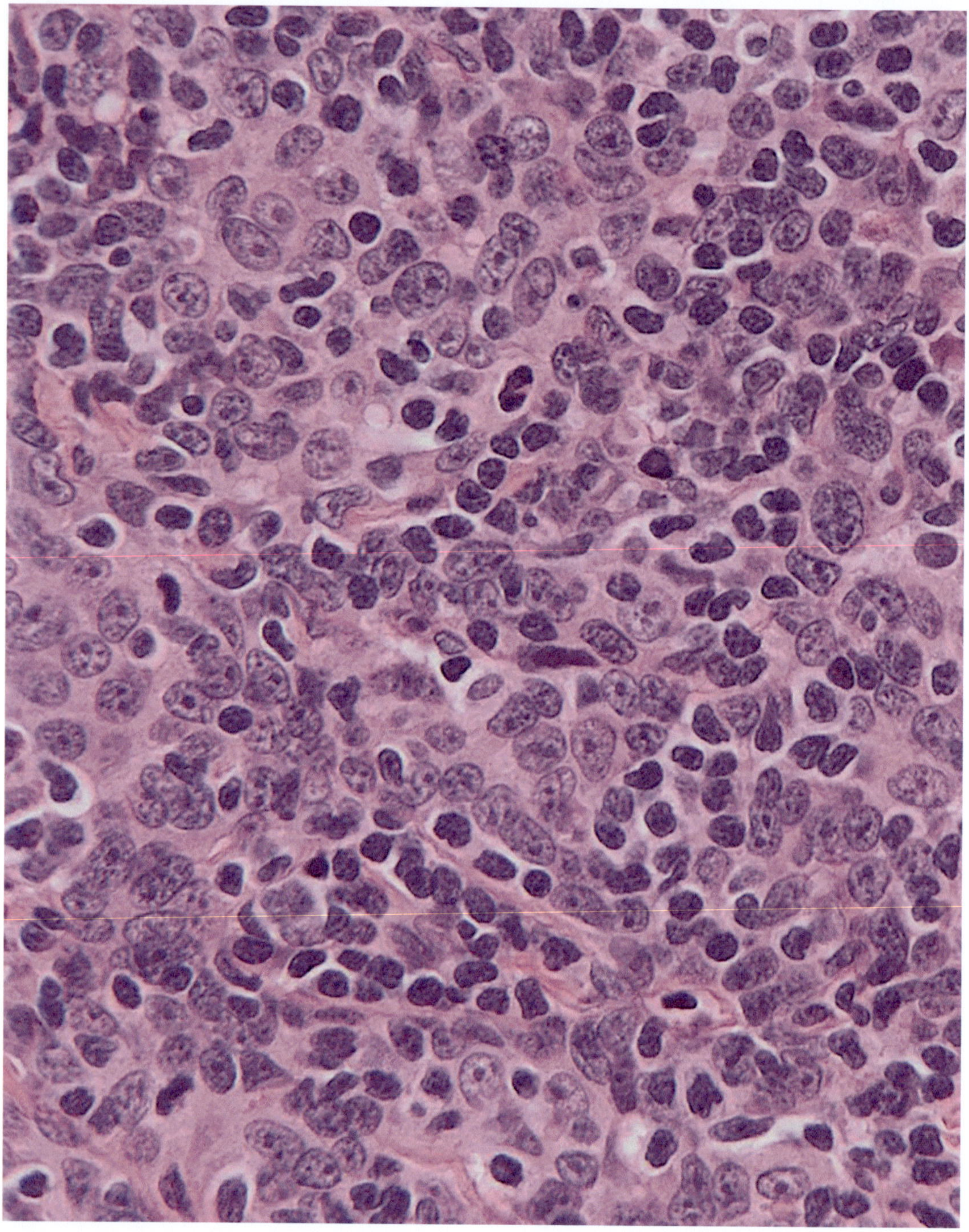

Fig. 4.25 HPV-mediated nonkeratinizing squamous carcinoma. Note the B-cell immunoblast-like morphology with a prominent amphophilic nucleolus and minimal cytoplasm. The chromatin pattern is coarse, and there is variation in nuclear shape. Many nuclei are larger than three lymphocytes in diameter

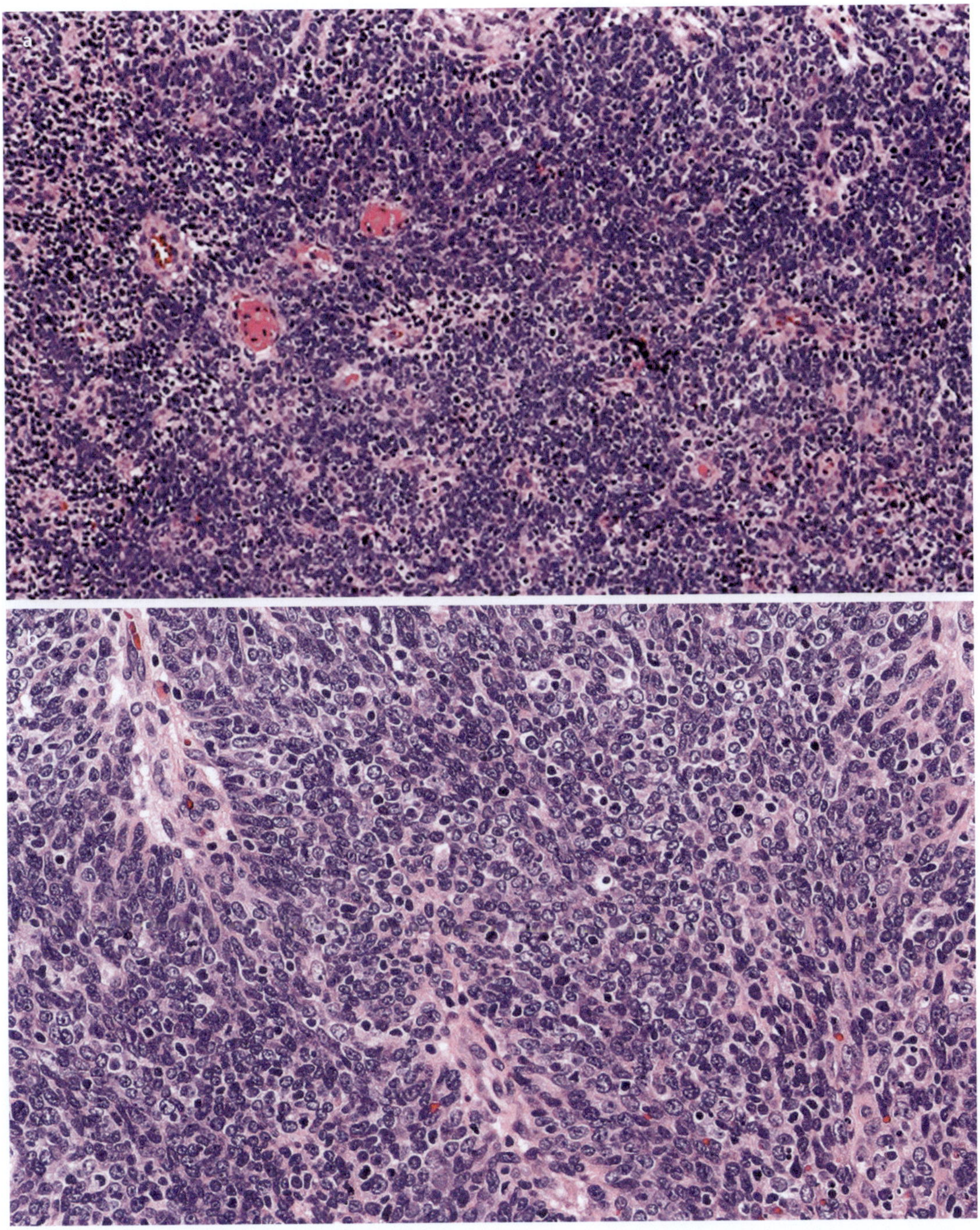

Fig. 4.26 **a** At low-power, you can appreciate a subtle reticulated pattern of the infiltrating carcinoma. **b** Rounded and spindled tumor cells infiltrating tonsillar tissue

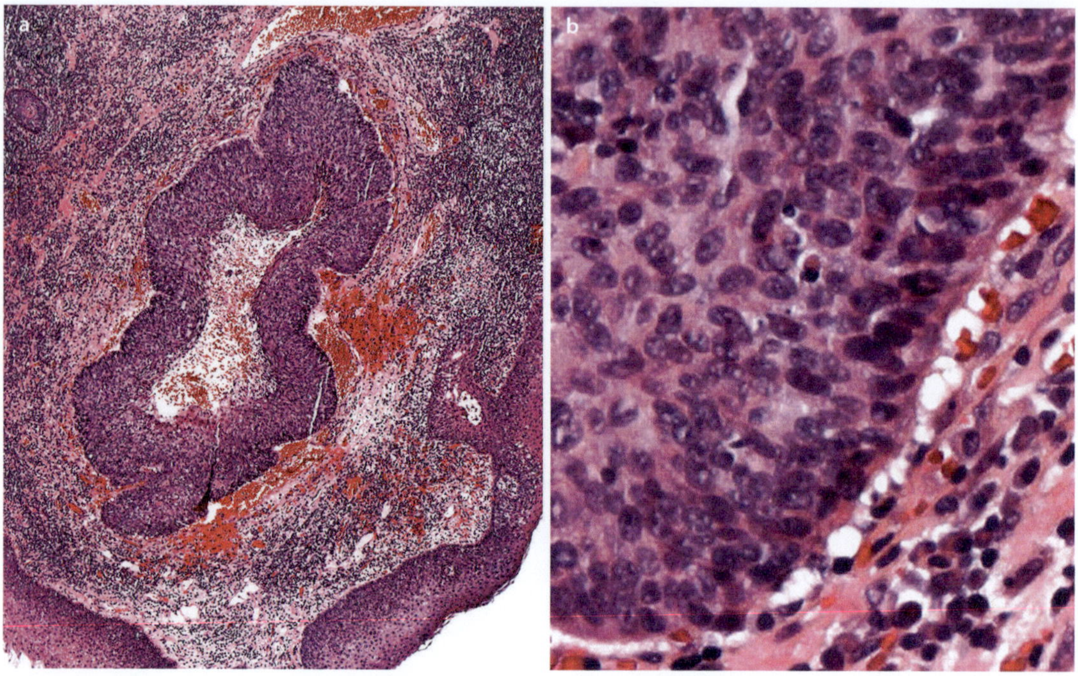

▣ **Fig. 4.27** **a** Tonsillar crypt replaced by oropharyngeal squamous carcinoma with maturation. This smooth contour (transitional pattern) is a common phenotype. It should not be confused with *carcinoma-in-situ,* which does not occur in tonsillar crypts. The lack of infiltrating lymphocytes seen at low-power serves as a hint that this area represents carcinoma. **b** These cells can be recognized as malignant by their size (>4× lymphocytes) and nuclear pleomorphism when compared to normal reticulated epithelium

Other morphologies which for HPV-mediated oropharyngeal cancers include "true" basaloid carcinomas with prominent nuclear palisading and basement membrane deposition (▣ Fig. 4.32), papillary variant of squamous carcinoma (▣ Fig. 4.33), and the lymphoepithelial variant of squamous carcinoma (▣ Fig. 4.34). ▣ Figures 4.35 and 4.36 illustrate some interesting treatment related phenomena.

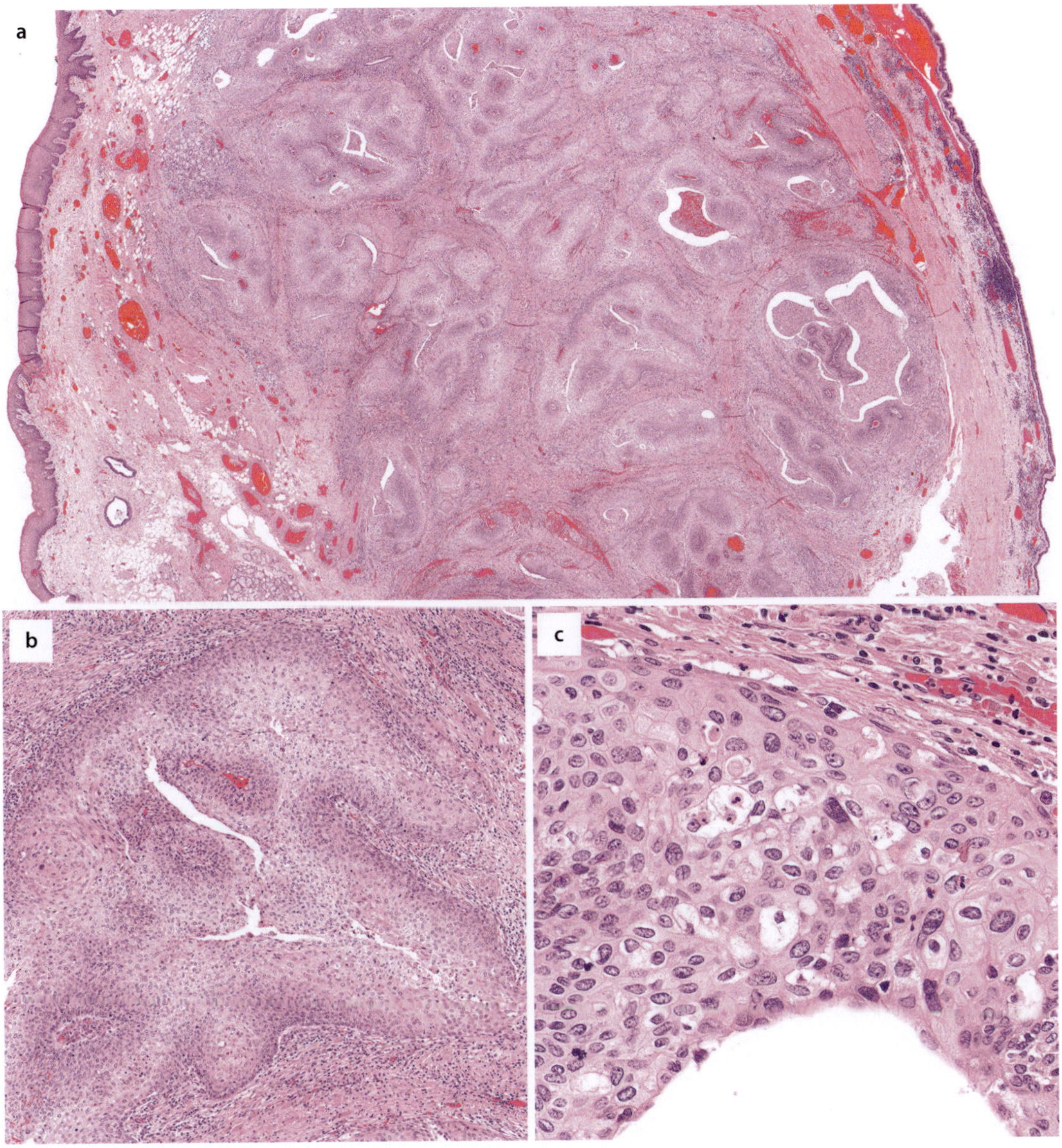

Fig. 4.28 **a** Transitional variant of squamous carcinoma of the soft palate. **b** This pattern refers to the formation of smooth ribbons of carcinoma. **c** An "up and down" polarity is obvious. The "down" refers to cells which mimic the basal reserve cells. The "up" refers to the cells opposite the basal reserve side, which demonstrate some maturation and flattening

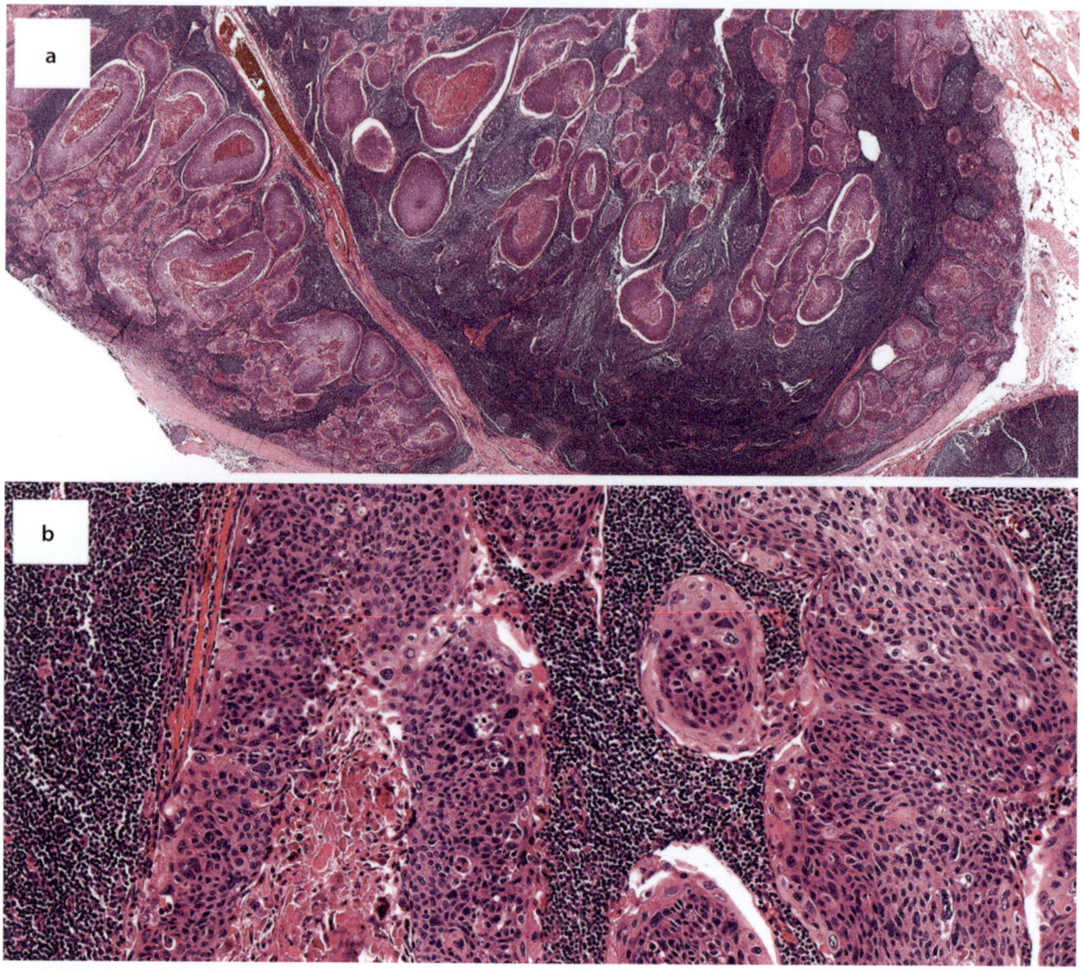

Fig. 4.29 **a**, **b** "Inside out" maturation – The peripheral rim of tumor the islands is composed of flattened keratinizing tumor cells. This is distinct from the usual non-HPV-mediated keratinizing squamous carcinoma, which reveals central keratinization

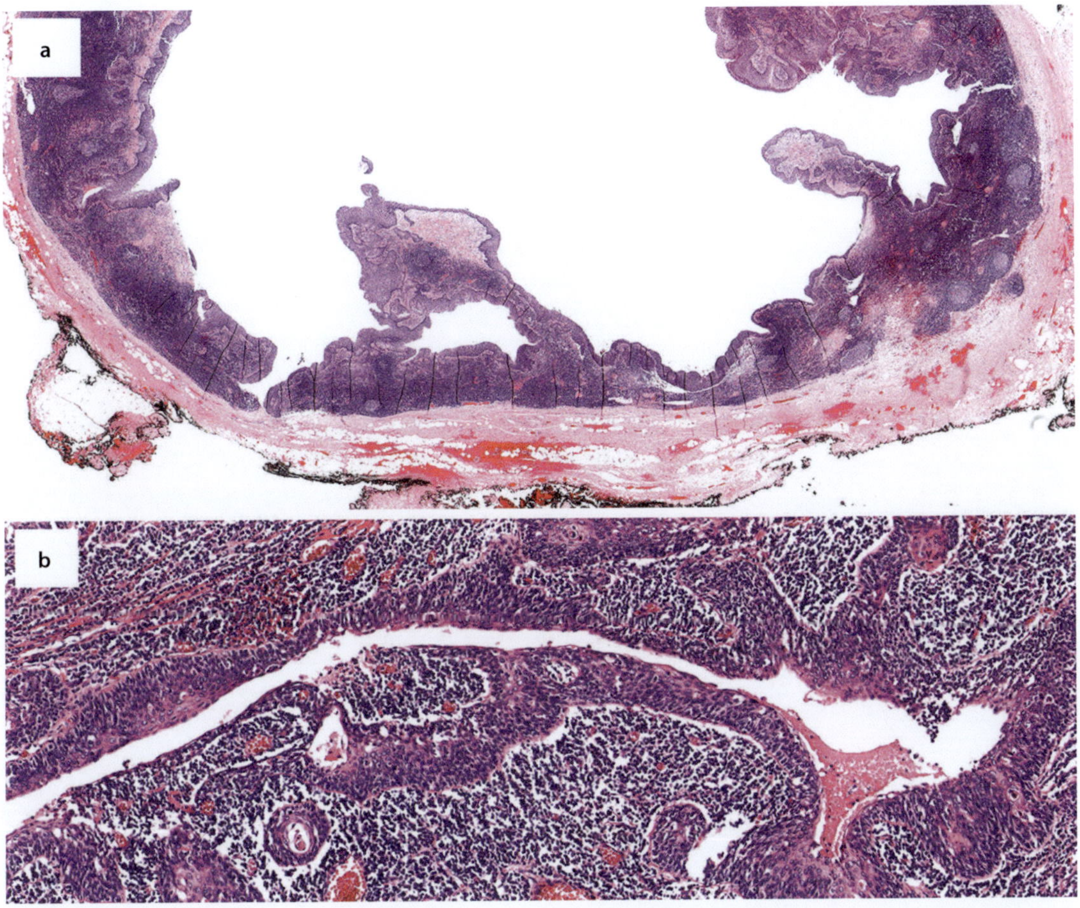

Fig. 4.30 HR-HPV-mediated oropharyngeal cancer can form cystic metastases in cervical lymph nodes, whereas the primary carcinoma is usually solid. It is unnecessary to document extranodal extension for p16 + oropharyngeal cancers. **a** Uniloculated cystic metastases. **b** The metastatic carcinoma forms a ribbon-like (transitional) pattern with variable tumor maturation appearing as flattened keratinizing cells

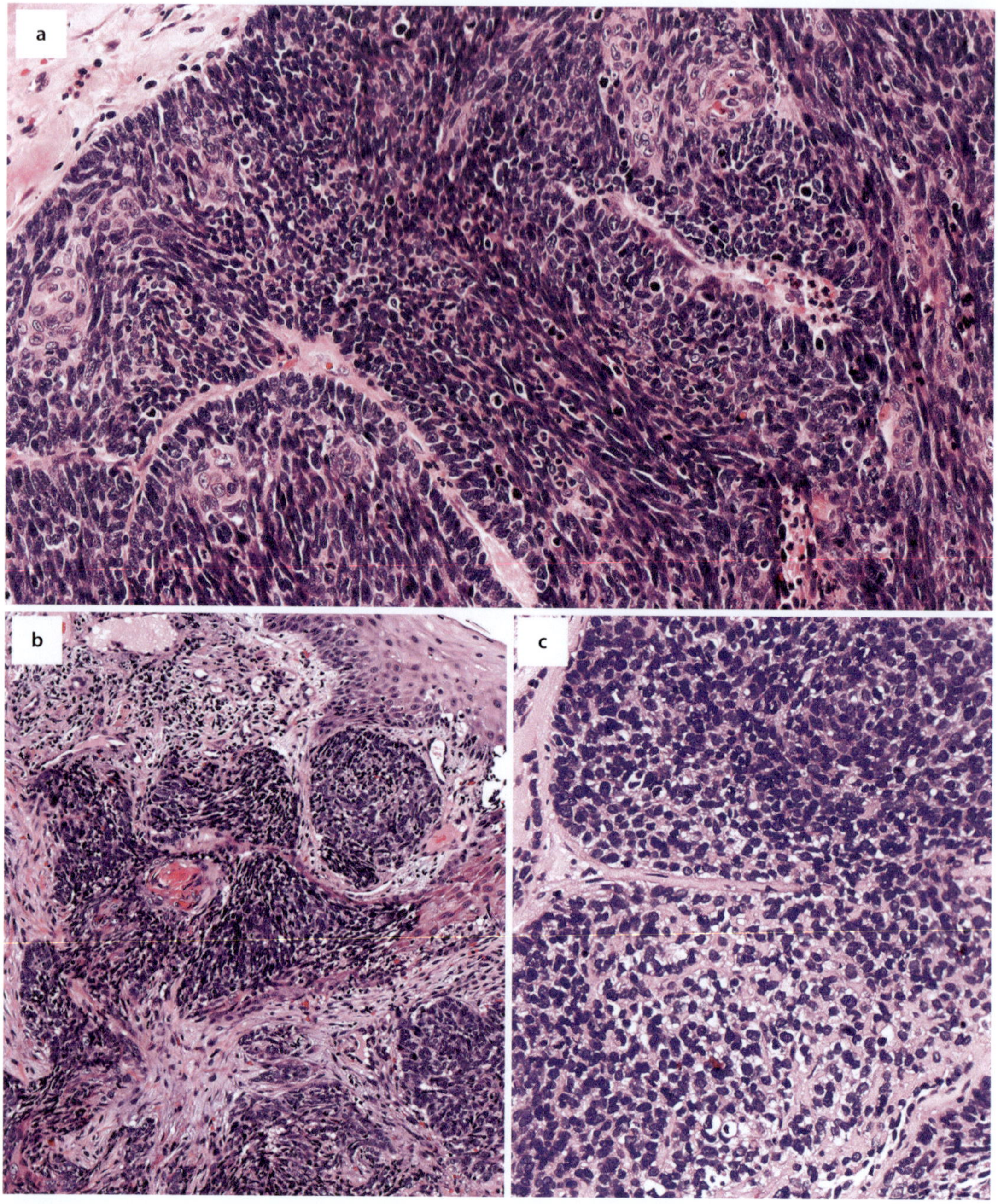

Fig. 4.31 The true basaloid variant of squamous carcinoma: The "basaloid" qualifier refers carcinomas composed of cells with high nuclear/cytoplasmic ration, with a tendency towards palisading and basement membrane production. **a** Prominent nuclear pallisading at the periphery of tumor islands. **b** An abrupt *in-situ* component is seen arising from the rete pegs. **c** Basement membrane deposits insinuating between individual tumor cells. This feature can be seen in the basaloid variant of squamous carcinoma, but is not a feature of adenoid cystic carcinoma or basal cell adenocarcinoma

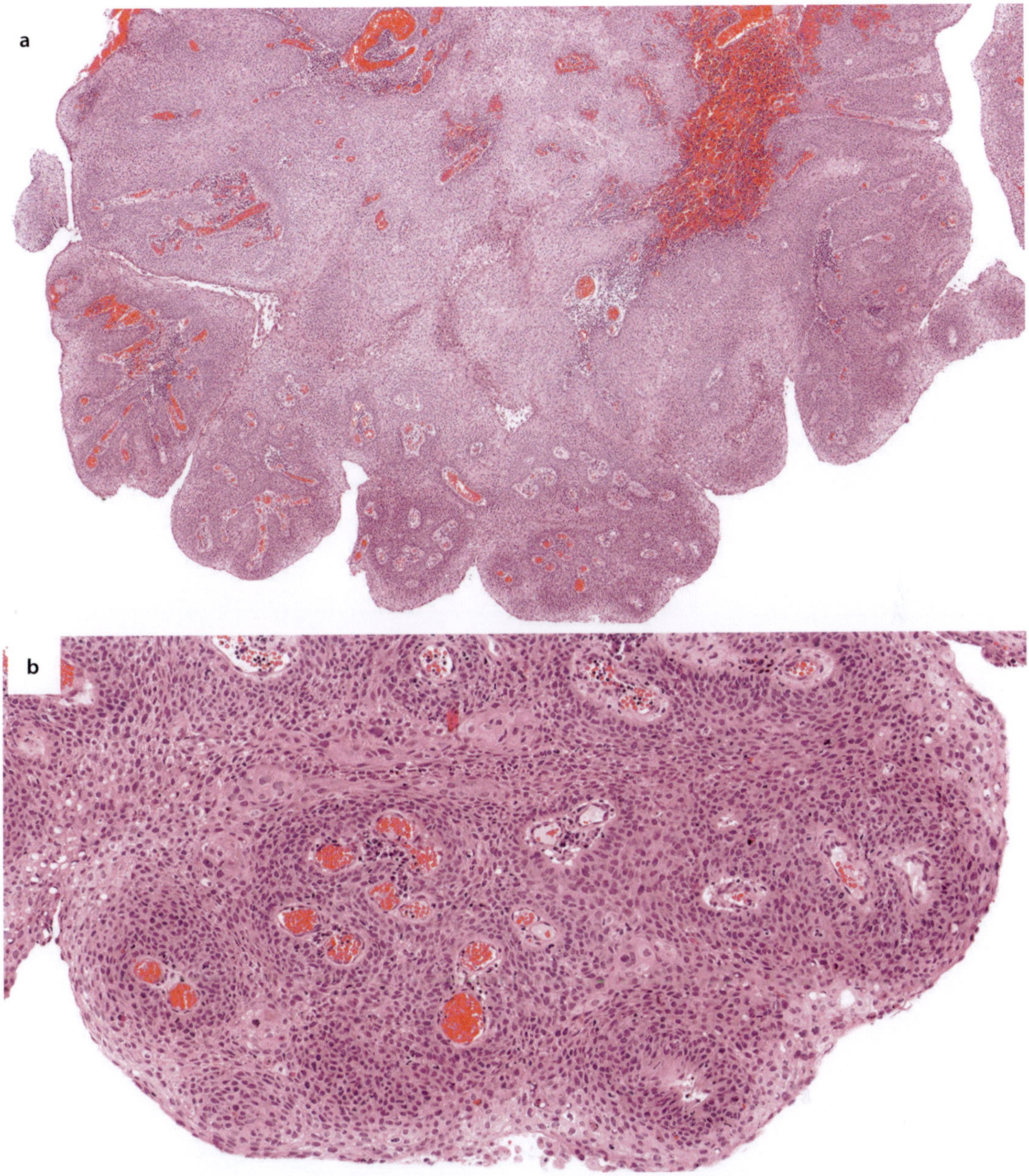

Fig. 4.32 **a** The papillary variant of squamous carcinoma: Notice the transition from papillary fibrovascular cores to a more confluent, transitional carcinoma-like pattern. **b** Increased cellularity and disordered maturation are present in this case

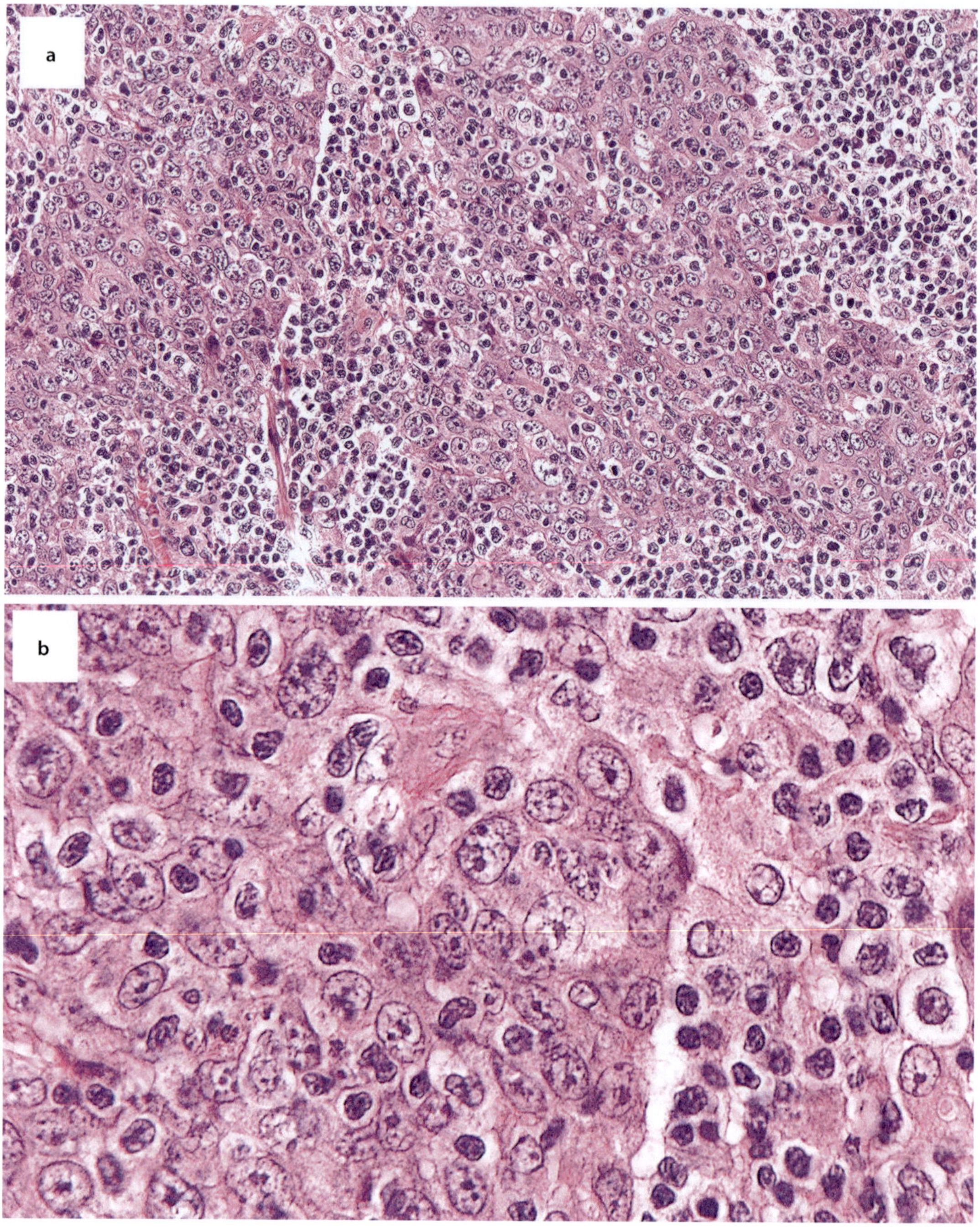

Fig. 4.33 **a** Lymphoepithelial variant of squamous carcinoma. Notice the syncytial pattern of epithelioid tumor cells within lymphoid tissue. **b** The syncytial pattern refers to the indistinct cell membranes between carcinoma cells. Again, notice the large tumor nuclei with prominent amphophilic nucleoli

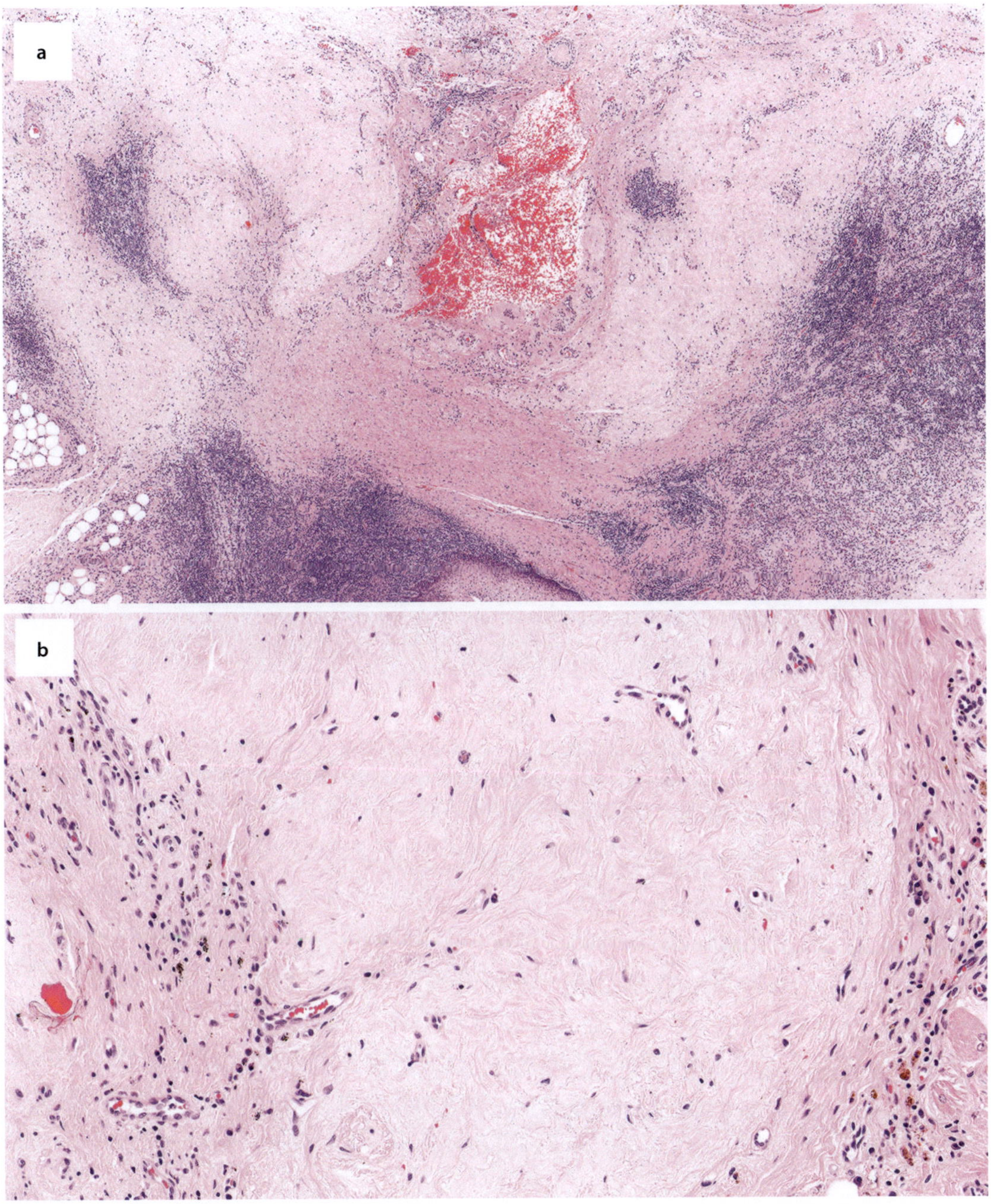

Fig. 4.34 a, b HPV-mediated tonsillar cancer with complete treatment response, post induction chemotherapy. Primary induction chemotherapy is one of a number of possible therapeutic approaches. Here we see complete response to induction chemotherapy alone, leaving a "loose" hyalinized scar and some residual chronic inflammation. By contrast, radiation alone, or chemoradiation, results in a more densely collagenized scar

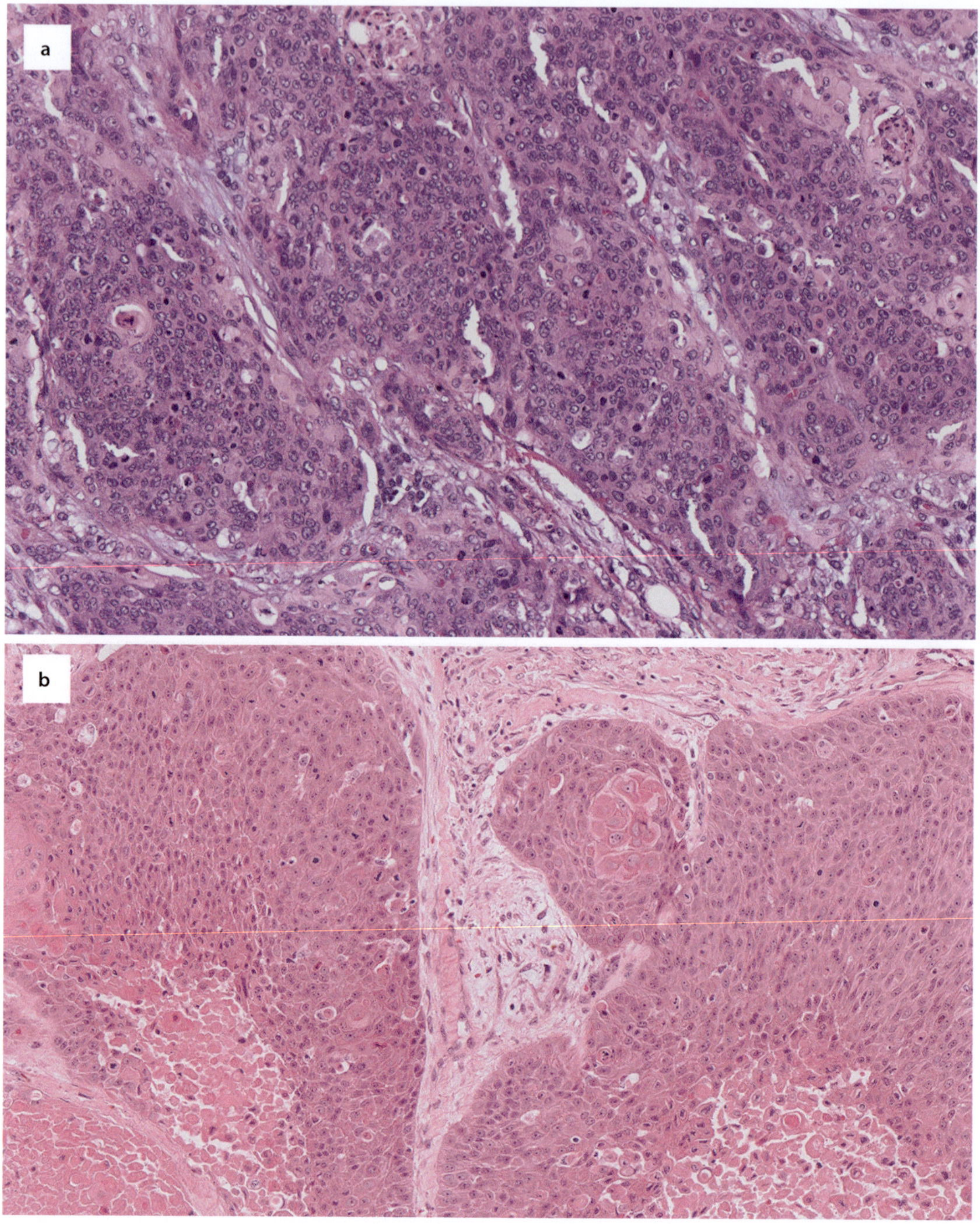

Fig. 4.35 HPV-mediated tonsillar cancer treated with cetuximab. **a** The response rate to Cetuximab, an EGFR targeted inhibitor is around 20–35% and associated with skin rash. Unfortunately, this skin rash remains the gold standard in predicting response. Functional labeled Cetuximab uptake studies have demonstrated increased uptake in phenotypically nonkeratinizing squamous carcinoma [81, 82]. **a** This patient presented in 2013 with an HPV-mediated oropharyngeal cancer which metastasized to an inguinal lymph node. He was treated with surgery and adjuvant radiation plus Cetuximab, then received maintenance Cetuximab. **b** When he presented in 2015 with recurrence in the inguinal bed, the morphology dramatically shifted to a Cetuximab-resistant, keratinizing squamous carcinoma. (Courtesy of Kathleen McGowan and Dr. Thom Loree, Erie County Medical Center, Buffalo, New York)

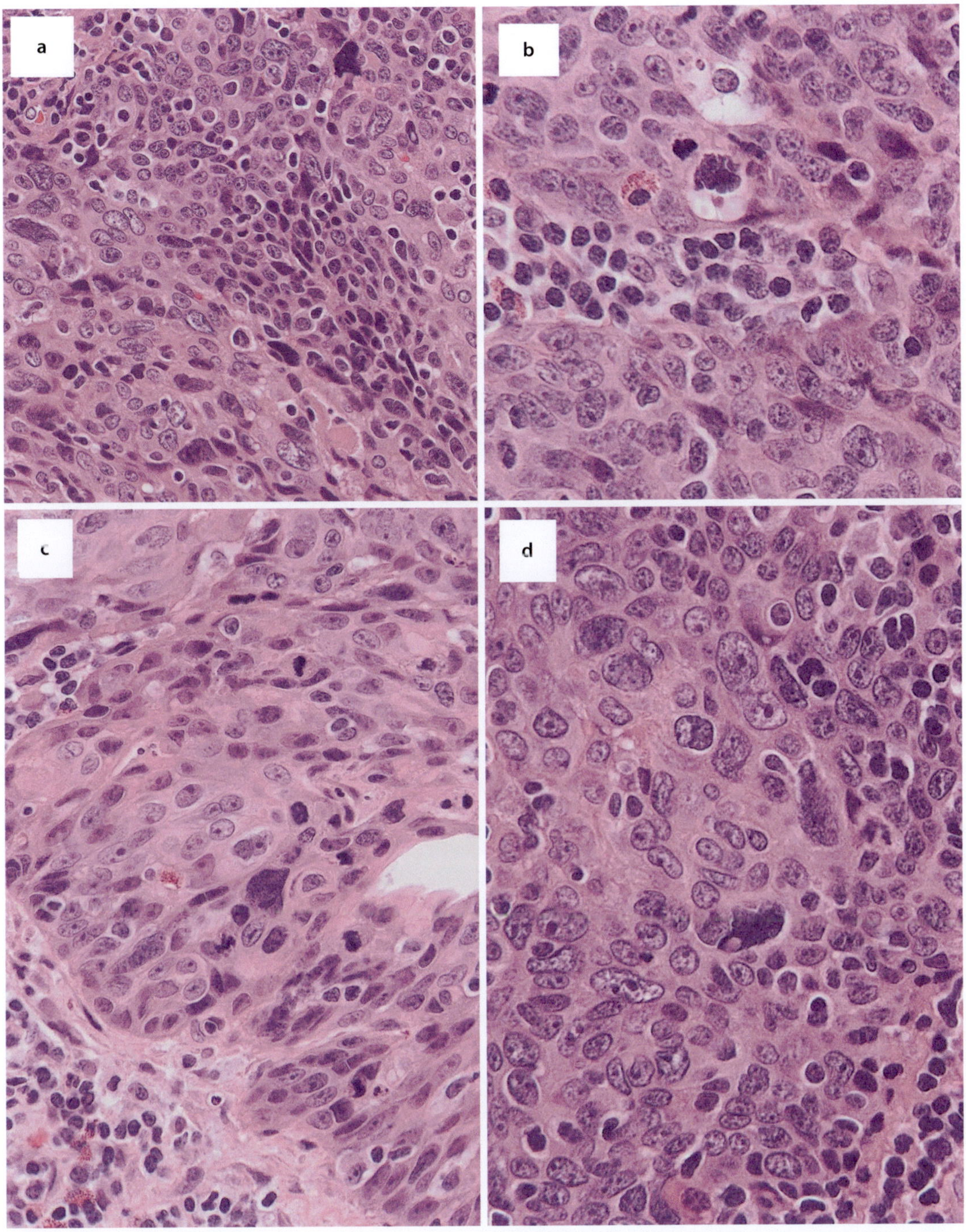

▣ **Fig. 4.36** **a–d** The many phenotypes of multinucleated and anaplastic tumor giant cells, another feature of HPV-mediated squamous carcinomas

4.18 Lymphoma of Waldeyer's Ring

Extranodal lymphomas often involve the head and neck, most commonly the mucosal associated lymphoid tissues (MALT) of Waldeyer's ring. Lymphomas of Waldeyer's ring are more common in Asian countries and the tonsil is the most commonly affected subsite. There is a wide age-rage at presentation including pediatric patients [113, 114]. Extranodal lymphomas more commonly are confined to one anatomic subsite. Patients usually present with painless masses; tonsillar lymphomas present as tonsillar asymmetries.

The vast majority of Waldeyer's ring lymphomas are high-grade, diffuse large B cell lymphomas (DLBCL) (66–75%) (■ Fig. 4.37) [115–118].

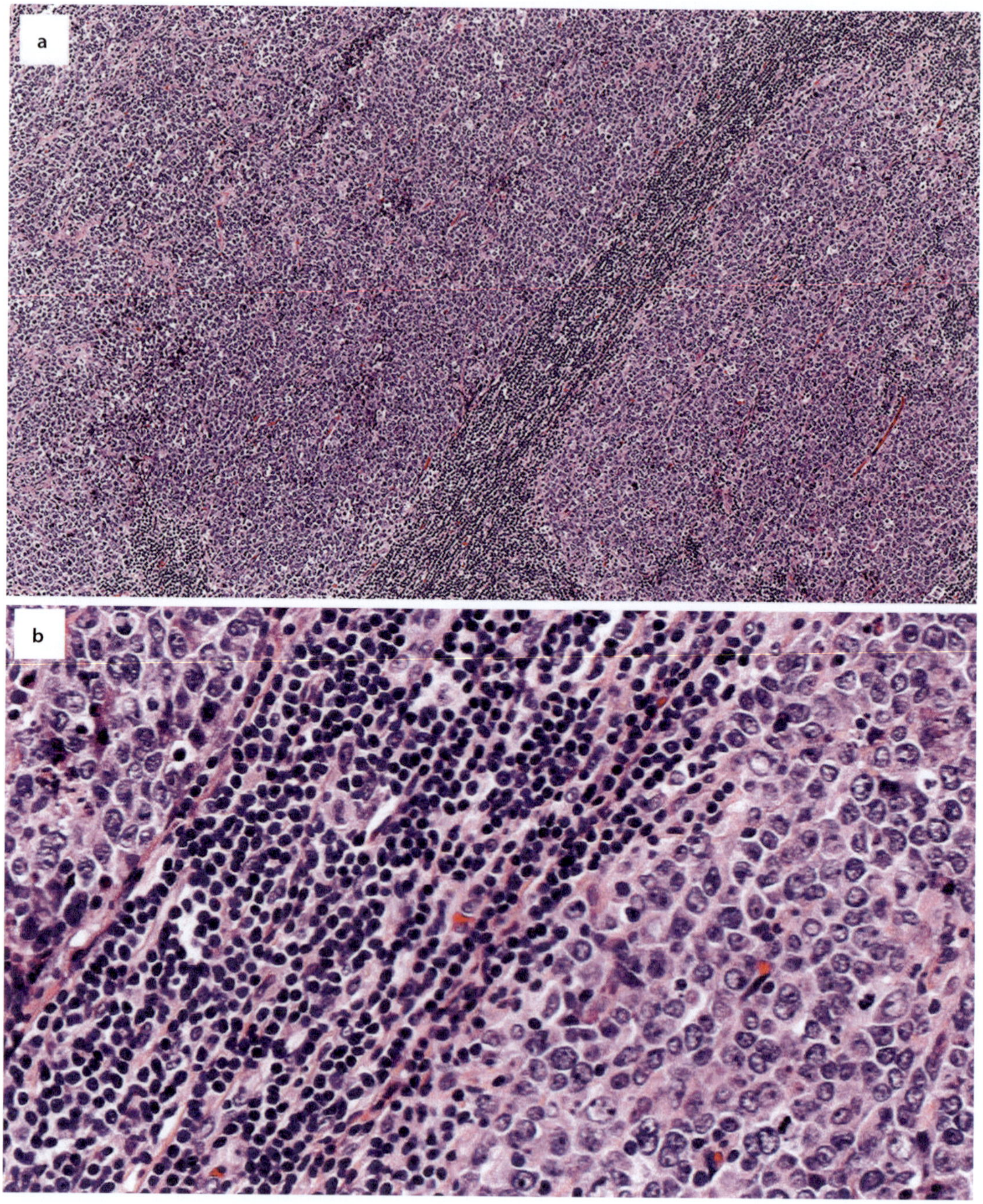

■ **Fig. 4.37** **a, b** Diffuse large B-cell lymphoma tongue base

DLBCL of Waldeyer's ring are associated with improved progression-free survival compared with matched nodal DLBCL [114]. The second most common phenotype is Pan-T/natural killer (PT/NK) (CD56+/CD8+/Granzyme B+) nasal type lymphoma, which is usually also EBV+ (4.3–19%) [115, 118]. The following phenotypes less commonly involve Waldeyer's ring: low-grade follicular lymphomas (6–9%), extraosseous plasmacytomas (3–10%), Burkitt's lymphoma (3–5%), and mantle cell lymphoma (3–4%) [115]. MALTomas (marginal zone lymphomas) are uncommon in Waldeyer's ring and associated with multiple organ involvement, usually gastrointestinal tract or eye [119].

Diagnostic pitfalls include confusing reactive diffuse paracortical T-cell zone hyperplasia with lymphoma [115]. Activated lymphocytes histologically stand out due to large nuclei and dispersed chromatin; pleomorphism should be minimal. Activated B-cells will demonstrate a spectrum of maturation including plasmacytic differentiation. Small mature lymphocytes should be seen scattered among transformed activated cells. Finally, immunohistochemistry should reveal mixed B-cell and T-cell lineage.

Acute infectious mononucleosis (IM) is well-known as a mimic of Hodgkin's lymphoma. Hodgkin's lymphoma will frequently involve contiguous lymph nodes. Both reactive immunoblasts of IM cells and Reed Sternberg cells express CD30+, but only the reactive immunoblasts express CD45/LCA. Hodgkin's disease will not reveal a maturation spectrum to plasmacytic differentiation. Finally, immunoblast-like lymphoma cells and lymphoepithelial-like carcinoma cells can mimic each other, replete with p16 overexpression (◘ Fig. 4.38). Don't let this happen on your watch.

4.19 Metastases to Waldeyer's Ring

Generally speaking, Waldeyer's ring is not a specific site for receiving metastatic disease. However, metastatic pulmonary neuroendocrine carcinoma, small cell type, to the tonsil is a known but rare phenomenon (◘ Fig. 4.39) [120–123]. Other malignancies which rarely metastasize to the tonsils include renal clear cell carcinoma, gastrointestinal carcinomas, seminomas, breast carcinomas, malignant phyloides tumor, pulmonary non-small cell carcinomas, and melanomas [120, 124, 125]. Bilateral tonsillar metastases is common in the context of metastatic melanoma (46%), seminoma (40%), gastric adenocarcinoma (40%), and breast adenocarcinoma (33%) [120]. Bilateral tonsillar metastases are uncommon in pulmonary non-small cell carcinoma (17%), and rare in renal clear cell carcinoma (8%) [120]. Not surprisingly, in some cases of tonsillar metastases of renal clear cell carcinoma, the metastases represented the index event [120].

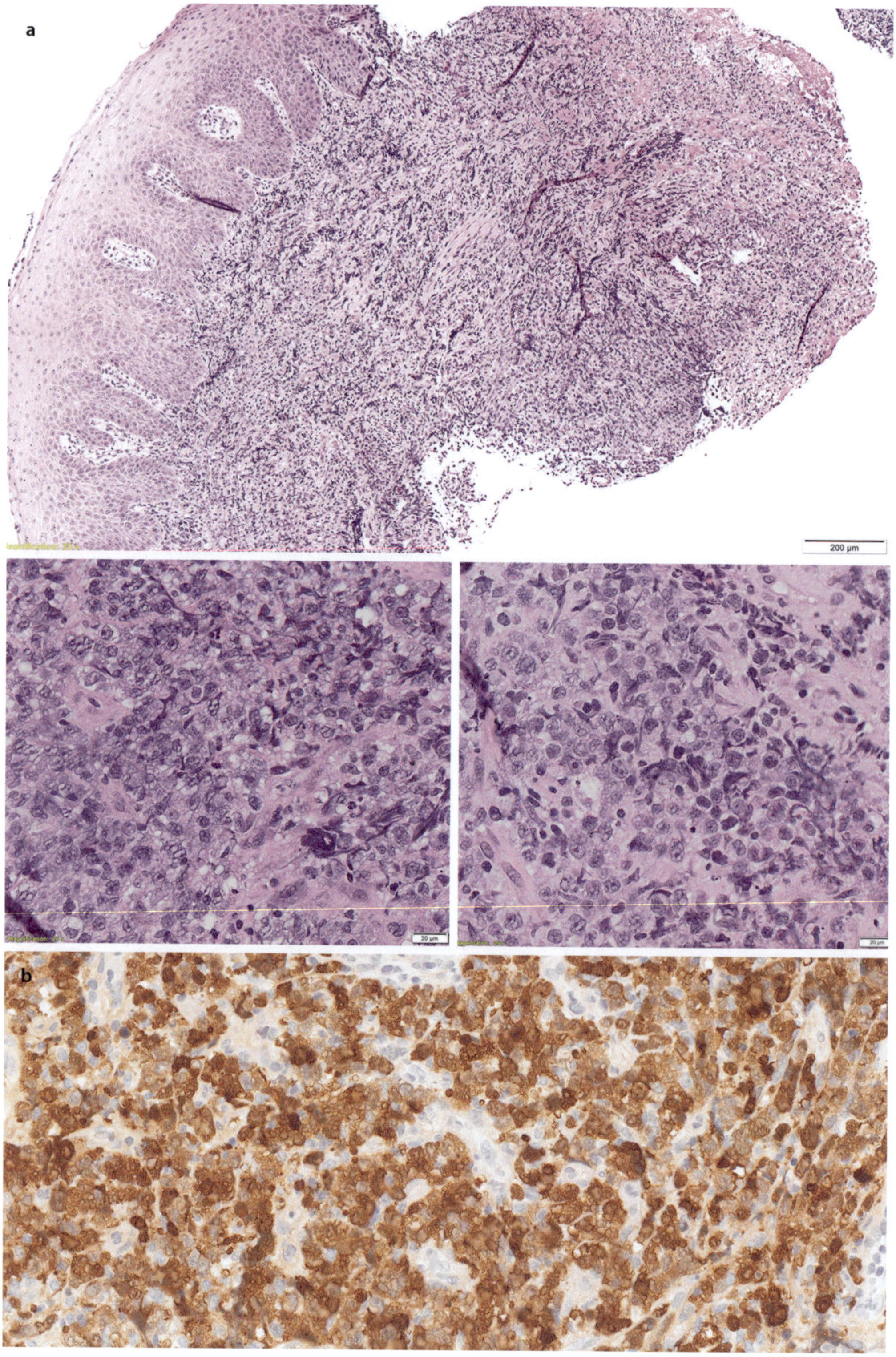

Fig. 4.38 **a**, **b** Tonsillar diffuse large B-cell lymphoma, overexpressing p16, originally diagnosed as an HPV-mediated squamous carcinoma. *Top*: Low power view of a dense submucosal infiltrate. *Middle left and right*: Discohesive large malignant cells. Notice the nuclei have an immunoblast-like appearence. Some of the nuclei have "popcorn" shapes. "Lymphoepithelioma-like carcinoma and diffuse large B-cell lymphoma should be considered. IHC for keratin and B-cell markers should have been performed. Instead, only IHC for p16 was performed, which was positive (*bottom*), leading to a misdiagnosis.

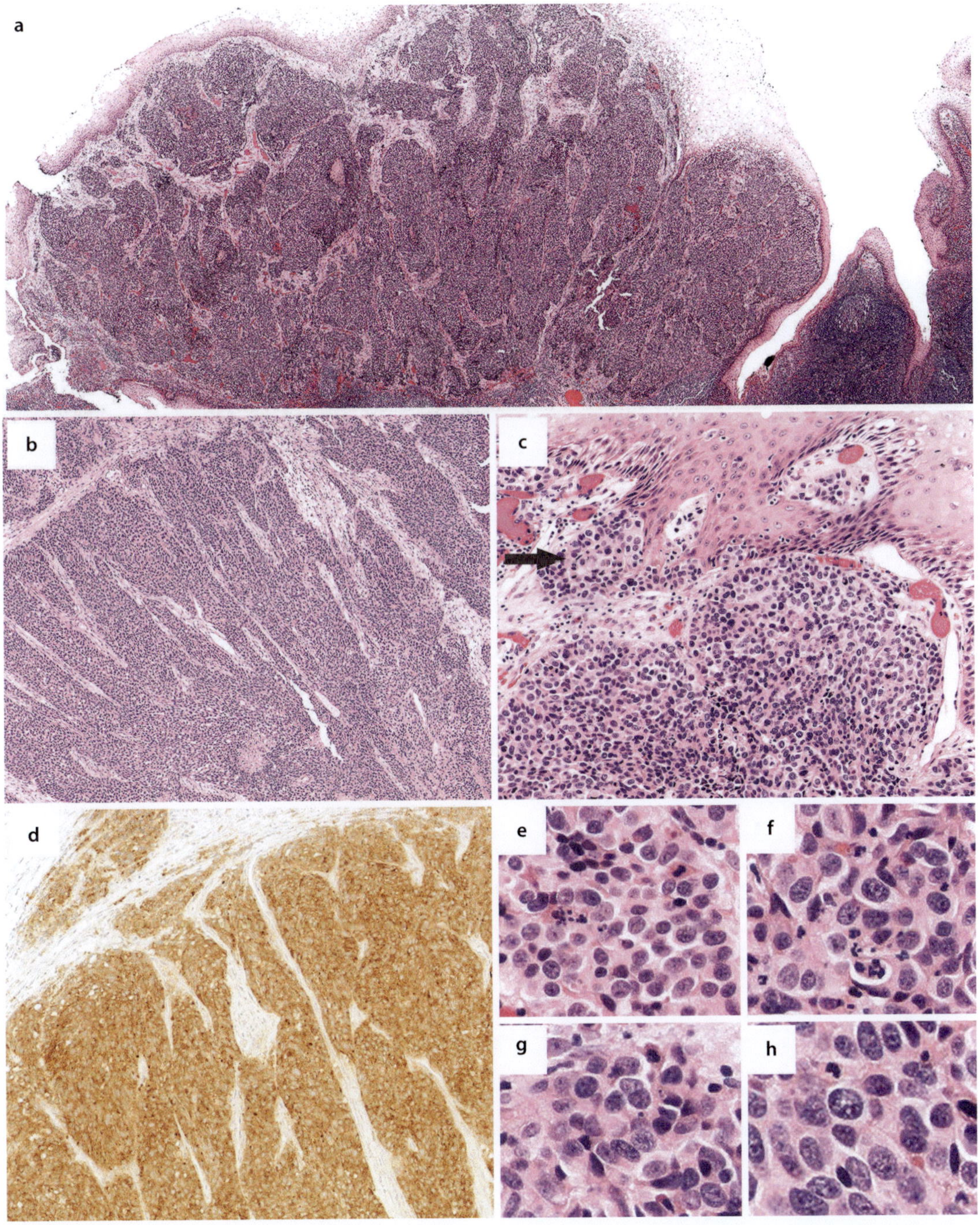

Fig. 4.39 Never forget that metastatic disease always lurks as a diagnostic confounder. **a**, **b** Low- and intermediate-power view of a metastatic pulmonary small cell neuroendocrine carcinoma presenting with metastasis to the tonsil. This was innocently diagnosed as a non-keratinizing squamous carcinoma, in the pre-p16 era. **c** The region interpreted as "in-situ" disease actually represents intramucosal extension (*arrow*). This patient also had a pulmonary mass and brain mass. The brain biopsy lead to the diagnosis of metastatic poorly-differentiated pulmonary neuroendocrine carcinoma, and re-examination of the tonsillar neoplasm. **d** Chromogrannin expression in tonsillar carcinoma. **e**, **f**, **g**, **h** In retrospect, look at these tumor nuclei. Fine "salt and pepper" chromatin, and small intranuclear bubbles hint at the neuroendocrine origin

Self-study

1. Study Fig. 4.40. Which of the following statements is true?
   A. If this originates from a hypopharyngeal cancer, then IHC for p16 is necessary for staging and prognostication.
   B. This benign papilloma is HPV-mediated.
   C. No cancer invasion is seen.
   D. If this originates from the oropharynx, then IHC for p40 is necessary for staging and prognostication.
   E. None of the above.

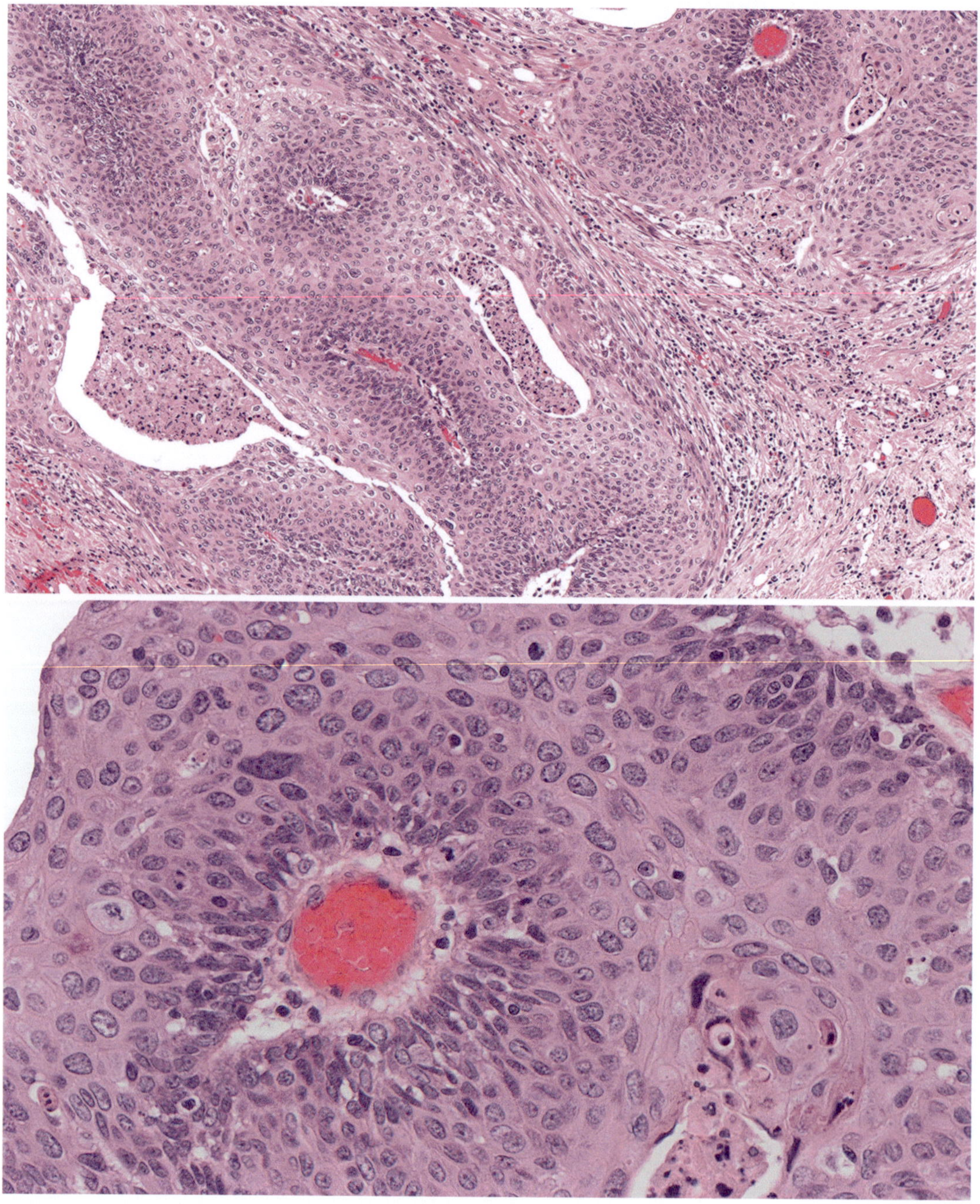

Fig. 4.40 Self study #1

2. Study ◘ Fig. 4.41. Which of the following is true regarding this tonsillar specimen, which overexpresses p16?
   A. This finding has been associated with significantly poorer outcomes when adjusted for confounders.
   B. The standard of care includes the following studies: ISH for HPV, EBV, and IHC for p16.
   C. If this patient has two positive lymph nodes under 3 cm, with extranodal extension, then he would be staged as pN2.
   D. This patient would benefit from radiosensitizers.

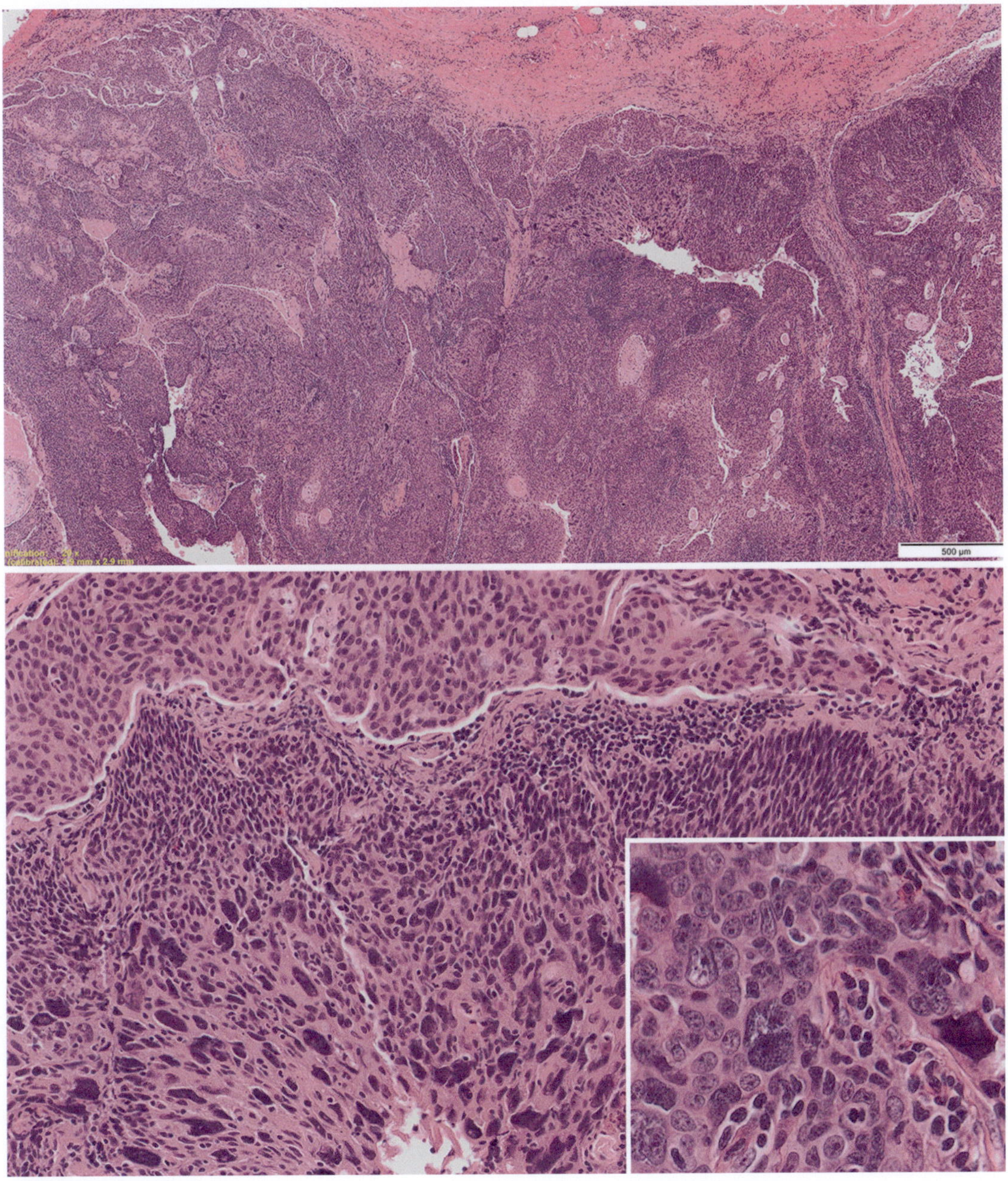

◘ **Fig. 4.41** Self study #2

3. Study ◘ Fig. 4.42, a sausage-shaped hypopharyngeal tumor. Which of the following statements is true?
   A. ◘ Figure 4.42 demonstrates a typical lipoma.
   B. ◘ Figure 4.42 demonstrates an atypical "fat-free" lipoma.
   C. This neoplasm is capable of multiple recurrences and locoregional metastases.
   D. FISH for *MDM2* is indicated.

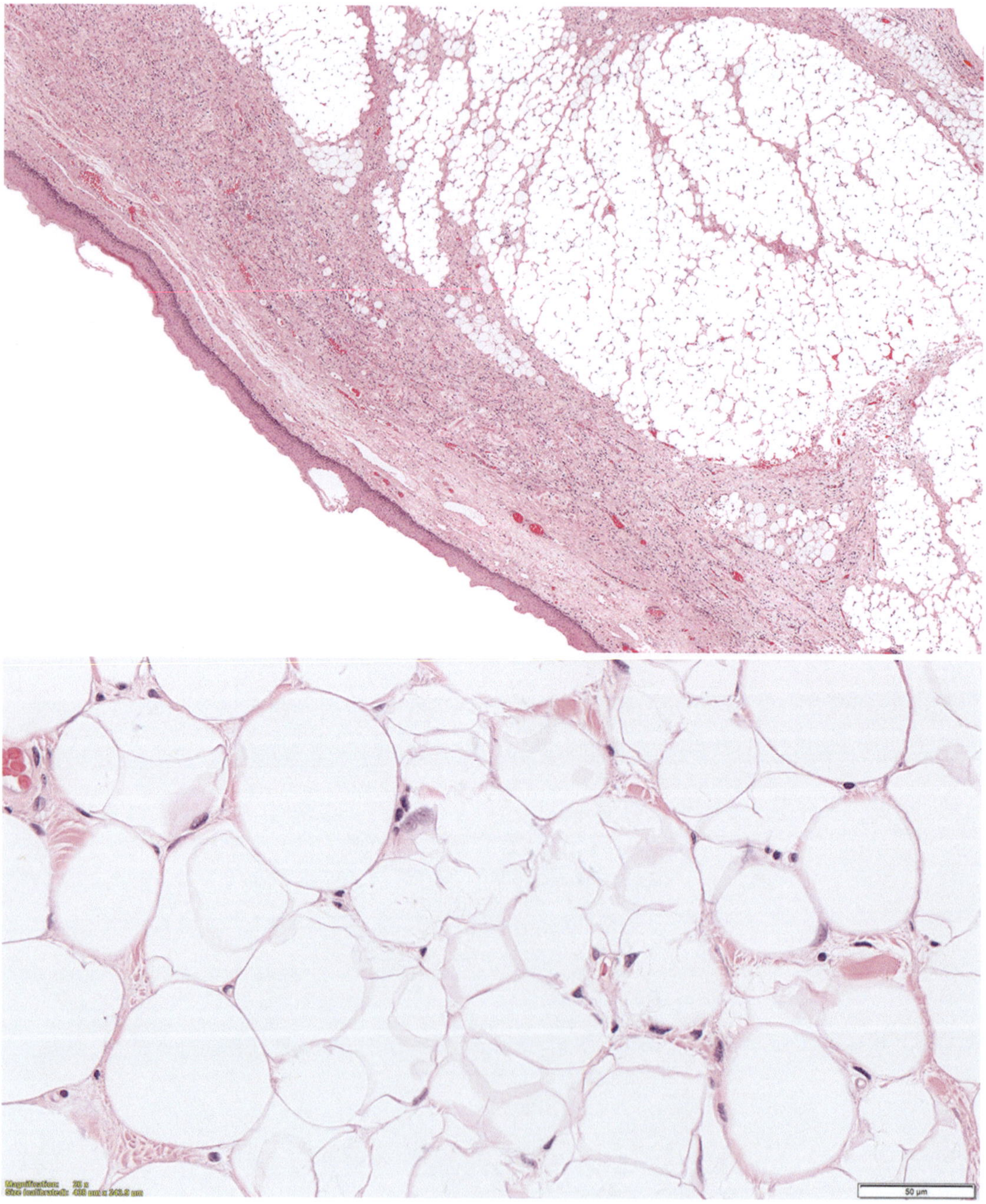

◘ **Fig. 4.42** Self study #3

4. Study ◘ Fig. 4.43, which is from a base of tongue biopsy. The inset represents CK5/6 IHC. IHC for p16 was negative. Which of the following statements is true?
   A. This is an HPV-mediated/p16 silenced carcinoma which requires staging as a p16 negative cancer.
   B. This is not HPV-mediated, and should be staged with the p16 negative cancers.
   C. This is an HPV-mediated oropharyngeal carcinoma, which should be staged with p16 positive cancers.
   D. This is a benign tonsillar crypt.
   E. The malignant potential cannot be assessed without knowledge of the lymph node status.

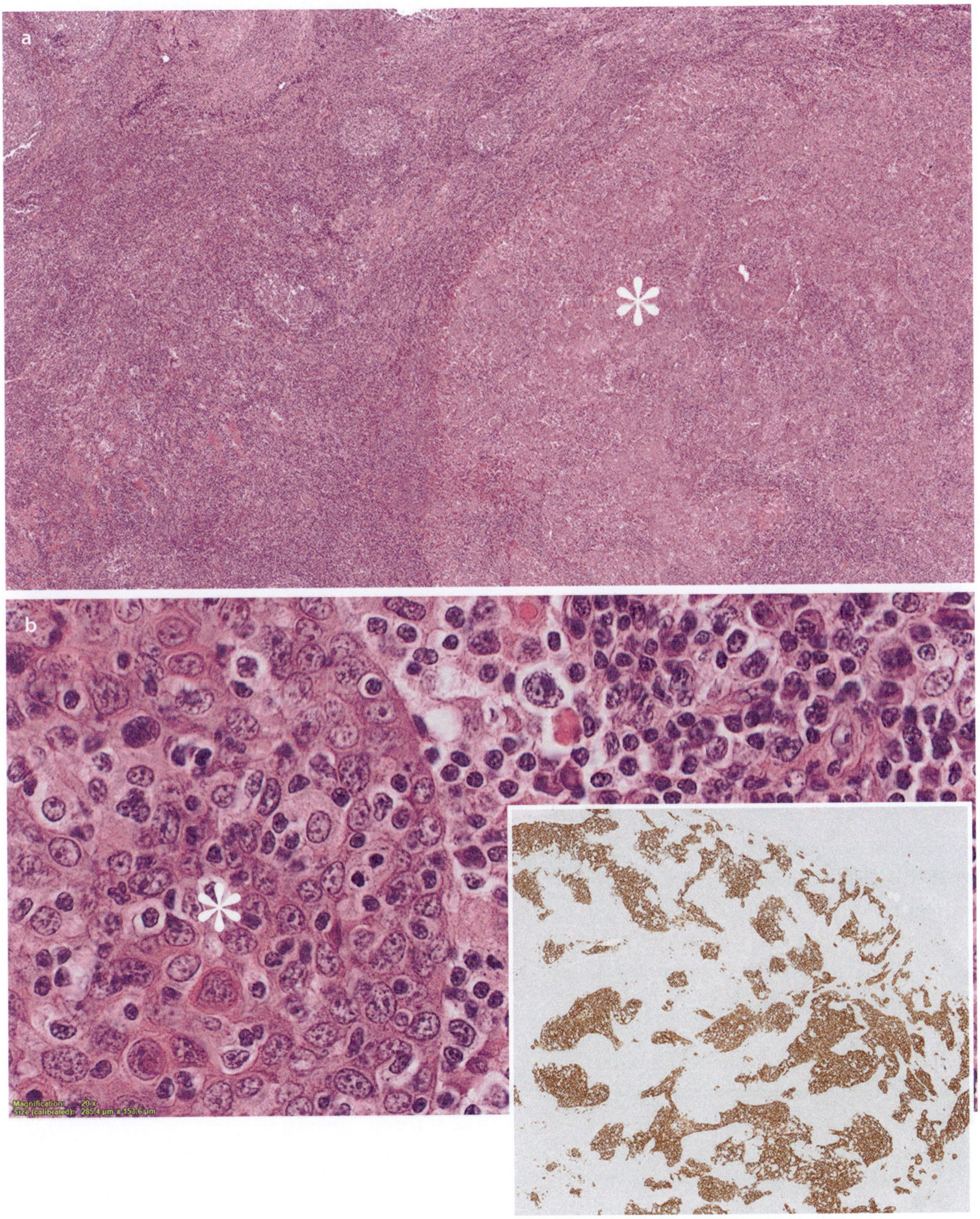

◘ **Fig. 4.43** Self study #4, **a** Low-power view of base of tongue biopsy. **b** Same specimen, high power. Notice the infiltrate at the asterisks. Inset represents IHC CK5/6

Answers

1. Study ◘ Fig. 4.40. Which of the following statements is true?
   A. If this originates from a hypopharyngeal cancer, then IHC for p16 is necessary for staging and prognostication. **False** – p16 expression is not included staging hypophaaryngeal cancers (See ◘ Table 4.3).
   B. This benign papilloma is HPV-mediated. **False** –The bottom image may correspond to a papillary structure, but the smooth ribbon of the upper panel corresponds to transitional type variant of squamous carcinoma. Even if you did not recognize this, the lower panel demonstrates significant pleomorphism and atypical mitotic figures.
   C. No cancer invasion is seen. **False** – the smooth ribbon of the upper panel corresponds to transitional type variant of squamous carcinoma. This represents a non-aggressive pattern of invasion.
   D. If this originates from the oropharynx, then IHC for p40 is necessary for staging and prognostication. **False** – p40 is a stem cell marker for epithelial cells, but irrelevant.
   E. None of the above. **TRUE** – This is a transitional type squamous carcinoma of the soft palate. However, you did not need to know this to answer the above questions.

2. Study ◘ Fig. 4.41. Which of the following is true regarding this tonsillar specimen, which overexpresses p16?
   A. This finding has been associated with significantly poorer outcomes when adjusted for confounders. **CORRECT.** See reference 109.
   B. The standard of care includes the following studies: ISH for HPV, EBV, and IHC for p16. **False** – If this specimen came from a metastatic lymph node with an unknown primary, then the above tests would have been useful to localize the cancer either to the nasopharynx or oropharynx. As you are told of the tonsillar location, EBV is no longer relevant.
   C. If this patient has two positive lymph nodes under 3 cm, with extranodal extension, then he would be staged as pN2. **False** – As you are told this is p16 overexpressing, the N staging criteria are 1–4 positive lymph nodes are N1. Lymph node size and extranodal extension do not modify N stage.
   D. This patient would benefit from radiosensitizers. **False.** See reference 85.

3. Study ◘ Fig. 4.42, a sausage-shaped hypopharyngeal tumor. Which of the following statements is true?
   A. ◘ Figure 4.42 demonstrates a typical lipoma. **False** –The distinction between lipoma and well-differentiated lipoma-like liposarcoma rests with the demonstration of *MDM2* amplification.
   B. ◘ Figure 4.42 demonstrates an atypical "fat-free" lipoma. **False** – Hahaha! No! This is not fat-free!
   C. This neoplasm is capable of multiple recurrences and locoregional metastases. **False** – well-differentiated lipoma-like liposarcoma may develop multiple local recurrences, but this tumor does not metastasize. The initial treatment of both lipomas and well-differentiated liposarcomas in this region is the same: conservative excision and close follow-up.
   D. FISH for *MDM2* is indicated. **CORRECT.** Amplification is sensitive and specific for well-differentiated lipoma-like liposarcoma.

4. Study ◘ Fig. 4.43, which is from a base of tongue biopsy. The inset represents CK5/6 IHC. IHC for p16 was negative. Which of the following statements is true?
   A. This is an HPV-mediated/p16 silenced carcinoma which requires staging as a p16 negative cancer. **CORRECT** – this is the most likely answer. The HPV-status is suggested by the

nonkeratinizing morphology. Panel A illustrates the potential diagnostic nightmare of HPV-mediated oropharyngeal cancers. This vague nodule seen at low-power (white asterisk) represents the cancer. From the surgeon's point of view, it is hardly palpable. From the pathologist's point of view, it hardly jumps out from the normal tonsillar tissue. A diagnosis of cancer can be made from panel B. Compare the size of the cells of interest with the tumor infiltrating lymphocytes. There is a greater skewing towards cells >4 times lymphocyte diameter. There is coarse chromatin, multiple nucleoli, and nuclear pleomorphism. The keratin expression is important in distinguishing this from large cell lymphoma. The lack of p16 overexpression should not exclude the possibility of there being transcriptionally active HR-HPV, as p16 promoter methylation due to smoking may be responsible for silencing. However, p16 silencing is important for prognostication and tumor staging.

B. This is not HPV-mediated, and should be staged with the p16 negative cancers. **False.** Cannot assume this based on p16 status.
C. This is an HPV-mediated oropharyngeal carcinoma, which should be staged with p16 positive cancers. **False.** It is p16 negative.
D. This is a benign tonsillar crypt. **False.** See the discussion above on morphology, panel B.
E. The malignant potential cannot be assessed without knowledge of the lymph node status. **False.** See the discussion above on morphology, panel B.

References

1. Perry ME. The specialised structure of crypt epithelium in the human palatine tonsil and its functional significance. J Anat. 1994;185:111–27.
2. Gloghini A, Colombatti A, Bressan G, Carbone A. Basement membrane components in lymphoid follicles: immunohistochemical demonstration and relationship to the follicular dendritic cell network. Hum Pathol. 1989;20:1001–7.
3. Jović M, Avramović V, Vlahović P, Savić V, Veličkov A, Petrović V. Ultrastructure of the human palatine tonsil and its functional significance. Romanian J Morphol Embryol. 2015;56:371–7.
4. Doorbar J. Latent papillomavirus infections and their regulation. Curr Opin Virol. 2013;3:416–21.
5. Doorbar J, Quint W, Banks L, Bravo IG, Stoler M, Broker TR, Stanley MA. The biology and life-cycle of human papillomaviruses. Vaccine. 2012;30:F55–70.
6. Israr M, Biryukov J, Ryndock EJ, Alam S, Meyers C. Comparison of human papillomavirus type 16 replication in tonsil and foreskin epithelia. Virology. 2016;499:82–90.
7. Chow W, Rotenberg BW. Discontinuing routine histopathological analysis after adult tonsillectomy for benign indication. Laryngoscope. 2015;125:1595–9.
8. Rokkjaer MS, Klug TE. Malignancy in routine tonsillectomy specimens: a systematic literature review. Eur Arch Otorhinolaryngol. 2014;271:2851–61.
9. Haughey BH, Sinha P, Kallogjeri D, Goldberg RL, Lewis JS Jr, Piccirillo J, Jackson RS, Moore EJ, Brandwein-Gensler M, Magnuson JS, Carroll WR, Jones TM, Wilkie MD, Lau A, Upile NS, Sheard J, Lancaster J, Tandon S, Robinson M, Husband D, Ganly I, Shah JP, Brizel DM, O'Sullivan B, Ridge JA, Lydiatt W. Pathology-based staging for HPV-positive squamous carcinoma of the oropharynx. Oral Oncol. 2016;62:11–9.
10. Carranza Leon BG, Turcu A, Bahn R, Dean DS. Lingual thyroid: 35-year experience at a tertiary care referral center. Endocr Pract. 2016;22:343–9.
11. Neinas FW, Gorman CA, Devine KD, Woolner LB. Lingual thyroid. Clinical characteristics of 15 cases. Ann Intern Med. 1973;79:205–10.
12. Meng Z, Lou S, Tan J, Jia Q, Zheng R, Liu G, Zhu M, He Q, Li D. Scintigraphic detection of dual ectopic thyroid tissue: experience of a chinese tertiary hospital. PLoS One. 2014. https://doi.org/10.1371/journal.pone.0095686.
13. Jain A, Pathak S. Rare developmental abnormalities of thyroid gland, especially multiple ectopia: a review and our experience. Indian J Nucl Med. 2010;25:143–6.
14. Castro PH, Volpato LE, Tramujas J, Borges AH. Ectopic thyroid at the base of the tongue of a young patient. Case Rep Dent. 2016;2016:9174970. Epub 2016
15. Sturniolo G, Vermiglio F, Moleti M. Thyroid cancer in lingual thyroid and thyroglossal duct cyst. Endocrinol Diabetes Nutr. 2017;64:40–3.
16. Mardekian S, Karp JK. Lymphangioma of the palatine tonsil. Arch Pathol Lab Med. 2013;137:1837–42.
17. Cengiz BP, Acar M, Giritli E. A pedunculated lymphangiomatous polyp of the palatine tonsil: a case report. Braz J Otorhinolaryngol. 2013;79:402.
18. Iliadou E, Papapetropoulos N, Karamatzanis E, Saravakos P, Saravakos K. Primary lymphangioma of the palatine tonsil in a 9-year-old boy: a case presenta-

tion and literature review. Case Rep Otolaryngol. 2016;2016:1505202. Epub 2016
19. Khatib Y, Gite V, Patel R, Shoeb M, Oraon A. Lymphangiomatous polyp of palatine tonsil in a child presenting with dysphagia and dysarthria. J Clin Diagn Res. 2015;9(5):ED01-2. https://doi.org/10.7860/JCDR/2015/11296.5877. Epub 2015
20. Chen HH, Lovell MA, Chan KH. Bilateral lymphangiomatous polyps of the palatine tonsils. Int J Pediatr Otorhinolaryngol. 2010;74:87–8.
21. Devi RS, Rajsekhar B, Srinivas GV, Moon NJ. Unusual length of pedicle: pedunculated squamous papilloma of uvula causing unusual dysphagia of long duration in a child of 10 years. Case Rep Dent. 2014;2014:313506. https://doi.org/10.1155/2014/313506.
22. Zhao M, Yu J, Li C. Lymphoid papillary hyperplasia of the palatine tonsil: a Chinese case report. Int J Clin Exp Pathol. 2013;6:1957–60.
23. Dias EP, Alfaro SE, De Piro SC. Lymphoid papillary hyperplasia: report of a case. Oral Surg Oral Med Oral Pathol Oral Radiol Endod. 2003;95:77–9.
24. Peitz U, Vieth M, Evert M, Arand J, Roessner A, Malfertheiner P. The prevalence of gastric heterotopia of the proximal esophagus is underestimated, but preneoplasia is rare – correlation with Barrett's esophagus. BMC Gastroenterol. 2017;17:87.
25. Di Nardo G, Cremon C, Bertelli L, Oliva S, De Giorgio R, Pagano N. Esophageal inlet patch: an under-recognized cause of symptoms in children. J Pediatr. 2016;176:99–104.
26. Rodríguez-Martínez A, Salazar-Quero JC, Tutau-Gómez C, Espín-Jaime B, Rubio-Murillo M, Pizarro-Martín A. Heterotopic gastric mucosa of the proximal oesophagus (inlet patch): endoscopic prevalence, histological and clinical characteristics in paediatric patients. Eur J Gastroenterol Hepatol. 2014;26:1139–45.
27. Sahin G, Adas G, Koc B, Akcakaya A, Dogan Y, Goksel S, Yalcin O. Is cervical inlet patch important clinical problem? Int J Biomed Sci. 2014;10:129–35.
28. Govani SM, Metko V, Rubenstein JH. Prevalence and risk factors for heterotopic gastric mucosa of the upper esophagus among men undergoing routine screening colonoscopy. Dis Esophagus. 2015;28:442–7.
29. Bingöl F, Balta H, Bingöl BÖ, Mazlumoğlu RM, Kılıç K. Lymphoepithelial cyst in the palatine tonsil. Case Rep Otolaryngol. 2016;2016:6296840. Epub 2016 Sep 18
30. Castro JG, Ferreira GM, Mendonça EF, Castro LA. A rare occurrence of lymphoepithelial cyst in the palatine tonsil: a case report and discussion of the etiopathogenesis. Int J Clin Exp Pathol. 2015;8:4264–8.
31. White JR, Weiss S, Anderson D, Mason SE, Schexnaildre MA, Nuss DW, Walvekar RR. Transoral resection of a retropharyngeal myxoma: a case report. Skull Base Rep. 2011;1:139–44.
32. Sinha SN, Yadav YC. Myxoma of the pharynx. Arch Otolaryngol. 1970;91:82–3.
33. Ayache S, Chatelain D, Tramier B, Strunski V. Oropharyngeal and hypopharyngeal myxoma: case report and literature review. J Laryngol Otol. 2007;121(5):e5.
34. Stratakis CA, Salpea P, Raygada M. Carney Complex. 2003 Feb 5 [Updated 2015 Jan 29]. In: Pagon RA, Adam MP, Ardinger HH, et al., editors. GeneReviews® [Internet]. Seattle (WA): University of Washington, Seattle; 1993–2017. Available from: https://www.ncbi.nlm.nih.gov/books/NBK1286/
35. Pereira GW, Pereira VD, Pereira Junior JA, da Silva RM. Cartilaginous choristoma of the tongue with an immunohistochemical study. BMJ Case Rep. 2012;2012. pii: bcr2012006752. https://doi.org/10.1136/bcr-2012-006752.
36. Kannar V, Prabhakar K, Shalini S. Cartilaginous choristoma of tonsil: a hidden clinical entity. J Oral Maxillofac Pathol. 2013;17:292–3.
37. Rossi-Schneider TR, Salum FG, Cherubini K, Yurgel LS, Figueredo MA. Cartilaginous choristoma of the tongue. Gerodontology. 2009;26:78–80.
38. Norris O, Mehra P. Chondroma (cartilaginous choristoma) of the tongue: report of a case. J Oral Maxillofac Surg. 2012;70:643–6.
39. Iglesias-Moreno MC, López-Salcedo MA, Gómez-Serrano M, Gimeno-Hernández J, Poch-Broto J. Parapharyngeal space tumors: fifty-one cases managed in a single tertiary care center. Acta Otolaryngol. 2016;136:298–303.
40. Locketz GD, Horowitz G, Abu-Ghanem S, Wasserzug O, Abergel A, Yehuda M, Fliss DM. Histopathologic classification of parapharyngeal space tumors: a case series and review of the literature. Eur Arch Otorhinolaryngol. 2016;273:727–34.
41. Caldarelli C, Bucolo S, Spisni R, Destito D. Primary parapharyngeal tumours: a review of 21 cases. Oral Maxillofac Surg. 2014;18:283–92.
42. Shi X, Tao L, Li X, Wu H, Huang W, Chen X, Li C, Shen Y, Chen Q, Tang D, Wei C, Wang D, Zhou L. Surgical management of primary parapharyngeal space tumors: a 10-year review. Acta Otolaryngol. 2017; 137(6):656–61.
43. Grilli G, Suarez V, Muñoz MG, Costales M, Llorente JL. Parapharyngeal space primary tumours. Acta Otorrinolaringol Esp. 2017;68:138–44.
44. Li G, Xin X, Wang X, Ren C. Dysphagia caused by giant schwannoma of the supraglottic oropharynx: a case report and review of the literature. Ann Med Surg (Lond). 2017;20:84–6.
45. Zheng Z, Jordan AC, Hackett AM, Chai RL. Pediatric desmoid fibromatosis of the parapharyngeal space: a case report and review of literature. Am J Otolaryngol. 2016;37:372–5.
46. Garcia-Perla A, Belmonte-Caro R, Infante-Cossio P, Muñoz-Ramos M, Esteban-Ortega F. Upper airway distress due to an oropharyngeal infantile myofibroma. J Craniomaxillofac Surg. 2012;40:e112–4.
47. Lin HW, Jung D, Lee LN, Sadow PM, Rocco JW. Solitary myofibroma of the oropharynx causing airway obstruction in an adult. Ear Nose Throat J. 2014;2014(93):410–7.
48. Smith MH, Reith JD, Cohen DM, Islam NM, Sibille KT, Bhattacharyya I. An update on myofibromas and myofibromatosis affecting the oral regions with report of 24 new cases. Oral Surg Oral Med Oral Pathol Oral Radiol. 2017;124:62–75.

49. Panja S, Champaka G, Shenoy AM. Infantile myofibroma of the pharynx presenting with severe upper airway obstruction in a child. Indian J Cancer. 2010;47:78–9.
50. Venkatesh V, Kumar BP, Kumar KA, Mohan AP. Myofibroma-a rare entity with unique clinical presentation. J Maxillofac Oral Surg. 2015;14:64–8.
51. Lopes RN, Alves Fde A, Rocha AC, Suassuna TM, Kowalski LP, de Castro JF, Perez DE. Head and neck solitary infantile myofibroma: Clinicopathological and immunohistochemical features of a case series. Acta Histochem. 2015;117:431–6.
52. Lu DY, Chang S, Cook H, Alizadeh Y, Karam AK, Moatamed NA, Dry SM. Genital rhabdomyoma of the urethra in an infant girl. Hum Pathol. 2012;43: 597–600.
53. Pichi B, Manciocco V, Marchesi P, Pellini R, Ruscito P, Vidiri A, Covello R, Spriano G. Rhabdomyoma of the parapharyngeal space presenting with dysphagia. Dysphagia. 2008;23:202–4.
54. Saini AT, Hernandez-Prera JC, Teng MS. Pyriform sinus soft-tissue mass recurring in esophagus after excision. JAMA Otolaryngol Head Neck Surg. 2015;141:573–4.
55. Helmberger RC, Stringer SP, Mancuso AA. Rhabdomyoma of the pharyngeal musculature extending into the prestyloid parapharyngeal space. AJNR Am J Neuroradiol. 1996;17:1115–8.
56. Papaspyrou G, Werner JA, Roessler M, Devaney KO, Rinaldo A, Ferlito A. Adult rhabdomyoma in the parapharyngeal space: report of 2 cases and review of the literature. Am J Otolaryngol. 2011;32:240–6.
57. Wang CP, Kwan PC, Ho CY. Lipoma of the palatine tonsil. J Formos Med Assoc. 2007;106:673–5.
58. Navaneetham A, Rao A, Gandhi A, Jeevan CA. Lipoma involving the masticator space. Ann Maxillofac Surg. 2011;1(1):93–4. https://doi.org/10.4103/2231-0746.83147.
59. Iwai K, Tomoda K, Nakai T, Kimura HA. Hypopharyngeal lipoma resulting in obstructive sleep apnea. Intern Med. 2015;54(21):2789–90. https://doi.org/10.2169/internalmedicine.54.4287. Epub 2015
60. Acquaviva G, Varakliotis T, Badia S, Casorati F, Eibenstein A, Bellocchi G. Lipoma of piriform sinus: a case report and review of the literature. Case Rep Otolaryngol. 2016;2016:2521583. Epub 2016
61. Zhu H, Sun J, Wei S, Wang D, Brandwein M. Well-differentiated laryngeal/hypopharyngeal liposarcoma in the MDM2 era report of three cases and literature review. Head Neck Pathol. 2017;11(2):146–51. https://doi.org/10.1007/s12105-016-0747-0. Epub 2016 Aug 4
62. Wenig BM, Heffner DK. Liposarcomas of the larynx and hypopharynx: a clinicopathologic study of eight new cases and a review of literature. Laryngoscope. 1995;105:747–56.
63. Gardner JM, Dandekar M, Thomas D, Goldblum JR, Weiss SW, Billings SD, Lucas DR, McHugh JB, Patel RM. Cutaneous and subcutaneous pleomorphic liposarcoma: a clinicopathologic study of 29 cases with evaluation of MDM2 gene amplification in 26. Am J Surg Pathol. 2012;36(7):1047–51. https://doi.org/10.1097/PAS.0b013e3182517b96.
64. Davis EC, Ballo MT, Luna MA, Patel SR, Roberts DB, Nong X, Sturgis EM. Liposarcoma of the head and neck: the University of Texas M. D. Anderson Cancer Center experience. Head Neck. 2009;31(1):28–36. https://doi.org/10.1002/hed.20923.
65. Golledge J, Fisher C, Rhys-Evans PH. Head and neck liposarcoma. Cancer. 1995;76(6):1051–8. Review. PubMed PMID: 8625207
66. Cheah A, Billings S, Goldblum J, Hornick J, Uddin N, Rubin B. Spindle cell/pleomorphic lipomas of the face: an under-recognized diagnosis. Histopathology. 2015;66:430–7.
67. Sachdeva MP, Goldblum JR, Rubin BP, Billings SD. Low-fat and fat-free pleomorphic lipomas: a diagnostic challenge. Am J Dermatopathol. 2009;31:423–6.
68. Frisch M, Hjalgrim H, Jaeger AB, Biggar RJ. Changing patterns of tonsillar squamous cell carcinoma in the United States. Cancer Causes Control. 2000;11: 489–95.
69. Dahlstrom KR, Adler-Storthz K, et al. HPV type 16 infection and squamous cell carcinoma of the head and neck in never-smokers: a matched pair analysis. Clin Cancer Res. 2003;9:2620–6.
70. D'Souza G, Kreimer AR, Viscidi R, et al. Case-control study of HPV and oropharyngeal cancer. N Engl J Med. 2007;356:1944–56.
71. El-Mofty SK, Lu DW. Prevalence of HPV type 16 DNA in squamous cell carcinoma of the palatine tonsil, and not the oral cavity, in young patients: a distinct clinicopathologic and molecular disease entity. Am J Surg Pathol. 2003;11:1463–70.
72. El-Mofty SK, Patil S. HPV-related oropharyngeal nonkeratinizing squamous cell carcinoma: characterization of a distinct phenotype. Oral Surg Oral Med Oral Pathol Oral Radiol Endod. 2006;101:339–45.
73. Furniss CS, McClean MD, Smith JF, et al. HPV 16 and head and neck squamous cell carcinoma. Int J Cancer. 2007;120:2386–92.
74. Gillison ML, Koch WM, Capone RB, et al. Evidence for a causal association between HPV and a subset of head and neck cancers. J Natl Cancer Inst. 2000;92:709–20.
75. Hansson BG, Rosenquist K, Antonsson A, et al. Strong association between infection with HPV and oral and oropharyngeal squamous cell carcinoma: a population-based case-control study in southern Sweden. Acta Otolaryngol. 2005;125:1337–44.
76. Kreimer AR, Clifford GM, Snijders PJ, et al. HPV16 semiquantitative viral load and serologic biomarkers in oral and oropharyngeal squamous cell carcinomas. Int J Cancer. 2005;115:329–32.
77. Mork J, Lie AK, Glattre E, et al. HPV infection as a risk factor for squamous-cell carcinoma of the head and neck. N Engl J Med. 2001;344:1125–31.
78. Nemes JA, Deli L, Nemes Z, Marton IJ. Expression of p16(INK4A), p53, and Rb proteins are independent from the presence of HPV genes in oral squamous cell carcinoma. Oral Surg Oral Med Oral Pathol Oral Radiol Endod. 2006;102:344–52.
79. Ringstrom E, Peters E, Hasegawa M, et al. HPV type 16 and squamous cell carcinoma of the head and neck. Clin Cancer Res. 2002;10:3187–92.

80. Schlecht NF, Burk RD, Adrien L, et al. Gene expression profiles in HPV-infected head and neck cancer. J Pathol. 2007;213:283–93.
81. Schwartz SR, Yueh B, McDougall JK, et al. HPV infection and survival in oral squamous cell cancer: a population-based study. Otolaryngol Head Neck Surg. 2001;125:1–9.
82. Weinberger PM, Yu Z, Haffty BG, et al. Molecular classification identifies a subset of HPV-associated oropharyngeal cancers with favorable prognosis. J Clin Oncol. 2006;24:736–47.
83. Lydiatt WM, Patel SG, O'Sullivan B, Brandwein MS, Ridge JA, Migliacci JC, Loomis AM, Shah JP. Head and neck cancers-major changes in the American Joint Committee on cancer eighth edition cancer staging manual. CA Cancer J Clin. 2017;67:122–37.
84. Black CC, Ogomo C. Does pTis exist in HPV-driven tonsillar carcinomas? An ultrastructural review and examination of two cases. Ultrastruct Pathol. 2017;41:55–61.
85. Lassen P, Eriksen JG, Hamilton-Dutoit S, Tramm T, Alsner J, Overgaard J, Danish Head and Neck Cancer Group (DAHANCA). HPV-associated p16-expression and response to hypoxic modification of radiotherapy in head and neck cancer. Radiother Oncol. 2010;94:30–5.
86. Schlecht NF, Brandwein-Gensler M, Nuovo GJ, Li M, Smith RV, Burk RD, Prystowsky MB. A comparison of clinically utilized human papillomavirus detection methods in head and neck cancer. Mod Pathol. 2011;24:1295–305.
87. Isayeva T, Xu J, Dai Q, Whitley AC, Bonner J, Nabell L, Spencer S, Carroll W, Jones G, Ragin C, Brandwein-Gensler M. African Americans with oropharyngeal carcinoma have significantly poorer outcomes despite similar rates of human papillomavirus-mediated carcinogenesis. Hum Pathol. 2014;45:310–9.
88. Hong A, Jones D, Chatfield M, Lee CS, Zhang M, Clark J, Elliott M, Harnett G, Milross C, Rose B. HPV status of oropharyngeal cancer by combination HPV DNA/p16 testing: biological relevance of discordant results. Ann Surg Oncol. 2013. https://doi.org/10.1245/s10434-012-2778-4.
89. Liu SZ, Zandberg DP, Schumaker LM, Papadimitriou JC, Cullen KJ. Correlation of p16 expression and HPV type with survival in oropharyngeal squamous cell cancer. Oral Oncol. 2015;51:862–9.
90. Liu JC, Parajuli S, Blackman E, Gibbs D, Ellis A, Hull A, Beck JR, Giri V, Iherjirka P, Khurana JS, Ragin CR. High prevalence of discordant human papillomavirus and p16 oropharyngeal squamous cell carcinomas in an African American cohort. Head Neck. 2016;38(Suppl 1):E867–72.
91. Koncar RF, Feldman R, Bahassi EM, Hashemi Sadraei N. Comparative molecular profiling of HPV-induced squamous cell carcinomas. Cancer Med. 2017;6:1673–85.
92. Faraji F, Zaidi M, Fakhry C, Gaykalova DA. Molecular mechanisms of human papillomavirus-related carcinogenesis in head and neck cancer. Microbes Infect. 2017. https://doi.org/10.1016/j.micinf.2017.06.001.
93. Seiwert TY, Zuo Z, Keck MK, Khattri A, Pedamallu CS, Stricker T, Brown C, Pugh TJ, Stojanov P, Cho J, Lawrence MS, Getz G, Brägelmann J, DeBoer R, Weichselbaum RR, Langerman A, Portugal L, Blair E, Stenson K, Lingen MW, Cohen EE, Vokes EE, White KP, Hammerman PS. Integrative and comparative genomic analysis of HPV-positive and HPV-negative head and neck squamous cell carcinomas. Clin Cancer. 2015. https://doi.org/10.1158/1078-0432.CCR-13-3310.
94. Cancer Genome AtlasN. Comprehensive genominc characterization of head nd neck squamous carcinomas. Nature. 2015;517:576–82.
95. Keck MK, Zuo Z, Khattri A, Stricker TP, Brown CD, Imanguli M, Rieke D, Endhardt K, Fang P, Brägelmann J, DeBoer R, El-Dinali M, Aktolga S, Lei Z, Tan P, Rozen SG, Salgia R, Weichselbaum RR, Lingen MW, Story MD, Ang KK, Cohen EE, White KP, Vokes EE, Seiwert TY. Integrative analysis of head and neck cancer identifies two biologically distinct HPV and three non-HPV subtypes. Clin Cancer Res. 2015;21:870–81.
96. Morris LG, Chandramohan R, West L, Zehir A, Chakravarty D, Pfister DG, Wong RJ, Lee NY, Sherman EJ, Baxi SS, Ganly I, Singh B, Shah JP, Shaha AR, Boyle JO, Patel SG, Roman BR, Barker CA, McBride SM, Chan TA, Dogan S, Hyman DM, Berger MF, Solit DB, Riaz N, Ho AL. The molecular landscape of recurrent and metastatic head and neck cancers: insights from a precision oncology sequencing platform. JAMA Oncol. 2016. https://doi.org/10.1001/jamaoncol.2016.1790.
97. Sepiashvili L, Bruce JP, Huang SH, O'Sullivan B, Liu FF, Kislinger T. Novel insights into head and neck cancer using next-generation "omic" technologies. Cancer Res. 2015;75:480–6.
98. Nulton TJ, Olex AL, Dozmorov M, Morgan IM, Windle B. Analysis of the cancer genome atlas sequencing data reveals novel properties of the human papillomavirus 16 genome in head and neck squamous cell carcinoma. Oncotarget. 2017;8:17684–99.
99. Walline HM, Goudsmit CM, McHugh JB, Tang AL, Owen JH, Teh BT, McKean E, Glover TW, Graham MP, Prince ME, Chepeha DB, Chinn SB, Ferris RL, Gollin SM, Hoffmann TK, Bier H, Brakenhoff R, Bradford CR, Carey TE. University of Michigan Head and Neck Specialized Program of Research Excellence (SPORE) Program. Integration of high-risk human papillomavirus into cellular cancer-related genes in head and neck cancer cell lines. Head Neck. 2017;39:840–52.
100. Gao G, Johnson SH, Vasmatzis G, Pauley CE, Tombers NM, Kasperbauer JL, Smith DI. Common fragile sites (CFS) and extremely large CFS genes are targets for human papillomavirus integrations and chromosome rearrangements in oropharyngeal squamous cell carcinoma. Genes Chromosomes Cancer. 2017;56:59–74.
101. Walline HM, Komarck CM, McHugh JB, Bellile EL, Brenner JC, Prince ME, McKean EL, Chepeha DB, Wolf GT, Worden FP, Bradford CR, Carey TE. Genomic integration of high-risk HPV alters gene expression in oropharyngeal squamous cell carcinoma. Mol Cancer Res. 2016;14:941–52.
102. Kelly JR, Husain ZA, Burtness B. Treatment de-intensification strategies for head and neck cancer. Eur J Cancer. 2016;68:125–33.

103. Bonner JA, Harari PM, Giralt J, Azarnia N, Shin DM, Cohen RB, et al. Radiotherapy plus cetuximab for squamous-cell carcinoma of the head and neck. N Engl J Med. 2006;354(6):567e78.
104. Marur S, Lee J-W, Cmelak A, Zhao W, Westra WH, Chung CH, et al. ECOG 1308: a phase II trial of induction chemotherapy followed by cetuximab with low dose versus standard dose IMRT in patients with HPV-associated resectable squamous cell carcinoma of the oropharynx (OP). In: ASCO Annual Meeting Proceedings, vol. 2012; 2012. p. 5566.
105. Cmelak A, Li S, Marur S, Zhao W, Westra WH, Chung CH, et al. Symptom reduction from IMRT dose deintensification: results from ECOG 1308 using the Vanderbilt Head and Neck Symptom Survey version 2 (VHNSS V2). In: ASCO Annual Meeting Proceedings, vol. 2015; 2015. p. 6021.
106. Lewis JS Jr, Khan RA, Masand RP, Chernock RD, Zhang Q, Al-Naief NS, Muller S, McHugh JB, Prasad ML, Brandwein-Gensler M, Perez-Ordonez B, El-Mofty SK. Recognition of nonkeratinizing morphology in oropharyngeal squamous cell carcinoma - a prospective cohort and interobserver variability study. Histopathology. 2012;60:427–36.
107. Gondim DD, Haynes W, Wang X, Chernock RD, El-Mofty SK, Lewis JS Jr. Histologic typing in oropharyngeal squamous cell carcinoma: a 4-year prospective practice study with p16 and high-risk HPV mRNA testing correlation. Am J Surg Pathol. 2016;40:1117–24.
108. Carpenter DH, El-Mofty SK, Lewis JS Jr. Undifferentiated carcinoma of the oropharynx: a human papillomavirus-associated tumor with a favorable prognosis. Mod Pathol. 2011;24:1306–12.
109. Lewis JS Jr, Scantlebury JB, Luo J, Thorstad WL. Tumor cell anaplasia and multinucleation are predictors of disease recurrence in oropharyngeal squamous cell carcinoma, including among just the human papillomavirus-related cancers. Am J Surg Pathol. 2012; 36:1036–46.
110. Lewis JS Jr, Ali S, Luo J, Thorstad WL, Madabhushi A. A quantitative histomorphometric classifier (QuHbIC) identifies aggressive versus indolent p16-positive oropharyngeal squamous cell carcinoma. Am J Surg Pathol. 2014;38:128–37.
111. Bishop JA, Westra WH. Ciliated HPV-related carcinoma: a well-differentiated form of head and neck carcinoma that can be mistaken for a benign cyst. Am J Surg Pathol. 2015;39:1591–5.
112. Radkay-Gonzalez L, Faquin W, McHugh JB, Lewis JS Jr, Tuluc M, Seethala RR. Ciliated adenosquamous carcinoma: expanding the phenotypic diversity of human papillomavirus-associated tumors. Head Neck Pathol. 2016;10:167–75.
113. Chen L, Al-Kzayer LF, Liu Y, Liu T. B-cell lymphomas involving Waldeyer's ring characterized by distinctive clinical and histopathological features: a comparison of pediatric to adult patients. Oncotarget. 2017;8:11544–54.
114. Guimarães AC, de Carvalho GM, Bento LR, Correa C, Gusmão RJ. Clinical manifestations in children with tonsillar lymphoma: a systematic review. Crit Rev Oncol Hematol. 2014;90:146–51.
115. Tan LH. Lymphomas involving Waldeyer's ring: placement, paradigms, peculiarities, pitfalls, patterns and postulates. Ann Acad Med Singap. 2004;33:15–26.
116. Laskar S, Mohindra P, Gupta S, Shet T, Muckaden MA. Non-Hodgkin lymphoma of the Waldeyer's ring: clinicopathologic and therapeutic issues. Leuk Lymphoma. 2008;49:2263–71.
117. Jing XM, Yu JR, Luo YK, Zhang SC, Liu JF, Li L, Wu P, Zhang ZH. Clinical characteristics and prognosis of primary Waldeyer's ring and lymph node diffuse large B-cell lymphoma in the rituximab era. Leuk Res. 2017;60:89–93.
118. Lee SJ, Suh CW, Lee SI, Kim WS, Lee WS, Kim HJ, Choi CW, Kim JS, Shin HJ, Consortium for Improving Survival of Lymphoma. Clinical characteristics, pathological distribution, and prognostic factors in non-Hodgkin lymphoma of Waldeyer's ring: nationwide Korean study. Korean J Intern Med. 2014;29:352–60.
119. Oh SY, Kim WS, Kim JS, Kim SJ, Lee S, Lee DH, Won JH, Hwang IG, Kim MK, Lee SI, Chae YS, Yang DH, Kang HJ, Choi CW, Park J, Kim HJ, Kwon JH, Lee HS, Lee GW, Eom HS, Kwak JY, Lee WS, Suh C, Kim HJ. Multiple mucosa-associated lymphoid tissue organs involving marginal zone B cell lymphoma: organ-specific relationships and the prognostic factors. Consortium for improving survival of lymphoma study. Int J Hematol. 2010;92:510–7.
120. Brownson RJ, Jaques WE, LaMonte SE, Zollinger WK. Hypernephroma metastatic to the palatine tonsils. Ann Otol Rhinol Laryngol. 1979;88:235–40.
121. D'Antonio C, Lombardini A, Onesti CE, Falcone R, Romiti A, Lombardi M, Lauro S, Marchetti P. A rare case of palatin tonsillar metastasis from small cell lung cancer. Transl Lung Cancer Res. 2016;5:709–11.
122. Unsal M, Kutlar G, Sullu Y, Yurtlu S. Tonsillar metastasis of small cell lung carcinoma. Clin Respir J. 2016;10:681–3.
123. Tajima S, Koda K. Palatine tonsillar metastasis of a small pulmonary adenocarcinoma showing an invasive micropapillary carcinoma pattern and Pagetoid spread at the tonsil: a case suggesting retrograde lymphatic metastasis from bulky lymph node metastases of the neck. Int J Clin Exp Pathol. 2015;8:13601–5.
124. Niu FY, Zhou Q, Yang JJ, Zhong WZ, Chen ZH, Deng W, He YY, Chen HJ, Zeng Z, Ke EE, Zhao N, Zhang N, Sun HW, Zhang QY, Xie Z, Zhang XC, Wu YL. Distribution and prognosis of uncommon metastases from non-small cell lung cancer. BMC Cancer. 2016. https://doi.org/10.1186/s12885-016-2169-5.
125. Sera T, Kashiwagi S, Takashima T, Asano Y, Goto W, Iimori N, Noda S, Onoda N, Ohsawa M, Hirakawa K, Ohira M. Multiple metastatic malignant phyllodes tumor of the breast with tonsillar metastasis: a case report. BMC Res Notes. 2017. https://doi.org/10.1186/s13104-017-2375-5.

Larynx: Anatomy, Nonneoplastic, Benign, and Malignant

M. S. Brandwein-Weber, *Textbook of Head and Neck Pathology*,
https://doi.org/10.1007/978-3-319-76106-0_5

Key Points

- Vocal nodules and vocal polyps are histologically identical, vocal nodules are usually bilateral, vocal polyps can be unilateral and are usually larger.
- Laryngeal oncocytic lesions are usually papillocystic, never solid. Consider the diagnoses of well-differentiated neuroendocrine carcinoma or oncocytoid mucoepidermoid carcinoma when facing a ***solid oncocytoid laryngeal lesion***.
- Florid aggressive papillomatosis can develop in up to 25% of patients. Around 3% of juvenile-onset recurrent respiratory papillomatosis patients develop pulmonary disease. Most juvenile-onset recurrent respiratory papillomatosis resolve by puberty, but 20% persist into adulthood. Less than 1% of patients with juvenile-onset florid tracheobronchial disease develop carcinomas of the lung, or unusual head and neck sites.
- Granular cell tumors can potentially be misdiagnosed as squamous carcinomas on superficial biopsies. Make yourself a habit of always searching the submucosa for islands of granular cells when you encounter squamous pseudoepitheliomatous hyperplasia.
- Functional staging of low T stage carcinomas is now replaced with the extent of anatomic involvement as a T stage determinant.
- The 2017 WHO criteria for laryngeal precursor lesions is now collapsed into low-grade versus high-grade schema. Carcinoma-*in-situ* is rolled in with high-grade dysplasia.
- Spindle cell variant of squamous carcinoma is more likely to be encountered in the larynx than a true spindle cell sarcoma.
- Chondrosarcoma is the most common laryngeal sarcoma and is usually low-grade; it hardly ever contains a spindle cell component.
- Laryngeal neuroendocrine carcinomas is the most common non-squamous carcinoma of the larynx; the small cell variant of poorly-differentiated neuroendocrine carcinoma is most common, followed by intermediate-grade neuroendocrine carcinoma

5.1 Anatomy and Histology

Anatomically, the larynx commences at the tip of the epiglottis and extends to the lower border of the cricoid cartilage (◘ Fig. 5.1). The anterior/superior boundaries of the larynx are the hyoepiglottic and thyrohyoid membranes, which separate the endolarynx from the pre-epiglottic space. The posterior laryngeal boundaries include the posterior commissure mucosa, the arytenoids, and the interarytenoid space. The inferior limit of the supraglottis is defined by an imaginary horizontal line joining the middle of the two ventricles. The supraglottis includes the epiglottis (◘ Fig. 5.2) saccular cyst, aryepiglottic folds, the vestibule (introitus, the space below the epiglottis and above the vestibular folds), and vestibular folds (false cords) extending to the superior half of the ventricle. The ventricle is the "pocket" between the vocal fold (true cord) and the vestibular fold (◘ Fig. 5.3). The lateral superior extension or "cul-de-sac" of the ventricle is variably sized, and referred to as the saccule (◘ Table 5.1).

The glottis compartment contains the vocal folds; it commences from the mid-point of the ventricle to 1.0 cm below the vocal fold (◘ Fig. 5.4). It is readily recognized by the segment of vocalis muscle. The superior surface of the vocal cord is usually covered by stratified squamous epithelium, the medial surface is invariably covered by stratified squamous epithelium. As an aside, the term "infraglottic" is often misused; neoplasia of the inferior aspect of the vocal fold are still classified as glottis. The subglottis extends from the inferior boundary of the glottis compartment to the inferior aspect of the cricoid ring. The term "transglottic" refers to a tumor involving both supraglottic and glottic compartments.

The hypopharynx is in continuity with the oropharynx, and is situated posterior to the larynx. Its superior border is represented by a plane at the level of the floor of the valleculae and hyoid bone. The inferior boundary is represented by a plane at the level lower border of the cricoid. The hypopharynx includes the pyriform sinuses, lateral and posterior hypopharyngeal walls and posterior cricoid mucosa. The paraglottic space refers to the hypopharyngeal region which is lateral to the thyroid lamina and cricoid, within the piriform sinuses (◘ Fig. 5.5). The paraglottic space is contiguous, superiorly, with the pre-epiglottic space. Tumor involvement of the paraglottic space

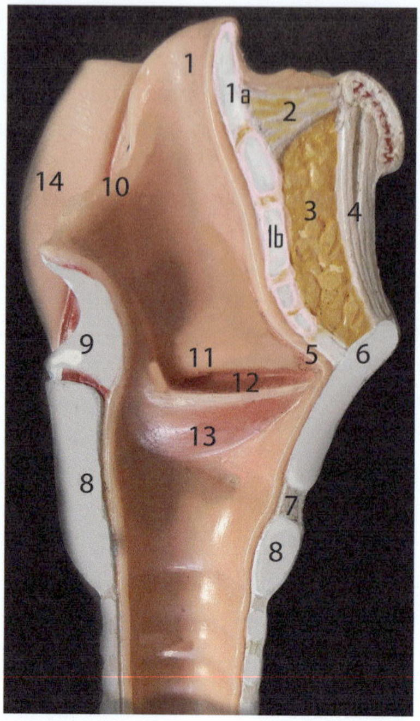

Fig. 5.1 **Epiglottis:** shaped like a leaf and composed of fenestrated elastic cartilage. 1a: Suprahyoid epiglottis 1b: Infrahyoid epiglottis **Hyoepiglottic membrane**: connects lingual aspect of epiglottis to hyoid bone; elevates larynx during swallowing. **Pre-epiglottic space** (Boyer's space): bordered superiorly by the hyoepiglottic ligament, anteriorly by the thyrohyoid membrane and the thyroid cartilage, and posteriorly by the epiglottis and thyroepiglottic ligament, and contains connective tissues and lymphatic vessels. Epiglottic fenestrations allow for the spread of cancer into this space. **Thyrohyoid membrane:** attaches superior thyroid lamina to posterior hyoid bone and elevates larynx during swallowing. **Petriole:** Stem like attachment of the epiglottis **Thyroid cartilage (thyroid lamina):** Supporting structure of larynx which articulates with the cricoid ring and protects the vocal cords. It is composed of hyaline cartilage; endochondral ossification occurs after the third decade of life and is more extensive in men. The pattern of ossification follows muscle insertions, i.e. the posterior cricoid ring and the oblique line of the posterior thyroid lamina. **Cricothyroid membrane**: composed of median and lateral elements. The median cricothyroid membrane connects the cricoid ring and thyroid lamina. The lateral membranes (conus elasticus) extend from the upper lateral cricoid to the lower margin of the vocal ligaments. **Cricoid ring:** major mechanical support of the larynx, as it is the only structure forming a closed ring. Provides attachments to numerous intrinsic laryngeal muscles responsible for phonation and respiration. **Arytenoid cartilage**: pyramidal-shaped ("pitcher-like") cartilages which articulate with the vocal folds. **Left ariepiglottic fold:** mucosal fold which stretches between the epiglottis and the arytenoid. **Vestibular fold** (ventricular fold, false cord): protects the upper airway during swallowing. **Ventricle** (Morgagni's sinus) is a pocket between the vestibular and vocal folds. Anteriorly, it leads into a variable sized diverticulum (saccule or Hilton's pouch). The abundant minor salivary glands of the ventricle and vestibular fold serve to lubricate the vocal folds. **Vocal cord:** The vocalis muscles originate from the inner thyroid lamina and insert on the arytenoids and the anterior commissure through the vocal ligaments. They are surrounded by distensible lamina propria and covered with stratified squamous epithelium at the plane of impact. **Piriform sinus:** these paired gutters lead into the esophagus. The cricopharyngeus (upper esophageal sphincter) is situated posterioinferior to the cricoid

may occur through cancer invasion of the ossified thyroid lamina, either inferiorly via the cricothyroid ligament and inferior aspect of thyroid lamina, or superiorly, extending over the superior aspect of the thyroid lamina. For the purposes of staging, paraglottic involvement is a radiographic, preoperative finding.

The anterior larynx is bordered anteriorly by the pre-epiglottic space, which is part of the oropharynx. The anterior border of the pre-epiglottic

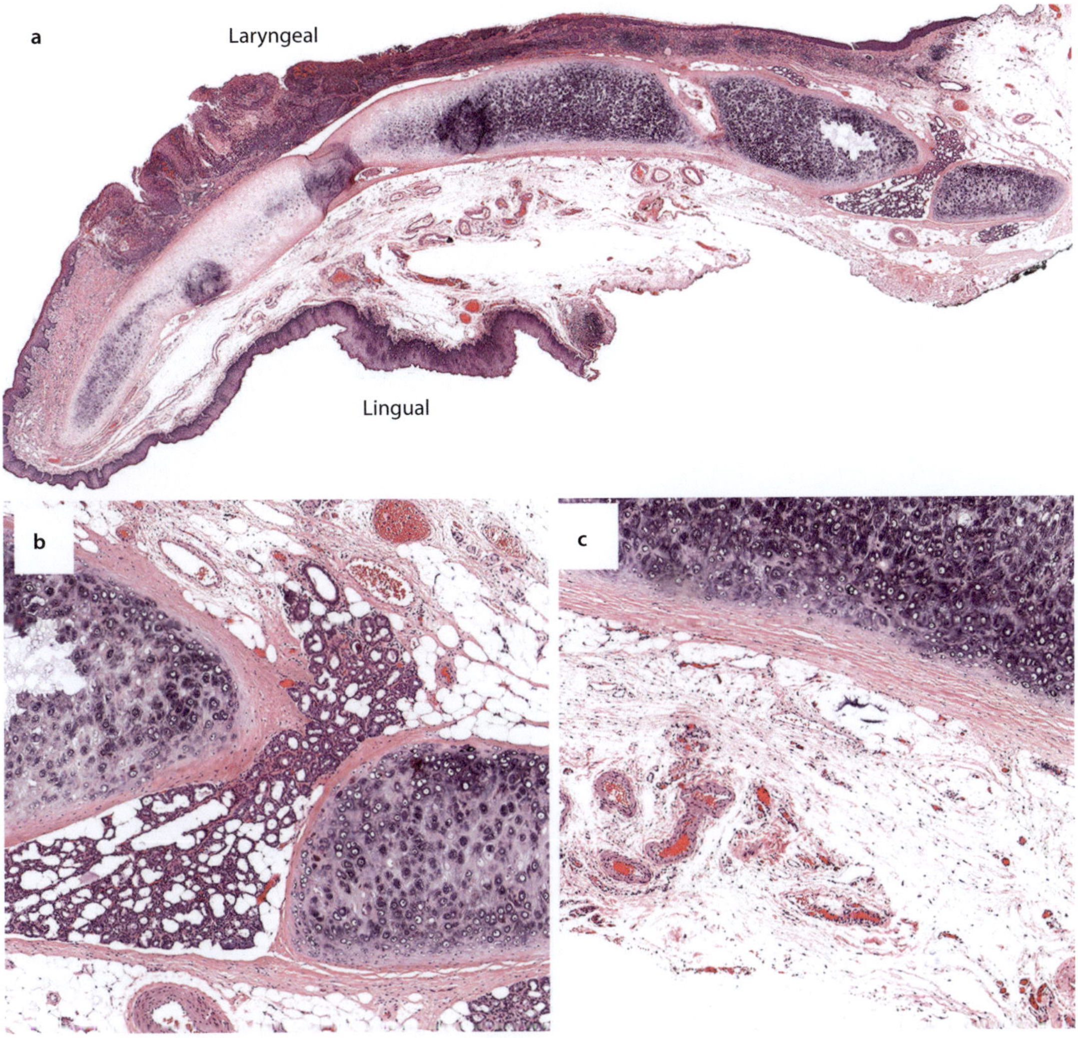

■ **Fig. 5.2** **a** The curved epiglottis points towards the tongue base. It has a laryngeal surface and a lingual side. Here we see a superficial carcinoma on the laryngeal surface. **b** Epiglottic fenestrations **c** Pre-epiglottic soft tissue

space is the thyrohyoid membrane, the superior border is the hyoepiglottic ligament, and the inferior border is the thyroepiglottic ligament.

Histologically, the epiglottis is recognized by its unique fenestrated pattern (■ Fig. 5.2). The fenestrae may contain minor salivary glands. They become a conduit for the spread of cancer in either direction. The epiglottic is covered with keratinizing stratified squamous mucosa. The keratinizing stratified squamous mucosa of the false cord is contiguous with the ciliated respiratory mucosa lining the ventricle (■ Fig. 5.3). Occasionally, Waldeyer's ring can extend into the supraglottic compartment. Supraglottic tissue can generally be distinguished from glottis tissue by the density of supraglottic minor salivary glands. Glottic tissue is distinguished from the supraglottis by the sizable vocalis muscle (■ Fig. 5.4). There is a paucity of minor salivary glands on the superior surface of the cord, greater gland density is seen on the inferior cord surface. The vocal folds are covered with keratinizing stratified squamous mucosa. All tissues thin out anteriorly at the anterior commissure. Here one may see the transfor-

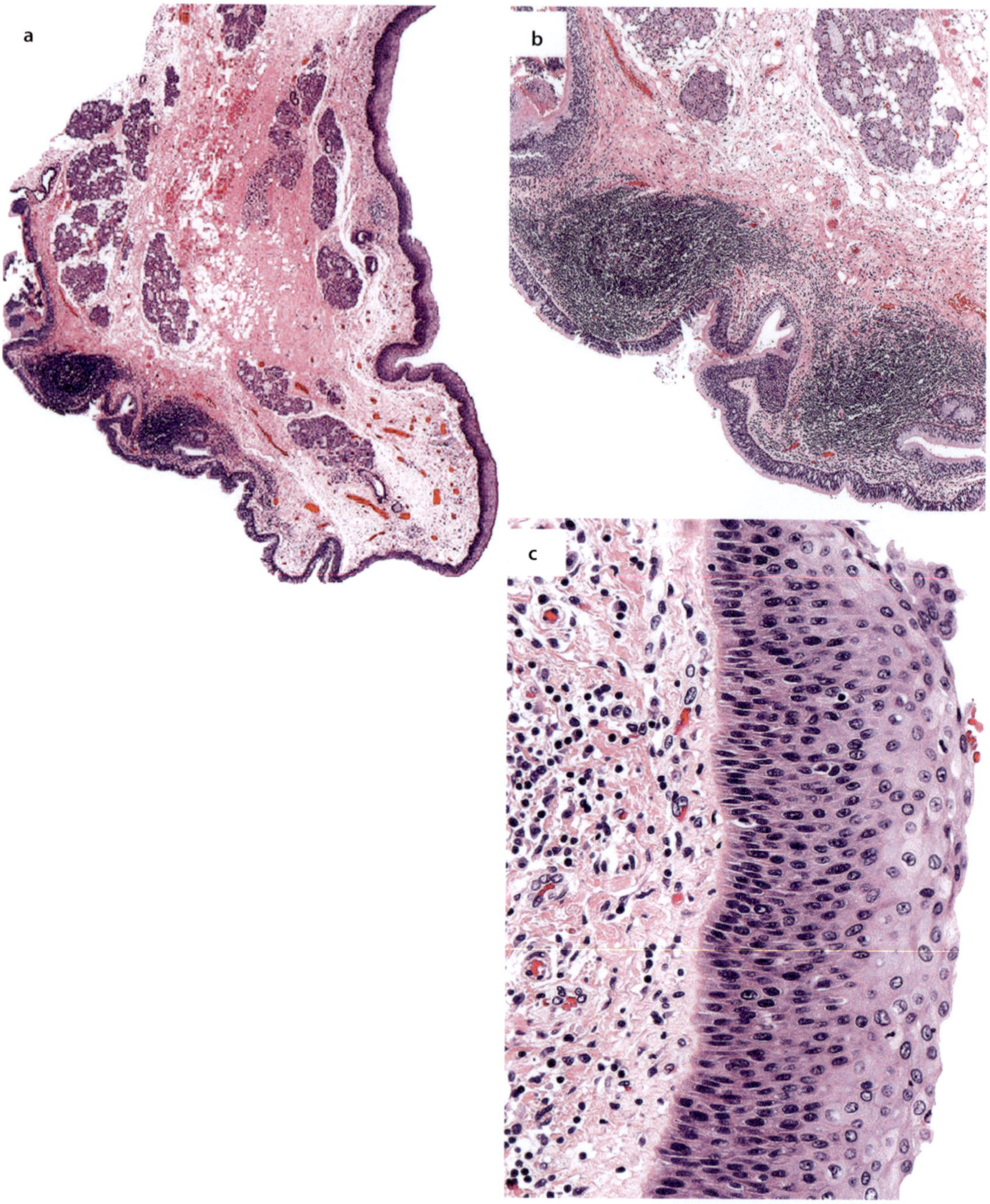

Fig. 5.3 **a** The ventricular fold or false cord contains abundant minor salivary glands, compared to the vocal folds. **b** The ventricle forms a pocket between the vestibular and vocal folds; it may contain mucosal associated lymphoid tissue. The ventricle is usually covered with respiratory mucosa **c** The ventricular fold is usually covered with stratified squamous epithelium

Table 5.1 Anatomic definitions

Supraglottis	Suprahyoid epiglottis
	Infrahyoid epiglottis
	Aryepiglottic folds
	Arytenoids
	Ventricular bands (false cords)
Glottis	Superior and inferior surfaces of the true vocal cords extending from anterior to posterior commissures, commencing at the lateral margin of the ventricle and extending 1 cm inferiorly to include the inferior surfaces of the true vocal cords
Subglottic	Inferior boundary of glottis to the inferior aspect of the cricoid ring

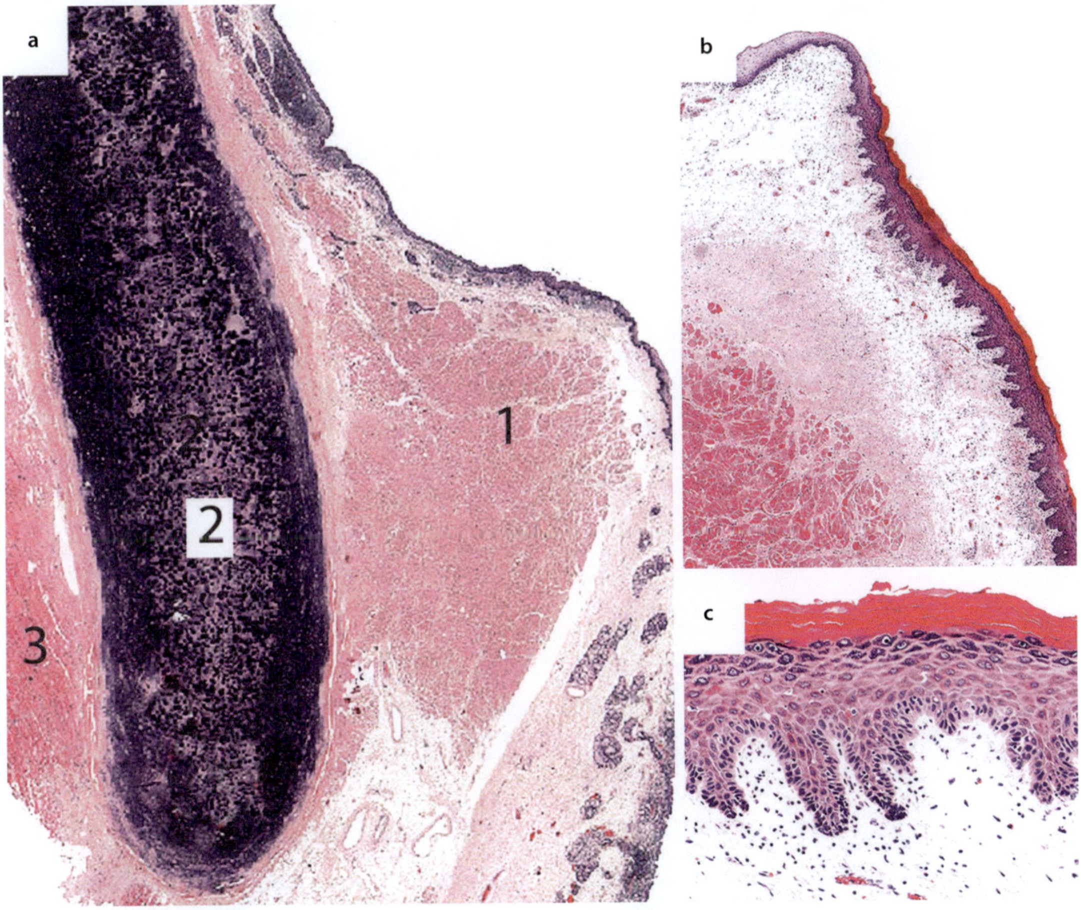

Fig. 5.4 **a** The glottis starts from an imaginary horizontal line through the middle of the ventricle, and extends to 1.0 cm below the vocal fold. 1. Vocalis muscle. 2. Thyroid lamina, 3. Strap muscles. **b** Superior and medial vocal cord. **c** Here the vocal mucosa is hyperkeratotic and hyperplastic

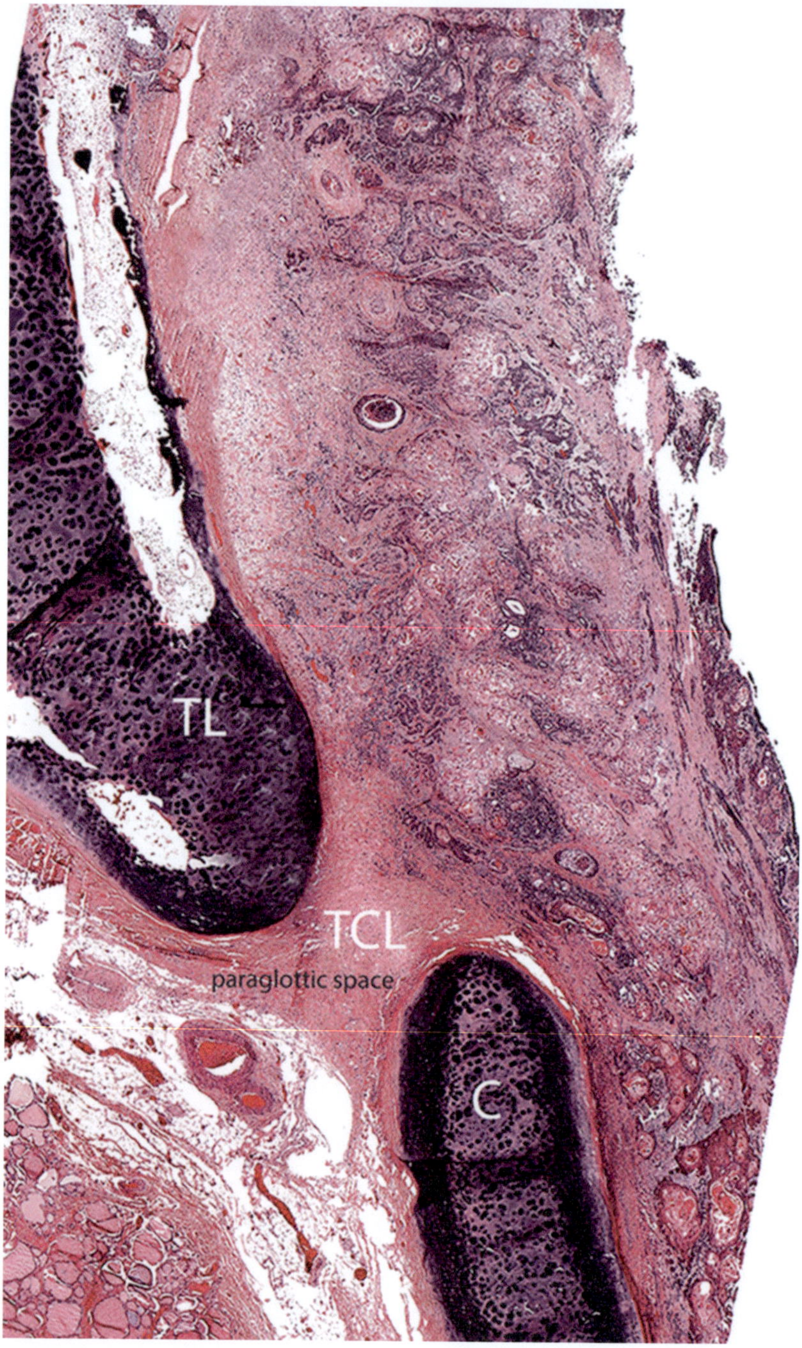

Fig. 5.5 The paraglottic space refers to the region lateral to the thyroid lamina and cricoid. TL: Thyroid lamina, C: Cricoid ring. TCL: thyroicricoid ligament. The thyroicricoid ligament is the gateway to the paraglottic region. For the purposes of staging, paraglottic involvement is a radiographic, preoperative finding

mation zone from stratified squamous mucosa to ciliated respiratory mucosa. The arytenoid tower is composed of the accessory arytenoid cartilages (Fig. 5.6). The cuneiform cartilage is long, the corniculate is comma shaped. These cartilages appear as submucosal bumps in the posterior supraglottis [1]. Do not confuse them, histologically, with a pathological finding.

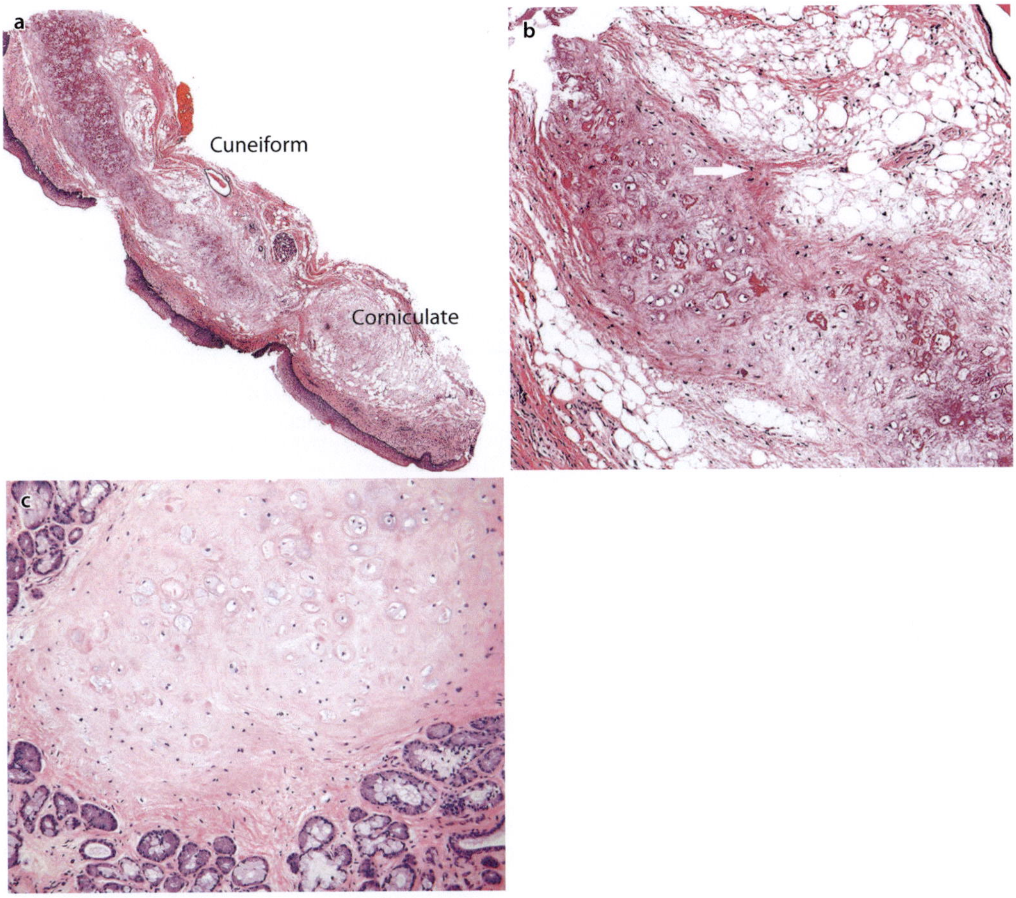

Fig. 5.6 **a** Low-power view of accessory arytenoid cartilages ("arytenoid tower"): The cuneiform is long, the corniculate is comma shaped. **b** Notice the irregular condensations of perichondrium. **c** Another accessory cartilage which "blends" into surrounding connective tissue

5.2 Vocal Nodules, Polyps, Contact Ulcers and Laryngeal Cysts

Vocal nodules (laryngeal nodules, singer's nodes, preacher's nodes, screamer's nodes) represent stromal reactions within Reinke's space, a gelatin-like potential space in the vocal fold subepithelium containing loose fibers and extracellular matrix. Reinke's space is devoid of vessels and lymphatics, making it susceptible to accumulation of fluids and proteins. The nodules develop after repetitive trauma from vocal misuse or excess vocal abuse; smoking may also play some role [2]. Vocal nodules are usually bilateral and symmetrical with a female predisposition [3]. Vocal nodules occur on the vibratory surface of the true vocal cord, usually the junction of the anterior and middle third, which is the point of maximum vibratory impact (Fig. 5.7). The presenting complaint is hoarseness.

Vocal polyps occur on the anterior one-third of the vocal fold. They are usually unilateral, with a male predisposition. The polyps can be sessile or pedunculated. Vocal cord polypoid degeneration, or Reinke's edema causes bilateral diffuse vocal polyps in middle aged to elderly population; it is unrelated vocal abuse, but associated with smoking. Occasionally polyps may originate from adjacent ventricular fold and rarely may they be associated with hypothyroidism. Polyps appear gray or white, translucent, sessile or polypoid lesions, and usually measure a few millimeters in

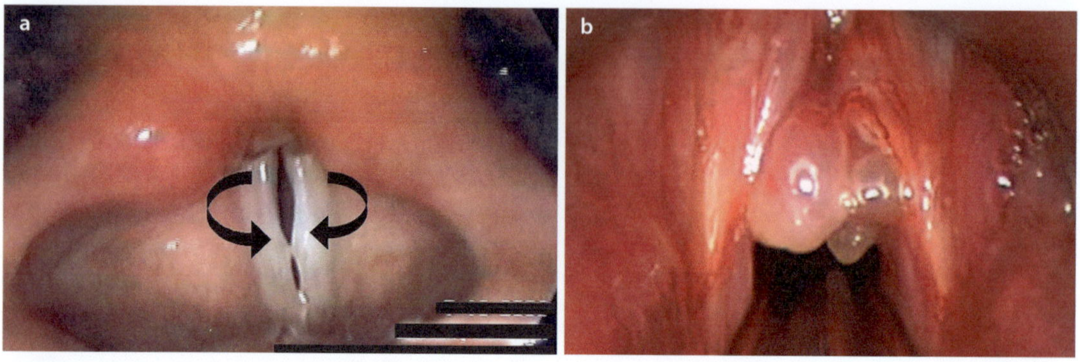

Fig. 5.7 **a** Bilateral vocal nodules at the mid-cord (*arrows*). Typical nodules like these are rarely biopsied, whereas unilateral vocal nodules are biopsied for diagnostic confirmation. (Courtesy of Greta Fries). **b** Large translucent vocal polyps at the anterior commissure. Vocal polyps tend to be larger than vocal nodules

diameter. The most frequent complaint is hoarseness or voice change.

Histopathologically, vocal nodules and polyps can be indistinguishable. Only the size of the lesion may support the particular process: biopsies smaller than 3 mm suggests a vocal nodule, whereas a biopsy greater than 3 mm supports a polyp.

Collectively, nodules and polyps are characterized by stroma which may appear myxoid, edematous, fibrous, vascular, or fibrinous stroma [4, 5] (Fig. 5.8). The basement membrane is thickened; this can be a nice diagnostic hint in a limited biopsy. Vascular spaces can be dilated; foci of hemorrhage may be seen. An important diagnostic finding is amyloid-like stromal change. Atypical stromal cells can be observed. The squamous epithelium may be normal, atrophic, hyperkeratotic, or dysplastic. Ulceration is infrequent in vocal polyps. On the other hand, vocal nodules may be ulcerated.

The differential diagnosis includes myxoma, which is extremely rare in the larynx. A myxoma is an expansile, hypovascular tumor. In contrast, a myxomatous laryngeal polyp contains increased vascularity, hemorrhage and fibrin deposition. Hypothyroidism and mucopolysaccharidosis may cause diffuse, edematous laryngeal thickening with deposition in the lamina propria. One might also consider the possibility of laryngeal amyloid. Amyloid deposits are nodular and may be associated with foreign body-type granulomatas. On hematoxylin and eosin stained slides, a characteristic "cracking" may be seen within the amyloid. Congo red, crystal violet or thioflavine T stains will be negative in vocal cord nodules or polyps.

Contact ulcers (contact granulomas) are distinguished from vocal cord nodules and polyps by their anatomic location. Contact ulcers develop posteriorly, on the vocal process of the arytenoids, as a result of forceful apposition during vocalization. They may be unilateral or bilateral. There is a male predominance, characteristically in lawyers, salesmen, managers and preachers ("preacher's nodules") who must affect a "deep" low frequency forceful voice. They may also develop with gastroesophageal reflux, and resolve when the underlying reflux is addressed [6]. Grossly, these lesions appear tan, yellow or red, polypoid with or without ulcerated surface (Fig. 5.9).

Histopathologically, contact granulomas are associated with nonspecific findings. One may see polypoid granulation tissue, +/− ulceration. The overlying epithelium may appear hyperplastic but not dysplastic. A ***splayed radial distribution*** of capillaries can be seen, emanating from a central core. No granulomas are seen, hence the name "contact granuloma" is a clinically derived misnomer. The differential diagnosis includes capillary hemangioma/pyogenic granuloma, which has a ***lobular*** rather than radial arrangement of blood vessels.

Laryngeal cysts can be categorized as either: **laryngocele**, **saccular cyst**, **ductal cyst**, or fall into a "**miscellaneous**" category.

Laryngoceles represent air-filled pulsion diverticulae of the saccule. The laryngeal ventricle (sinus of Morgagni) is the space between the vocal fold (true cord) and the ventricular fold (false cord). The bilateral upward extension or "cul-de-sac" of the ventricle is the laryngeal sac-

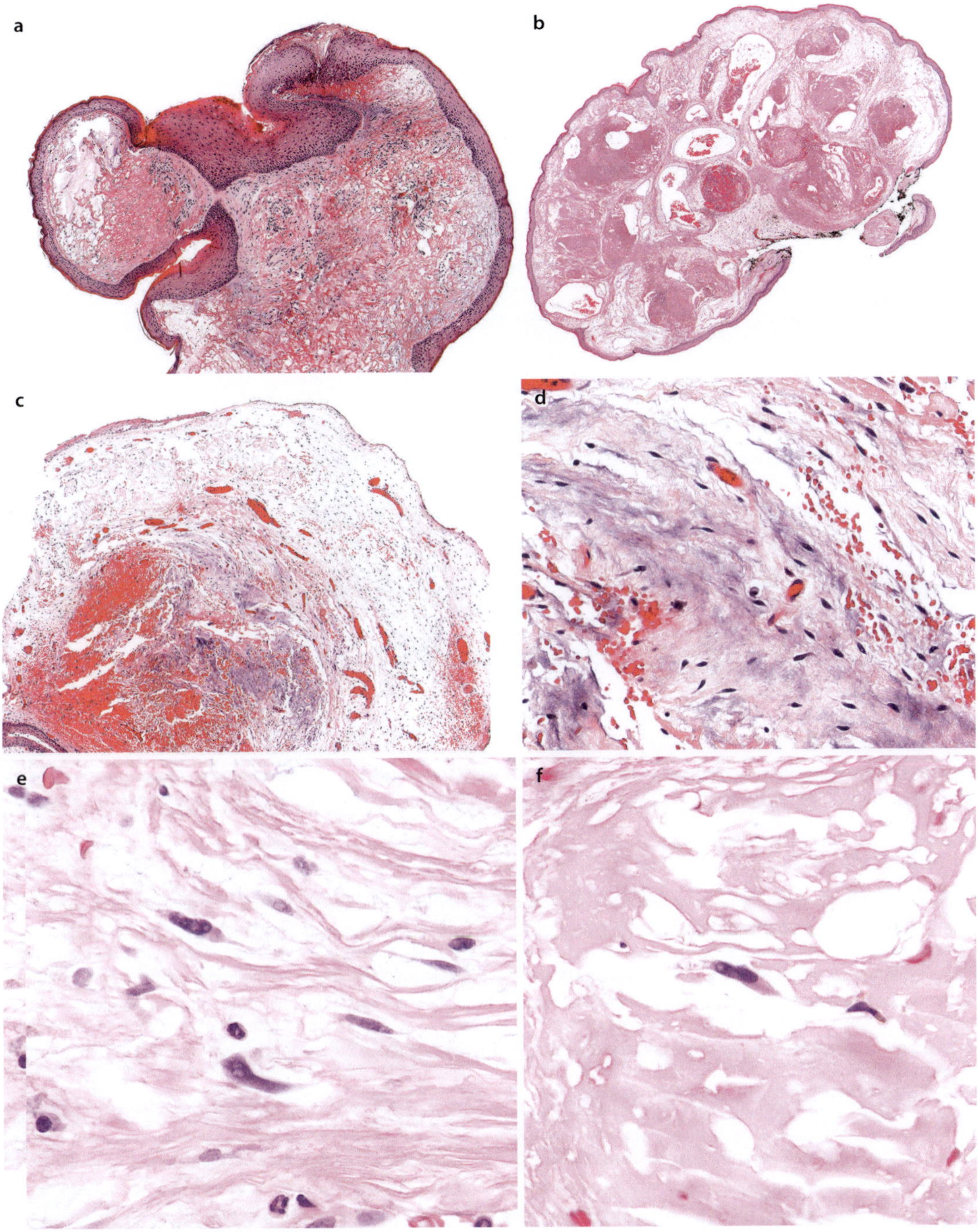

Fig. 5.8 **a, b** Low-power views of two vocal polyps. There's a range of possible phenotypes, varying with respect to vascularity, inflammation, and stromal deposition. Amyloid-like stromal deposition can be seen. **c, d** Low-, and high-power view of cartilaginous metaplasia within a vocal polyp **e, f** Fear not the occasional reactive stromal fibroblast. As a general rule of thumb, single dispersed spindled cells with smudgey blue chromatin and cytoplasm with a blue tinge are reactive in nature. The bluish cytoplasm indicates mRNA translation

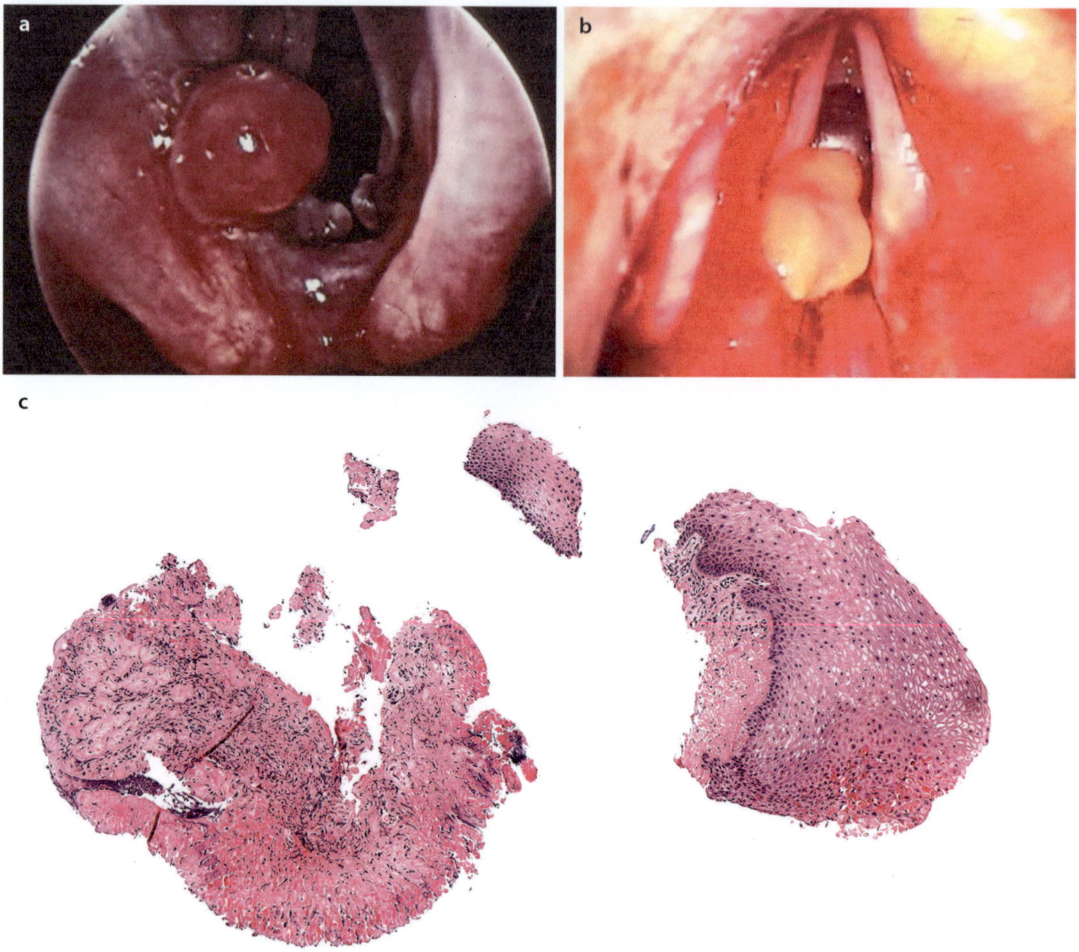

Fig. 5.9 **a** Reflux granuloma – the clinical term "laryngeal granuloma" refers to plump, active granulation tissue due to trauma such as endotracheal intubation, vocal abuse, and laryngopharyngeal reflux. Reflux granulomas are relatively common. The diagnosis is confirmed with (1) symptomatic relief with dietary changes and gastric acid inhibitors, (2) endoscopic observation of injury of the posterior larynx ("posterior laryngitis"), and (3) demonstration of reflux by pH-monitoring studies and barium swallow esophagram. Reflux granulomas are rarely biopsied. (Courtesy of Dr. Richard V Smith). **b** Contact granuloma – polypoid saucer-like lesion projecting from the arytenoid process secondary to vocal abuse. Contact ulcers also tend to develop in the posterior larynx; they may become large and can be bilateral ("kissing ulcers"). (Courtesy of Dr. Peak Woo). **c** Posterior laryngeal ulcer bed demonstrating fibrinous, suppurative exudate

cule. A laryngocele is the symptomatic dilation of the laryngeal saccule by entrapped air, i.e. a pulsion diverticulum, which still communicates with the laryngeal lumen. A laryngocele may remain confined to the endolarynx, (internal laryngocele) as a supraglottic submucosal bulge. It may also undermine the paraglottic space superiorly, protrude over the superior rim of the thyroid lamina, and herniate through the thyrohyoid membrane via the foramen of the superior laryngeal neurovascular bundle. This type of laryngocele (mixed external/internal, or foramina cyst) presents as an anterior neck mass. External laryngoceles must have some internal component, and for that reason may be termed "mixed" laryngoceles. Patients with internal and mixed laryngoceles complain of hoarseness, dyspnea and chronic cough. Newborn infants with laryngoceles present with a feeble cry, difficulty in feeding, cough and a neck mass. The air-filled nature of laryngoceles is easily confirmed on radiographic examination (Fig. 5.10). Sometimes, laryngoceles undergo intermittent obstruction, and secretions will result in a mucus filled sac. Coughing may clear the obstruction, dispelling the secretions. If communication

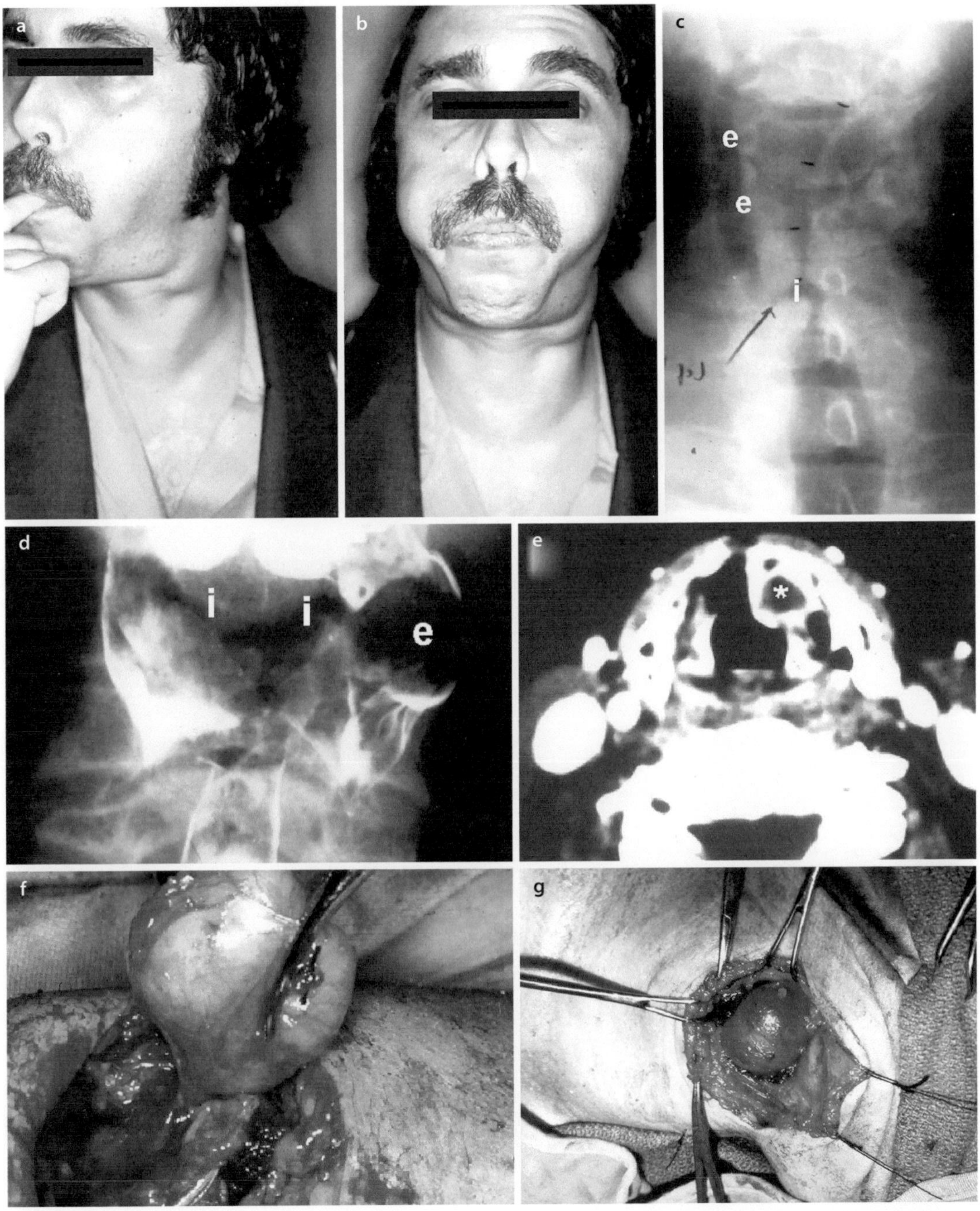

Fig. 5.10 **a, b** Bilateral upper neck masses are seen on forceful expiration with an opened glottis represent laryngoceles **c, d** Plain X-rays demonstrate the internal (i) and external (e) air-filled components **e** This air-filled cyst, in a different patient, is confined to the endolarynx (*) and therefore is an internal laryngocele **f, g** "Delivery" of two laryngoceles from an external cervical approach. The neck of the cyst may be seen in the bottom left (*arrow*). (Courtesy of Dr. Hugh Biller)

exists between the sac and the laryngeal lumen, this can still be classified as a laryngocele. A laryngopyocele is an obstructed laryngocele, or a saccular cyst, which has become secondarily infected.

Laryngoceles are usually unilateral, less often bilateral, and may be seen over a wide age range, from neonates to incidental autopsy findings in the middle aged and elderly. A small subset of patients with laryngoceles are involved with activities involving increased intralaryngeal pressure (e.g. glass blowers, trumpet blowers).

A **saccular cyst** results from the obstruction of the saccule. It is a mucin-filled dilatation of the laryngeal saccule secondary to obstruction, either acquired or congenital [7] (◘ Fig. 5.11). Congenital laryngeal cysts are uncommon, and present dramatically with neonatal stridor and respiratory distress. Congenital laryngeal cysts are most often of the saccular type, but rarely can be classified as ductal cyst or laryngeal duplication cysts (see below).

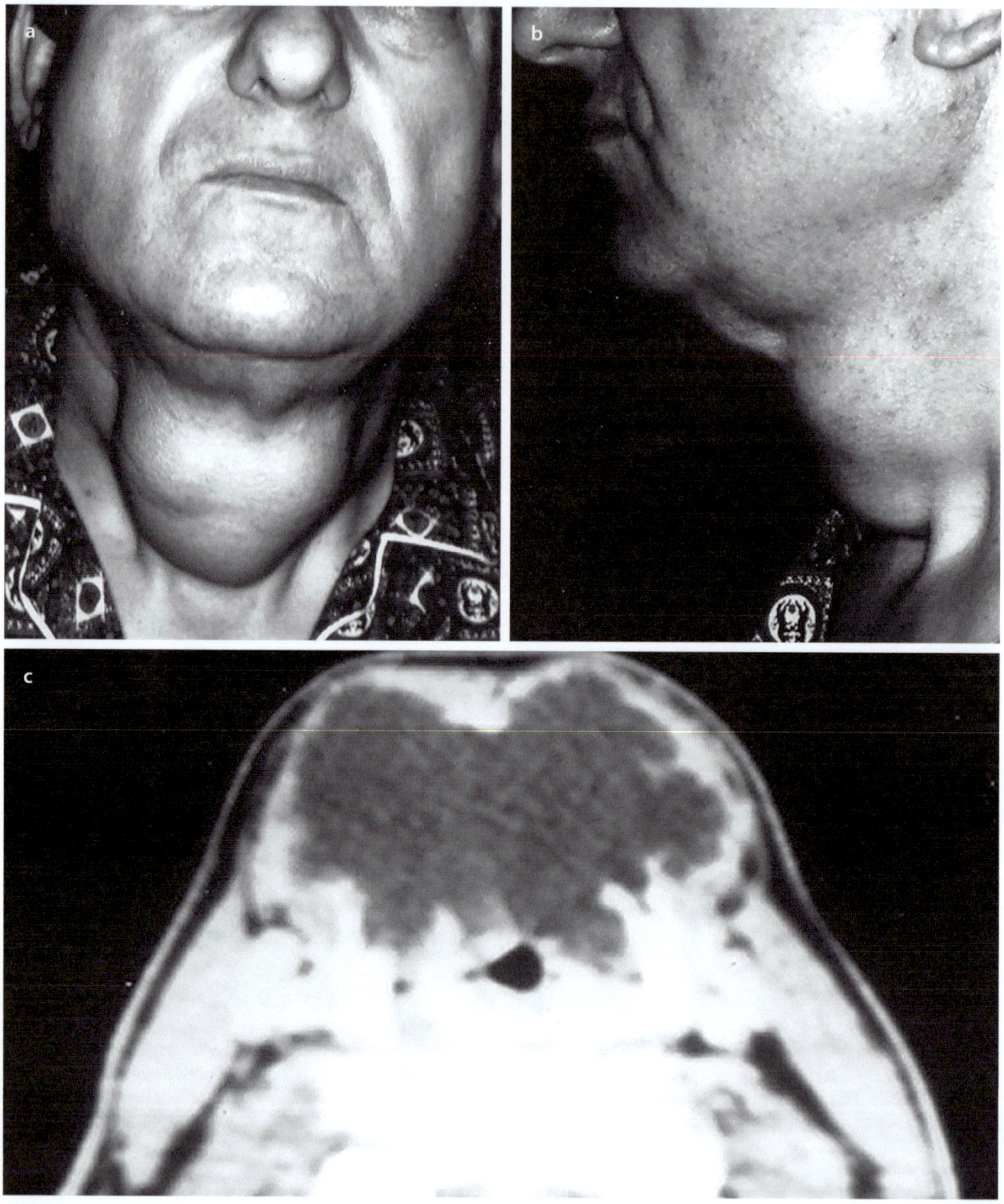

◘ **Fig. 5.11** **a, b** Saccular cyst forming a bulky cyst in the anterior neck. **c** CT scan reveals a mucous filled cyst of the anterior neck. The distinction between a saccular and thyroglossal duct cyst (TDC) during surgery by the tract location. A TDC tracks back to the hyoid bone, while a saccular cyst herniates through the thyrohyoid membrane. (Courtesy of Dr. Hugh Biller)

Saccular cysts may extend either medially or laterally. Medial saccular cysts obscure the anterior vocal fold, but are limited in size and extension by the anterior commissure. Lateral saccular cysts, point superior-laterally, and like external laryngoceles may herniate through the thyrohyoid membrane and reach massive proportions if neglected. Histopathologically, saccular cysts are lined respiratory mucosa, or occasionally squamous or oncocytic mucosa - and filled with mucinous material (◘ Fig. 5.12). The differential diagnosis may include laryngocele, which would not be mucin-filled, as it represents an air-filled "pocket". A **thyroglossal duct** cysts may extend into the larynx, and mimic saccular cysts [8, 9]. The distinguishing factor is the fact that the stalk or tract of a thyroglossal duct cyst is midline and leads to the hyoid bone, whereas the stalk of a large saccular cyst is lateral, and herniates through the thyrohyoid membrane. Branchial cleft cyst might also enter into the differential diagnosis. Here the tract will not lead through the thyrohyoid membrane, but will continue superiorly along the anterior border of the sternocleidomastoid muscle and may end at the angle of the mandible or in the tonsillar bed. Lastly, squamous cell carcinomas have been known to obstruct the saccule resulting in a secondary mucocele, or laryngocele.

Ductal cysts are the most commonly encountered form of laryngeal cysts; they arise from obstructed minor salivary ducts [10, 11]. Ductal cysts can be seen in the lingual epiglottis (◘ Fig. 5.13). Curiously, the superior aspect of the vocal cord has also been cited as a region for ductal cyst formation, despite the paucity of minor salivary glands at this site [12].

Histopathologically, a ductal cyst is composed of dilated ductal epithelium, which may be squamous, or oncocytic (◘ Fig. 5.14), or contain surrounding lymphoid tissue, in which case it may be referred to as a "tonsillar" cyst. Squamous and oncocytic ductal cysts have a predisposition for supraglottic sites. Tonsillar cysts have a predisposition for the vallecula, which contains Waldeyer's ring.

Other types of endolaryngeal cysts include epidermal inclusion cysts, dermoid cysts, thyroglossal duct cysts, and branchial cleft cysts. An epidermoid cyst, a keratin-filled cyst lined by stratified squamous mucosa, may be the result of a traumatic mucosal inclusion, or a congenital rest. Rarer still are dermoid cysts, which contain skin adnexal structures and are purely mature benign growths of presumed congenital rests.

Branchial cleft anomalies of the supraglottis are extremely rare. The supraglottis is derived from branchial arches 3 and 4; the glottis is derived from arches 5 and 6. Fourth branchial pouch sinuses manifest as sinus tracts leading from the pyriform sinus to skin, or may follow the course of the left recurrent laryngeal nerve, into the mediastinum, and back to the cricothyroid joint ending in the

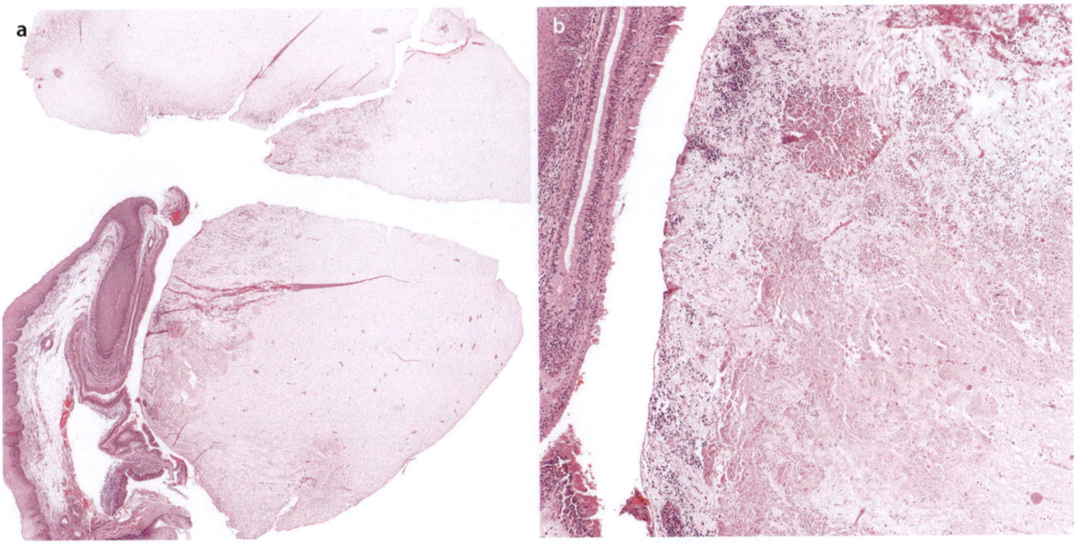

◘ **Fig. 5.12** **a, b** A saccular cyst is caused by mucinous secretions expanding the saccule; the diagnosis requires clinicoradiographic correlation. Here is an inspisated mucin cast from the cyst, and adjacent ventricular/saccular tissue

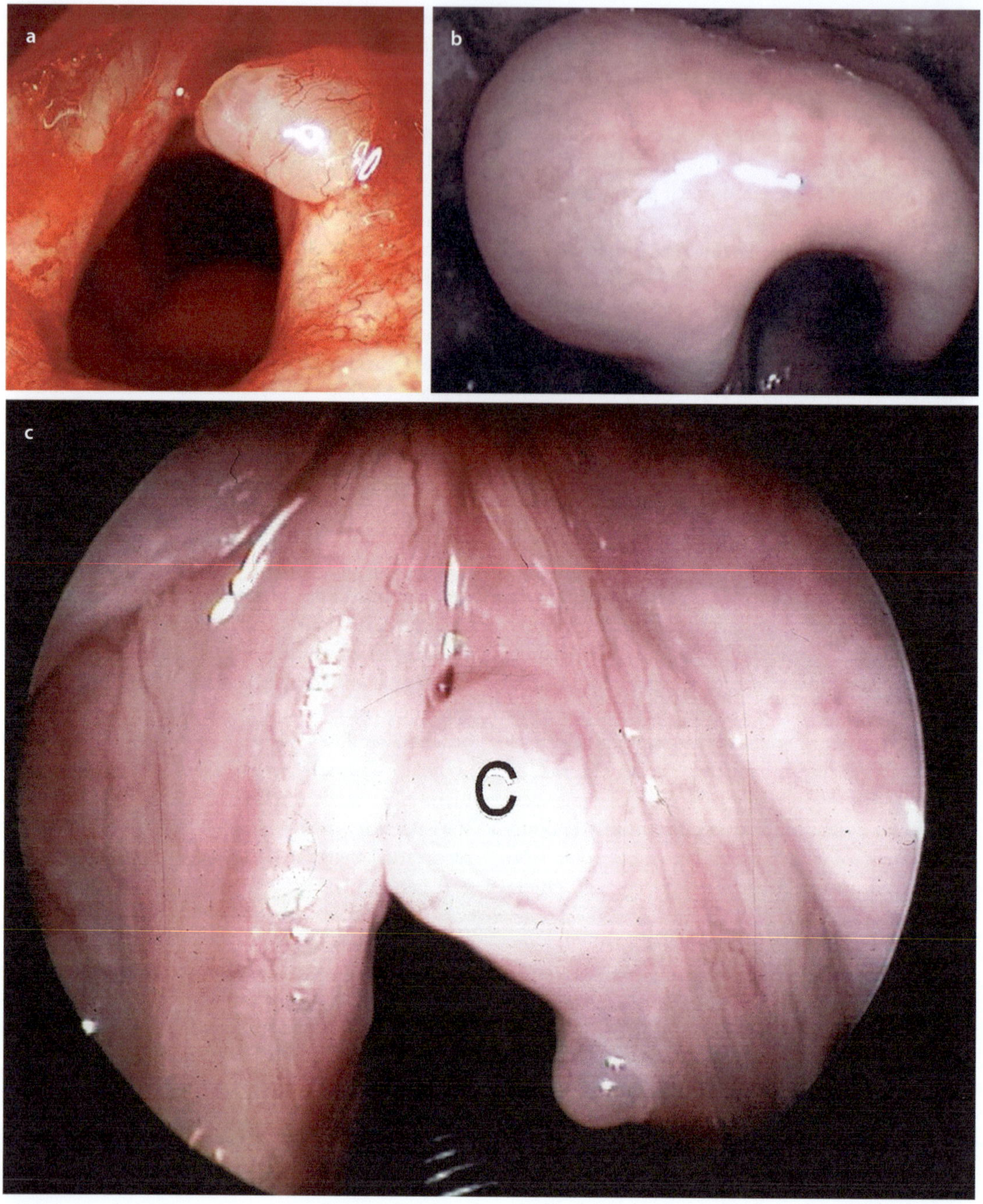

Fig. 5.13 **a** Endoscopic view right anterior vocal fold cyst forming a well-circumscribed submucosal lesion. **b** Congenital epiglottic cyst: Saccular cysts represent the most common congenital laryngeal cyst, followed by duplication-type cysts. Here is a rare congenital ductal cyst. **c** Vocal fold ductal cyst. (All courtesy of Dr. Richard V Smith)

pyriform sinus. Branchial cleft cysts can be lined by columnar epithelium and/or squamous mucosa, or a combination of both. Foamy histiocytes, cholesterol clefts, and inflammatory cells may be present within the cyst; a prominent lymphoid stroma usually accompanies the cyst lining.

Lastly, **congenital laryngeal duplication cyst** is a rarely encountered event. The lining mucosa of a duplication cyst is contiguous with the endolarynx. A duplication cyst also contains variable degree of mesodermal elements, such as cartilaginous and muscularis [13–16].

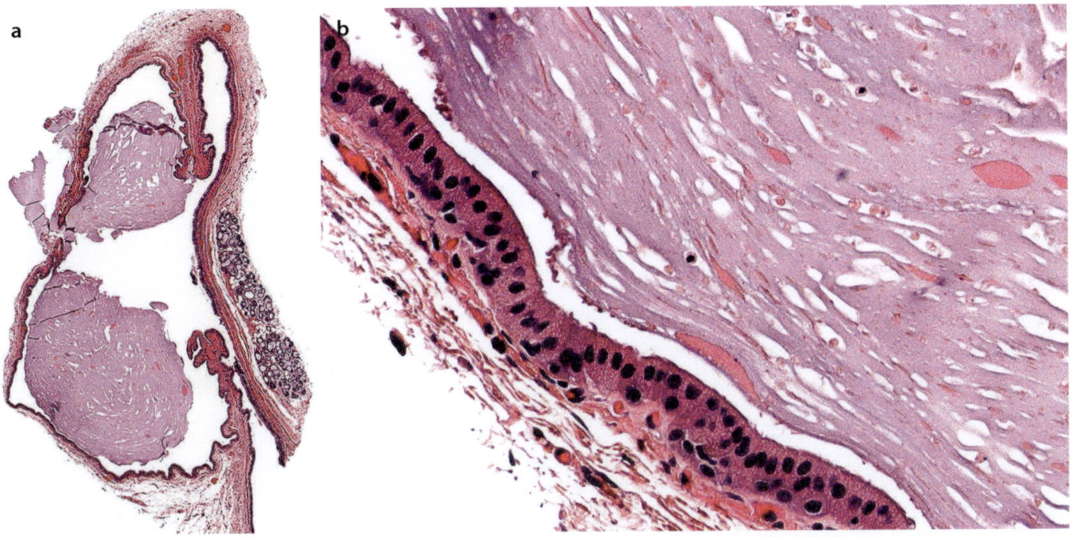

Fig. 5.14 a, b Low-, and high-power view of simple ductal cyst lined by oncocytic ductal epithelium

5.3 Oncocytic Cystadenoma

Laryngeal oncocytic cystadenoma represents the so-called, "extraparotid Warthin's tumor". It is presented after the discussion on ductal cysts, as this is a logical extension of the oncocytic ductal cyst. These lesions occur predominantly in older individuals in supraglottic locations. Patients present with upper airway symptoms, such as dysphonia, and may be the cause extreme upper airway obstruction [17]. Histologically, one sees a unicystic or microcystic oncocytic proliferation composed of a double layer of lumenal tall oncocytes over cuboidal cells [17, 18] (Fig. 5.15). The luminal tall oncocytes are frequently ciliated. A variable degree of papillocystic proliferation can be seen. Lymphocytic infiltrate from persistent Waldeyer's ring may be prominent, bringing to mind an "extraparotid" Warthin's tumor. Oncocytic metaplasia could be seen in adjacent large and small minor salivary ducts. Laryngeal oncocytic cystadenoma are cured with conservative excision. The differential diagnosis for any ***solid*** oncocytic laryngeal lesion should include laryngeal neuroendocrine carcinoma and oncocytic variant of mucoepidermoid carcinoma.

Interestingly, oncocytic papillary cystadenoma has been reported coincidental to laryngeal squamous carcinoma; no causal relationship was suggested [19].

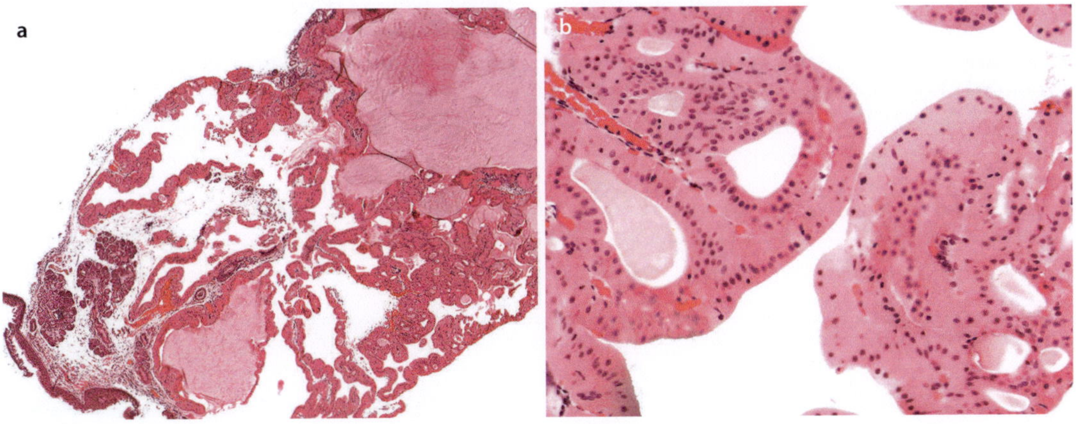

Fig. 5.15 Oncocytic cystadenoma ("extraparotid 'Warthin's-like tumor.") has a supraglottic predisposition **a** This papillocystic lesion is composed of cuboidal and columnar oncocytes forming cystic cribriform spaces. **b** The abundant cytoplasm is granular and intensely eosinophilic

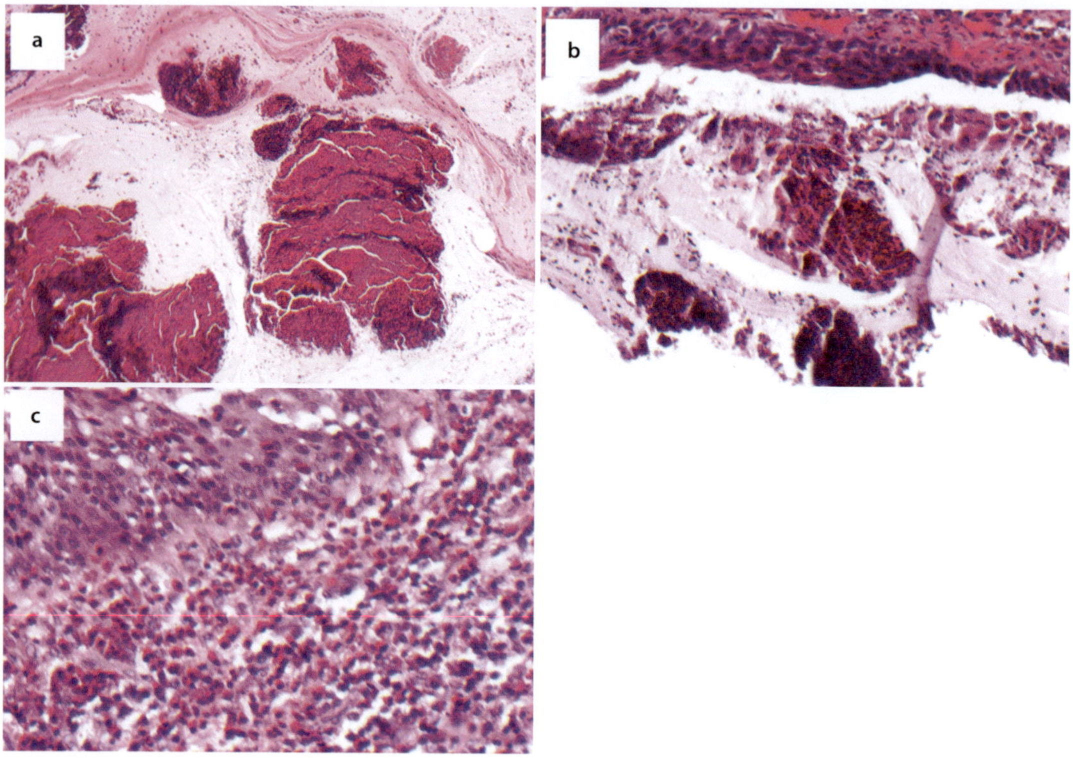

Fig. 5.16 **a, b** Low- and high-power view of cystically dilated duct with allergic mucin, within a laryngeal polyp. The dense pink and blue ripples represent degranulating eosinophils and other inflammatory cells. **c** Tissue eosinophilia

5.4 Allergic Laryngitis

The concept of allergic laryngitis is relatively new, but certainly "connects the dots", so to speak, between Ig E mediated allergic rhinosinusitis and allergic bronchitis [20–24]. Patients present with cough, throat clearing, and foreign body sensation. There is seasonal variation to the symptoms, and association with rhinitis. It is rare to receive specimens from allergic laryngitis, but one can expect to see findings identical to allergic rhinosinusitis, namely allergic mucin and Charcot Leydin crystals. (Fig. 5.16).

5.5 Fungal Infection

Laryngeal fungal infections are extremely uncommon. Yeast-forming fungi such as *Histoplasma, Coccidiodomycosis, Blastomyces,* are regionally endemic and may cause granulomatous laryngitis in either immunocompetent or immunocompromised individuals [25]. *Cryptococcus* and *Candida glabrata* are *ubiquitous* yeast-forming fungi that can cause granulomatous laryngitis in diabetics or individuals using steroid inhalants [26, 27]. *Aspergillus* or *Mucormycosis* can cause invasive laryngeal fungal infection in diabetics or neutropenic individuals [28–31] (Fig. 5.17).

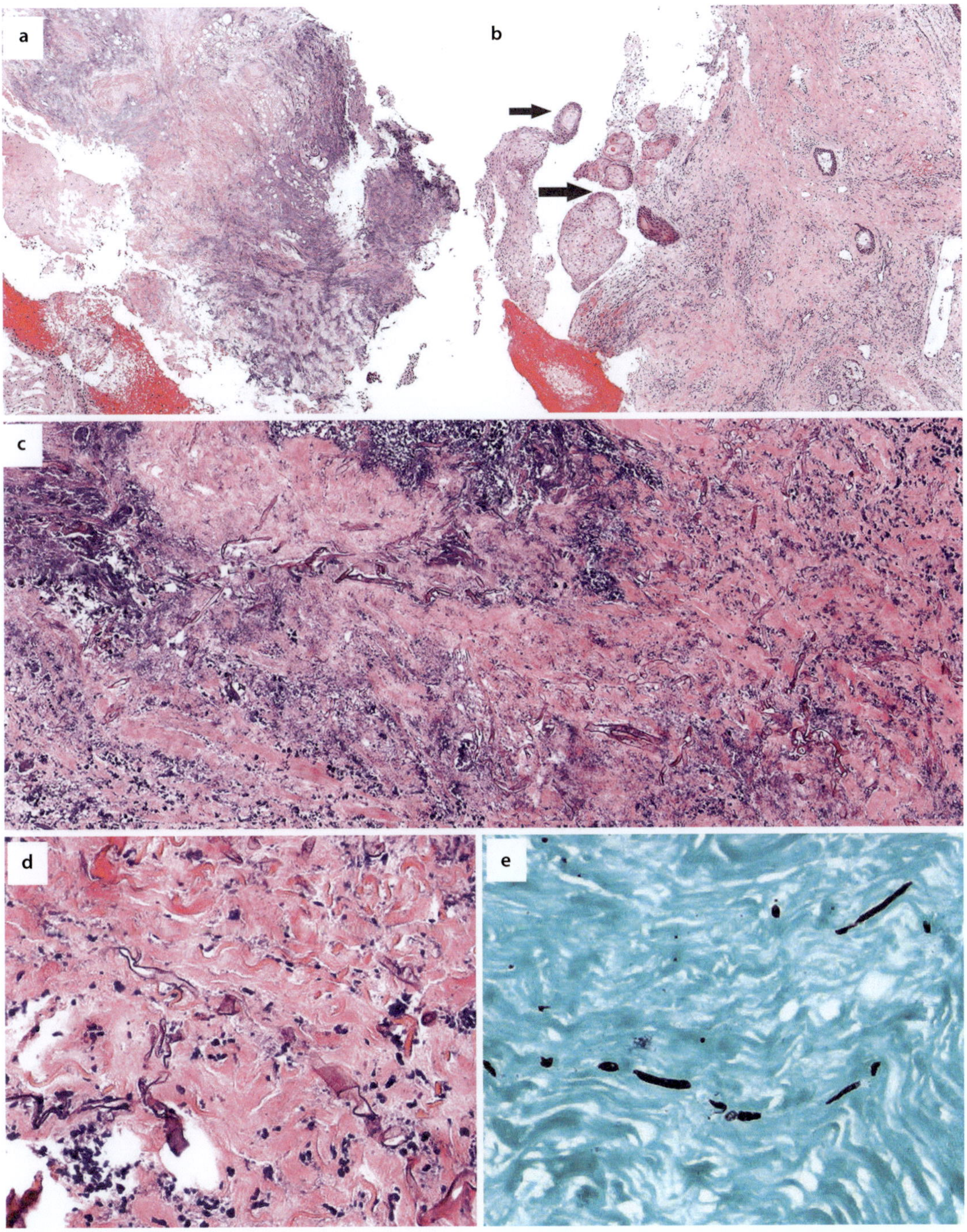

Fig. 5.17 **a, b** Low power view of necrotic laryngeal tissues in a patient with poorly-controlled diabetes. The squamous metaplasia (*arrows*) indicates that this process has been evolving over time. **c** The fungal hyphae can be seen on H + E slides. **d** The "bent cellophane tube: appearance refers to the irregular oblique contours of the hyphal walls. **e** Hyphae on GMS stain

5.6 Autoimmune Diseases

The laryngeal manifestations of autoimmune diseases such as lupus erythematosus, rheumatoid arthritis, and Sjogren's syndrome are varied, and may be the initial presenting symptoms or develop during the course of known disease. Manifestations include diffuse laryngeal edema, vocal paresis or paralysis due to neuritis or vasculitis, cricoarytenoid joint arthritis, and corditis [32–37]. "Bamboo joints" have been described, which refers to bilateral corditis forming raised yellow white band-like lesions at the mid- or posterior vocal folds, at a point of maximum mechanical stress. These bamboo joints are different from rheumatoid nodules, which appear as smooth, rounded, submucosal nodules.

Histologically, the bamboo nodes have revealed deposition of amorphous eosinophilic material, surrounded by granulomas and palisading histiocytes. This is distinct from rheumatoid nodules which demonstrate **fibrinoid necrosis** – a denser shade of pink embedded with ghost nuclei, the hallmark of necrosis (Fig. 5.18). Lupus erythematosus can demonstrate **LE bodies,** which represent engulfed nuclei with denatured DNA (Fig. 5.19).

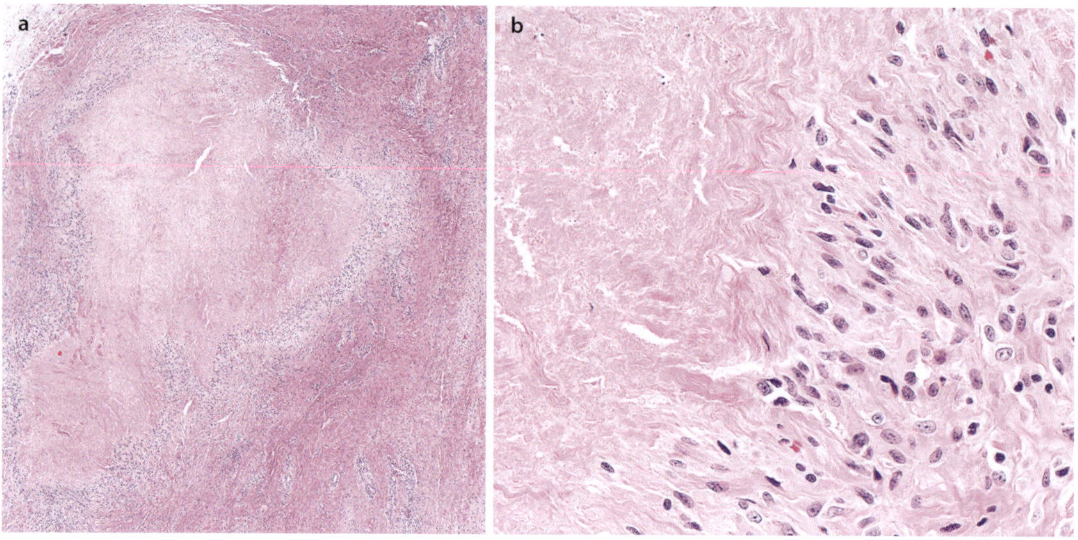

Fig. 5.18 **a** Rheumatoid nodule demonstrating irregular shaped granuloma with fibrinoid necrosis. **b** The granuloma is rimmed by pallasading epithelioid histiocytes

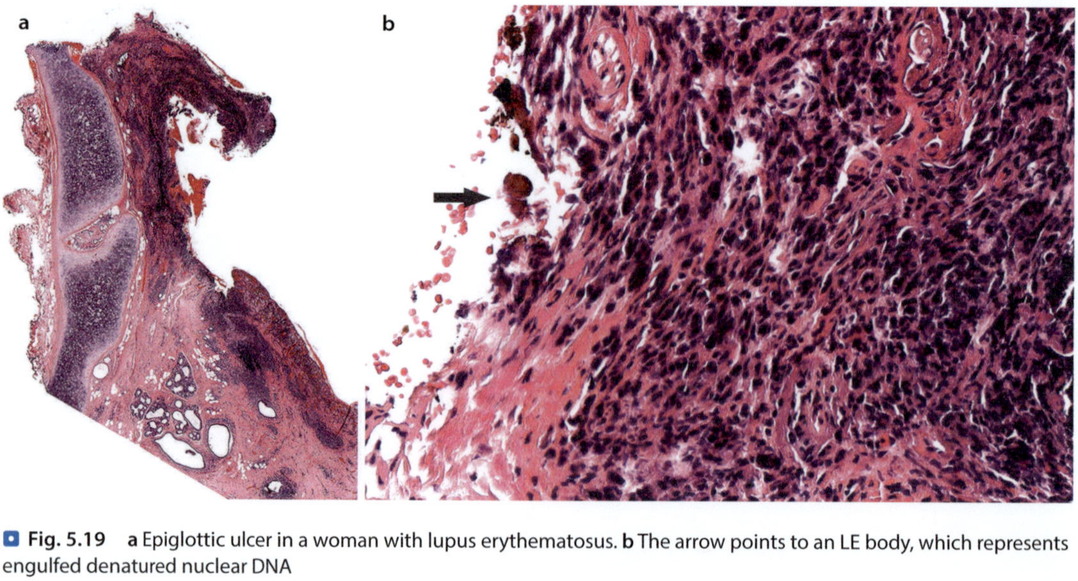

Fig. 5.19 **a** Epiglottic ulcer in a woman with lupus erythematosus. **b** The arrow points to an LE body, which represents engulfed denatured nuclear DNA

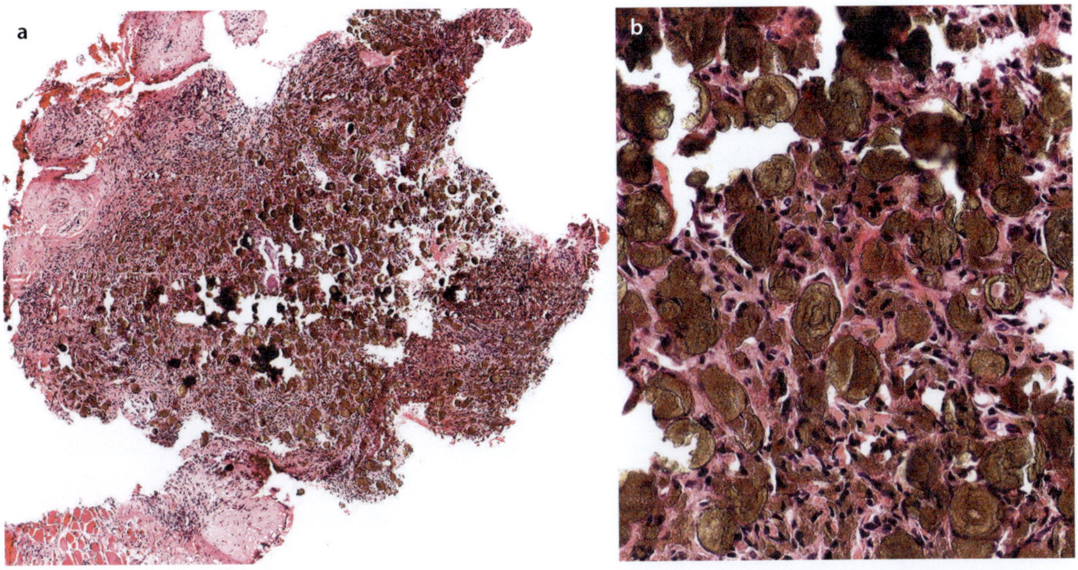

■ **Fig. 5.20** Injection laryngoplasty to medialize a paralyzed vocal cord is a strategy for improving the "breathy voice" associated with paralysis. The medialized cord decreases air escape during phonation. **a, b** Low- and high-power views of hydroxyapatite granulomas. The inorganic material appears as brown lamellations of crystalline material

5.7 Vocal Cord Injectables

The numerous approaches to improving vocal quality for patients with unilateral vocal cord paralysis hinge upon paralyzed cord medialization via injection of materials (e.g. Teflon, calcium hydroxylapatite, collagen, hyaluronic acid, methylcellulose) which may show up on subsequent vocal biopsies (■ Fig. 5.20) [38–43].

5.8 Amyloidoma

Amyloidosis refers to the deposition of β-pleated proteins, most commonly kappa or lamda immunoglobulin light chains (Type AL) secreted by plasma cells. Amyloidosis can be classified as either **systemic**, which is the more common form and usually related to plasma cell dyscrasias, chronic inflammatory processes (also known as secondary amyloidosis which is associated with deposition of hepatic-derived AA [amyloid associated immunoglobulin]), or more rarely, autosomal recessive familial amyloidosis. The less commonly encountered form is **localized amyloidosis,** which does not progress to systemic disease. The larynx represents the most common head and neck site for an amyloidoma which only rarely represents part of a systemic process [44–47]. However, medical workup is always recommended to rule out systemic amyloidosis and plasma cell dyscrasias after a diagnosis of a localized amyloidoma.

Patients with laryngeal amyloidoma may complain of hoarseness. Clinically, laryngeal amyloidomas appear as either solitary or multiple submucosal masses. Histopathogically, one can see the characteristic deposition of pink fibrillary material which has varying hue densities and "cracks" (■ Fig. 5.21). Periductal or perivascular deposition can be seen. On brightfield microscopy, amyloid stains red with Congo red stain. Polarized light will reveal a light green birefringence, as opposed to collagen, which shows white birefringence. Patients with laryngeal amyloidomas are treated by local conservative excision. Local re-accumulation of laryngeal amyloid may develop.

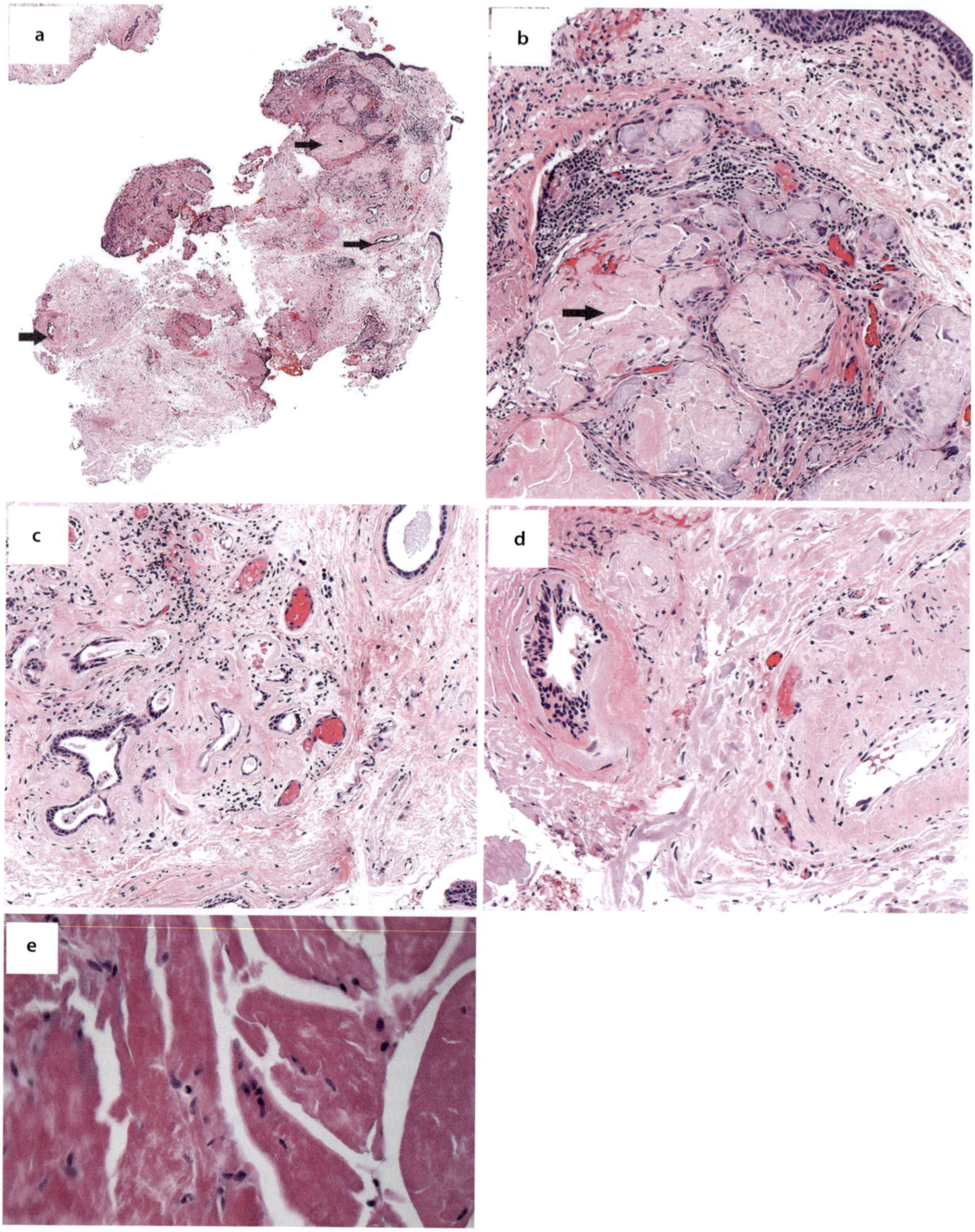

Fig. 5.21 Laryngeal amyloid **a** Polypoid laryngeal tissue: at low-power you can already spot dense eosinophilic depositions (*arrows*). **b** The pink hue of amyloid has variable intensity. The cracks (*arrow*) is characteristic **c, d** Dense periductal amyloid deposition causing acinar atrophy. **e** Brightfield microscopy of positive Congo red staining

5.9 Langerhans Cell Histiocytosis

Langerhans cell histiocytosis is the current terminology for a group of diseases formally classified as **Letter-Siwe disease** (multisystem), **Hand-Schuller-Christian disease** (unisystem multiorgan), **eosinophilic granuloma** (unifocal disease), **and Hashimoto-Pritzker congenital self-healing histiocytosis.** It represents a rare clonal proliferative disorder of Langerhans cells which com-

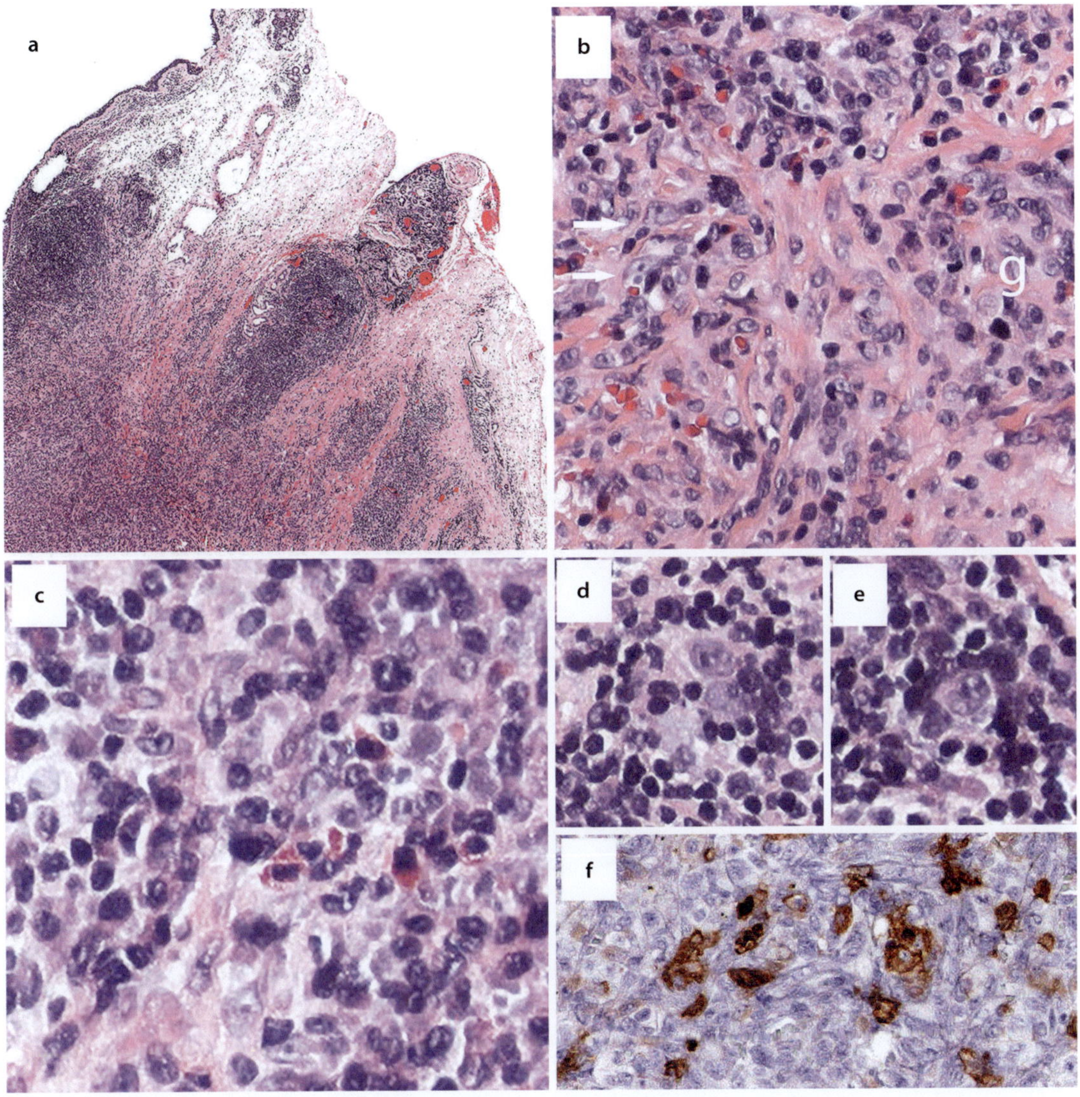

Fig. 5.22 Langerhan's histiocytosis **a** Low power view of inflamed laryngeal tissue from a young woman. **b** Vague granulomatous pattern is seen (g). **c** Numerous eosinophils are present in the inflammatory background. **d, e** Scattered large atypical cells are seen with prominent nucleoli and nuclear grooves **f** CD1a expression

monly harbor the *BRAF*V600E mutation [48]. Langerhans cells are **S100+/CD1a +** antigen presenting cells with characteristic ultramicroscopic **Birbeck inclusions**. **Langerhans cell sarcoma** represents the malignant form of Langerhans cell histiocytosis.

Laryngeal Langerhans cell histiocytosis is an extraordinarily rare phenomenon and an unifocal event (Fig. 5.22) [49–52]. Histopathologically, it might be the eosinophils embedded within dense inflammation that first cues you into considering Langerhans cell histiocytosis. Look for the Langerhans cells which appear as dispersed large atypical single cells with folded grooved nuclei which can taper like an Oriental slipper. These cells are **S100+/CD1a +** which seals the diagnosis. "Atypical Langerhans cell histiocytosis" refers to non-classical morphology; eosinophils may be absent. In fact, atypical Langerhans cell histiocytosis can appear as a solid proliferation of epithelioid cells entirely devoid of inflammation.

5.10 Lymphoma

Primary **laryngeal lymphomas** are extremely rare [53–57]. An extensive search through English language publications yielded only 57 patients with laryngeal lymphomas [53]. The mean age at diagnosis is 53 years. As the caudal aspect of Waldeyer's ring can extend to the supraglottic larynx, it is not surprising to see that 63% of laryngeal lymphomas are supraglottic. Twelve percent of laryngeal lymphomas are confined to the subglottis and 25% are transglottic. Patients may present with the symptoms of a laryngeal mass and may also manifest "B symptoms" (low-grade fever, chills, night sweats, unexplained weight loss). Association with autoimmune syndromes has also been reported. The majority (85%) of laryngeal lymphomas are either diffuse large B-cell, which is generally an aggressive lymphoma, or marginal B-cell (MALT) lymphoma, which is an indolent B-cell lymphoma. T-cell or natural killer cell phenotypes comprise the remaining 15% (◘ Fig. 5.23).

Histopathologically, diffuse large B-cell lymphomas are composed of medium to large atypical lymphocytes with scanty cytoplasm, fine chromatin, and multiple nucleoli (centroblastic),

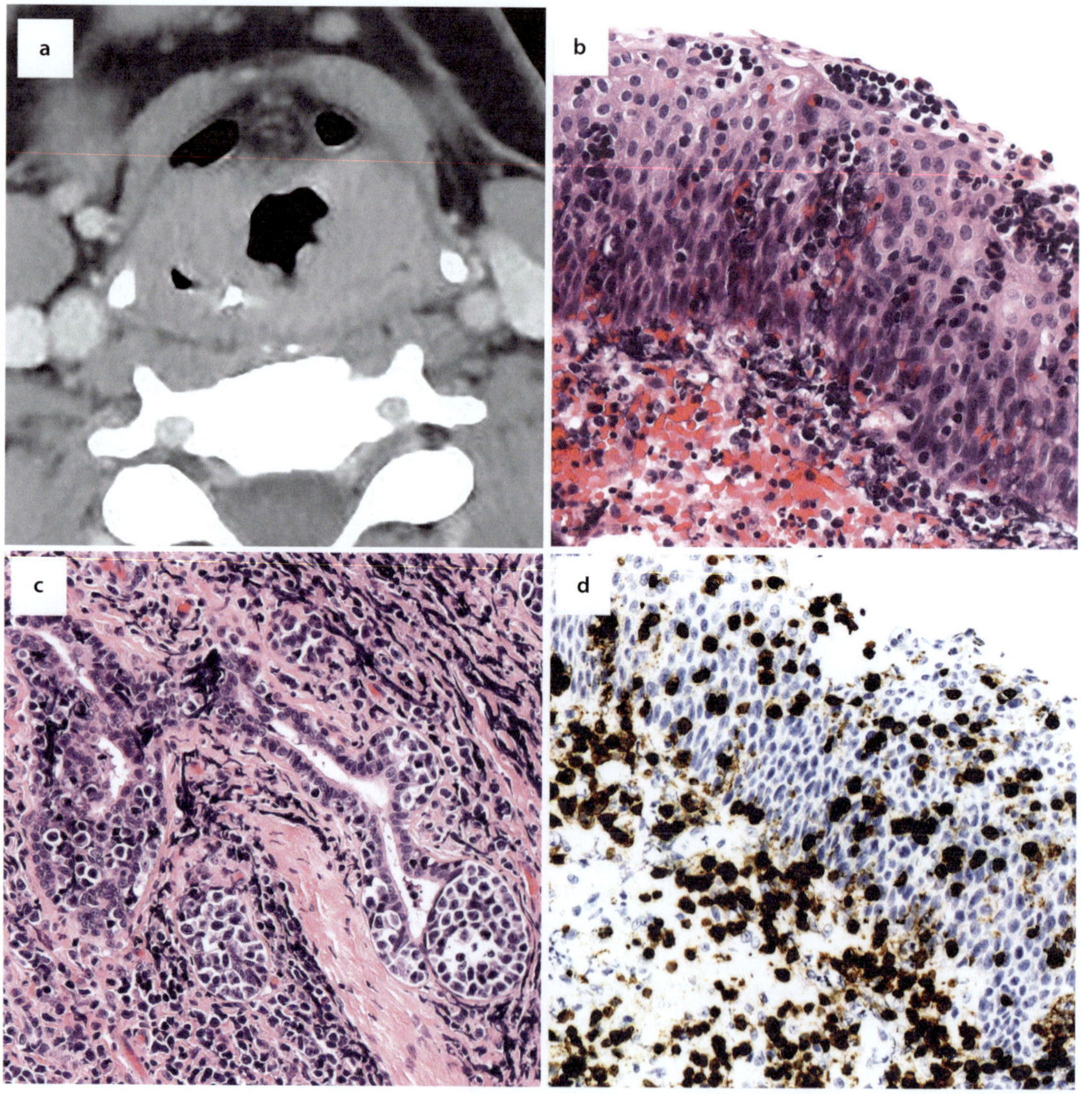

◘ **Fig. 5.23** T-cell lymphoma **a** Hypopharyngeal/supraglottic homogeneous mass. **b** The original superficial biopsy revealed a T-cell infiltrate forming intraepithelial microabscesses. **c** A subsequent deeper biopsy demonstrated periductal T-cell infiltrate **d** CD3 expression. PCR studies revealed diagnostic T-cell receptor clonality or large nuclei with single large nucleoli (immunoblastic). **Anaplastic diffuse large B-cell lymphoma appears as** discohesive infiltrate of round or polygonal cells which are highly pleomorphic. The IHC profile of diffuse large B-cell lymphomas are **CD20+ / CD19+ / CD22+ / CD79a+ / PAX5+ / BCL6+ / CD10+.** Ki67 proliferative index is between **30–90%. Anaplastic diffuse large B-cell lymphoma** is also **CD30+,** and the **Ki67** proliferative index is around **100%.**

Marginal zone lymphomas are composed of monocytoid B cells, centrocytes-like cells, small lymphocytes, plasma cells, scattered immunoblasts, and centroblast-like cells. "Lymphoepithelial islands", which refers to lymphocytes infiltrating minor salivary glands, can be seen. Marginal zone lymphomas express **CD19+ / CD20+ / CD79a +** with **variable CD43** expression. They are **negative** for **BCL6** and **CD10. T-cell/natural killer cell** lymphomas may demonstrate intramucosal extension and Pautrier's microabscess formation (■ Fig. 5.23). Lymphoepithelial islands may also be seen. The atypical lymphocytes range from medium to large with angulated nuclei. These cells are typically **CD2+ / CD56+** and lack membranous CD3 but may express **cytoplasmic CD3. EBER is typically +.** The following stains are also usually positive: TIA1, granzyme, CD43, CD45RO, CD25, CD95.

5.11 Laryngeal Papillomatosis: Juvenile Onset, Adult Onset, and Aggressive Papillomatosis

Juvenile onset laryngeal papillomatosis is an extremely rare condition (4.3/100,000 children) caused by HPV6/11, which is the result of vertical maternal fetal transmission. Maternal genital condylomas during pregnancy increases the relative risk of juvenile-onset recurrent respiratory papillomatosis 200 fold [58–61]. In general, vertical HPV transmission from mother to infant is not uncommon. Maternal HPV significantly increases the risk of recovering HPV from neonatal oral and genital swabs [62, 63]. However, the clinical significance of neonatal HPV recovery is unknown, as neonates will clear infection. It has been hypothesized that early HPV exposure may contribute to immune tolerance and inability to clear subsequent infections. Patients with recurrent respiratory papillomatosis demonstrate dampened Langerhan's cell response to proinflamatory IL-36Ɣ, supporting immune tolerance [64].

Juvenile-onset recurrent respiratory papillomatosis is usually diagnosed before 2 years of age. Children can present with hoarseness, coughing, stridor, and dyspnea. Airway patency is maintained by laser excisions; about 60% of children require multiple (≤ 5) excisions. Florid aggressive papillomatosis refers to severe diffuse laryngotracheal papillomatosis which can develop in up to 25% of patients [65]. A more aggressive course has been associated with HPV11 [66–68]. Around 3% of juvenile-onset recurrent respiratory papillomatosis patients develop pulmonary disease [68]. In general, most cases of juvenile-onset recurrent respiratory papillomatosis resolve by puberty, but 20% of patients experience disease persistence into adulthood. Less than 1% of patients with juvenile-onset florid tracheobronchial disease will develop carcinomas of the lung, or unusual head and neck sites [67–69]. These cases are associated with low risk HPV6/11, and usually lack risk factors such as radiation, alcohol, smoking, and immunosuppression [69–71].

Adult onset laryngeal papillomatosis is presumably transmitted by sexual contact. Patients with adult onset laryngeal papillomatosis have greater numbers of lifetime sexual partners than control patients. Adult onset laryngeal papillomas are usually diagnosed in the third or fourth decades of life, with a strong male predominance. These lesions are usually single and amenable to endoscopic excision, but a subset of adult patients can also go on to develop florid disease. The rates of malignant transformation for adult onset papillomatosis is on the order of 5–10%, and may affect either the upper or lower respiratory tract [72–74]. Malignant degeneration is usually related to long disease duration, may occur in the setting of known promoters (irradiation, cigarette smoking), or may rarely develop de-novo.

As mentioned above, recurrent respiratory papillomatosis is managed symptomatically by laser excisions. VEGF inhibitors have demonstrated promise in significantly increasing symptoms-free periods for patients with florid disease [75–77].

Clinically, respiratory papillomas appear as single or multiple exophytic, pedunculated, sessile, friable "pebbly" or cauliflower-like growths. Histopathologically, exophytic papillomas are composed of epithelial proliferations scaffolded upon the *sine qua non fibrovascular cores,* which produce the characteristic fungiform architecture (■ Fig. 5.24). (These fibrovascular cores may explain responsiveness to VEGF inhibitors). The squamous mucosa is

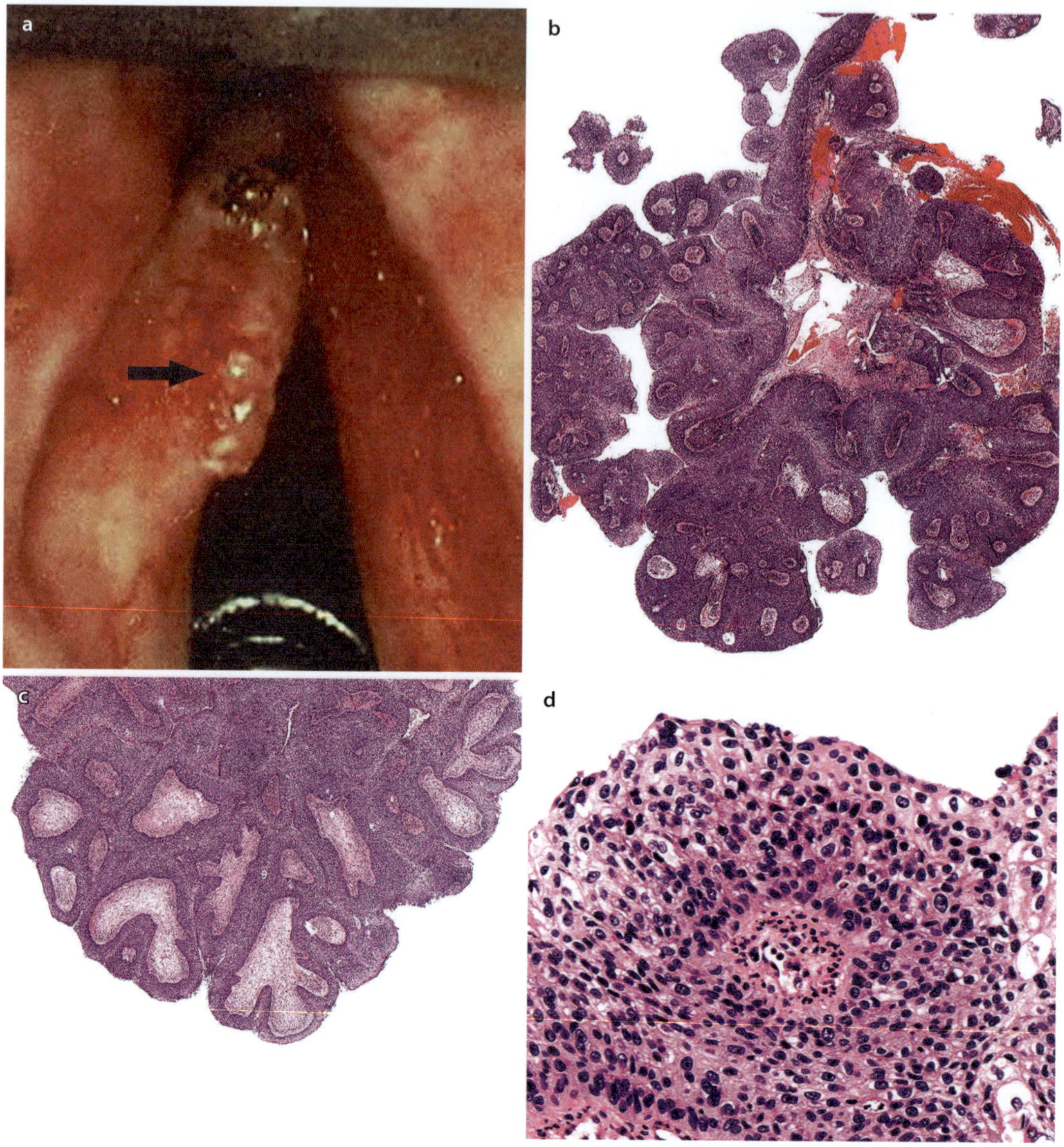

Fig. 5.24 **a** Endoscopic view of recurrent papillomatosis (*arrow*). (Courtesy of Dr. Richard V Smith). **b, c** Exophytic papillomas have finger-like projections of fibrovascular cores covered by maturing stratified squamous mucosa. **d** This dysplastic papilloma demonstrated variation in nuclear shape and size, plus disturbed maturation

usually glycogenated, without significant keratinization. On the other hand, orderly epithelial maturation (increased epithelial cytoplasm, flattening of nuclei) should be observed. Intraepithelial inflammation is common; finding high mitotic figures and nuclear pleomorphism signify dysplasia and should not be "written–off" as an inflammation-related change. Classic "viropathic" changes such as koilocytes may be observed but are not diagnostically requisite.

The differential diagnosis includes **condylomas**, which are sessile and broad based, and the **papillary variant of squamous cell carcinoma** which is exophytic with either broad or slender papillae. The papillary fronds have more crowded, complicated, unsmooth silhouettes. Intraepithelial keratin pearls are not routinely seen in exophytic papillomas and should raise the suspicion of either malignant progression of a papilloma, or papillary variant of squamous cell carcinoma. **Verruca vulgaris** might also come into consideration; it lacks complex branching fibrovascular cores of exophytic papillomas, has a thick hyperkeratosis and parakeratosis, and prominent keratohyaline granules. The rete pegs of verruca vulgaris are thin, non-clubbed shape, and do not push into underlying deep tissues. Also, the fibrovascular cores of verruca vulgaris frequently radiate from a central focus.

5.12 Granular Cell Tumor

Granular cell tumor is a benign tumor first described by Abriskoff in 1926; Schwannian derivation is supported by ultrastructural similarities between tumor cytoplasmic granules and myelin, detection of lipoproteins and sphingomyelin, and tendency for this tumor to concentrate around nerves [78–82]. The head and neck is the most common site for granular cell tumor, most often the oral cavity. Laryngeal location comprises 3–10% of all granular cell tumors. Patients can present with stridor, dysphonia, and hemoptysis. The most common site for laryngeal granular cell tumor is the posterior larynx; other sites include vocal folds, anterior glottis, arytenoids, supraglottis, and subglottis. Pediatric laryngeal granular cell tumors have been reported, most commonly affecting the anterior subglottis. The usual appearance is that of a small, firm, sessile nodule, with a smooth yellow/pink/grey surface and distinct circumscribed borders.

Clinically, granular cell tumors of hollow organs appear as submucosal nodule; the surface mucosa is invariably intact and grey/white. Histopathology, the cells of a granular cell tumor form small nests and cords with an infiltrative growth pattern (◘ Fig. 5.25). The tumor cells have a syncytial "histiocytoid" appearance with small eccentric nuclei, abundant, granular cytoplasm

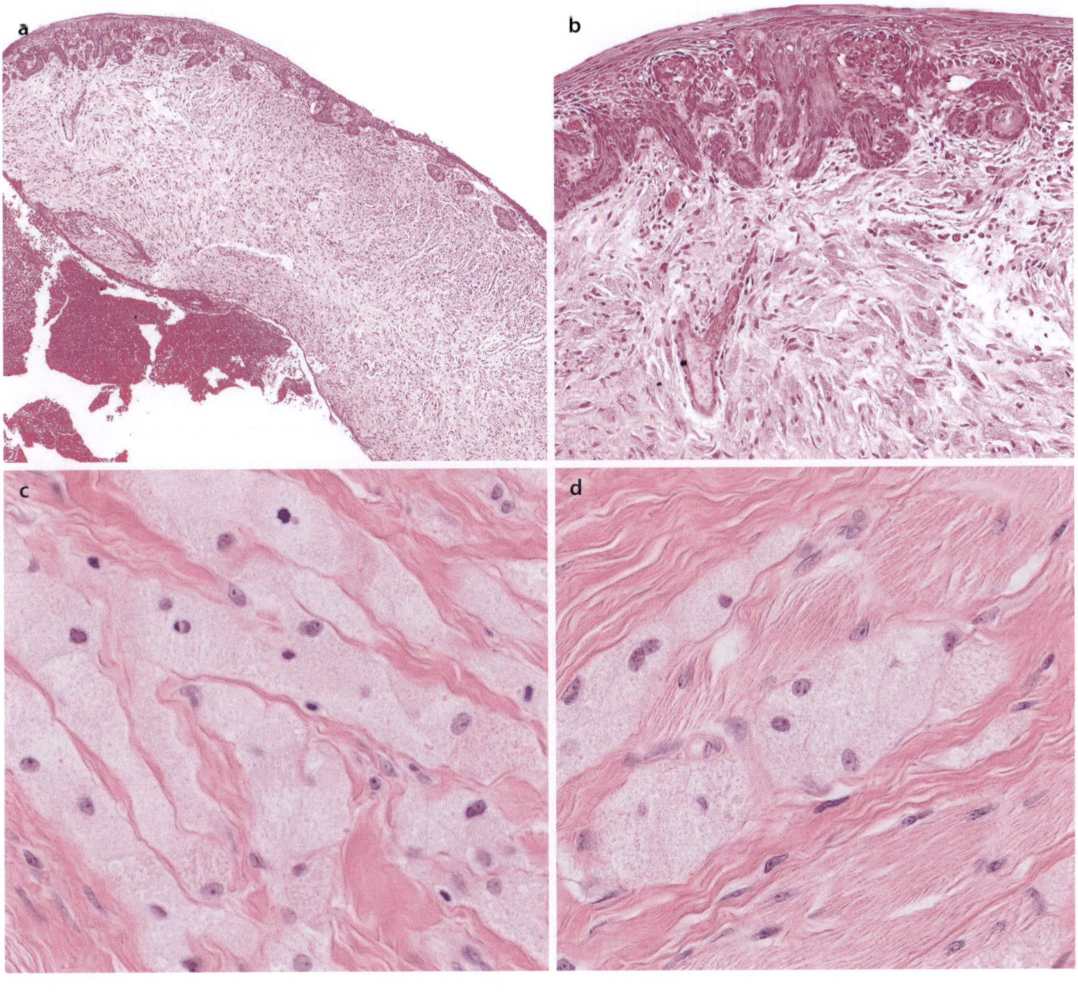

◘ **Fig. 5.25** Granular cell tumor **a, b** Laryngeal biopsies demonstrating pseudoepitheliomatous hyperplasia and submucosal infiltrate **c, d** The nest of granular cells mimic histiocytes. Tumor cells have small, condensed, peripheral nuclei and abundant, granular cytoplasm

and indistinct cytoplasmic membranes. Nuclear pleomorphism and mitotic figures are usually absent. The cytoplasmic granules are PAS positive, and diastase resistant. S-100 is usually strongly positive. However, S100 negative noncongenital granular cell tumors have been reported, thus emphasizing the adage that H + E trumps (so to speak) IHC. Pseudoepitheliomatous hyperplasia is common present in the overlying mucosa. Thus, there is the potential for misdiagnosing granular cell tumors as squamous carcinomas especially on superficial biopsies. Make yourself a habit of always searching the submucosa for islands of granular cells when you encounter squamous pseudoepitheliomatous hyperplasia.

The great majority of granular cell tumors are benign. Three malignant and one atypical laryngeal granular cell tumors have been previously reported [83–86]. Malignant granular cell tumors come in two flavors: (1) Histologically benign, yet metastatic, or (2) Histologically malignant and metastatic. In general, malignancy is associated with tumors larger than 4 cm (average 9 cm). [87, 88] Histologically malignant granular cell tumors are marked by ***spindled tumor cells, vesicular nuclei with prominent nucleoli, > 2 mitoses/10 fields*** (@ 200× total magnification), ***high nuclear cytoplasmic ratio, pleomorphism, and necrosis***. By IHC, p53 expression is seen in >10% of tumor cells, and the Ki 67 index is increased (normally <1%).

5.13 Paraganglioma

Paraganglia cells are derived from the neural crest, they are found adjacent to sympathetic or parasympathetic nerves. In the head and neck, paraganglia are normally present along ***parasympathetic*** nerves in the ear, along the glossopharyngeal and vagus nerves, at the carotid bifurcation, and along the superior and inferior laryngeal nerves. Carotid body tumors (chemodectoma), and middle ear paraganglia ("glomus tumor") are the most common head and neck paragangliomas. Paraganglia adjacent to the superior sympathetic cervical ganglia give rise to rare sympathetic paragangliomas, ***an exception to the head and neck parasympathetic rule***.

Superior laryngeal paragangliomas are more common than inferior laryngeal paragangliomas with a ratio of 6:1 [89–92]. Superior laryngeal paragangliomas are polypoid, submucosal intralaryngeal tumors (◘ Fig. 5.26). Inferior laryngeal paraganglioma are usually dumbbell shaped, with intra- laryngeal and extra-laryngeal extension. There is a female to male ratio of 3:1 and a right to left ratio of 2.3:1. Laryngeal paragangliomas may be associated with paragangliomas elsewhere, or with a family history of paragangliomas. Supraglottic paragangliomas cause hoarseness, dyspnea and hemoptysis. Infraglottic tumors may also cause dyspnea and hoarseness is due to nerve palsy of the recurrent laryngeal nerve. Infraglottic tumors may also mimic thyroid tumors.

Histopathologically, paraganglioma is characteristized as a hypervascular, epithelioid tumor forming "balls of cells" (zell-ballen); this refers to a compact arrangement of ball-like nests separated by fibrovascular tissue (◘ Fig. 5.27). Zell ballen can be highlighted by reticulin stain. Two different cell types can be discerned: chief cells and sustentacular cells. The chief cells are polygonal with abundant granular cytoplasm, round nuclei and "salt and pepper" stippled of chromatin. Cellular pleomorphism can be present, may be marked, but has no independent prognostic value. The sustentacular cells are spindled cells scattered at the periphery of the cell balls.

By immunohistochemistry, paragangliomas express neuron specific enolase, synaptophysin, and chromogranin. S-100 highlights the Schwann-like sustentacular cells that ensheathe the "zell-ballen". Epithelial markers (cytokeratin, carcinoembryonic antigen and epithelial mem-

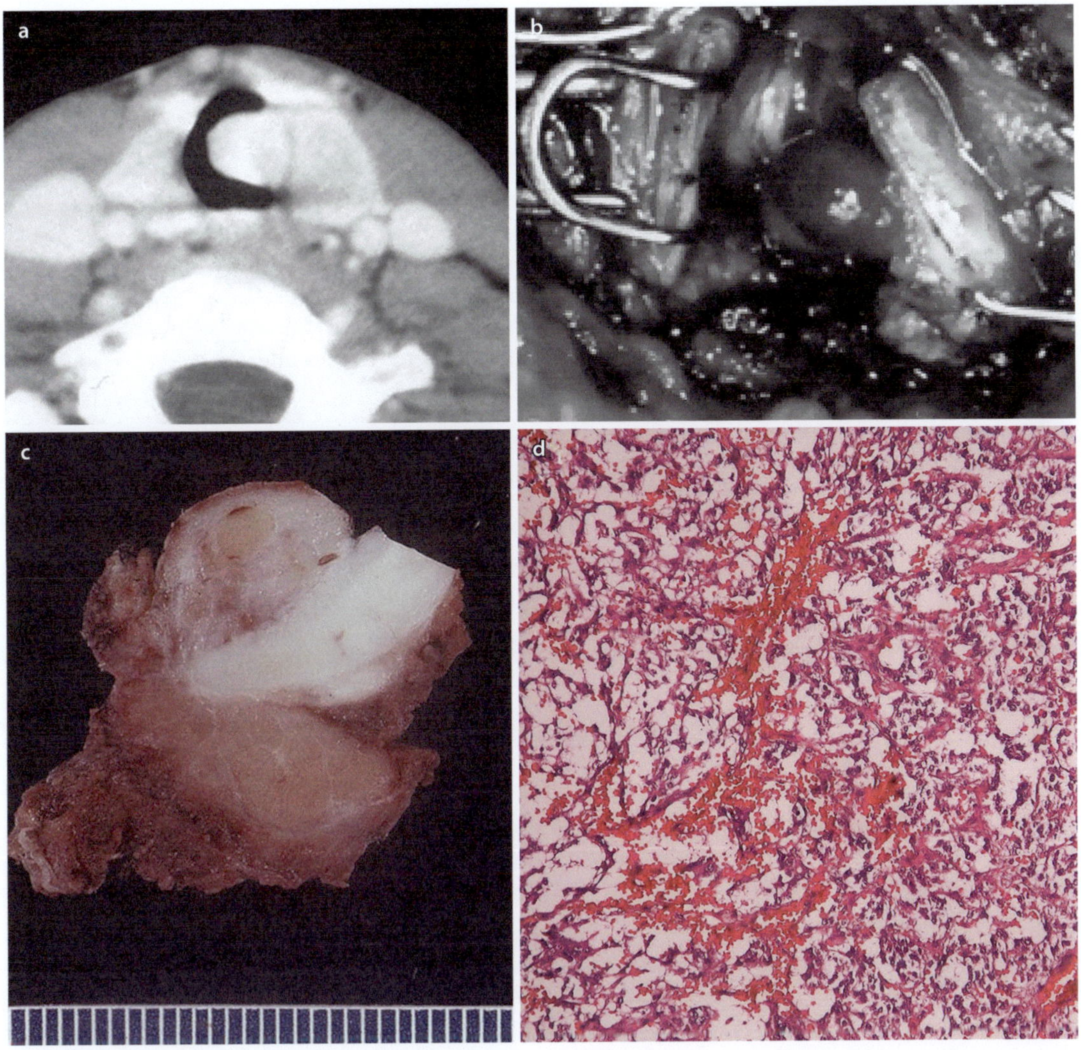

Fig. 5.26 Paraganglioma **a** Inferior laryngeal paraganglioma: the radiograph demonstrates an intratracheal component. **b** Intraoperative view: the cricoid has been cut and retracted. The intratracheal tumor component is seen as a vascular polypoid tumor **c** Dumbbell- shaped subcricoid mass protruding between the inferior cricoid and the first tracheal ring **d** Highly vascular tumor forming organoid nests

brane antigen) and calcitonin are negative. The differential diagnosis is with a typical carcinoid tumor (well-differentiated neuroendocrine carcinoma (NEC)) and atypical carcinoid tumor (moderately-differentiated NEC). Moderately-differentiated NEC has a higher nuclear/cytoplasmic ratio than paraganglioma. Infiltration, necrosis, or mitotic figures may be appreciated. Neuroendocrine carcinoma will express epithelial markers whereas paragangliomas will not.

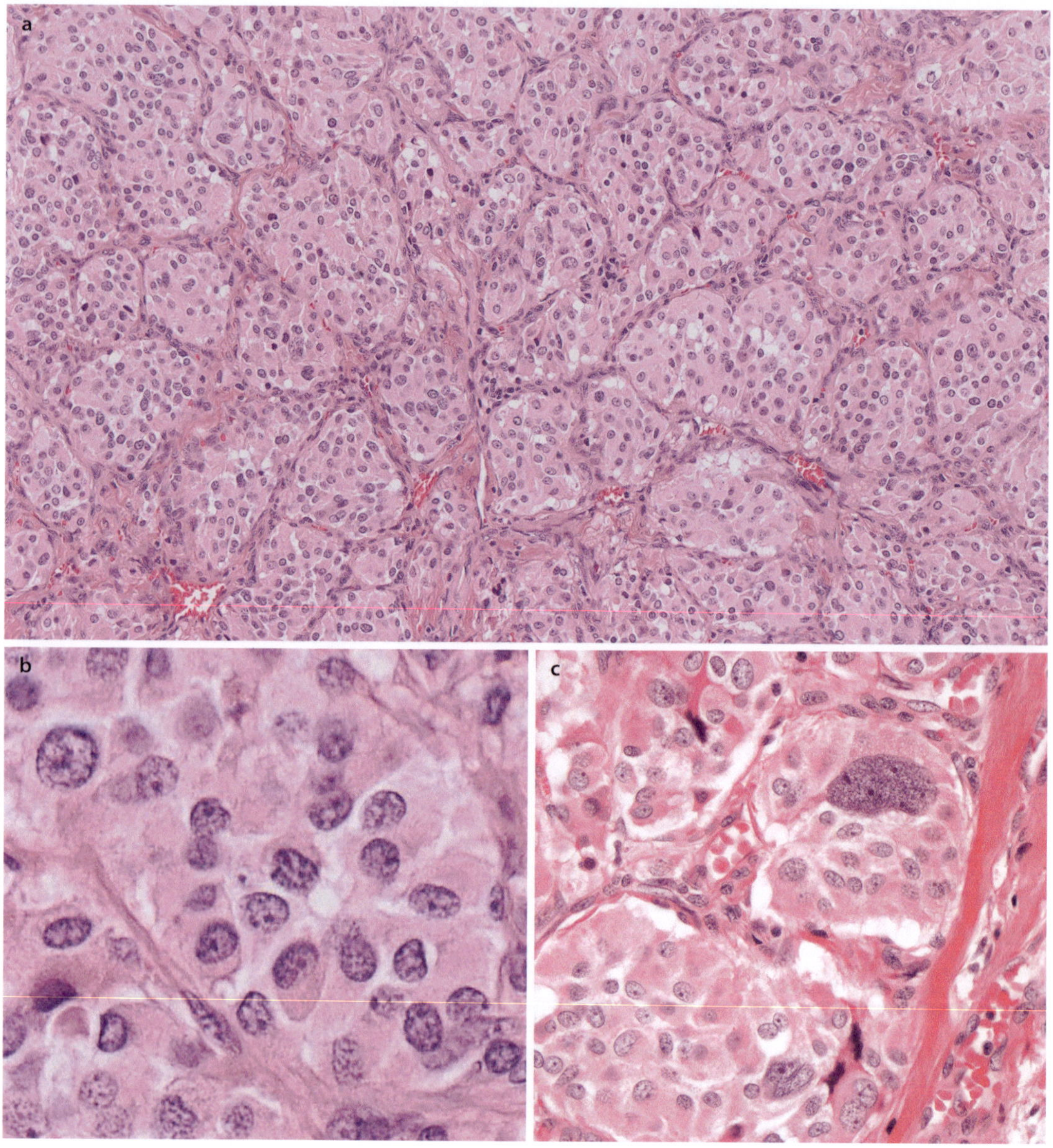

Fig. 5.27 Paraganglioma **a, b** These organoid nests of epithelioid cells produce the typical "zell-ballen" pattern. Note the round nuclei, stippled chromatin, and abundant cytoplasm. **c** Cellular pleomorphism can be seen in any endocrine tumor, and does not predict oncological behavior

5.14 Hamartoma

A hamartoma is defined as a benign growth composed of mature tissues indigenous to that region. (In distinction, a collection of nonindigenous mature tissue is classified as a choristoma.) Laryngeal hamartomas are rare and have been reported in both children and adults [93–100]. Some pediatric laryngeal hamartomas are associated with cleft larynges; adult hamartomas have not been associated with laryngeal defects. A laryngeal hamartoma may form either a submucosal "septum-like" mass in the posterior larynx, or a polypoid tumor. Upper airway symptoms are common to all patients.

Histopathologically, hamartomas can be classified as either epithelial or mesenchymal. The term "mesenchymoma" has also been

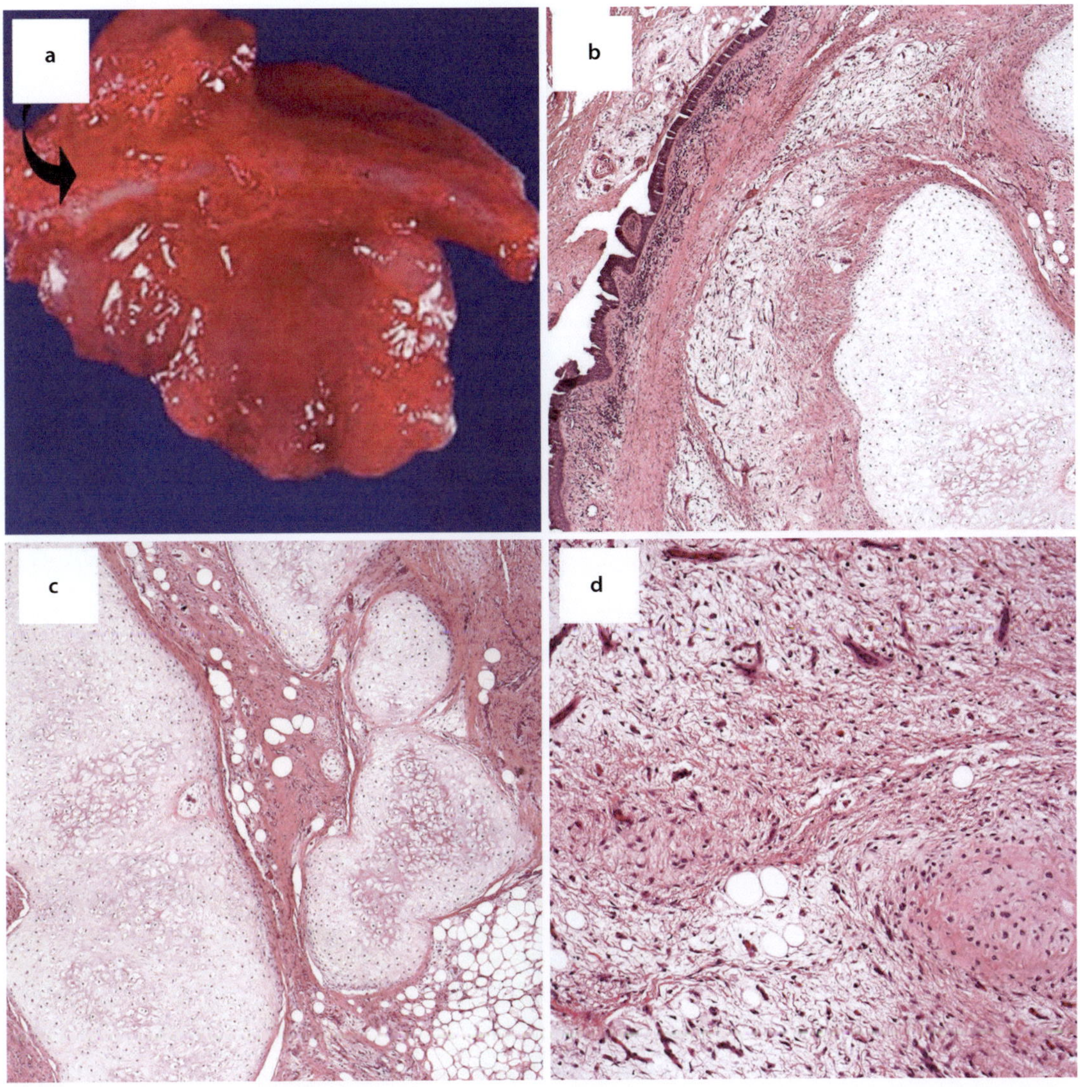

Fig. 5.28 **a** Endotracheal polypoid hamartoma. The arrow indicates tracheal cartilage **b–d** This tumor contains disorganized maturing cartilage fibroadipose and vascular tissue

applied to benign mesenchymal hamartomas. Histopathologically, multiple mature but disorganized mesenchymal elements are seen, usually skeletal muscle, cartilage, fat, vessels, nerves, and fibroconnective tissue (Figs. 5.28 and 5.29). The cartilaginous component can "blend " or "merge" into the surrounding stroma. Epithelial hamartomatous elements are mucinous minor salivary tissue.

The differential diagnosis of hamartoma includes **vocal cord chondrometaplasia** (Fig. 5.30), which refers to benign, metaplastic cartilage with limited growth potential (see below). The cartilage is bland and typically "blends" into the surrounding soft tissue rather than pushes against it. Chondrometaplasia has no direct attachment to underlying cartilaginous structures, and is not admixed with other tissue types (muscle, glands, etc). The differential diagnosis also includes the rare **laryngeal teratoma,** which is comprised of **immature** and **maturing** tissues of ectodermal, mesodermal and endodermal origin [101].

Low-grade cartilaginous tumors may also enter into the differential diagnosis.

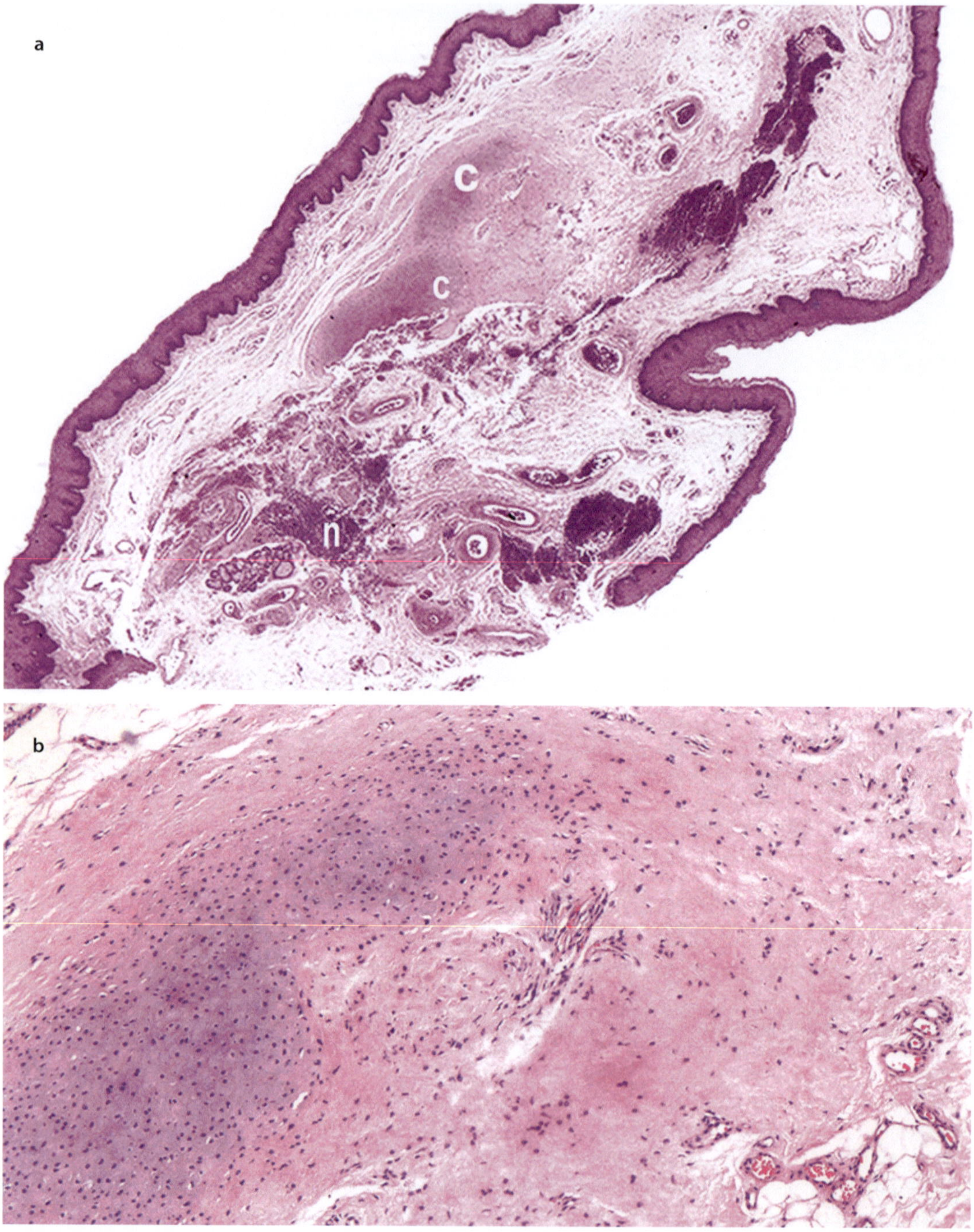

Fig. 5.29 **a** Another laryngeal hamartoma from the ventricle. Cartilage (C), neural (n) tissue, and other connective tissue elements are present. **b** Immature fibrocartilaginous tissue

Chondrosarcomas arise either from the thyroid lamina or cricoid ring, and are composed solely of cartilaginous tissue, no admixture of other tissue types are present. Similarly, laryngeal adult rhabdomyomas are composed solely of large mature skeletal muscle cells and no additional mesenchymal elements [102, 103]. Lastly, low-grade liposarcoma can mimic a mesenchymal hamartoma as it may have a prominent fibroblastic component. Other mesenchymal elements (thick walled vessels, smooth or skeletal muscle, etc) will point to a hamartoma.

5.15 Laryngeal Nodular Chondrometaplasia

This unusual condition is characterized by tissue transformation into nodular mature cartilage. These lesions are small, usually less than one centimeter. Chondrometaplasia may occur in the posterior or mid-vocal cords or the false cords. A history of prior trauma may be elicited [104]. Histologically, chondrometaplasia appears as mature cartilage **smoothly rimmed by fibroblasts** (◘ Fig. 5.30) which appears to blend into the surrounding tissues. By contrast, a low-grade chondrosarcoma growth in a lobulated fashion with borders sharply demarcated from surrounding tissues.

Tracheopathia chondro-osteoplastica is an extraordinarily rare disorder of unknown etiology marked by cartilaginous and bony submucosal nodules of the tracheal rings causing a "rock garden" effect [105, 106]. The posterior tracheal wall is spared (◘ Fig. 5.31).

Lastly, **osseous metaplasia** refers to benign bone growth within soft tissue, commonly skeletal muscle; laryngeal osseous metaplasia has been reported [107].

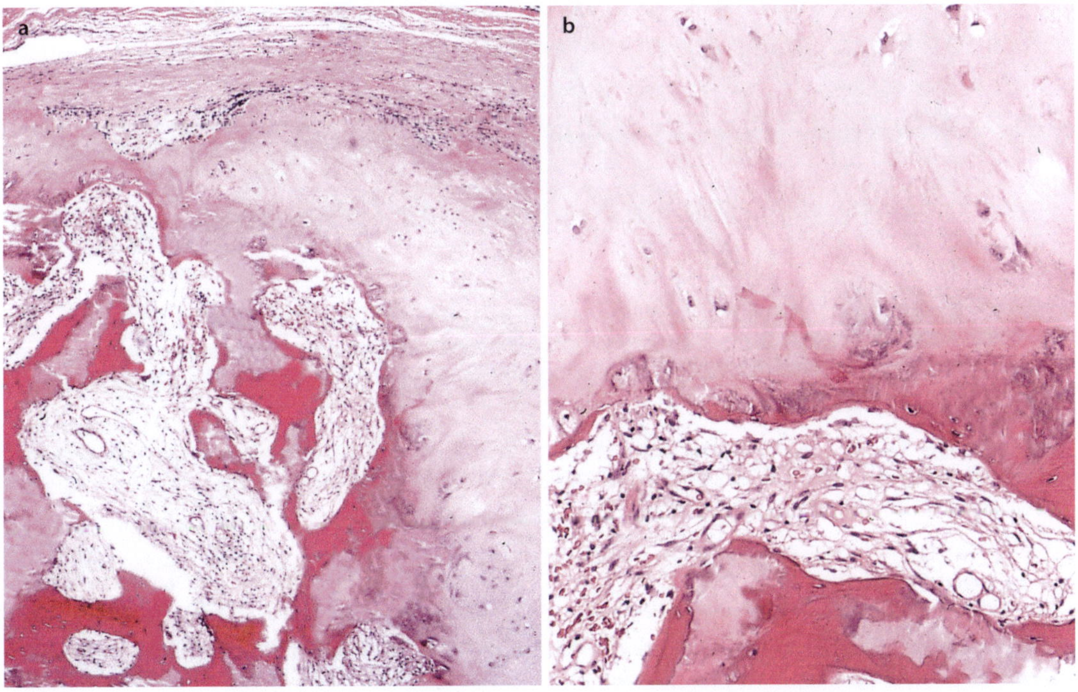

◘ **Fig. 5.30** **a, b** Chondrometaplasia of the vocal fold. Here, central ossification is seen. The periphery reveals mature chondroid matrix which "blends" into the surrounding fibroconnective tissue. This diagnosis requires confirmation that the lesion originates within the vocal fold, away from the arytenoid tower

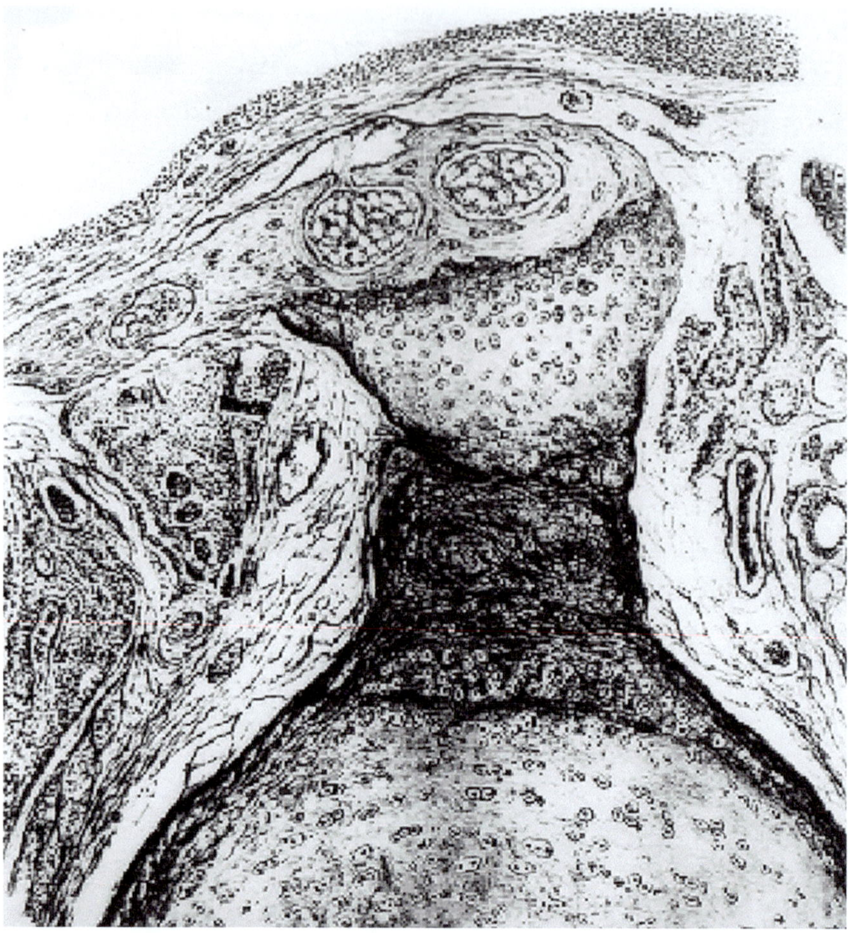

Fig. 5.31 Tracheopathia chondro-osteoplastica (TPCO) is characterized by heterotopic calcification and ossification. This image is from the original illustration by Muckleston 1909 demonstrating disorganized cartilage contiguous with underlying tracheal cartilage

5.16 Leiomyoma

Approximately 95% of all leiomyomas arise in the uterus. Head and neck smooth muscle neoplasia are extremely rare, and thought to arise from pluripotential mesenchymal stem cells within blood vessels. In 1994, Hellquist identified 33 cases of laryngeal leiomyomas in the published literature, and found a male to female ratio of 2:1, and the mean age at diagnosis in the fifth decade [108]. The majority of laryngeal leiomyomas arise in the supraglottis [108–114]. They can be entirely submucosal or polypoid.

Histopathologically, they can be classified as either simple, epithelioid, or vascular (angioleiomyoma or angiomyoma). At low-power, leiomyomas produce cellular bundles and swirled fascicles. One can find tumor spindle cells originating from muscular vessels. Cytologically. they are characterized by blunt cigar-shaped nuclei and abundant pink cytoplasm (Fig. 5.32). No cellular crowding, necrosis, or mitotic activity should be present. Occasionally, atypical but benign degenerative cells can be seen (symplastic cells) which do not express p53. Epithelioid leiomyoma are composed of nests and sheets of non-spindled cells with abundant cytoplasm; perinuclear clearing can be seen. Epithelioid leiomyomas are usually intermixed with typical spindle cell regions. One quarter of laryngeal leiomyomas can be classified as vascular leiomyoma. These tumors have abundant capillary, cavernous, or venous-type vessels. Leiomyoma cells express actin, desmin, and vimentin, and are negative for S100.

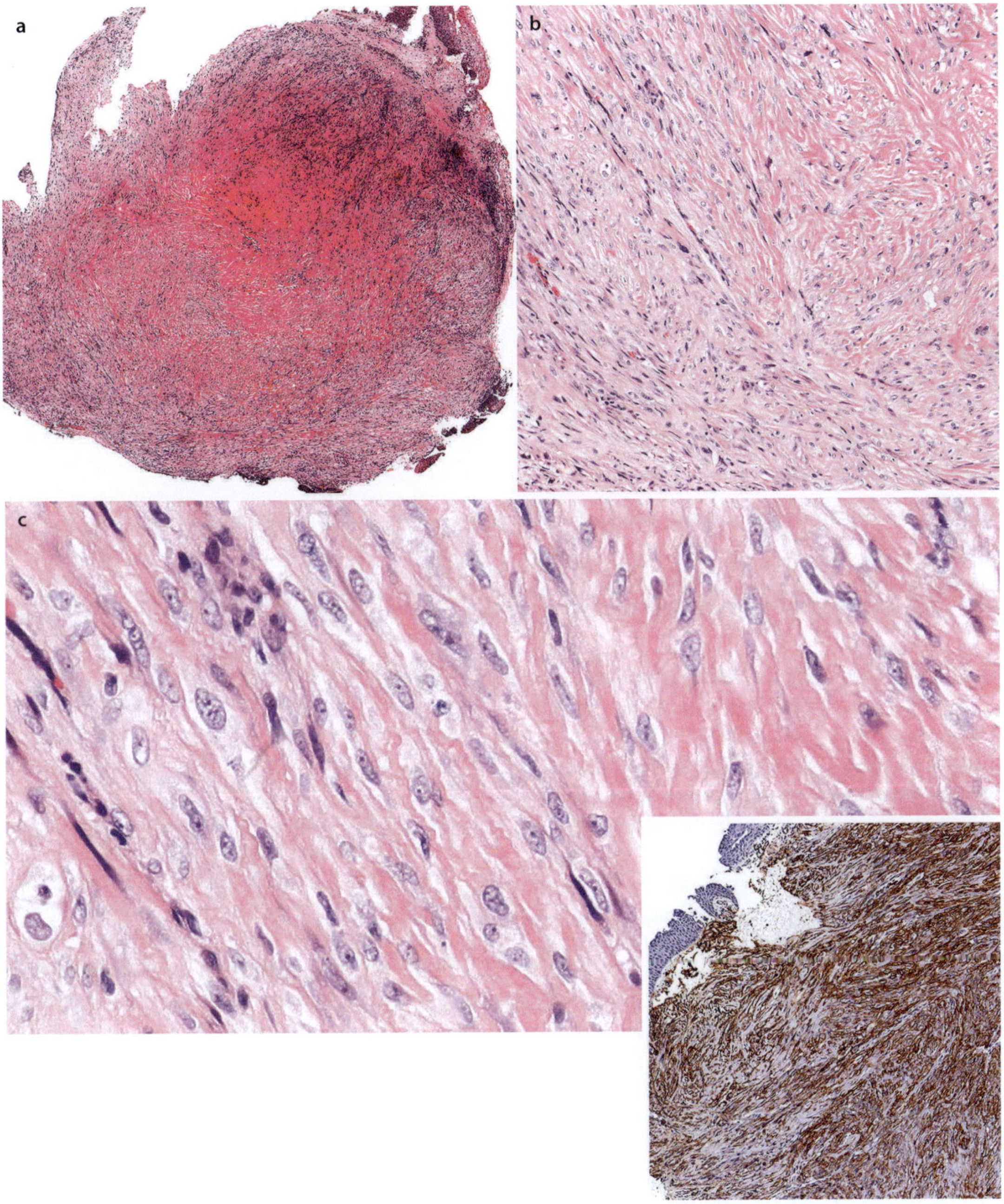

Fig. 5.32 Laryngeal leomyoma **a** Polypoid laryngeal tumor. **b** At low-power, you can see that spindled tumor cells are spaced apart from one another, and red bands of hyalinization **c** At higher-power, the spindle cells have "cigar-shaped" nuclei (rounded ends) with fine chromatin. **Inset:** Smooth muscle actin

5.17 Laryngeal Cancer

Over 13,000 new laryngeal cancers were diagnosed in the United States in 2017, and over 3600 disease specific mortalities were attributed to laryngeal cancer [115]. The overall age standardized incident rates of laryngeal cancer have been decreasing; the National Cancer Institute Surveillance, Epidemiology, and End Results (SEER) data demonstrate that the average annual percent change from 2002–2013 was −1.85 (−2.28 to 1.42) [116]. There is a pronounced male predilection; the male to female ratio is 4.8 to 1 [116]. The risk of developing laryngeal cancer

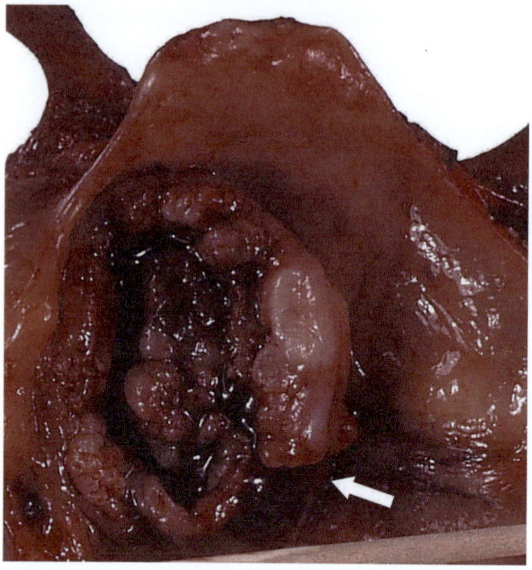

Fig. 5.33 This exophytic and ulcerated supraglottic carcinoma hangs over, but does not extend into, the glottis. The arrow points to the level of the ventricle

significantly increases with tobacco use, which is potentiated with concomitant heavy alcohol usage [117, 118]. Other occupational exposures which promote laryngeal carcinoma include asbestos, polycyclic aromatic hydrocarbons, and textile dust [117].

The exact laryngeal tumor site will influence presenting symptoms, stage at presentation, treatment options, and prognosis. Vocal cord tumors present with changes in voice quality, i.e. hoarseness; patients tend to seek medical care when these tumors are relatively small. Large or bilateral glottic tumors may present with worsening upper airway obstruction and stridor. Epiglottic tumors may cause a change in vocal quality (a muffled or "hot potato voice") (Fig. 5.33). Primary ventricular carcinomas are rare, and the majority of tumors encountered here result from the direct spread of glottic primaries. Primary ventricular carcinomas are noteworthy in that they remain hidden from the observer on laryngeal examination, merely forming a bulge under the intact vestibular fold mucosa. Most tumors that appear "infraglottic" actually arise from the undersurface of the vocal fold. Infraglottic tumors have a more insidious course of onset with patients complaining of increasing exertional dypsnea. Primary tracheal malignancies are extremely rare - it is more likely to encounter a primary carcinoma of the esophagus eroding into the trachea rather than finding a primary neoplasm. Pyriform sinus tumors are not endolaryngeal; they don't cause any vocal or respiratory symptoms. The pyriform sinuses are extralaryngeal gutters flanking the thyroid lamina. The lateral wall of the pyriform is the thyroid lamina; the medial wall is the cricoid ring. On swallowing, the larynx is raised and the epiglottis moves inferiorly partially covering the endolarynx, and the vocal folds close. Fluids are deflected laterally and inferiorly down the pyriform sinuses into the opened cricopharyngeaus - the esophageal inlet. Tumors of the pyrifom sinuses become symptomatic only after reaching considerable size; patients may complain of pain on swallowing radiating to the ear.

Glottic carcinomas may spread by undermining the tissue around the ventricles (paraglottic region), and escape the endolarynx by spreading laterally to invade the cricothyroid ligament and the inferior aspect of the thyroid lamina. The perichondrium and avascular cartilage are effective barriers against tumor invasion. By contrast, ossified thyroid lamina is more vulnerable to tumor invasion. The epiglottis is composed of fenestrated cartilage, which allows for early tumor spread from the laryngeal surface to the lingual surface and into the pre-epiglottic space. The latter contains abundant lymphatics; tumor spread into this space increases the risk for cervical metastasis and worsens prognosis.

The TMN staging criteria are presented below (Table 5.2):

5.17.1 Treatment of Laryngeal Cancers

Early stage glottis and supraglottic cancers may be treated with transoral laser excision. Transoral laser resections have replaced many of the traditional partial laryngectomy techniques such as supraglottic laryngectomy. Local disease-control

Table 5.2 8th AJCC staging criteria: laryngeal neoplasia

Supraglottis	
T Stage	**Criteria**
Tx	Primary tumor cannot be accessed
Tis	Carcinoma-in-situ
T1	Limited to one supraglottic subsite, normal cord mobility
T2	Invades one adjacent subsite of supraglottis or glottis or region beyond supraglottis (tongue base, vallecular, medial piriform sinus) without fixation of larynx
T3	Limited to larynx with vocal cord fixation and/or invades postcricoid region, pre-epiglottic space, paraglottic region, inner cortex thyroid lamina.
T4a	Moderately advanced local disease invading through outer cortex thyroid lamina, or beyond larynx (trachea, soft tissue neck, deep muscle tongue, strap muscles, thyroid, esophagus)
T4b	Very advanced local disease, invading prevertebral space, encases carotid, mediastinal structures
Glottis	
T Stage	**Criteria**
Tx	Primary tumor cannot be accessed
Tis	Carcinoma-*in-situ*
T1a	Limited to one vocal cord
T1b	Limited to both vocal cords
T2	Extends to supraglottis and/or subglottis, and/or impaired cord mobility
T3	Limited to larynx with vocal cord fixation and/or invades paraglottic region and/or inner cortex thyroid lamina
T4a	Moderately advanced local disease invading through outer cortex thyroid lamina, or beyond larynx (trachea, cricoid, soft tissue neck, deep muscle tongue, strap muscles, thyroid, esophagus)
T4b	Very advanced local disease, invading prevertebral space, encases carotid, mediastinal structures
Subglottic	
T Stage	**Criteria**
Tx	Primary tumor cannot be accessed
Tis	Carcinoma-*in-situ*
T1	Limited to subglottis
T2	Extends to vocal folds with normal/impaired cord mobility
T3	Limited to larynx with vocal cord fixation and/or invades paraglottic region and/or inner cortex thyroid lamina
T4a	Moderately advanced local disease invading through cricoid, or thyroid lamina, or beyond larynx (trachea, soft tissue neck, deep muscle tongue, strap muscles, thyroid, esophagus)
T4b	Very advanced local disease, invading prevertebral space, encases carotid, mediastinal structures

Table 5.2 (continued)

N Category	Number and Size	ENE
Nx	Cannot be assessed	
N0	No metastases	
N1	One ipsilateral lymph node ≤ 3 cm	No
N2a	One ipsilateral lymph node ≤ 3 cm	Yes
N2b	One ipsilateral lymph node > 3 cm but ≤ 6cm	No
N2c	Multiple ipsilateral, bilateral or contralateral lymph nodes ≤ 6cm	No
N3a	One lymph node > 6 cm	No
N3b	One ipsilateral lymph node > 6 cm, or any multiple ipsilateral, contralateral or bilateral lymph nodes	Yes

Stage Grouping

If T..	And N...	And M...	Then Stage
Tis	N0	M0	0
T1	N0	M0	I
T2	N0	M0	II
T3	N0	M0	III
T1, T2, T3	N1	M0	III
T4a	N0, N1	M0	IVA
T1, T2, T3, T4a	N2	M0	IVA
Any T	N3	M0	IVB
T4b	Any N	M0	IVB
Any T	Any N	M1	IVC

rates are similarly favorable for low-stage laryngeal cancers treated by either transoral laser excision or primary radiotherapy. Evaluating resection margins for transoral laser resections may be challenging; in some cases the surgeon will laser through the tumor as a way of assessing tumor spread. In these cases, it is preferable for the surgeon to harvest mucosa from the defect to assess margin status. This is an exception to the rule of thumb that specimen-directed margin assessment is superior to defect-directed margin assessment. A resection margin distance of 2 mm is still considered appropriate [116]. Involvement of the anterior commissure is a known predictors of local recurrence.

Treatment options for patients with T3 disease include chemoradiation (organ sparing protocol), radiation alone, transoral laser resection and open partial laryngectomy. The organ-sparing induction chemotherapy protocols came out of Radiation Therapy Oncology Group (RTOG) study 91–11, published in 2003 [116]. The rationale of this approach was that the larynx could be preserved in a majority of patients, and failure after chemoradiotherapy requiring salvage laryngectomy did not adverse disease-specific survival. Larynx preservation, though, did not always equate with functional preservation. The declining 5-year relative survival rates in the late 1980's to 1990's indirectly implicated the rise of primary "organ sparing" approaches [119]. A recent systematic literature review on patient outcomes for T3 disease concluded that induction chemotherapy "seemed to worsen" survival rates when compared to either primary open partial laryngectomy or transoral laser resection. Heterogeneity with respect to staging schemata, tumor subsite, preoperative, and postoperative therapies, limited the conclusions of this analysis [120]. The standard approach for T4 laryngeal cancer is total laryngectomy. Aggressive features which are indications for postoperative radiotherapy include perineural invasion, lymphovascular invasion, margins <1 mm, thyroid cartilage invasion, ≥1.1 cm subglottic extension, extension into soft tissues of neck, bone invasion, and multiple positive lymph nodes.

5.17.2 HPV and Laryngeal Cancer

The original Danish Head and Neck Cancer Group (DAHANNCA) clinical trials, which demonstrated superior outcomes for p16 overexpressing cancers was composed of oropharyngeal and non-oropharyngeal carcinomas; this latter group included laryngeal cancers. It is then logical to ask if these survival benefits extend to p16 overexpressing laryngeal cancers? In a recent subgroup analysis of DAHANNCA trial patients (1992–2012), p16 overexpression was present in 13.7% of 321 patients with laryngeal cancers [121]. As expected, this frequency was much lower in laryngeal cancers compared with oropharyngeal cancers (52%). Overexpression of p16 had no impact on outcome for the combined laryngeal and hypopharyngeal patients. Recent studies have also confirmed that p16 overexpression cannot be used as a surrogate HR-HPV biomarker for laryngeal cancer [122, 123]. Furthermore, no significant survival differences were observed for a group of 674 laryngeal cancer patients stratified by HPV status [123].

5.18 Laryngeal Precursor Lesions

The 2017 World Health Organization (WHO) classification of laryngeal precursor lesions collapses dysplasia into a two-tiered system, based on modifications of the Ljubljana classification [124–126]. The Ljubljana experience with laryngeal dysplasia is quite impressive as over 1400 patients have been followed for up to 25 years. ◘ Table 5.3 presents the two-tiered low-grade versus high-grade schema. Carcinoma-*in-situ* is rolled in with high-grade dysplasia. However, features of carcinoma-in-situ are detailed, in the event that clinical nuances warrant distinction between these two categories.

A systemic review and meta-analysis of 940 patients with laryngeal precursor lesions demonstrated an overall rate of malignant transformation of 14%, mean time of 5.8 years. The rate of progression to invasive cancer significantly cor-

◘ **Table 5.3** 2017 WHO criteria for laryngeal precursor lesions

	Architecture	Cytology
Low-grade dysplasia	Preserved stratification	No atypia
	Preserved transition of nuclear orientation from perpendicular to horizontal	Parabasal cells may have larger nuclei than basal cells
	Preserved prickle cells in upper layers	Mitotic figures regular, rare, low
	Parabasal cells may extend to midepithelium	Few dyskeratotic cells
High-grade dysplasia	Abnormal maturation, disordered stratification and polarity	Marked cellular and nuclear atypia
	Disordered cells half to full thickness	Variation of cell shapes and sizes
	Rete ridges may be irregular	Nuclear hyperchromasia
		Nucleoli increased in number and size
		Mitotic figures increased throughout, with/without atypical mitotic figures
		Dyskeratotic/apoptotic cells throughout

Table 5.3 (continued)

Carcinoma-*in-situ*	Complete loss of stratification and polarity throughout	Severe cellular and nuclear atypia
	Uppermost layer may have thin, compressed, horizontally oriented cells	Severe pleomorphism
	Intact basement membrane, irregular rete pegs	Frequent nuclear hyperchromasia
		Nucleoli increased number and size
		Mitotic figures increased throughout, with atypical mitotic figures
		Dyskeratotic/apoptotic cells throughout
		High nuclear/cytoplasmic ratio

related with degree of dysplasia: 10.6% for low-grade dysplasia (mild/moderate-dysplasia) versus 30.4% for high-grade dysplasia (severe dysplasia/carcinoma-*in-situ*) [127]. In the largest published retrospective study of laryngeal precursor lesions, comprised of 1444 patients with laryngeal SILs, classified according to the Ljubljana classification, the rates of malignant progression were 1.6% (19/1204 patients within 2–15 years) for low-grade dysplasia and 12.5% (30/240 patients within 2–26 years) for high-grade dysplasia.

5.19 Spindle Cell Variant Squamous Cell Carcinoma

Spindle cell variant of squamous carcinoma (spindled squamous carcinoma) refers to squamous carcinoma with prominent malignant spindle cell component. These tumors are invariably described as polypoid. The SEER database reveals that ***the larynx is the most common head and neck site*** for the spindle cell variant (46.6%) followed by oral cavity [128]. Glottic tumors are more common (72%) than supraglottic (16%), or subglottic (4%) tumors [129]. As compared to conventional laryngeal squamous carcinomas, spindled squamous carcinoma is significantly more likely to be as T1 N0 [128, 130]. It follows, then that laryngeal spindled squamous carcinoma has a significantly more favorable prognosis than conventional laryngeal carcinoma. In comparison, oral cavity spindled squamous carcinoma is associated with a worse prognosis than conventional oral cavity carcinoma ($p = 0.008$) [128, 130].

Histopathologically, recognition that spindle cell variant is actually a squamous carcinoma comes from finding either typical keratinizing squamous carcinoma within the tumor, or overlying squamous carcinoma *in-situ*, or demonstrating cytokeratin or p63 expression. These conditions are not necessary for this diagnosis. ***Sometimes all that may guide you in making this diagnosis is the knowledge that spindled squamous carcinoma is significantly more common than true sarcomas in the head and neck*** (Figs. 5.34, 5.35, 5.36, 5.37, and 5.38). Many times, one can suspect a spindle cell variant of squamous carcinoma from the obser-

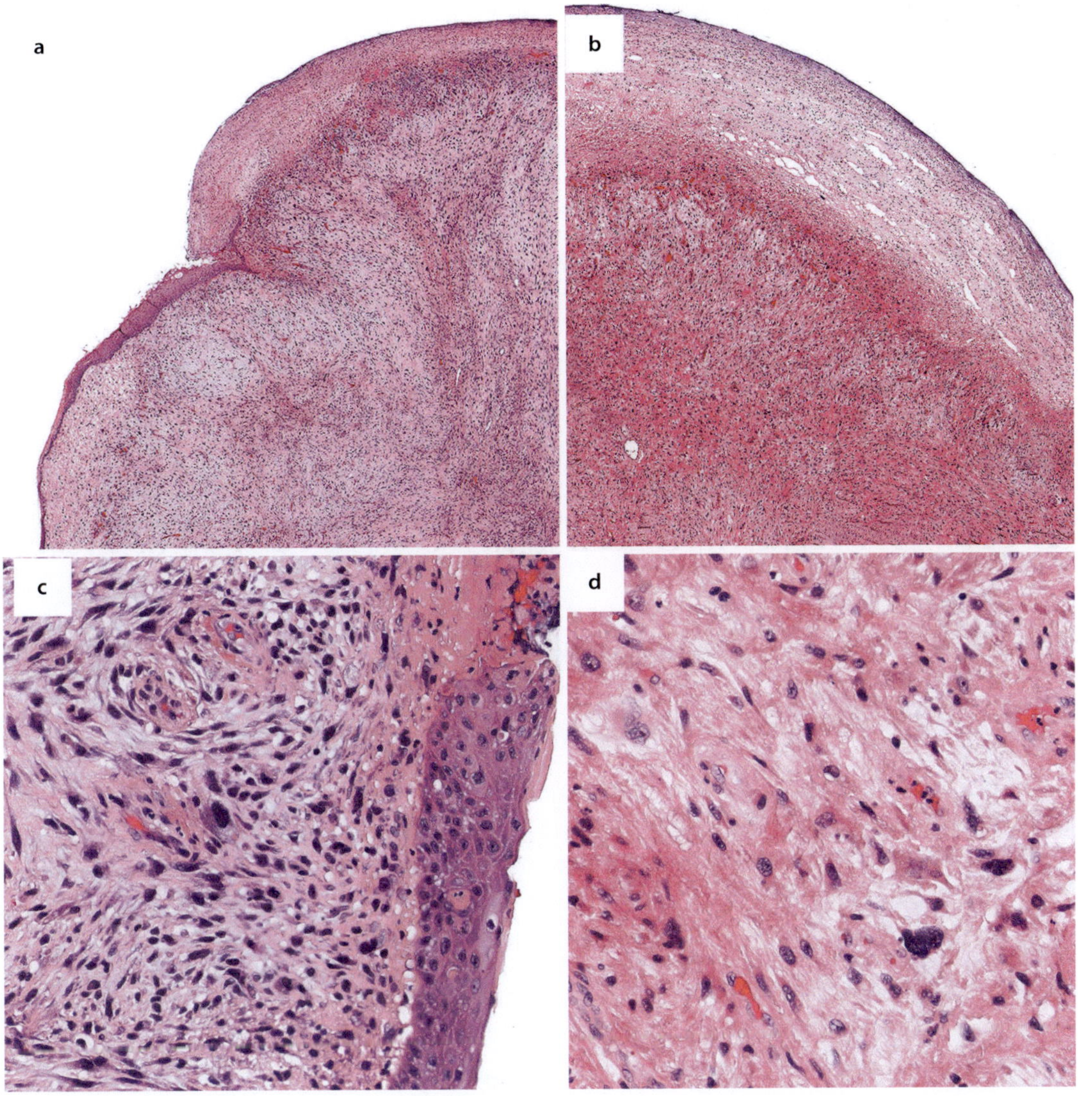

Fig. 5.34 **a, b** Polypoid squamous carcinomas, spindle cell variant. **c, d** Cellular, pleomorphic malignant spindle cells

vation that the malignant spindled cells are more plump and epithelioid than true sarcomas. This is not always the case, as other spindled squamous carcinomas are composed of densely packed elongated nuclei with high nuclear/cytoplasmic ratio.

A unique feature of laryngeal spindled squamous carcinoma is the production of collagenized osteoid-like matrix, which can be extensive and also mineralize [131]. Thus, the concept of extraosseous "laryngeal osteosarcoma" is dubious [132].

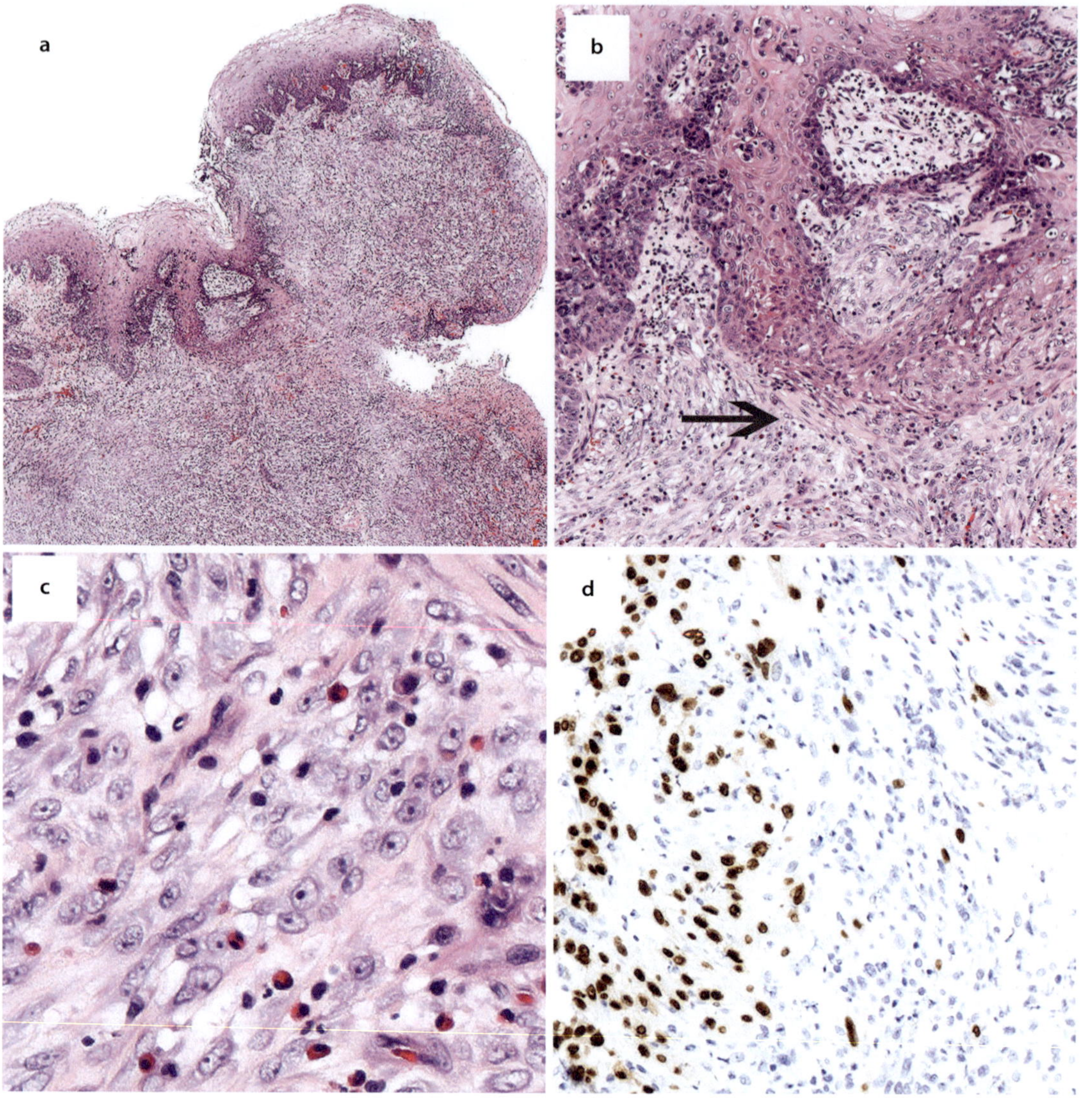

Fig. 5.35 **a** Low power view of another polypoid squamous carcinomas, spindle cell variant. **b** One way to make this diagnosis is finding a zone of squamous – sarcomatoid transition (*arrow*). **c** The spindle cell tumor nuclei here still resemble squamous carcinoma, with respect to shape and chromatin quality. **d** Another way to make this diagnosis is by finding keratin or p63 expression (shown here)

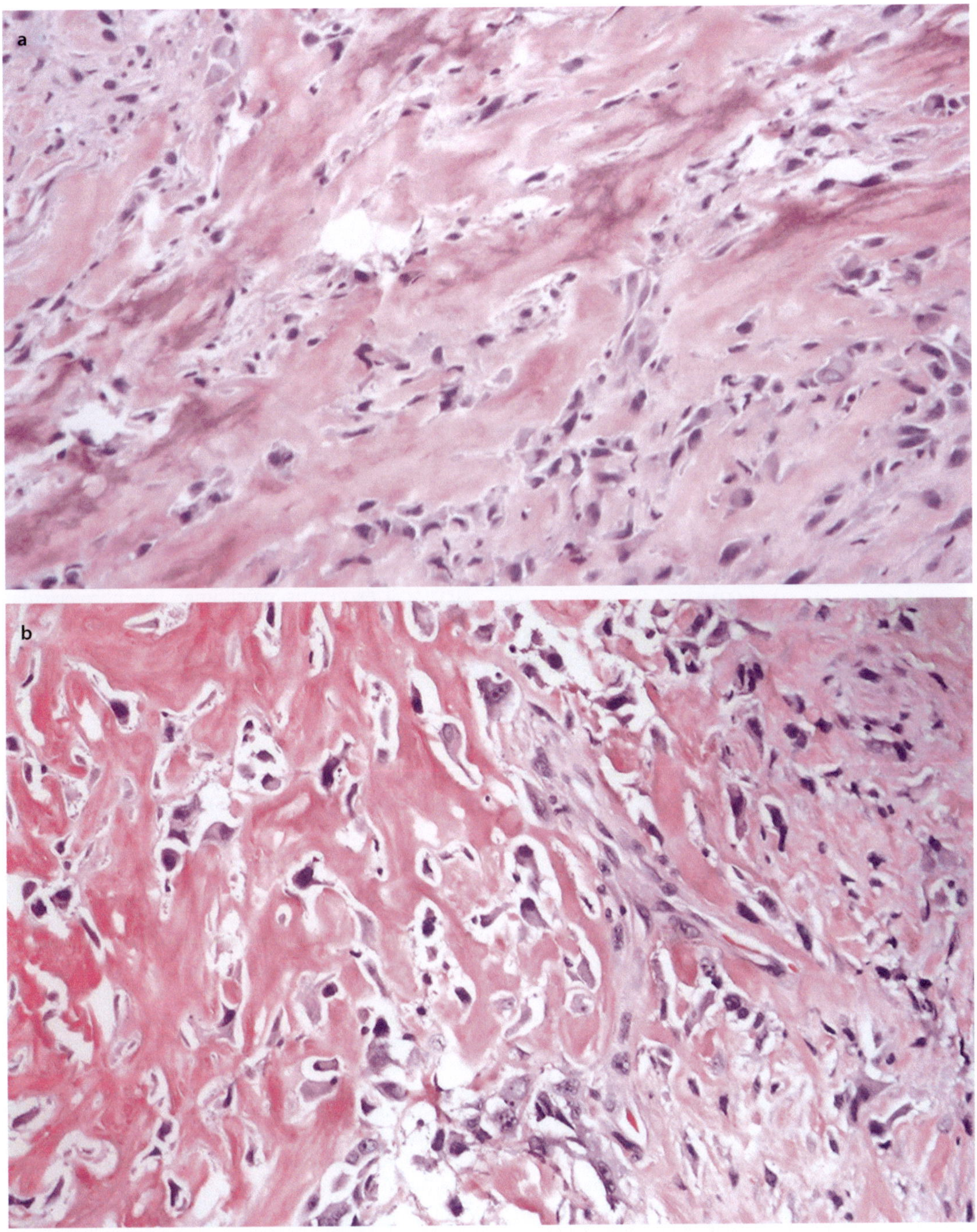

Fig. 5.36 a, b A unique aspect of laryngeal sarcomatoid carcinomas is the ability to produce osteoid-like matrix which can mineralize, thus mimicking "extraskeletal osteosarcoma"

5.20 Papillary Variant Squamous Cell Carcinoma

The papillary variant of squamous carcinoma refers a predominantly exophytic carcinoma forming a papillary architecture. The larynx and oropharynx are the most common anatomic sites [133, 134]. The glottis is the most common laryngeal subsite followed by the supraglottis [135].

The prognosis of laryngeal papillary variant squamous carcinoma, for all stages, is significantly better than that of conventional laryngeal squamous carcinoma [135]. This relates to the fact that the majority of patients present with T1/T2 disease (78.6%) versus T3/T4 (21.4%), and are N0 (74%) versus N+(22.6%).

Although this squamous variant is unrelated to exophytic papillomas, tumor architecture begs the question regarding relationship to HR-HPV. *In-situ* studies revealed HR-HPV in 26.3% (5/19) [133] and 55% (6/11) [134] laryngeal papillary squamous carcinomas by using RNA and DNA probes, respectively.

Histopathologically, this tumor may be either well-differentiated, or pleomorphic, with the common theme of fibrovascular cores. The cores may be slender or more bulbous. Cytologically pleomorphic papillary squamous carcinomas are easily recognized as malignant (◘ Fig. 5.37). In the absence of pleomorphism, the diagnosis can be more challenging. Remember that the larynx represents a relatively confined, limited space. Here, more than any other head and neck subsite, the amount of tissue submitted in a biopsy can also guide you. ◘ Figures 5.38a, b are true to size regarding a "normal" amount of laryngeal tissue biopsied. Compare that to the slide inset on ◘ Fig. 5.38c. More tissue submitted already hints at a squamo-proliferative process. If cytological pleomorphism is absent, this may represent a well-differentiated papillary variant of squamous carcinoma.

It is probably unwarranted to discuss invasion in a biopsy report. As the majority of these tumors are exophytic, leave classification of degree of invasion for the resection specimen report.

The differential diagnosis is with a benign laryngeal exophytic papilloma. The fibrovascular cores of an benign exophytic papilloma are uniform and slender. The overlying epithelium demonstrates regular maturation. Carcinoma-in-situ-ex-papilloma may also enter into the differential diagnosis of a cytologically pleomorphic papillary variant of squamous carcinoma. If there is a clinical history of laryngeal papillomatosis,

◘ Fig. 5.37 The papillary variant of squamous carcinoma is not difficult to diagnose, if cytologic pleomorphism is present. In its absence, the crucial clinicopathologic issues then become those of quantity and function. With respect to quantity: (1) Does the specimen consist of more epithelial tissue than expected for a vocal cord stripping? (See ◘ Figs. 5.10–5.38). Does the biopsy represent *all* the lesional tissue, or just a sampling? If there is more tissue than "normal", and this does not represent the whole lesion, then classification as "squamoproliferative process" may be in order. Diagnoses such as verrucous carcinoma, papillary variant of squamous carcinoma, or well-differentiated keratinizing squamous carcinoma, can be appropriately rendered in the absence of cytological plemorphism, ***with clinico-pathological correlation***. With respect to function: "Is vocal cord mobility impaired"? Decreased vocal mobility correlates with invasion into, or beyond, lamina propria. Here, the distinction between papillary variant of squamous carcinoma **a, c** and exophytic papilloma **b, d** is subtle. Both specimens revealed increased amount of tissue (insets). However, compare the fibrovascular cores for both lesions. In this papillary variant of squamous carcinoma, the fibrovascular cores give way to a broader proliferative pattern (*arrows*). Fibrovascular cores are seen throughout the exophytic papilloma. At higher power, epithelial maturation is present in the carcinoma **e.** Thus this diagnosis depends on clinicopathologic correlation. The exophytic papilloma lacks maturation. **f** and was diagnosed as diffuse carcinoma-in-situ-ex papilloma

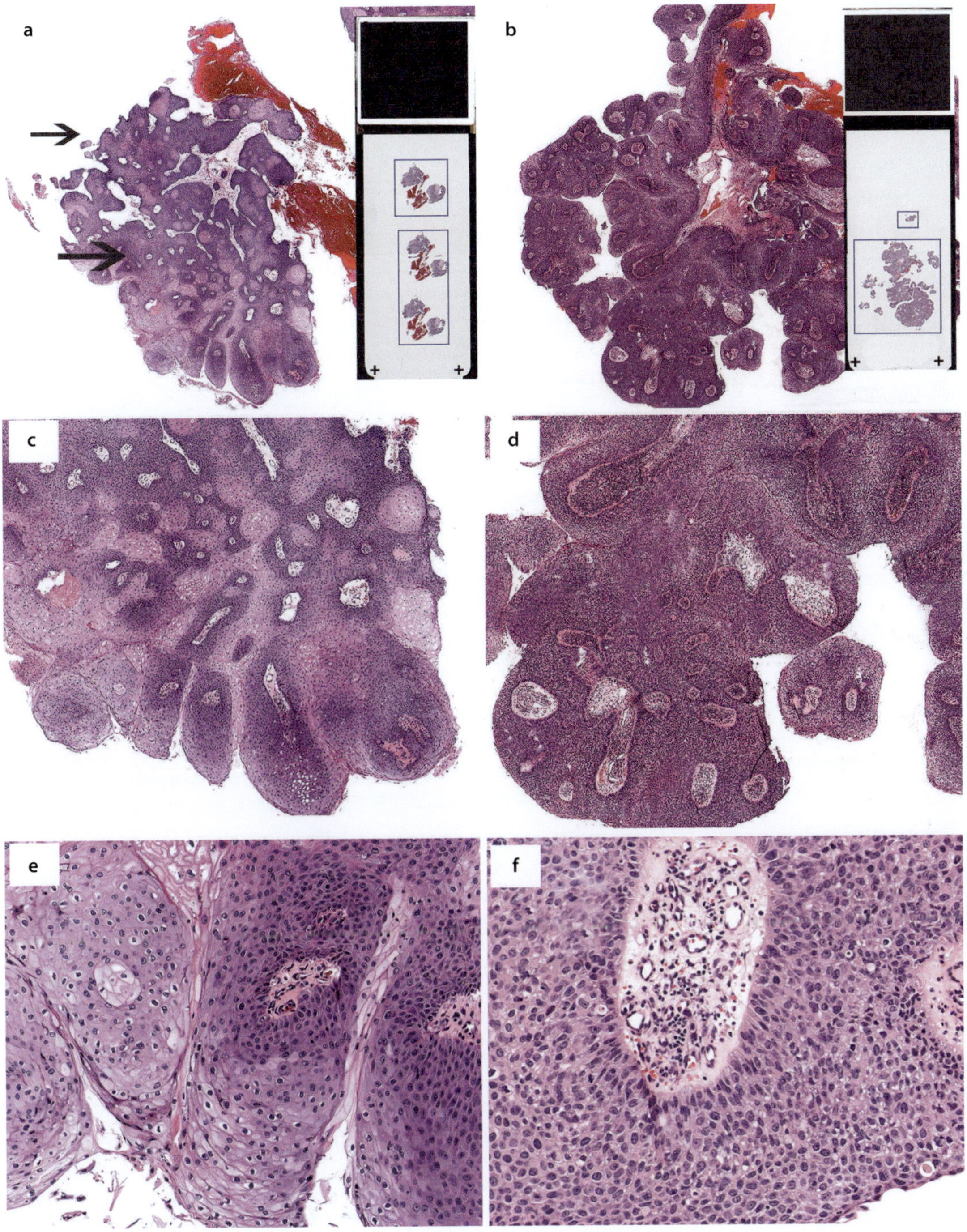
a
b
c
d
e
f

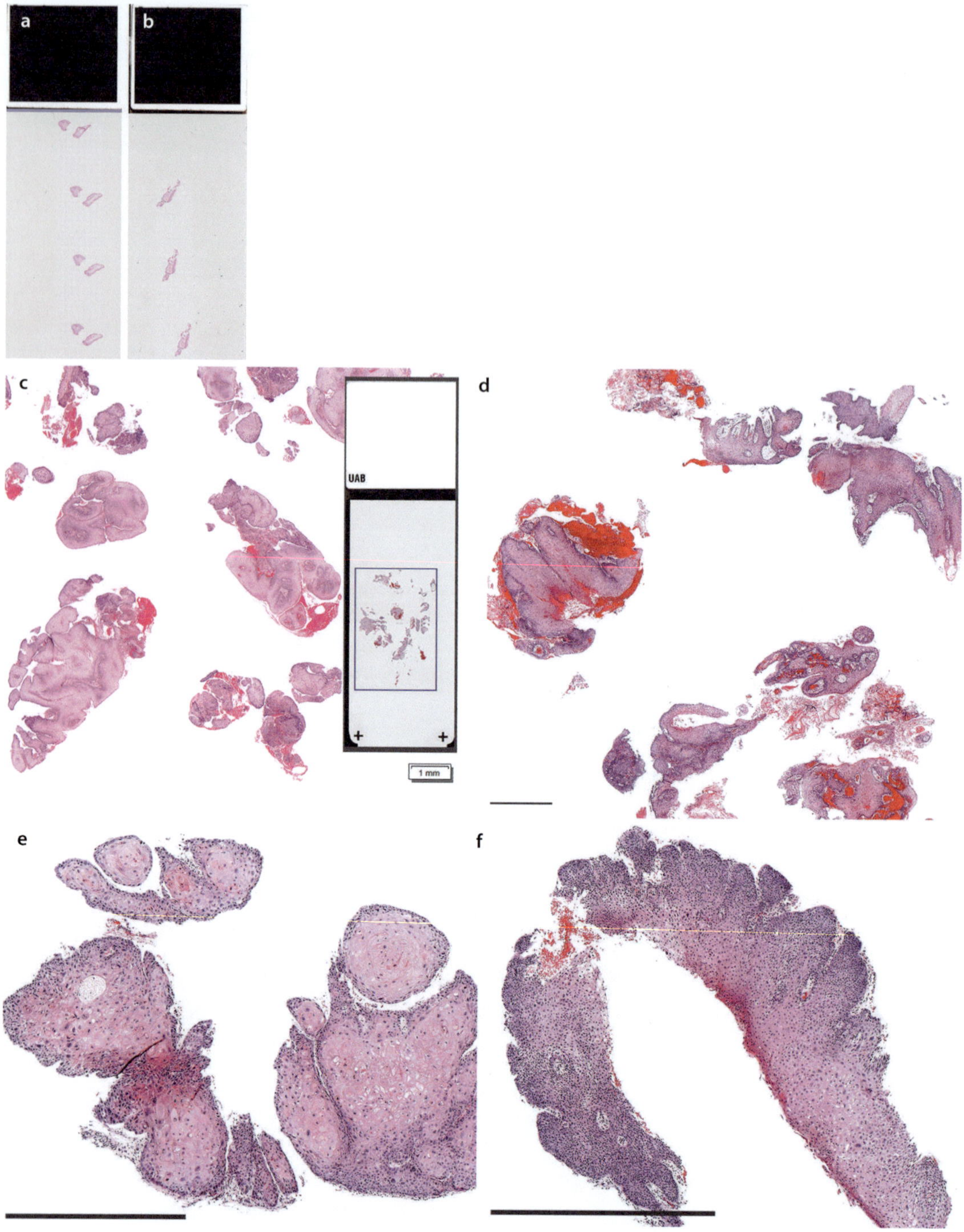

■ **Fig. 5.38** "Too much" It's important to get a *feel* for how much tissue from a laryngeal biopsy represents "too much". Remember that the vocal cords have relatively small real estate holdings. **a, b** are biopsy slides, true to size, demonstrating the expected, normal amount of tissue from a vocal cord. **c–f** Each panel represents "too much tissue" from a squamoproliferative process. The glass slide is also true to size, and each black bar here represents 1 mm at magnification

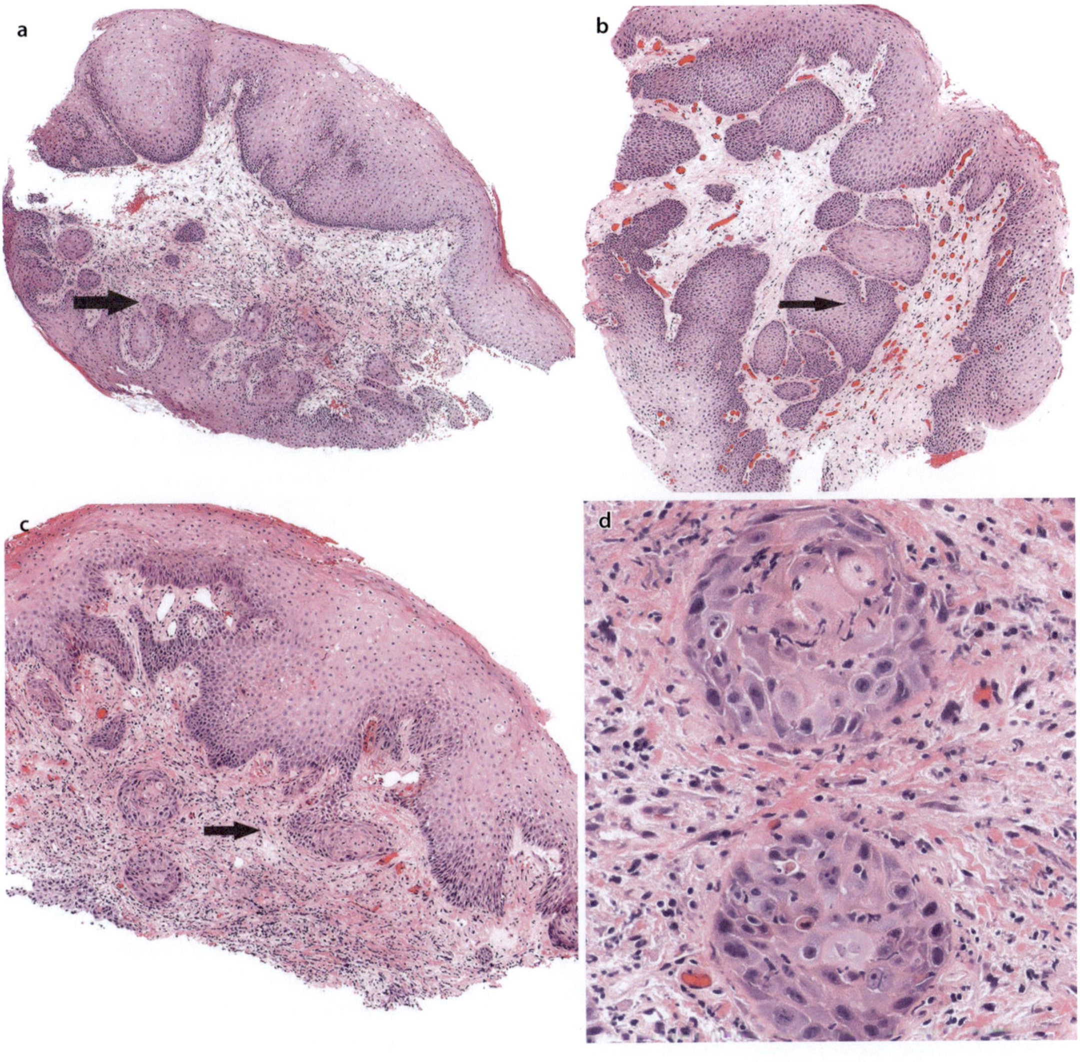

Fig. 5.39 Sialometaplasia It's equally important to think about sialometaplasia before pulling the trigger on a diagnosis of carcinoma **a, b** and **c** The arrows point to expanded ducts with a "kinked tube" appearance. Imagine trying to bend a long balloon that is not fully inflated. This is the first hint of sialometaplasia. The second hint would be the find ductal lumena. **d** The last hint is to confirm the lack of nuclear pleomorphims, and presence of neutrophils. The ductal cells in **D** are reactive in nature, not dysplastic

then opt for the classification of carcinoma-*in-situ-ex*-papilloma. Laryngeal carcinoma-*in-situ-ex*-papilloma is more likely to develop in long-standing florid respiratory papillomatosis. There are no practical aspects to the distinction between the laryngeal carcinoma-*in-situ-ex*-papilloma and papillary variant of squamous carcinoma.

On a limited biopsy, one might need to distinguish sialometaplasia (Fig. 5.39) from a histologically benign squamous proliferative process. Remember the "kinked tube" appearance of the metaplastic ducts, the residual duct lumena, and the likelihood of acute inflammation, these findings point to sialometaplasia.

5.21 Verrucous Carcinoma

Verrucous carcinoma represents an unusual squamous carcinoma variant which can be locally aggressive yet never metastasizes. The oral cavity is the most common site for verrucous carcinoma, followed by the larynx, where it comprises less than 1% of laryngeal malignancies. A SEER database search yielded 516 laryngeal verrucous carcinomas (1973–2011) [136]. The age-adjusted incidence of this tumor decreased (annual-percentage change −5.42%, 2000–2011), which is significantly in excess of the same incidence change for other laryngeal malignancies (−0.91%). Laryngeal verrucous carcinomas have a significantly greater male predominance (88.4%) and predilection for Whites (88.4%) as compared to other laryngeal malignancies. The vast majority of tumors involve the glottis (79.7%). Clinically, these tumors present as exophytic, white, grey, warty, or cauliflower-like growths.

The standard of care for treating verrucous carcinoma is primary surgery with negative resection margins. Patients may be treated with primary radiotherapy if they be poor surgical candidates. The fear of anaplastic transformation after irradiation is unfounded [137]. A rare subset of verrucous carcinomas can progress to develop conventional squamous carcinoma ("hybrid tumors"), however this is unrelated to prior irradiation. It is these rare hybrid tumors which account for the unusual metastatic cases.

The five-year disease-free survival rates are excellent (88%) [136]. The survival advantage for laryngeal verrucous carcinomas is quite pronounced when high-stage (III/IV) patients are compared with stage-matched counterparts with other laryngeal malignancies (90.0% versus 34.0%, respectively).

Histopathologically, there are well-known sagas on the historical difficulties associated with establishing the correct diagnosis on superficial biopsies [138–142]. The two architectural elements of verrucous carcinoma are (1) ***surface papillations with thick hyperkeratosis and parakeratosis***, and (2) **broad, pushing rete pegs** (◘ Figs. 5.40 and 5.41). The reason for the potential delayed diagnoses is, typically, verrucous carcinomas are cytologically well-differentiated and indistinguishable from benign processes. If you only receive a superficial biopsy, you can still suggest the diagnosis after clinical correlation: if there a large mass, then likely this is verrucous carcinoma. You can advise your clinicians, the next time they encounter a verrucous carcinoma, to take a biopsy from the periphery of the keratotic lesion, aiming deeply towards the center of the tumor. This approach is likely to capture some deep pushing rete pegs.

Pseudoepitheliomatous hyperplasia is frequently observed adjacent to verrucous carcinoma. The bulbous pushing rete pegs of verrucous carcinoma can be distinguished from those of pseudoepitheliomatous hyperplasia as the former are more fused, broad, and push deeper. As mentioned, the surface papillations of verrucous carcinoma are covered by thick, piled-up hyperkeratosis/parakeratosis. However, "keratin clefts", characteristic of verrucoid hyperplasia, are not part of verrucous carcinoma. Cytologically, the tumor cells have abundant glassy pink cytoplasm and prominent intercellular bridges. Atypical mitotic figures and pleomorphic cells are not part of the usual morphology of this tumor.

The differential diagnosis includes "hybrid tumors" (conventional squamous carcinomas-ex-verrucous carcinoma), and verruca vulgaris. Ten to 20% of verrucous carcinomas may contain a component of conventional squamous carcinoma. However, there seems to be a tendency to over diagnose hybrid tumors. Make certain that any apparent deviation from the pattern of broad, pushing rete pegs, is not merely tangential sectioning through a disorganized expanding verrucous carcinoma. Laryngeal verruca vulgaris can occur on rare occasion in immunosuppressed individuals. This differential diagnosis can be more difficult (◘ Fig. 5.42). Ascertain that the

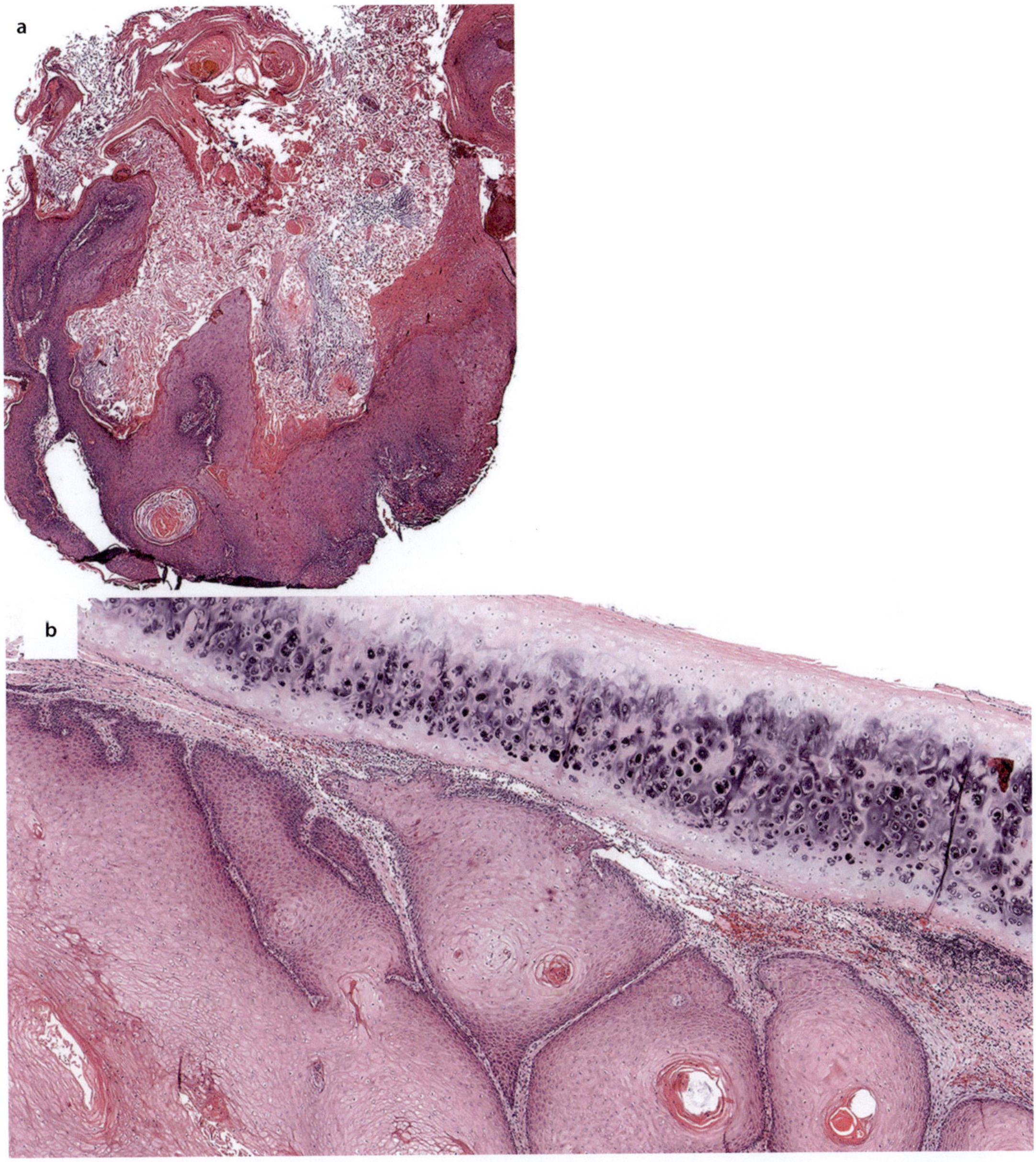

Fig. 5.40 Verrucous carcinoma is architecturally characterized by a densely hyperkeratotic papillary surface **a**, and broad pushing advancing edge **b**

specimen at hand represents the ***entire*** lesion, and there is no decreased vocal mobility. The surface of a verruca demonstrates spikey parakeratotic spires, rather than the smoother papillations, and the rete pegs of a verruca do not extend as deeply as in verrucous carcinoma.

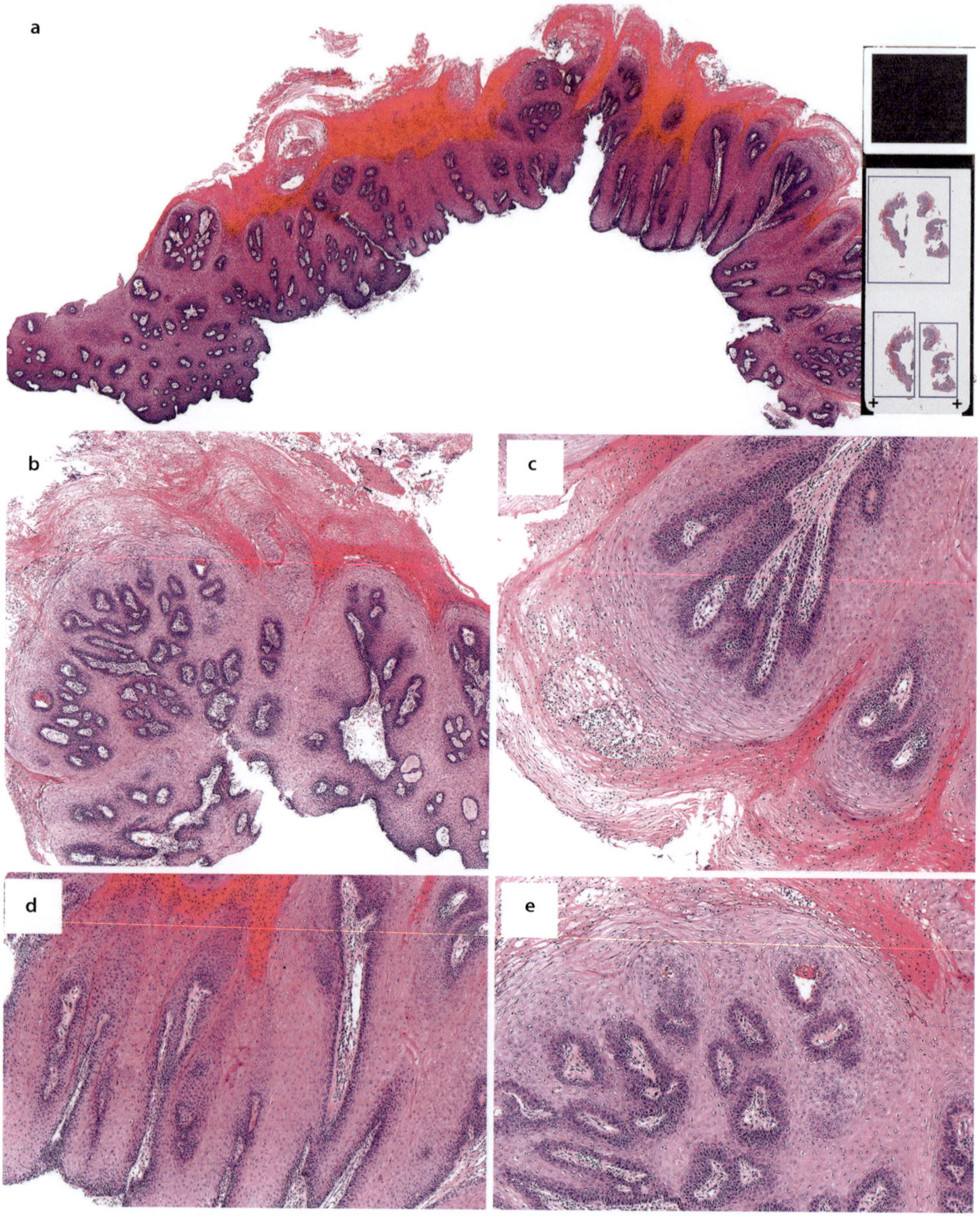

Fig. 5.41 **a** Low-power view of verrucous carcinoma from a vocal cord striping. (Inset is glass slide, true to size). **b, c** Papillary formation with dense hyperkeratosis.**d** Broad, fused, rete pegs. **e** The lack of cytologic pleomorphism is characteristic

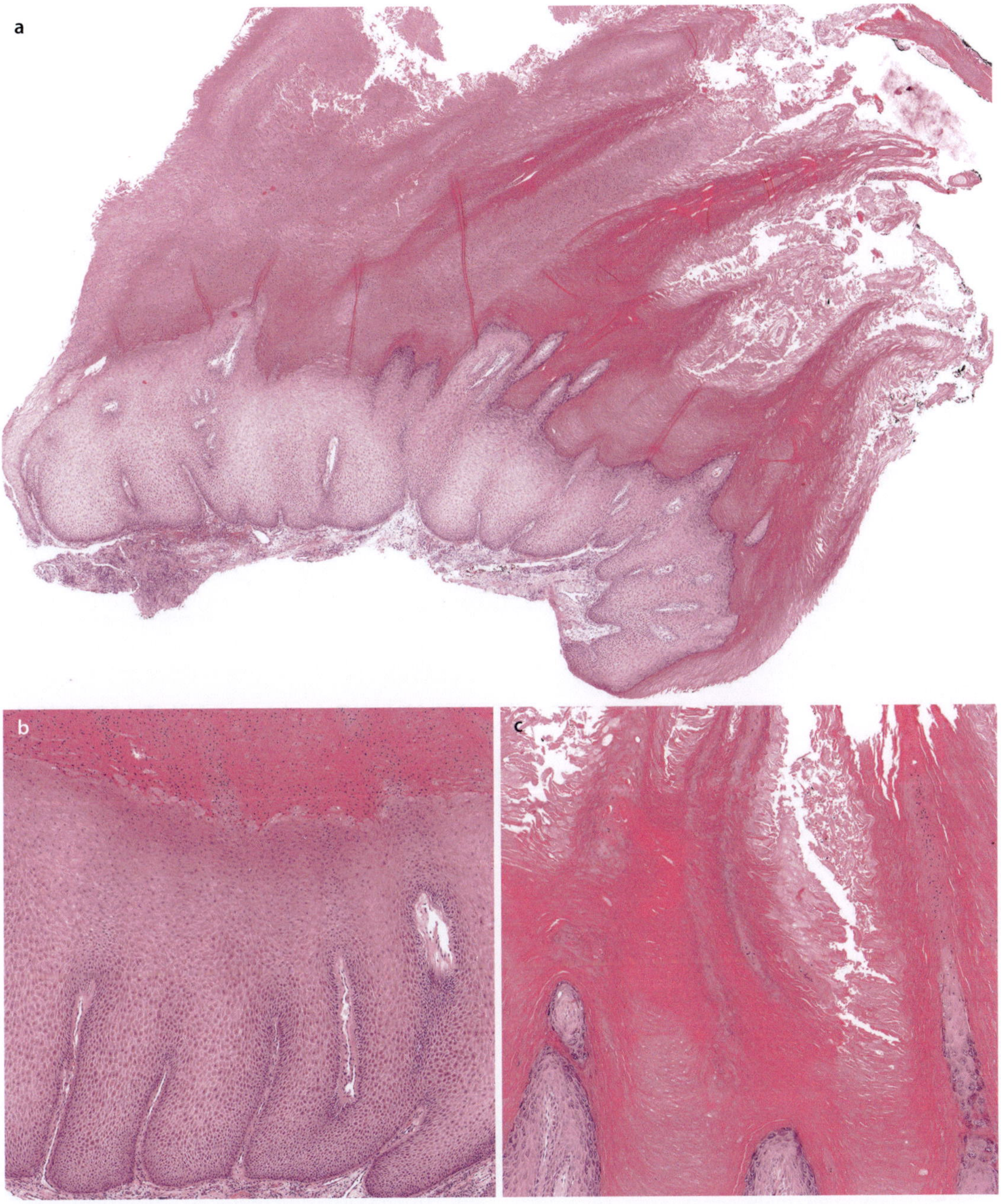

Fig. 5.42 **a** Laryngeal verruca vulgaris may be seen in immunosuppressed individuals. Before rendering this diagnosis, you should ascertain that the specimen represents the entire lesion, and there is no decreased vocal mobility. **b** The rete pegs do not extend as deeply as in verrucous carcinoma. **c** The surface demonstrates spikey parakeratotic spires, rather than papillations

Table 5.4 Classification of Laryngeal Neuroendocrine Tumors

CLINICAL ASPECTS	Well-differentiated neuroendocrine carcinoma (Carcinoid)	Moderately- differentiated neuroendocrine carcinoma (Atypical Carcinoid)	Poorly-differentiated neuroendocrine carcinoma (Small Cell and Large Cell)
Mean age	61.9 [143]		
Sex (M:F)	3:1 [144]		
Location	Most commonly supraglottic, submucosal		
Frequency	5%	37%	42% small cell, 7% large cell [144]
5-year DSS	50% – 80%		20.5%
Growth pattern	Trabecular, glandular, rosettes	Cribriform, ribbons, solid sheets	
Crush artifact	Absent		Prominent
Necrosis	Usually absent	Present	Prominent
Mitoses	**<2/10 hpf**	**2–10/10 hpf**	**>10/10 hpf**
Nuclear pleomorphism	Absent	Mild to marked	Prominent
Nuclear shape	Round/oval, vesicular, central	Round/oval, hyperchromatic	Oval/spindle +/– eccentric
Nucleoli	Absent	Variable	Absent
Cytoplasm	Eosinophilic, oncocytic	Variable	Absent
N/C ratio	Low	Variable	High

Hpf high-power fields

5.22 Neuroendocrine Carcinoma

Laryngeal neuroendocrine carcinomas are uncommon and account for less than 1% of laryngeal malignancies. However, the larynx is the most common head and neck site for neuroendocrine carcinomas, and this is the second more common laryngeal malignancy after squamous cell carcinoma. A SEER database search yielded 257 laryngeal neuroendocrine carcinomas (1973–2011), with an age adjusted incidence of 0.012/100,000 [143]. There is a male predisposition (63%) and the mean age at diagnosis was 61.9 years. There is a strong association with smoking. The most frequent presenting symptom is hoarseness; patients may also complain of laryngeal pain/discomfort and dysphagia. The majority of tumors affect the supraglottis (62.6%), followed by the glottis (12.5%). They are typically polypoid, submucosal tumors ranging from a few millimeters up to over 5.0 cm in greatest dimension. Table 5.4 details the current classification schema and diagnostic criteria for laryngeal neuroendocrine carcinomas.

A recent met-analysis of 436 laryngeal neuroendocrine carcinomas found that small cell variant of poorly-differentiated neuroendocrine carcinoma is most common, followed by intermediate-grade neuroendocrine carcinoma [144]. In practice, the large cell variant of poorly-differentiated neuroendocrine carcinoma is the least common subtype, although it may be over-represented in the literature [144].

Treatment has always been defined by the histological grade. Well- and moderately-differentiated neuroendocrine carcinomas are treated with primary surgery, most commonly supraglottic laryngectomy with neck dissection.

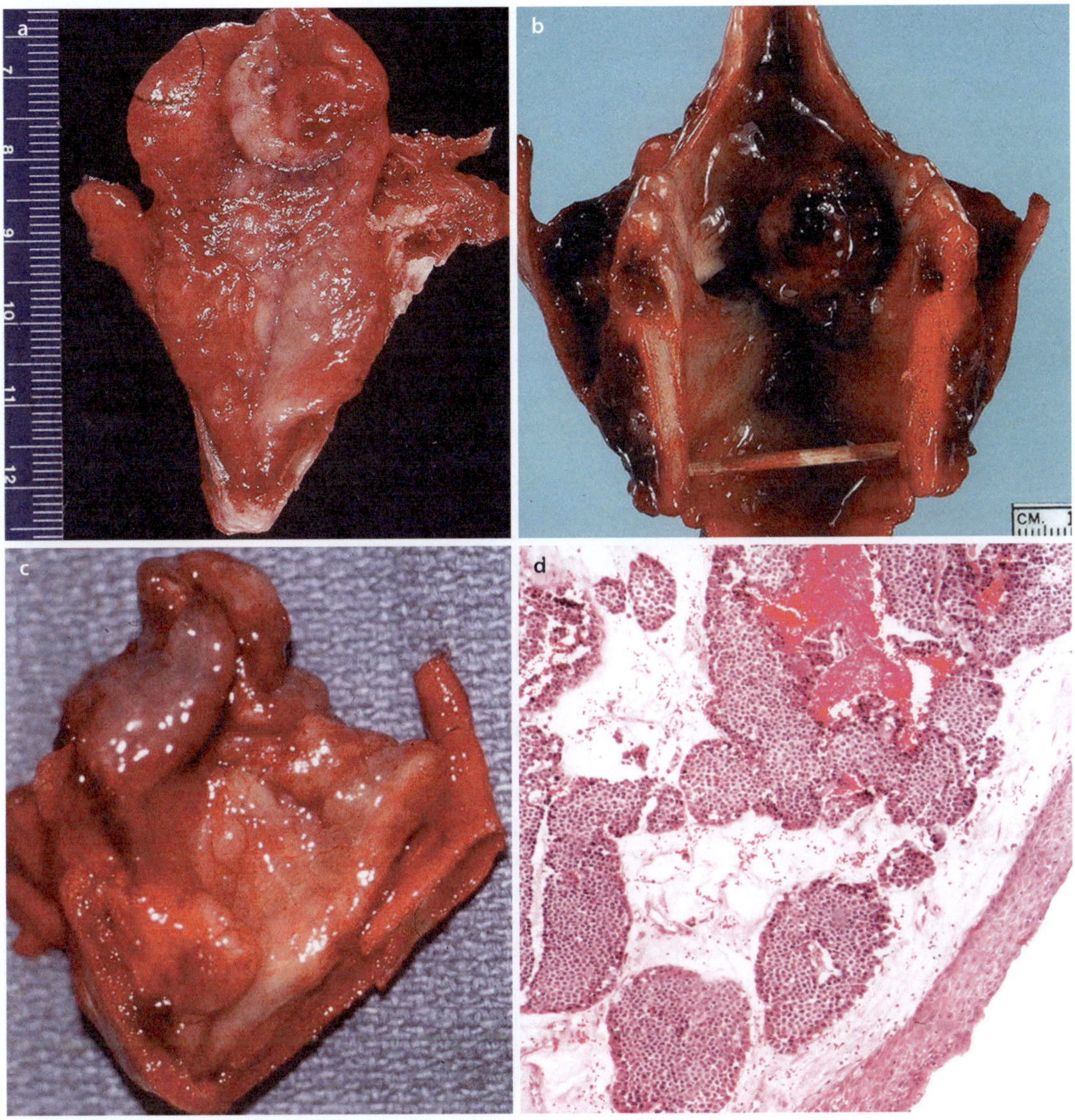

■ **Fig. 5.43** **a–c** The most common presentation of a laryngeal neuroendocrine carcinoma is that of a soft, polypoid supraglottic mass. **d** Well-differentiated neuroendocrine carcinoma forming an organoid pattern

Moderately-differentiated neuroendocrine carcinoma can metastasize to cervical lymph nodes in up to 66% of cases [145]. Poorly-differentiated neuroendocrine carcinomas commonly present with distant metastases and are usually treated with combined chemoradiation. Survival will follow grade: the 5-year disease specific survival for well- and moderately differentiated neuroendocrine carcinomas is 50–80% [143, 145] whereas the same for poorly-differentiated carcinoma is 20.5%.

Histopathologically, **well-differentiated neuroendocrine carcinoma** is characterized as epithelioid neoplasm forming nests, sheets, glands, trabeculae, and rosettes. A tumor-free zone in the immediate submucosa, on low-power examination of non-ulcerated tumor, can be the first diagnostic hint encountered (■ Fig. 5.43). Cytologically, the tumor cells are bland, uniform, round to spindled-shaped with eosinophilic cytoplasm. Tumor nuclei are round to oval, with stippled or vesicular chromatin, inconspicuous or absent nucleoli (■ Fig. 5.44). Occasional oncocytic differentiation may be seen. There should be no cellular pleomorphism or necrosis. Mitoses usually absent but occasionally present (<2 mitoses/ 10 high power fields).

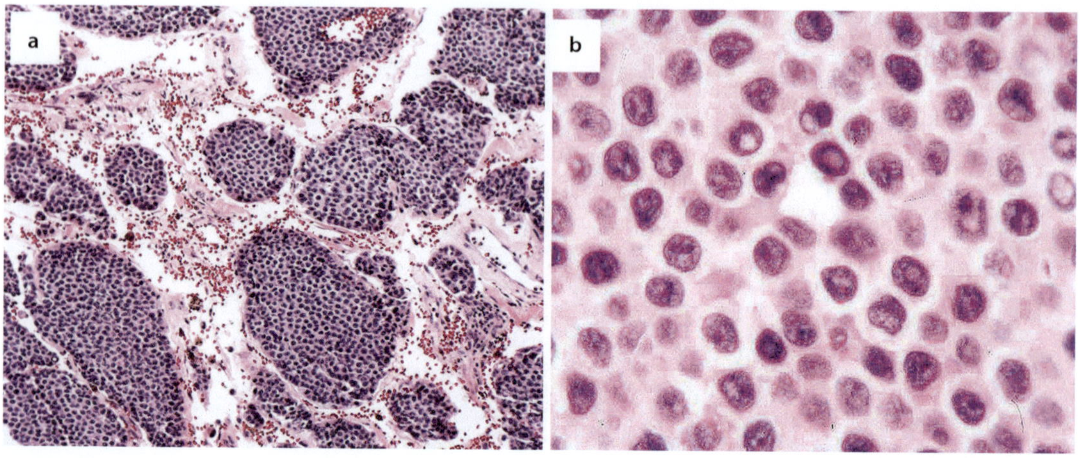

Fig. 5.44 **a** Well-differentiated neuroendocrine carcinoma forming an organoid pattern. The similarity of tumor nuclear size and shape can be appreciated at this power. **b** Tumor nuclei demonstrate a fine chromatin pattern ("salt and pepper") and are relatively round

Here the differential diagnosis would be with paraganglioma, and the two can best be distinguished by Immunohistochemistry. Paragangliomas and well-differentiated neuroendocrine carcinoma express neuron specific enolase, synaptophysin, and chromogranin. However, epithelial markers (cytokeratin, carcinoembryonic antigen and epithelial membrane antigen) and calcitonin are not expressed in paragangliomas.

Moderately-differentiated neuroendocrine carcinoma has a definitive infiltrative growth pattern. It can also form various patterns which overlap with the well-differentiated counterpart, such as glandular, organoid, acinar, trabecular, solid, and nests. "Zellballen-type" pattern and sustentacular cells occasionally seen. Cytologically, the tumor cells are generally larger than well-differentiated neuroendocrine carcinoma and at least twice the size of the small cell variant. Cytoplasm is eosinophilic and occasionally oncocytic. The tumor nuclei are round to oval, with stippled or vesicular chromatin and **prominent nucleoli. Tumor nuclei are eccentric, with a range of pleomorphism** (Fig. 5.45). Necrosis and mitotic activity separate this tumor from the well-differentiated counterpart. The mitotic index is between **2–10 mitotic figures/10 high power fields**. Vascular invasion can be seen. Mucinous differentiation may also be seen (Fig. 5.46).

One might consider squamous carcinoma in the differential diagnosis, however, the growth patterns are uniquely neuroendocrine features.

Poorly-differentiated neuroendocrine carcinoma is subclassified into the small cell variant (which includes the intermediate cell variant) and the large cell variant. The small cell variant is quite identical to the pulmonary counterpart. It is composed of sheets and interconnecting ribbons of undifferentiated small cells. The tumor cells are defined as smaller than 3 resting lymphocytes. Cytoplasm is minimal. The intermediate variant of small cell has slightly larger cells with minimal to moderate amounts of cytoplasm. Tumor nuclei are typically hyperchromatic, pleomorphic, oval, round, or spindled with delicate chromatin and absent or inconspicuous nucleoli (Fig. 5.47). Apoptosis or zones of necrosis are seen. Vascular and perineural invasion can be seen. Mitotic activity is brisk, **frequently > 10 mitotic figures/ 10 high power** fields. Other characteristic features are the DNA coating blood vessels walls and "crush artifact" (**Azzopardi phenomenon**). Glandular or squamous differentiation, and rosette formation can also be observed on occasion. These tumors should be classified as "**combined small cell carcinoma, neuroendocrine type, with *non*small cell carcinoma (squamous carcinoma, adeno-**

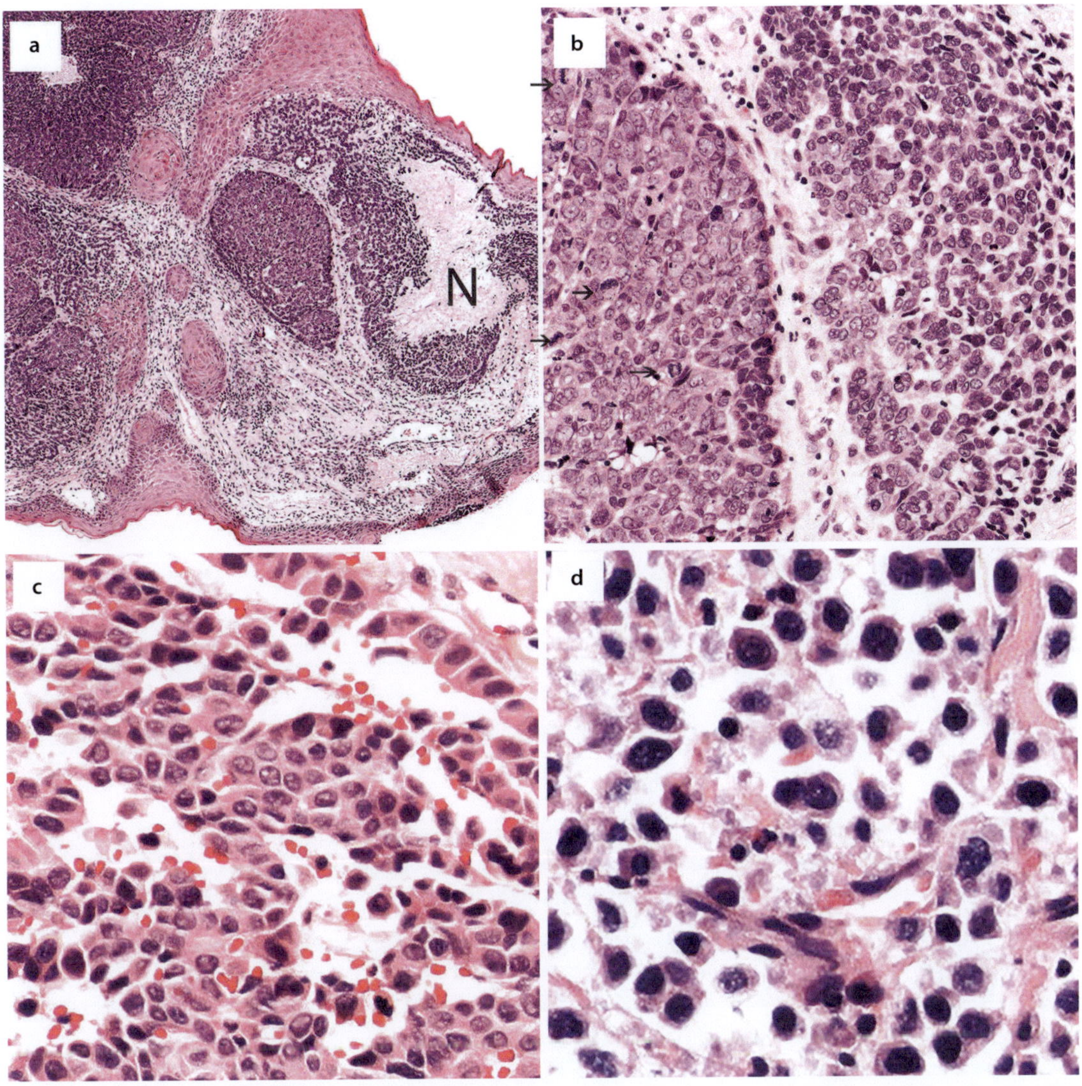

■ **Fig. 5.45** **a** Moderately-differentiated neuroendocrine carcinoma. Tumor necrosis (N) is present. **b** Mitotic activity can be appreciated (*arrows*). **c** This trabecular pattern suggests neuroendocrine origin. **c** and **d** The degree of nuclear pleomorphism is greater here than in ■ Fig. 5.44

carcinoma, etc) [146]. The nonsmall cell component can be distinct and obviously different from the small cell component. Alternatively, nonkeratinizing poorly-differentiated squamous carcinoma cells can be intermingled with the poorly-differentiated neuroendocrine small cells and sorted out only by immunohistochemistry. Again, the non-small cell component would not express neuroendocrine markers.

The large cell variant is least commonly encountered in practice. It forms a variety of patterns: organoid nesting, trabeculae, sheets, rosettes, or palisading. Tumor cells are larger than the small cell variant, with low nuclear to cytoplasmic ratio. **The nuclei are characteristically vesicular**, with coarse to fine chromatin and frequent nucleoli (■ Fig. 5.48). Necrosis is prominent. The mitotic rate is **≥ 11 mitoses/10 hpfs.**

All grades of neuroendocrine carcinoma will express chromogranin, neuron-specific enolase, synaptophysin, cytokeratin, epithelial membrane antigen, and carcinoembryonic antigen. **Calcitonin**

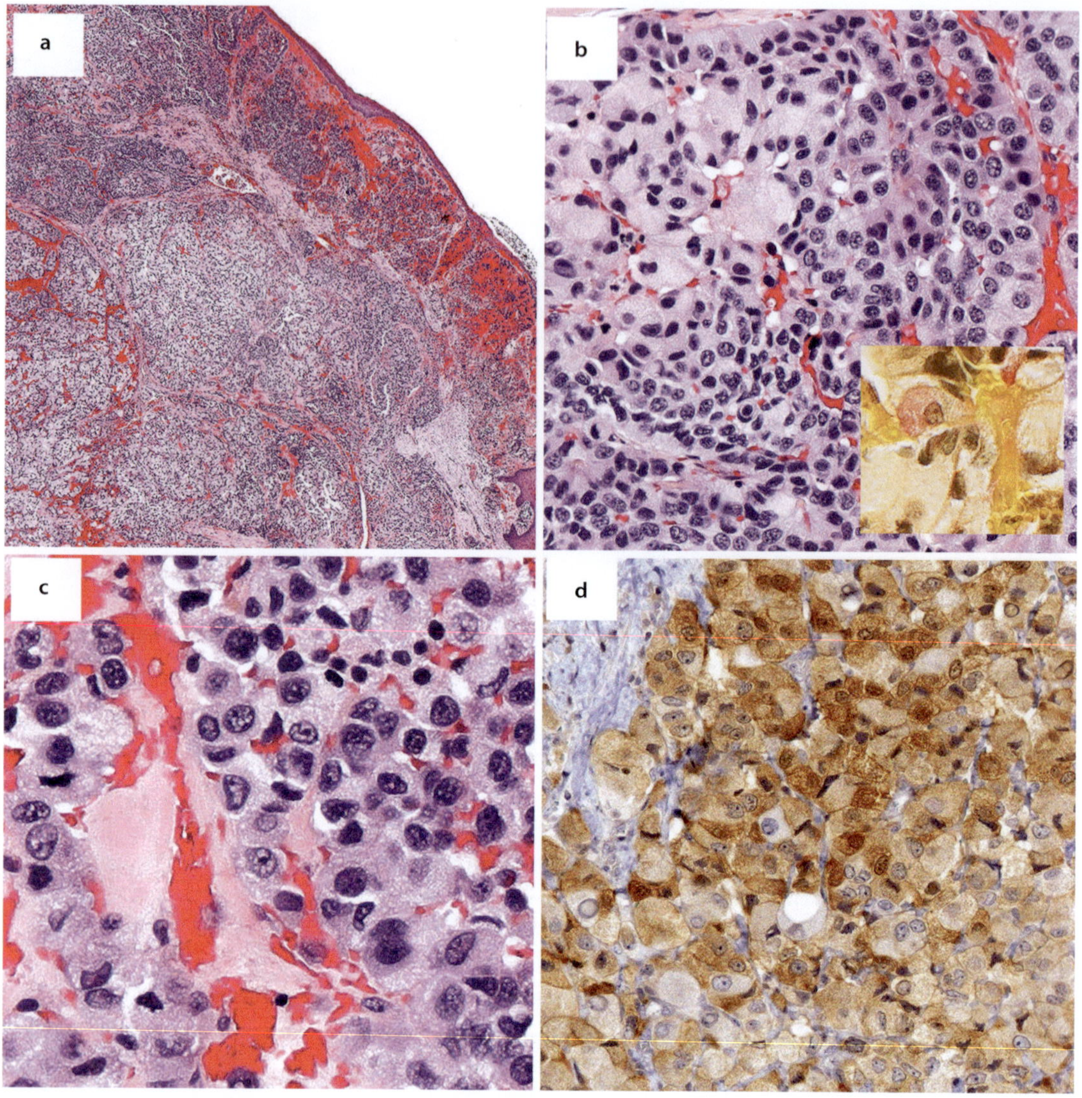

Fig. 5.46 **a, b** Laryngeal neuroendocrine carcinoma, moderately-differentiated, with goblet cell differentiation. The tumor cells with abundant cytoplasmic vacuole mucicarmine positive (**inset**). **c** Nuclear pleomorphism in the range for moderately differentiated. **d** Calcitonin expression is an unusual feature, which is known to happen

can also be expressed in all tumor grades. Large cell variants are largely p63 and Ck5/6 negative [147]. p16 can be overexpressed in high-grade neuroendocrine carcinomas unrelated to HR-HPV; take care not to fall into that pit! [148].

The differential diagnosis for poorly-differentiated neuroendocrine carcinoma includes melanoma, which will express melanoma markers. Medullary thyroid carcinoma might be a consideration, which will express TTF1. Large cell variant of poorly-differentiated neuroendocrine carcinoma is usually TTF1 negative, but occasionally can demonstrate focal TTF1 expression. The basaloid variant of squamous carcinoma or adenoid cystic carcinoma will not express chromogranin, synaptophysin, or calcitonin.

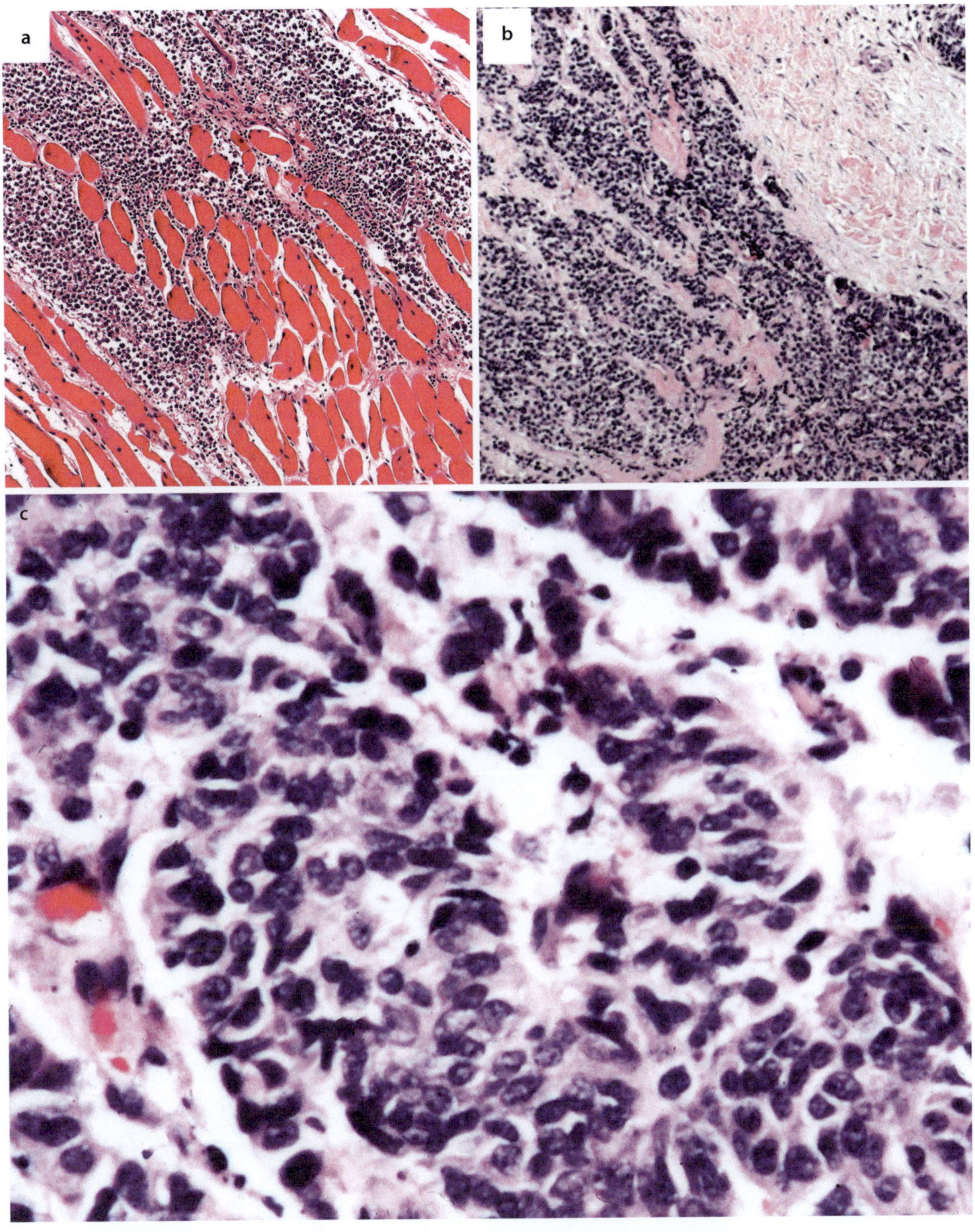

Fig. 5.47 **a, b** Poorly-differentiated neuroendocrine carcinoma, small cell type **c** Classification as poorly-differentiated neuroendocrine carcinoma is based on the degree of necrosis, pleomorphism, and mitotic activity. The "small cell" variant has minimal cytoplasm, and dark, yet fine chromatin. Nucleoli are inconspicuous or absent. Tumor cell size are generally smaller than the diameter of three resting lymphocytes

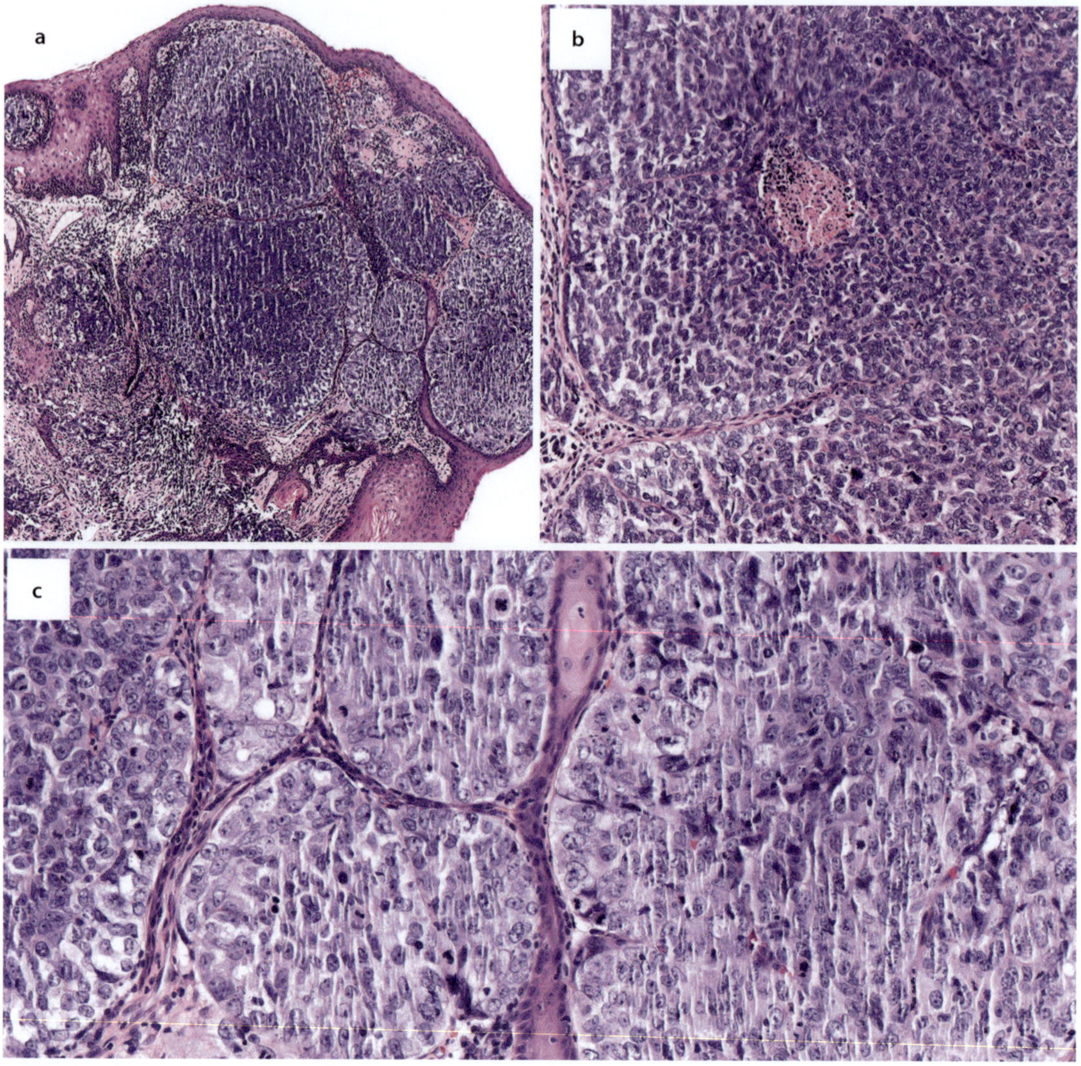

Fig. 5.48 a–c The large cell variant of poorly-differentiated neuroendocrine carcinoma is defined as large pleomorphic epithelioid tumor cells with vesicular nuclear chromatin pattern, necrosis, and mitotic rate greater than 10/10 hpf

5.23 Chondrosarcoma

Laryngeal chondrosarcomas have a pronounced male predisposition, probably relating to the fact that the larynx is a sexually dimorphic androgen sensitive organ. Laryngeal chondrosarcomas arise from the cricoid ring and thyroid lamina with a ratio of 3:1, respectively [149, 150]. Cricoid tumors are often expand posteriorly, causing slowly evolving dyspnea, or limited arytenoid adduction. Tumors of the thyroid lamina expand anteriolaterally, and can present as palpable neck masses (Fig. 5.49). Chondrosarcomas of the epiglottis and arytenoids are extremely rare [151, 152]. Chondrosarcomas of the hyoid bone are also uncommon [153–155].

The peak incidence of laryngeal chondrosarcomas is in the fifth to eighth decades, when the cartilages have already ossified. The process of laryngeal ossification follows muscle insertions, i.e. the posterior cricoid ring and the oblique line of the posterior thyroid lamina. The site preference for chondrosarcomas (posterior and posterior-lateral cricoid, and inferior-lateral thyroid lamina) closely follows the areas of laryngeal muscle insertion and hence patterns of ossification.

Laryngeal chondrosarcomas are generally indolent tumors; the vast majority are either Grade I

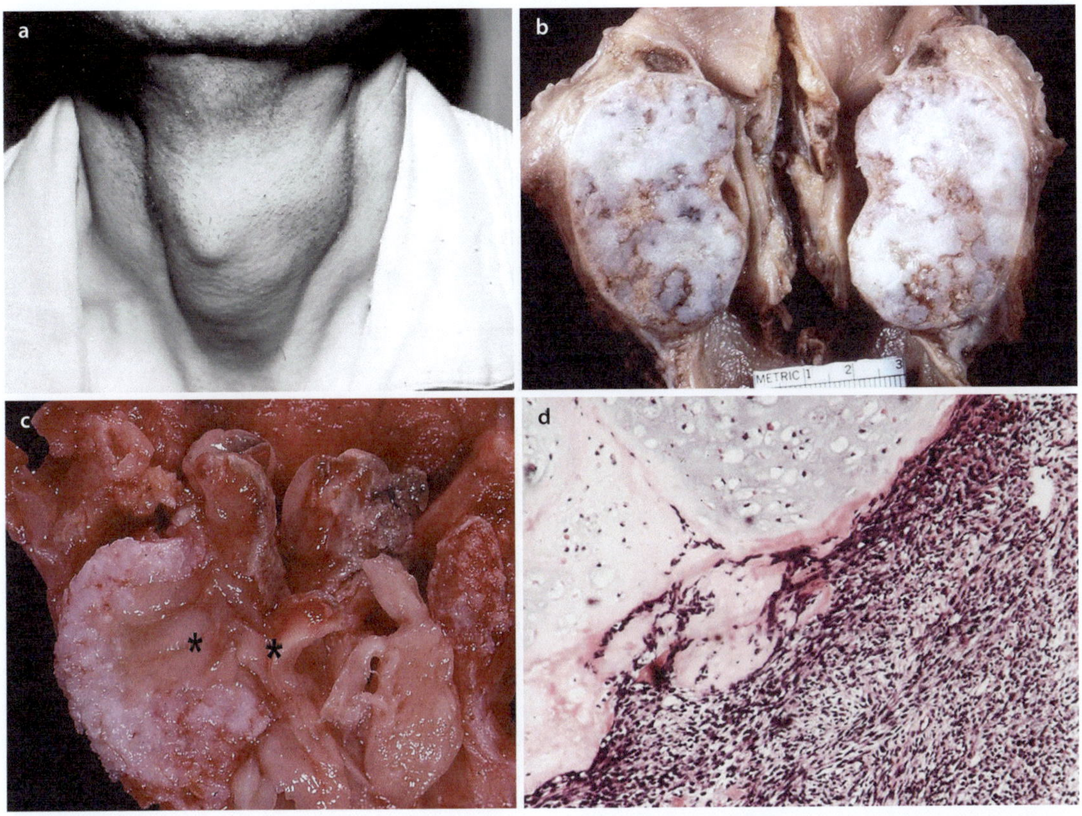

Fig. 5.49 **a** This left-sided laryngeal chondrosarcoma can be appreciated as a firm mass which moves with the larynx. **b**Typically, the cut surface of a chrondrosarcoma is white/blue, firm, and glistening. **c** An unusual case of "dedifferentiated" laryngeal chondrosarcoma. A soft tan polypoid tumor component can be seen arising from the center of the cartilaginous component (asterisks). **d** Dedifferentiated chondrosarcoma – note abrupt transition from low-grade chondrosarcoma to high-grade undifferentiated spindle cells

(67.8%) or Grade II (23.5%). The overall recurrence rate (all-grades) is 24.2% [150]. Disease-specific survival rates for 5, 10, and 20 years are 91.4%, 81.8%, and 68.0%, respectively. Disease recurrence does not generally compromise patient outcome. A metastatic rate of 8.5% has been estimated from reported cases, and metastatic potential correlates with histologic grade. The overall disease-related mortality rate (all grades) is 4.8%.

A tendency for local recurrence is noted for hyoid chondrosarcomas [153–155]. It may be that the marrow space of the hyoid is quite prone to harbor satellite foci of tumor. Recommendations are to remove the entire hyoid bone, rather than partial hyoid resection. "De-differentiated" laryngeal chondrosarcomas are rare, but are generally aggressive sarcomas [158, 159]. Lastly, laryngeal myxoid chondrosarcoma is associated with a distinctly poorer prognosis [160].

Grossly, laryngeal chondrosarcomas have a glassy firm white/gray cut surface and a gritty texture. Histopathologically, **grade I chondrosarcomas** have a lobulated growth pattern, and produce abundant cartilaginous matrix. Cluster disarray refers to the disorganized appearance of the malignant chondrocytes [156]. Chondrocytes are crowded chondrocytes with double nuclei within lacunae. Pleomorphism is minimal, but nucleoli are present. Chondrosarcomas of all grades can invade the ossified laryngeal framework.

The diagnosis of **chondromas** is reserved for small lesions under 2.0 cm. Chondromas are more cellular than normal cartilage, with a lobulated growth pattern and disorganized chondrocytes (cluster disarray). There is no nuclear pleomorphism, or **nucleoli**, or increased nuclear/cytoplasmic ratio. Chondromas do not invade bone [157]. The differential diagnosis also includes chondrometaplasia. This occurs in the true vocal fold, not in thyroid lamina or cricoid cartilage. Chondrometaplasia blends into the surrounding soft tissue and does not invade.

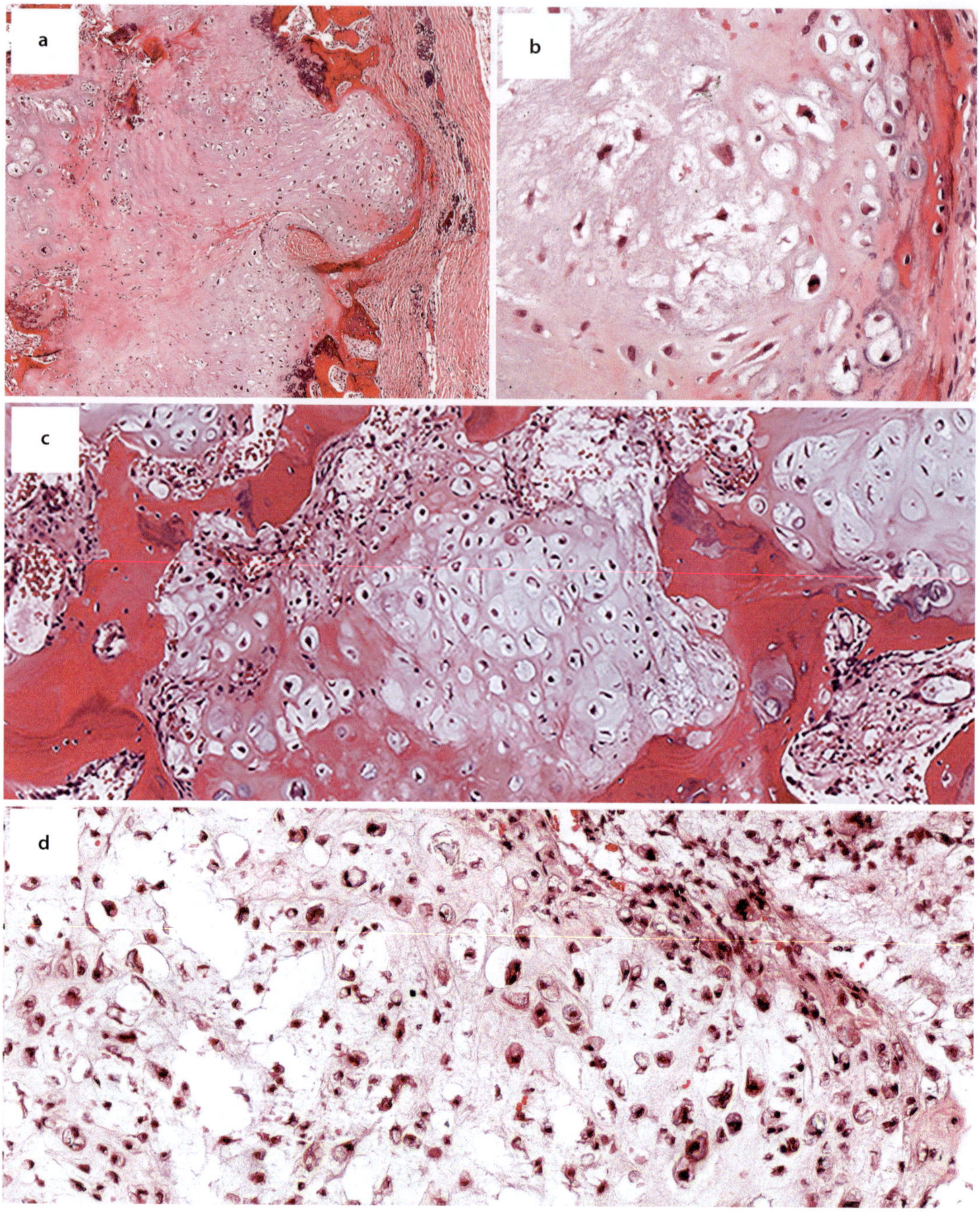

Fig. 5.50 **a, b** Grade I chondrosarcoma is an expansile tumor with greater cellularity than normal cartilage and evidence of mild chondrocyte nuclear atypia. The advancing edge of chondrosarcoma is well demarcated from the surrounding tissue **c** Mature ossification can be seen **d** Greater cellularity and pleomorphism is present in a Grade II chondrosarcoma

Grade II chondrosarcomas are characterized by greater cellularity and crowding than grade I tumors. Cytological pleomorphism and hyperchromatism is obvious and mitotic activity is seen (Fig. 5.50). Grade III tumors lose chondroblastic differentiation. Chondroid material is more sparse and there are greater areas of solid tumor cells. Mitotic activity is brisk.

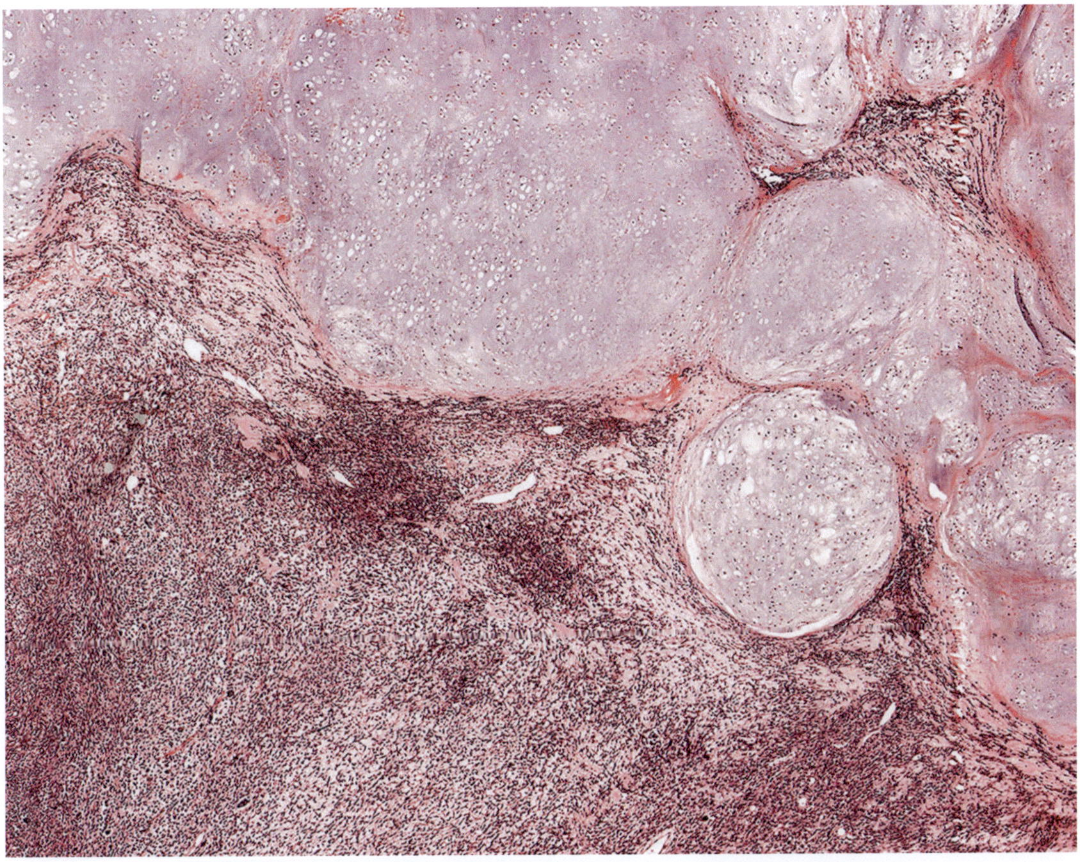

Fig. 5.51 By definition, "de-differentiated" chondrosarcoma has an abrupt transition between the chondrosarcoma, and the high-grade sarcomatous element

Dedifferentiated chondrosarcoma (Figs. 5.49, 5.50, and 5.51) refers to a high-grade sarcoma which arises, in a sharply demarcated manner, from a grade I-II chondrosarcoma. The sarcoma reveals no chondroid differentiation; it can have features of osteosarcoma, fibrosarcoma, rhabdomyosarcoma, leiomyosarcoma, or may be unclassifiable.

Myxoid chondrosarcoma is comprised of strands and trabeculae of small chondrocytes with a plasmacytoid rim of eosinophilic cytoplasm; these strands form "strings of pearls" within a basophilic and myxoid matrix, as compared to the eosinophilic hyaline chondroid matrix. Tumors with 10% or greater myxoid differentiation should be classified as myxoid chondrosarcomas.

Clear cell chondrosarcoma is comprised of balloon-like clear cells in excess of 20%, in addition to conventional chondrosarcoma [161]. Chondroid matrix is absent in clear cell regions.

5.24 "Blastoma"

A blastoma (embryoma) is a malignant neoplasm of mixed mesenchymal, epithelial, and nondifferentiated "blastemous" elements that mimics embryonic development of the particular organ. They can occur both in children and adults; pulmonary blastomas occur with a male predominance, usually in adults, hepatoblastomas and pancreaticoblastomas occur mostly in children. Eble and colleagues reported an exophytic tumor of the piriform sinus that developed in a 65-year man, an employee of a glass factory and smoker, which microscopically was analogous to a pulmonary blastoma [162].

Histopathologically, blastomas are composed of three endogenous laryngeal elements: mesenchymal, epithelial, and blastemous, in varying proportions. Transformation can be seen between elements. Mesenchymal elements

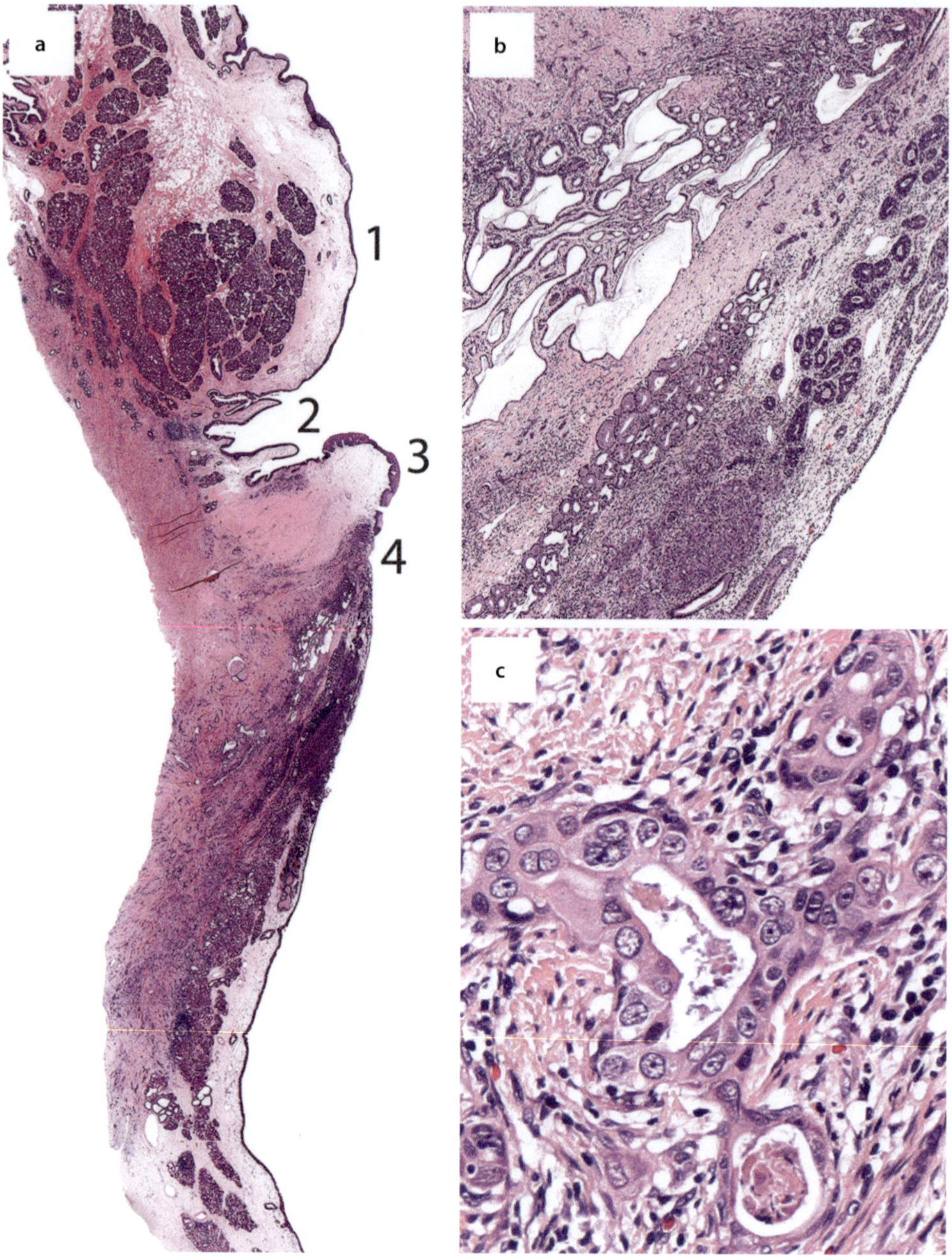

Fig. 5.52 **a** High-grade laryngeal adenocarcinoma, not otherwise specified. 1: false cord, 2: ventricle, 3: true vocal cord, 4: subglottis **b** This carcinoma arises from the inferior aspect of the vocal cord **c** No features of any specific salivary malignancy are seen

are comprised of primitive spindle cells, chondroid, and myxoid elements. The epithelial elements are composed of strands of primitive cells with glandular or squaumous differentiation. The blastemous elements appear as small, non-differentiated primitive cells, that are poorly cohesive and lack definite epithelial or mesenchymal characteristics. The differential diagnosis includes spindled squamous cell carcinoma, which lacks glandular differentiation or blastemous elements, and adenocarcinoma, not otherwise specified (Fig. 5.52). Malignant teratoma contains nonindigenous elements such as central nervous tissue and retina. In children, the diagnosis of metastatic Wilm's tumor should be considered.

Self Study

1. Figures 5.53, 5.54, 5.55, 5.56, 5.57, and 5.58 are all of laryngeal origin. Study the biopsy in Fig. 5.53. Which statement is correct?
   A. The best diagnosis here is "Squamoproliferative process. Clinical correlation necessary to rule out malignant process."
   B. The best diagnosis here is "Benign florid papillomatosis."
   C. The best diagnosis here is verruca vulgaris.
   D. The best diagnosis here is verrucous carcinoma.

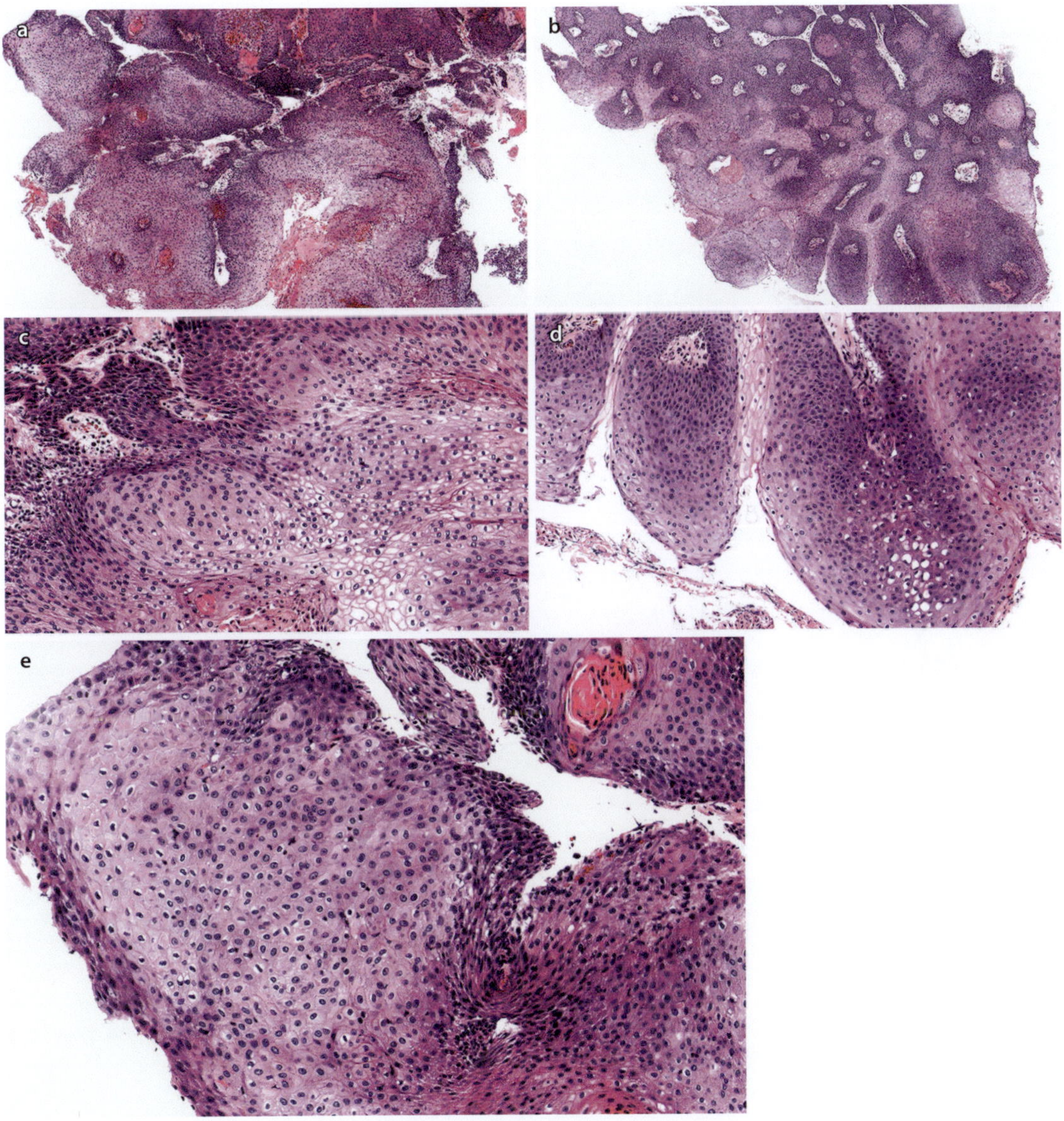

Fig. 5.53 Self study #1

2. Study ◘ Fig. 5.54. The inset represents vimentin IHC. Which statement is correct?
   A. This represents a true soft tissue osteosarcoma.
   B. This represents the most common true sarcoma of the larynx.
   C. This reactive process caused by acid reflux.
   D. The diagnosis of carcinoma can be made only with documentation of keratinization, or expression of epithelial markers.
   E. The larynx is one of the most common sites for this carcinoma.

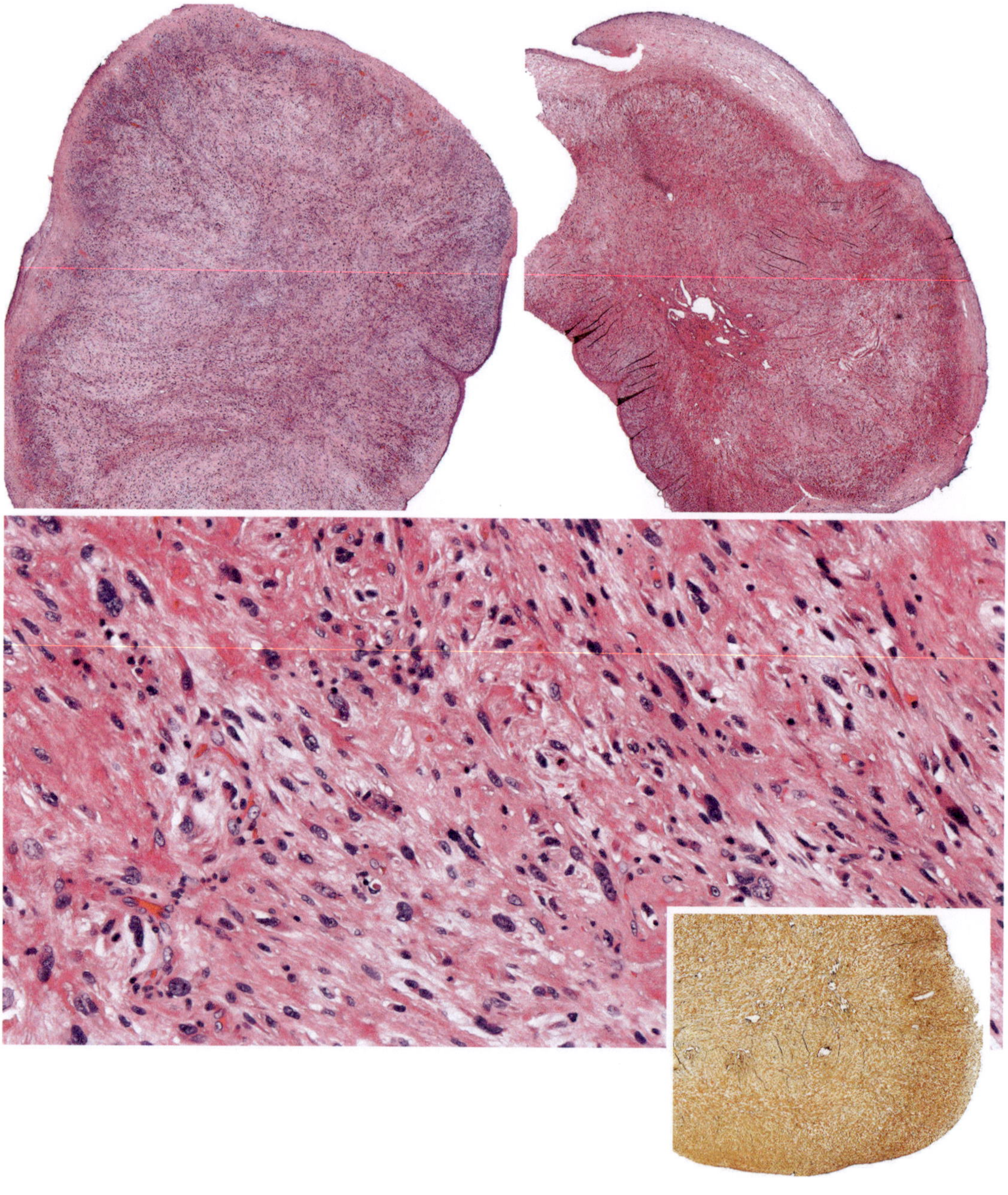

◘ **Fig. 5.54** Self study #2

3. Study ◘ Fig. 5.55. The IHC profile is as follows: Cam 5.2+/CD56+/Chromogranin+/Synaptosin - . The mitotic count is 15/10 high power fields. Which statement is correct?
   A. This is the most common form of neuroendocrine carcinoma encountered.
   B. Calcitonin expression can be expected from a laryngeal paraganglioma.
   C. Both neuroendocrine carcinomas and paragangliomas express epithelial markers.
   D. This most likely represents metastasis from pulmonary primary.
   E. Diagnostic features of this carcinoma include vesicular nuclei and high mitotic rate.

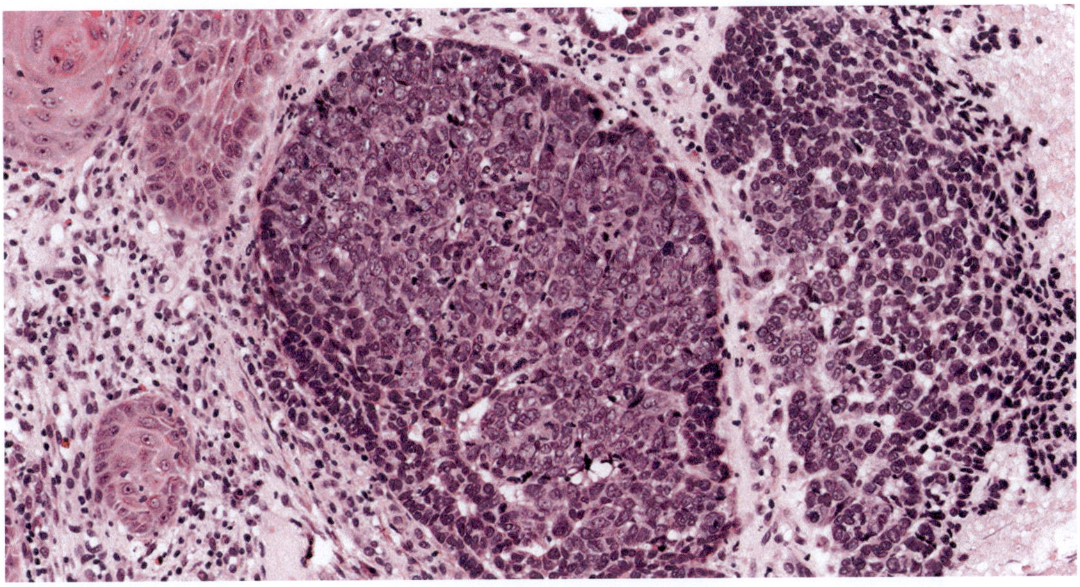

◘ **Fig. 5.55** Self study #3

4. Study ◘ Fig. 5.56. The IHC profile is as follows: Cam 5.2+/CD56+/ Chromogranin+/Synaptosin - . Which statement is correct?
   A. This represents metastatic melanoma to the glottis.
   B. This represents the most common laryngeal tumor of childhood.
   C. This represents the second most common laryngeal tumor of childhood.
   D. Supraglottic paraganglioma cannot be ruled out.
   E. No statement is correct.

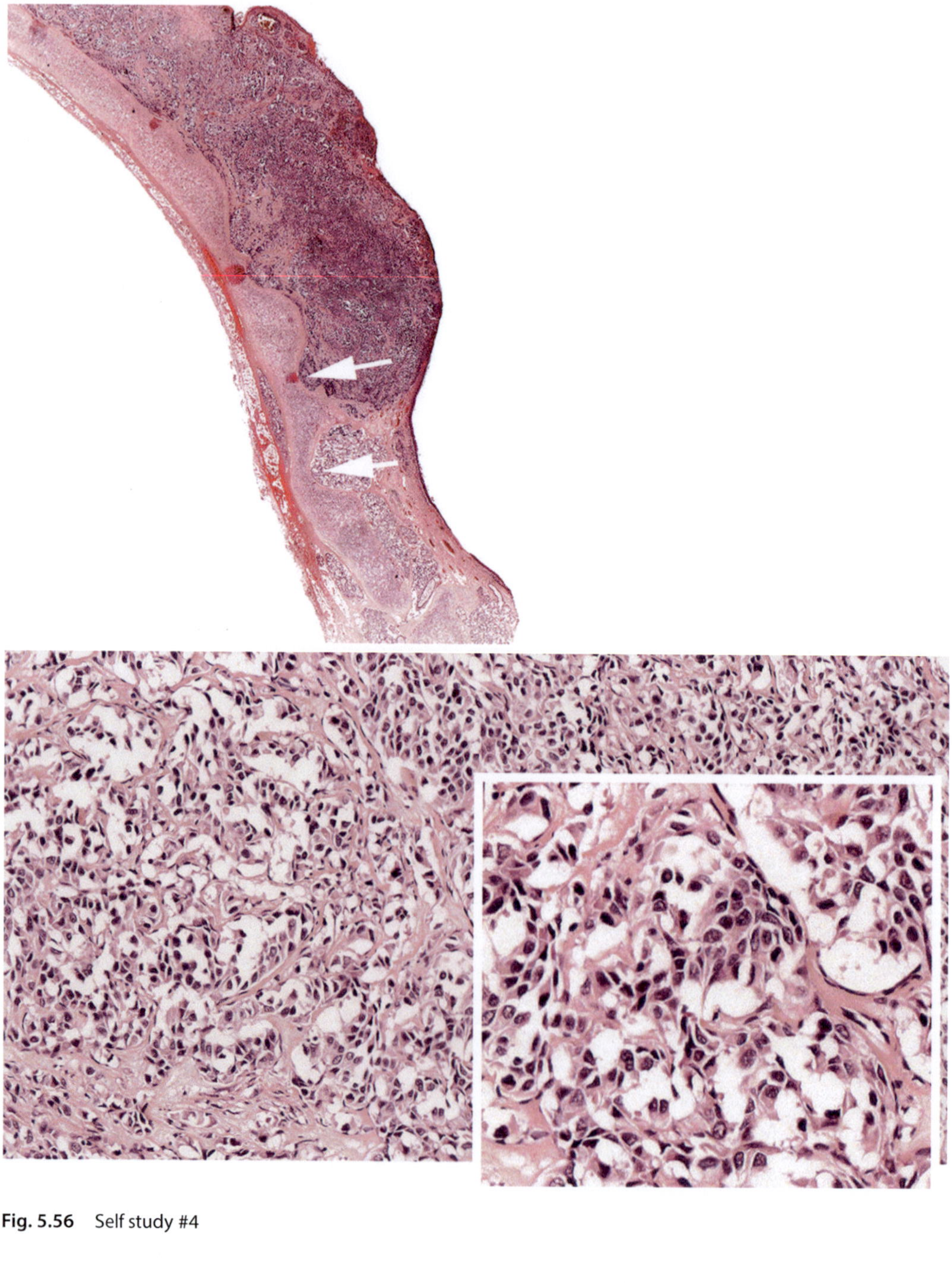

◘ **Fig. 5.56** Self study #4

5. Study ◘ Fig. 5.57. Which statement is correct?
   A. No statement is correct.
   B. This represents a non-squamous malignancy.
   C. Vocal cord mobility will be important to staging.
   D. This is a reactive process.
   E. If this is confined to one vocal cord, then it is staged as pT1.

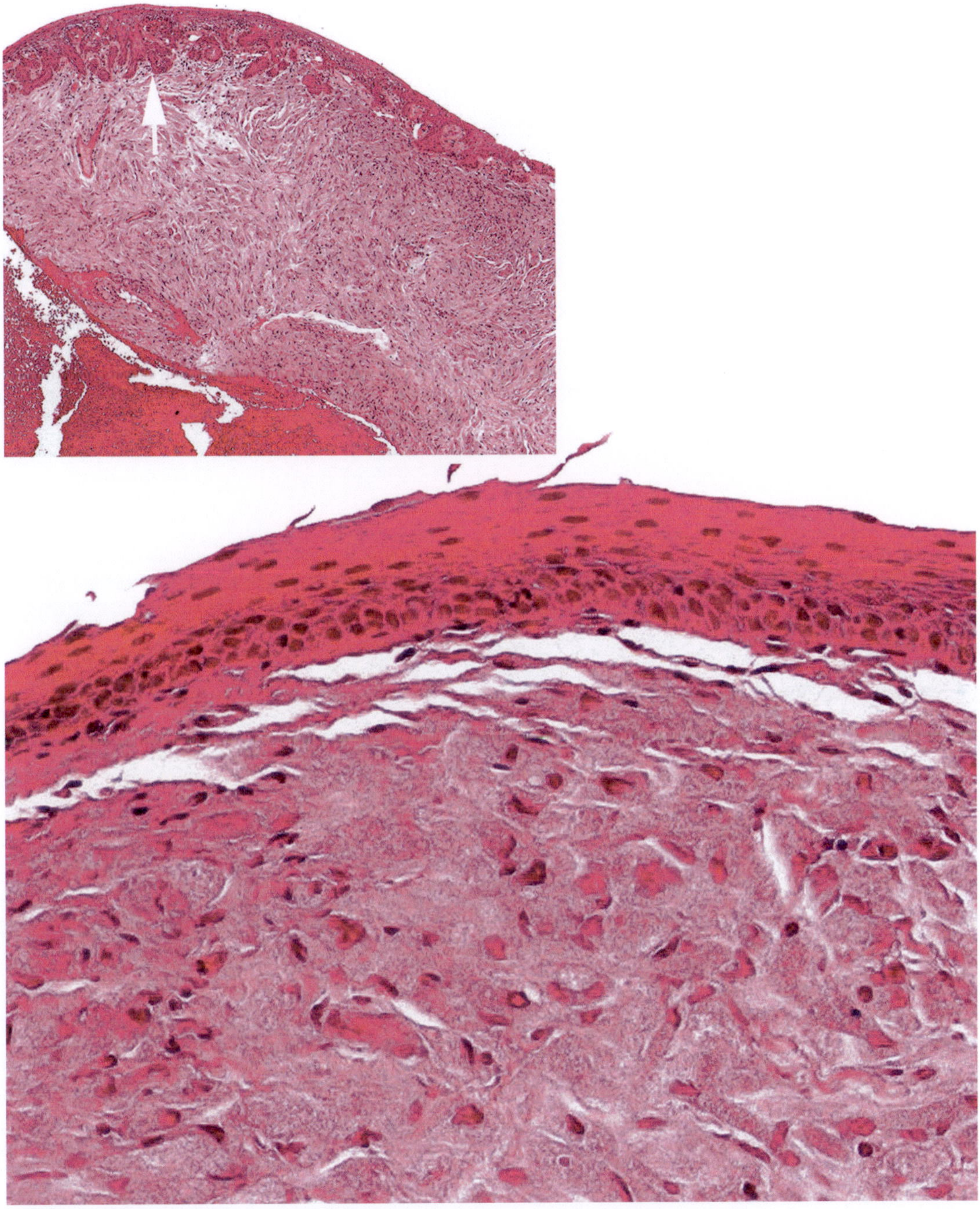

◘ **Fig. 5.57** Self study #5

6. Study ◘ Fig. 5.58. Which statement is correct?
   A. If this is confined to one vocal cord, then it is staged as pT1.
   B. Vocal cord mobility will be important to staging.
   C. This is caused by HPV1/2.
   D. The best diagnosis here is "Benign florid papillomatosis."
   E. The best diagnosis here is verruca vulgaris.

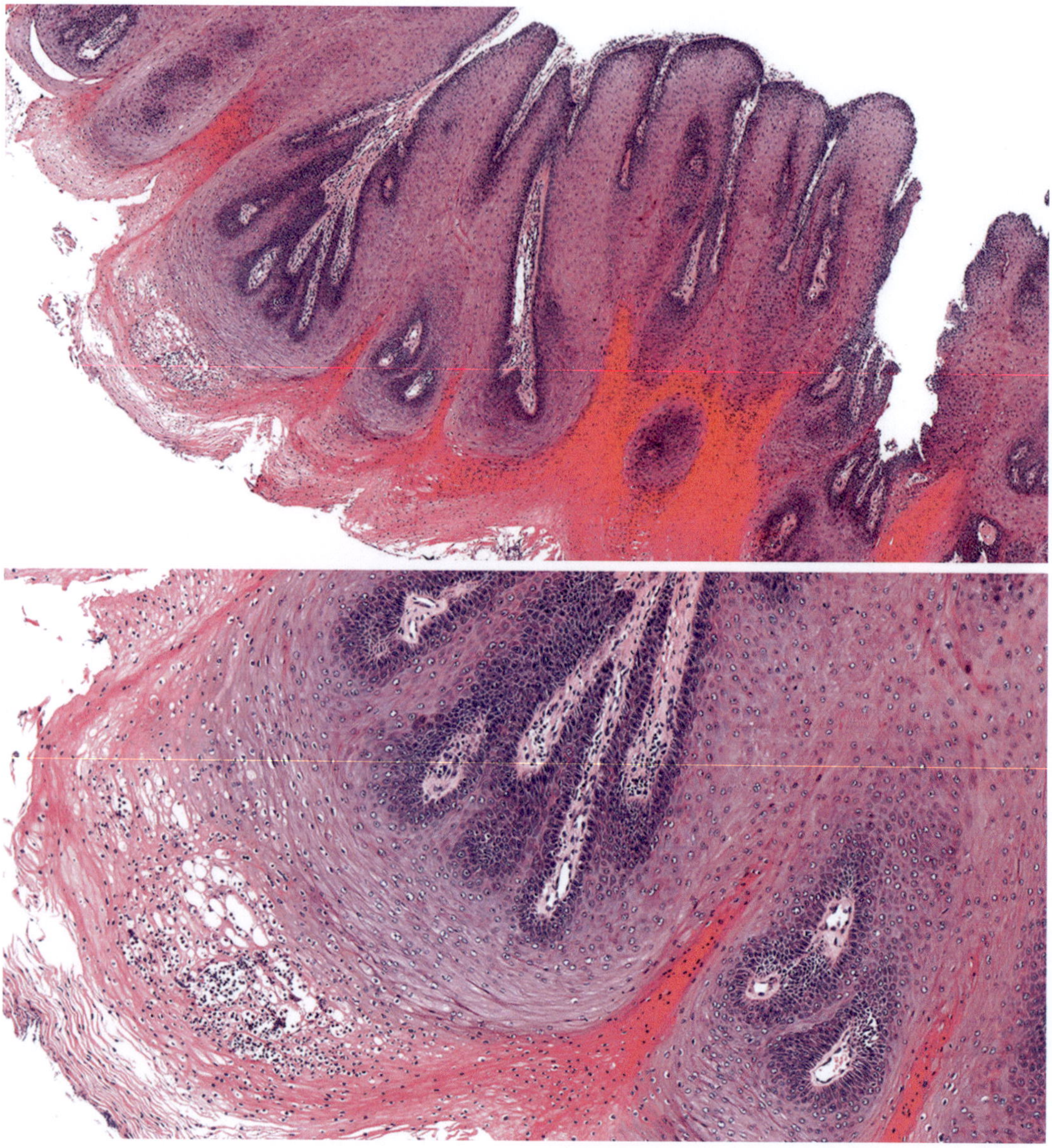

◘ **Fig. 5.58** Self study #6

Answers

1. Study the biopsy in ▫ Fig. 5.53. Which statement is correct?
   A. The best diagnosis here is *"Squamoproliferative process. Clinical correlation necessary to rule out malignant process."* **CORRECT** – here we see various different profiles, some exophytic papillary, but other areas which are too broad and proliferative for laryngeal papillomatosis. This likely represents a well-differentiated squamous carcinoma, although there is no pleomorphism or definite evidence of invasion to support that diagnosis. I make certain my surgeons understand that this could be a carcinoma, if suspect so, clinically.
   B. The best diagnosis here is "Benign florid papillomatosis." **False**. As above.
   C. The best diagnosis here is verruca vulgaris. **False**. No parakeratotic spires as would be expected in a verruca vulgaris. This is too much proliferation.
   D. The best diagnosis here is verrucous carcinoma. **False**. No dense hyperkeratosis as would be expected from superficial biopsies of verrucous carcinoma.
2. Study ▫ Fig. 5.54. The inset represents vimentin IHC. Which statement is correct?
   A. This represents a true soft tissue osteosarcoma. **False**. "Osteogenic sarcomas" of the larynx reported in the older literature likely represent spindle cell variant of squamous carcinoma.
   B. This represents the most common true sarcoma of the larynx. **False**. The most common true laryngeal sarcoma is a chondrosarcoma, which only rarely contains malignant spindle cells.
   C. This reactive process caused by acid reflux. **False**. This degree of nuclear pleomorphism speaks for malignancy.
   D. The diagnosis of carcinoma can be made only with documentation of keratinization, or expression of epithelial markers. **False**. These features support a diagnosis of spindle cell variant of squamous carcinoma, but are not requisite.
   E. The larynx is one of the most common sites for this carcinoma. **CORRECT** – Spindle cell variant of squamous carcinoma often presents as a polypoid tumor in the larynx or oral cavity. Vimentin expression here is not helpful. You do not know the status of epithelial markers. But you can deduce the diagnosis by the nuclear pleomorphism of the spindle cells and the knowledge that spindle cell variant of squamous carcinoma is most common in the larynx than a true laryngeal sarcoma.
3. Study ▫ Fig. 5.55. The IHC profile is as follows: Cam 5.2+/CD56+/ Chromogranin+/Synaptosin - . The mitotic count is 15/10 high power fields. Which statement is correct?
   A. This is the most common form of neuroendocrine carcinoma encountered. **False**. This represents large cell variant of laryngeal neuroendocrine carcinoma, which is *the least* common variant.
   B. Calcitonin expression can be expected from a laryngeal paraganglioma. **False**. Laryngeal neuroendocrine carcinomas, but not pragangiomas, can express calcitonin.
   C. Both neuroendocrine carcinomas and paragangliomas express epithelial markers. **False**. Expression of epithelial markers excludes laryngeal paraganglioma.
   D. This most likely represents metastasis from pulmonary primary. **False**.
   E. Diagnostic features of this carcinoma include vesicular nuclei and high mitotic rate. **CORRECT** – This represents large cell variant of laryngeal neuroendocrine carcinoma, which is *the least* common variant. Vesicular nuclear chromatin, seen here, is one of the distinguishing features of this variant.

4. Study ◘ Fig. 5.56. The IHC profile is as follows: Cam 5.2+/CD56+/ Chromogranin+/Synaptosin - . Which statement is correct?
   A. This represents metastatic melanoma to the *glottis*. **False**. My emphasis on glottis is your hint to confirm tumor site. This laryngeal structure has fenestrated cartilage, hence it represents the ***epiglottis***.
   B. This represents the most common laryngeal tumor *of childhood*. **False**. Laryngeal neuroendocrine carcinoma represents the most common laryngeal non-squamous carcinoma. There is no association with childhood.
   C. This represents the second most common laryngeal tumor of childhood. **False**. As above.
   D. Supraglottic paraganglioma cannot be ruled out. **False**. I tell you that Cam 5.2 is positive. This excludes the possibility of laryngeal paraganglioma.
   E. No statement is correct. **CORRECT** – This represents a laryngeal neuroendocrine carcinoma, which is supported by the given IHC profile and the light microscopic findings of a nested pattern. The "salt and pepper" chromatin can't really be appreciated here, but the IHC rules the day.
5. Study ◘ Fig. 5.57. Which statement is correct?
   A. No statement is correct. **CORRECT** – This is a granular cell tumor. The top panel demonstrates pseudoepitheliomatous hyperplasia (white arrow), which is not to be confused with squamous carcinoma. The bottom panel demonstrates densely packed cells with abundant granular cytoplasm and peripheral condensed nuclei. Look closely at the cytoplasm to appreciate this granularity. These findings are sufficient to make the diagnosis of granular cell tumor. None of the statements in B through E are then correct.
   B. This represents a non-squamous malignancy. **False**. See above.
   C. Vocal cord mobility will be important to staging. **False.** This is a benign tumor, staging is irrelevant.
   D. This is a reactive process. **False.** See above.
   E. If this is confined to one vocal cord, then it is staged as pT1. **False.** This is a benign tumor, staging is irrelevant.
6. Study ◘ Fig. 5.58. Which statement is correct?
   A. If this is confined to one vocal cord, then it is staged as pT1. **CORRECT** – This tumor is best diagnosed as verrucous carcinoma, in which case this statement is correct as per the 8th AJCC staging system (See ◘ Table 5.2). The top panel demonstrates the requisite features of verrucous carcinoma: a papillary surface covered by dense hyperkeratosis plus deep broad pushing rete pegs. Note the distinction between "a papillary surface" and discreet papillae with fibrovascular cores formed by exophytic papillomas.
   B. Vocal cord mobility will be important to staging. **False.** This was true according to the 7th AJCC.
   C. This is caused by HPV1/2. **False.** HPV1/2 causes verruca vulgaris. Verruca vulgaris enters the differential diagnosis of verrucous carcinoma. The surface silhouette of verruca vulgaris is spiky with parakeratotic spires (see ◘ Fig. 5.42). Pushing rete pegs are absent in verruca vulgaris.
   D. The best diagnosis here is "Benign florid papillomatosis." **False.** There are no discreet exophytic papillae (see ◘ Fig. 5.24). Pushing rete pegs are absent in papillomatosis.
   E. The best diagnosis here is verruca vulgaris. **False.** See above.

References

1. Reidenbach MM. Aryepiglottic fold: normal topography and clinical implications. Clin Anat. 1998; 11:223–35.
2. Bastian RW, Thomas JP. Do talkativeness and vocal loudness correlate with laryngeal pathology? A study of the vocal overdoer/underdoer continuum. J Voice. 2016;30:557–62.
3. Mattei A, Revis J, Giovanni A. Personality traits inventory in patients with vocal nodules. Eur Arch Otorhinolaryngol. 2017;274:1911–7.
4. Dikkers FG, Nikkels PG. Benign lesions of the vocal folds: histopathology and phonotrauma. Ann Otol Rhinol Laryngol. 1995;104:698–703.
5. Cipriani NA, Martin DE, Corey JP, Portugal L, Caballero N, Lester R, Anthony B, Taxy JB. The clinicopathologic spectrum of benign mass lesions of the vocal fold due to vocal abuse. Int J Surg Pathol. 2011;19:583–7.
6. Miko TL. Peptic (contact ulcer) granuloma of the larynx. J Clin Pathol. 1989;42:800–4.
7. Prowse S, Knight L. Congenital cysts of the infant larynx. Int J Pediatr Otorhinolaryngol. 2012;76:708–11.
8. Bando H, Uchida M, Matsumoto S, Ushijima C, Dejima K. Endolaryngeal extension of thyroglossal duct cyst. Auris Nasus Larynx. 2012;39:220–3.
9. Touati MM, Ammar H. Intralaryngeal thyroglossal duct cyst. Pan Afr Med J. 2015 Nov;24(22):294. https://doi.org/10.11604/pamj.2015.22.294.8264.
10. Aubry K, Kapella M, Ketterer S, Massri K, Bessede JP. A case of laryngeal ductal cyst: antenatal diagnosis and peripartum management. Int J Pediatr Otorhinolaryngol. 2007;71:1639–42.
11. Chang CC, Lee LA, Hsia SH, Hsueh C, Wang CJ. Huge epiglottic cyst: a rare cause of airway obstruction in an adolescent. Paediatr Int Child Health. 2016;36:305–7.
12. Kaur A, Kini U, Alva SK. Cysts of the larynx : a clinicopathologic study of nine cases. Indian J Otolaryngol Head Neck Surg. 1998;50:250–6.
13. Saha D, Sinha R, Pai RR, Kumar A, Chakraborti S. Laryngeal cysts in infants and children--a pathologist's perspective (with review of literature). Int J Pediatr Otorhinolaryngol. 2013;77:1112–7.
14. Kim JK, Park KK. Foregut duplication cyst of the hypopharynx: a rare cause of upper airway obstruction. J Pediatr Surg. 2007;42:E5–7.
15. Forte V, Warshawski J, Thorner P, Conley S. Unusual laryngeal cysts in the newborn. Int J Pediatr Otorhinolaryngol. 1996;37:261–7.
16. Nussenbaum B, McClay JE, Timmons CF. Laryngeal duplication cyst. Arch Otolaryngol Head Neck Surg. 2002;128:1317–20.
17. Brandwein M, Huvos A. Laryngeal oncocytic cystadenomas. Eight cases and a literature review. Arch Otolaryngol Head Neck Surg. 1995;121:1302–5.
18. Feinstein AJ, Peng KA, Bhuta SM, Abemayor E, Mendelsohn AH. Laryngeal oncocytic cystadenomas masquerading as laryngoceles. Am J Otolaryngol. 2016;37:17–21.
19. Stenner M, Müller KM, Koopmann M, Rudack C. Squamous cell carcinoma of the larynx arising in multifocal pharyngolaryngeal oncocytic papillary cystadenoma: a case report and review of the literature. Medicine (Baltimore). 2014;93(12):e70. https://doi.org/10.1097/MD.0000000000000070.
20. Stachler RJ, Dworkin-Valenti JP. Allergic laryngitis: unraveling the myths. Curr Opin Otolaryngol Head Neck Surg. 2017;25:242–6.
21. Platt MP, Brook CD, Kuperstock J, Krouse JH. What role does allergy play in chronic ear disease and laryngitis? Curr Allergy Asthma Rep. 2016;16:76.
22. Krouse JH. Allergy and laryngeal disorders. Curr Opin Otolaryngol Head Neck Surg. 2016;24:221–5.
23. Brook CD, Platt MP, Reese S, Noordzij JP. Utility of allergy testing in patients with chronic laryngopharyngeal symptoms: is it allergic laryngitis? Otolaryngol Head Neck Surg. 2016;154:41–5.
24. Randhawa PS, Nouraei S, Mansuri S, Rubin JS. Allergic laryngitis as a cause of dysphonia: a preliminary report. Logoped Phoniatr Vocol. 2010;35:169–74.
25. Jawale PM, Gulwani HV. Histoplasmosis presenting as laryngeal ulcer in a post-renal transplant male: an unusual case from India. J Mycol Med. 2017;27(4):573–6. doi.org/101016/jmycmed201706003
26. Bergeron M, Gagné AA, Côté M, Chênevert J, Dubé R, Pelletier R. Primary Larynx Cryptococcus neoformans Infection: a Distinctive Clinical Entity. Open Forum Infect Dis. 2015;2(4):ofv160. https://doi.org/10.1093/ofid/ofv160.
27. Jeng JY, Tomblinson CM, Ocal IT, Vikram HR, Lott DG. Laryngeal cryptococcosis: Literature review and guidelines for laser ablation of fungal lesions. Laryngoscope. 2016;126:1625–9.
28. Tao T, Zhang YH, Xue SL, Wu DP, Chen F. Fulminant Laryngeal-tracheobronchial-pulmonary Aspergillosis: a Rare and Fatal Complication in Allogeneic Hematopoietic Stem Cell Transplantation Recipients. Intern Med. 2017;56:347–51.
29. Saha A, Saha K, Chatterjee U. Primary aspergillosis of vocal cord: long-term inhalational steroid use can be the miscreant. Biom J. 2015;38:550–3.
30. Ohashi T, Mizuta K, Kuze B, Aoki M, Ito Y. Invasive epiglottic aspergillosis: a case report and literature review. Auris Nasus Larynx. 2015;42:501–4.
31. Schwartz JR, Nagle MG, Elkins RC, Mohr JA. Mucormycosis of the trachea: an unusual cause of acute upper airway obstruction. Chest. 1982;81:653–4.
32. Malinvaud D, Mukundan S, Crevier-Buchman L, Bonfils P, Laccourreye O. Glottic bamboo nodules from systemic lupus erythematosus. Ann Otol Rhinol Laryngol. 2013;122:496–9.
33. Murano E, Hosako-Naito Y, Tayama N, Oka T, Miyaji M, Kumada M, Niimi S. Bamboo node: primary vocal fold lesion as evidence of autoimmune disease. J Voice. 2001;15:441–50.
34. Woo P, Mendelsohn J, Humphrey D. Rheumatoid nodules of the larynx. Otolaryngol Head Neck Surg. 1995;113:147–50.
35. Iacovou E, Vlastarakos PV, Nikolopoulos TP. Laryngeal Involvement in Connective Tissue Disorders. Is it Important for Patient Management? Indian J Otolaryngol Head Neck Surg. 2014;66:22–9.
36. Yamashita H, Takahashi Y, Kano T, Mimori A. A case of systemic lupus erythematosus with bamboo joint-

like corditis as an antecedent symptom. Rheumatology (Oxford). 2013;52:759–61.
37. Lee JH, Sung IY, Park JH, Roh JL. Recurrent laryngeal neuropathy in a systemic lupus erythematosus (SLE) patient. Am J Phys Med Rehabil. 2008;87:68–70.
38. Wang CC, Chang MH, Jiang RS, Lai HC, De Virgilio A, Wang CP, Wu SH, Liu SA, Liang KL. Laryngeal electromyography-guided hyaluronic acid vocal fold injection for unilateral vocal fold paralysis: a prospective long-term follow-up outcome report. JAMA Otolaryngol Head Neck Surg. 2015;141:264–71.
39. Wen MH, Cheng PW, Liao LJ, Chou HW, Wang CT. Treatment outcomes of injection laryngoplasty using cross-linked porcine collagen and hyaluronic acid. Otolaryngol Head Neck Surg. 2013;149:900–6.
40. Lakhani R, Fishman JM, Bleach N, Costello D, Birchall M. Alternative injectable materials for vocal fold medialisation in unilateral vocal fold paralysis. Cochrane Database Syst Rev. 2012;10:CD009239. https://doi.org/10.1002/14651858.CD009239.pub2.
41. Cohen MS, Mehta DK, Maguire RC, Simons JP. Injection medialization laryngoplasty in children. Arch Otolaryngol Head Neck Surg. 2011;137:264–8.
42. Gillespie MB, Dozier TS, Day TA, Martin-Harris B, Nguyen SA. Effectiveness of calcium hydroxylapatite paste in vocal rehabilitation. Ann Otol Rhinol Laryngol. 2009;118:546–51.
43. Sulica L, Rosen CA, Postma GN, Simpson B, Amin M, Courey M, Merati A. Current practice in injection augmentation of the vocal folds: indications, treatment principles, techniques, and complications. Laryngoscope. 2010;120:319–25.
44. Rodríguez-Romero R, Vargas-Serrano B, Cortina-Moreno B, Fernández-Gallardo JM, Cervera-Rodilla JL. Calcified amyloidoma of the larynx. AJNR Am J Neuroradiol. 1996;17:1491–3.
45. Phillips NM, Matthews E, Altmann C, Agnew J, Burns H. Laryngeal amyloidosis: diagnosis, pathophysiology and management. J Laryngol Otol. 2017;131:S41–7.
46. Hazenberg AJ, Hazenberg BP, Dikkers FG. Long-term follow-up after surgery in localized laryngeal amyloidosis. Eur Arch Otorhinolaryngol. 2016;273:2613–20.
47. Wang Q, Chen H, Wang S. Laryngo-tracheobronchial amyloidosis: a case report and review of literature. Int J Clin Exp Pathol. 2014;7:7088–93.
48. Nakamine H, Yamakawa M, Yoshino T, Fukumoto T, Enomoto Y, Matsumura I. Langerhans Cell Histiocytosis and Langerhans Cell Sarcoma: Current Understanding and Differential Diagnosis. J Clin Exp Hematop. 2016;56:109–18.
49. Duynstee ML, Verwoerd-Verhoef HL, Monnier P, Mooi WJ. Langerhans cell histiocytosis of the larynx. Int J Pediatr Otorhinolaryngol. 2000;56:65–9.
50. Lhoták J, Dvorăcková I. Histiocytosis X of the larynx. J Laryngol Otol. 1975;1975(89):771–7.
51. Booth JB, Thomas RS. Histiocytosis X. J Laryngol Otol. 1970;84:1123–32.
52. Friedmann I, Ferlito A. Primary eosinophilic granuloma of the larynx. J Laryngol Otol. 1981;95:1249–54.
53. Kim KH, Kim RB, Woo SH. Individual participant data meta-analysis of primary laryngeal lymphoma: Focusing on the clinical characteristics and prognosis. Laryngoscope. 2015;125:2741–8.
54. Liu M, Liu B, Liu B, Cui X, Yang S, Wang Q, Dong L. Mucosa-associated lymphoid tissue lymphoma of the larynx: a case report and literature review. Medicine (Baltimore). 2015 May;94(17):e788. https://doi.org/10.1097/MD.0000000000000788.
55. Rahman B, Bilal J, Sipra QU, Riaz IB. All that Wheezes Is Not Asthma: a Case of Diffuse Large B-Cell Lymphoma of the Larynx. Case Rep Oncol Med. 2017;2017:7072615. https://doi.org/10.1155/2017/7072615.
56. Brown NA, Elenitoba-Johnson KS. Update from the 4th Edition of the World Health Organization Classification of Head and Neck Tumours: hematolymphoid Tumours. Head Neck Pathol. 2017;11:96–109.
57. Quimby AE, Caulley L, Rodin D, Purgina B, Eapen L, Shier L, Johnson-Obaseki S. Primary Burkitt lymphoma of the supraglottic larynx: a case report and review of the literature. J Med Case Rep. 2017 Mar 10;11(1):65. https://doi.org/10.1186/s13256-017-1209-3.
58. Derkay CS. Task force on recurrent respiratory papillomas. A preliminary report. Arch Otolaryngol Head Neck Surg. 1995;121:1386–91.
59. Silverberg MJ, Thorsen P, Lindeberg H, Grant LA, Shah KV. Condyloma in pregnancy is strongly predictive of juvenile onset recurrent respiratory papillomatosis. Obstet Gynecol. 2003;101:645–52.
60. Silverberg MJ, Thorsen P, Lindeberg H, Ahdieh-Grant L, Shah KV. Clinical course of recurrent respiratory papillomatosis in Danish children. Arch Otolaryngol Head Neck Surg. 2004;130:711–6.
61. Rodier C, Lapointe A, Coutlée F, Mayrand MH, Dal Soglio D, Roger M, Trottier H. Juvenile respiratory papillomatosis: risk factors for severity. J Med Virol. 2013;85:1447–58.
62. Merckx M, Liesbeth WV, Arbyn M, Meys J, Weyers S, Temmerman M, Vanden Broeck D. Transmission of carcinogenic human papillomavirus types from mother to child: a meta-analysis of published studies. Eur J Cancer Prev. 2013;22:277–85.
63. Chatzistamatiou K, Sotiriadis A, Agorastos T. Effect of mode of delivery on vertical human papillomavirus transmission - A meta-analysis. J Obstet Gynaecol. 2016;36:10–4.
64. DeVoti J, Hatam L, Lucs A, Afzal A, Abramson A, Steinberg B, Bonagura V. Decreased Langerhans cell responses to IL-36γ: altered innate immunity in patients with recurrent respiratory papillomatosis. Mol Med. 2014;20:372–80.
65. Wang J, Han DM, Ma LJ, Ye JY, Xiao Y, Yang QW. Risk factors of juvenile onset recurrent respiratory papillomatosis in the lower respiratory tract. Chin Med J. 2012;125:3496–9.
66. Fortes HR, von Ranke FM, Escuissato DL, Araujo Neto CA, Zanetti G, Hochhegger B, Souza CA, Marchiori E. Recurrent respiratory papillomatosis: a state-of-the-art review. Respir Med. 2017;126:116–21.
67. Lin HW, Richmon JD, Emerick KS, de Venecia RK, Zeitels SM, Faquin WC, Lin DT. Malignant transformation of a highly aggressive human papillomavirus type 11-associated recurrent respiratory papillomatosis. Am J Otolaryngol. 2010;31:291–6.

68. Snietura M, Chelmecka-Wiktorczyk L, Pakulo S, Kopec A, Piglowski W, Drabik G, Kosowski B, Wyrobek L, Stanek-Widera A, Balwierz W. Vertically transmitted HPV-dependent squamous cell carcinoma of the external auditory canal : case report of a child. Strahlenther Onkol. 2017;193:156–61.
69. Gelinas JF, Manoukan J, Cote A. Lung involvement in juvenile onset respiratory papillomatosis: a systematic review of the literature. Int J Pediatr Otorhinolaryngol. 2008;72:433–52.
70. Azadarmaki R, Lango MN. Malignant transformation of respiratory papillomatosis in a solid-organ transplant patient: case report and literature review. Ann Otol Rhinol Laryngol. 2013;122:457–60.
71. Huebbers CU, Preuss SF, Kolligs J, Vent J, Stenner M, Wieland U, Silling S, Drebber U, Speel EJ, Klussmann JP. Integration of HPV6 and downregulation of AKR1C3 expression mark malignant transformation in a patient with juvenile-onset laryngeal papillomatosis. PLoS One. 2013;8(2):e57207. https://doi.org/10.1371/journal.pone.0057207.
72. Gerein V, Rastorguev E, Gerein J, Draf W, Schirren J. Incidence, age at onset, and potential reasons of malignant transformation in recurrent respiratory papillomatosis patients: 20 years' experience. Otolaryngol Head Neck Surg. 2005;132:392–4.
73. Can NT, Tretiakova MS, Taxy JB. Natural history and malignant transformation in recurrent respiratory papillomatosis: Human Papillomavirus (HPV), dysplasia and an autopsy review. Fetal and Pediatric Pathol. 2015;34:80–90.
74. Karatayli-Ozgursoy S, Bishop JA, Hillel A, Akst L, Best SR. Risk factors for dysplasia in recurrent respiratory papillomatosis in an adult and pediatric population. Ann Otol Rhinol Laryngol. 2016;125:235–41.
75. Best SR, Mohr M, Zur KB. Systemic bevacizumab for recurrent respiratory papillomatosis: a national survey. Laryngoscope. 2017;127:2225–9.
76. Mohr M, Schliemann C, Biermann C, Schmidt LH, Kessler T, Schmidt J, Wiebe K, Müller KM, Hoffmann TK, Groll AH, Werner C, Kessler C, Wiewrodt R, Rudack C, Berdel WE. Rapid response to systemic bevacizumab therapy in recurrent respiratory papillomatosis. Oncol Lett. 2014;8:1912–8.
77. Best SR, Friedman AD, Landau-Zemer T, Barbu AM, Burns JA, Freeman MW, Halvorsen YD, Hillman RE, Zeitels SM. Safety and dosing of bevacizumab (avastin) for the treatment of recurrent respiratory papillomatosis. Ann Otol Rhinol Laryngol. 2012;121: 587–93.
78. Lazar RG, Younis RT, Kluka EA, Joyner RE, Storgion S. Granular cell tumor of the larynx. Report of two pediatric cases. Ear Nose Throat J. 1992;71:440–3.
79. Montojo J, Echarri R, Santana A, Mico A, Gamboa J, Cobeta I. A multifocal granular cell tumor of the upper airways. Acra Otorrinolaringol Esp. 1999;50: 498–501.
80. Sproat R, Wong G, Rubin J. Granular cell tumour of the larynx. Head Neck Pathol. 2016;10:538–40.
81. Santos S, Gutiérrez González IJ, Colmenero I, Domínguez González de Rivera MJ. Granular cell tumor of laryngeal location: description of 2 pediatric cases. Acta Otorrinolaringol Esp. 2014;65:126–8.
82. Scala WA, Fernandes AM, Duprat Ade C, Costa HO. Granular cell tumor of the larynx in children: a case report. Braz J Otorhinolaryngol. 2008;74:780–5.
83. Aksoy S, Abali H, Kilickap S, Harputluoglu H, Erman M. Metastatic granular cell tumor: a case report and review of the literature. Acta Oncol. 2006;45:91–4.
84. Chiang MJ, Fang TJ, Li HY, Chen IH, Lee KF. Malignant granular cell tumor in larynx mimicking laryngeal carcinoma. Am J Otolaryngol. 2004;25:270–3.
85. Brandwein M, Le Benger J, Strauchen J, Biller H. Atypical granular cell tumor of the larynx. Head Neck Surg. 1990;12:154–9.
86. McGuire LS, Yakoub D, Möller MG, Rosenberg A, Livingstone A. Malignant granular cell tumor of the back: a case report and review of the literature. Case Rep Med. 2014;2014:794648. https://doi.org/10.1155/2014/794648.
87. Meling TR, Fridrich K, Evensen JF, Nedregaard B. Malignant granular cell tumor of the skull base. Skull Base. 2008;18:59–66.
88. Morita S, Hiramatsu M, Sugishita M, Gyawali B, Shibata T, Shimokata T, Urakawa H, Mitsuma A, Moritani S, Kubota T, Ichihara S, Ando Y. Pazopanib monotherapy in a patient with a malignant granular cell tumor originating from the right orbit: a case report. Oncol Lett Aug. 2015;10:972–4.
89. Brandwein M, Levi G, Som P, Urken ML. Paraganglioma of the inferior laryngeal paraganglia. A case report. Arch Otolaryngol Head Neck Surg. 1992;118:994–6.
90. Zhou X, Jiang S, Li H. A case of laryngeal paraganglioma and literature review. Int J Clin Exp Med. 2015;8:16934–6.
91. Berta E, Camuzard O, Poissonnet G. A strange form of dysphonia… Laryngeal paraganglioma. Eur Ann Otorhinolaryngol Head Neck Dis. 2015;132:297–300.
92. Naik SM, Shenoy AM, Chavan P, Patil A, Gupta S. Laryngeal paraganglioma: a rare clinical entity managed by supraselective embolization and lateral pharygotomy. Indian J Otolaryngol Head Neck Surg. 2013;65:95–104.
93. Uçar Ş, Zorlu P, Yıldırım I, Metin Ö. Hamartoma of the larynx: an unusual cause of stridor. Balkan Med J. 2014;31:349–51.
94. Webb S, Richmond S, Wright C, Adair S. Laryngeal hamartoma causing polyhydramnios and lethal pulmonary hypoplasia. Aust N Z J Obstet Gynaecol. 2010;50:297–8.
95. García Rica E, Maza Solano JM, Herrero Salado T, Sánchez Gómez S. Chondroid hamartoma of the larynx: an exceptional case. Acta Otorrinolaringol Esp. 2016;67:117–9.
96. Leoncini G, Maio V, Mirabile L, Baggi R, Franchi A. Glandular hamartoma of the larynx: report of a case. Auris Nasus Larynx. 2008;35:149–51.
97. Yigitbasi OG, Guler G, Ozturk F, Guney E. Glandular hamartoma of the larynx. Int J Pediatr Otorhinolaryngol. 2002;65:163–6.
98. Mäkitie AA, Lehtonen H, Bäck L, Aaltonen LM, Leivo I. Hamartoma of the larynx: an unusual cause of dyspnea. Ann Otol Rhinol Laryngol. 2003;112:841–3.
99. Işik Gönül I, Asal K, Ceylan A, Akyol G. Hamartoma of the larynx: an unusual cause of upper airway obstruction. Eur Arch Otorhinolaryngol. 2004;261:435–8.

100. Rinaldo A, Mannarà GM, Fisher C, Ferlito A. Hamartoma of the larynx: a critical review of the literature. Ann Otol Rhinol Laryngol. 1998;107:264–7.
101. Cannon CR, Johns ME, Fechner RE. Immature teratoma of the larynx. Otolaryngol Head Neck Surg. 1987;96:366–8.
102. Carta F, Sionis S, Gerosa C, Puxeddu R. Endoscopic management of adult-type rhabdomyoma of the glottis: case report and review of the literature. Braz J Otorhinolaryngol. 2016;82:244–7.
103. Pinho MM, de Carvalho E, Castro J, Ramos RG. Adult rhabdomyoma of the larynx. Int Arch Otorhinolaryngol. 2013;17:415–8.
104. Orlandi A, Fratoni S, Hermann I, Spagnoli LG. Symptomatic laryngeal nodular chondrometaplasia: a clinicopathological study. J Clin Pathol. 2003;56:976–7.
105. Natt RS, Helliwell T, McCormick M. Tracheopathia chondro-osteoplastica—an unusual cause of stridor. J Laryngol Otol. 2009;123:1039–41.
106. Härmä RA, Suurkari S. Tracheopathia chondro-osteoplastica. A clinical study of thirty cases. Acta Otolaryngol. 1977;84:118–23.
107. Jones HA, Manjaly JG, Sandison A, Almeyda JS, Sandhu GS. Acute airway obstruction secondary to vocalfold heterotopic ossification. Head Neck Pathol. 2015;9:96–9.
108. Hellquist HB, Hellqvist H, Vejlens L, Lindholm CE. Epithelioid leiomyoma of the larynx. Histopathology. 1994;24:155–9.
109. Kleinsasser O, Glanz H. Myogenic tumours of the larynx. Arch Otorhinolaryngol. 1979;225:107–19.
110. Hirakawa K, Harada Y, Tatsukawa T, Nagasawa A, Fujii M. A case of vascular leiomyoma of the larynx. J Laryngol Otol. 1994;108:593–5.
111. McKiernan DC, Watters WR. Smooth muscle tumours of the larynx. J Laryngol Otol. 1995;109:77–9.
112. Xu Y, Zhou S, Wang S. Vascular leiomyoma of the larynx: a rare entity. Three case reports and literature review. ORL J Otorhinolaryngol Relat Spec. 2008;70:264–47.
113. Jun F, Li L, Ning L, Yan L, Siquan T, Shixi L. Giant laryngeal angioleiomyomas: a case report with review of literature. Am J Otolaryngol. 2009;30:2192–20.
114. Matsumoto T, Nishiya M, Ichikawa G, Fujii H. Leiomyoma with atypical cells (atypical leiomyoma) in the larynx. Histopathology. 1999;34:532–6.
115. Siegel RL, Miller KD, Jemal A. Cancer Statistics, 2017. CA Cancer J Clin. 2017;67:7–30.
116. Steuer CE, El-Deiry M, Parks JR, Higgins KA, Saba NF. An update on larynx cancer. CA Cancer J Clin. 2017;67:31–50.
117. Stell PM, McGill T. Asbestos and laryngeal carcinoma. Lancet. 1973; 2:416–417. 12. Paget-Bailly S, Cyr D, Luce D. Occupational exposures and cancer of the larynx systematic review and meta-analysis. J Occup Environ Med 2012;54:71–84.
118. Mourad M, Jetmore T, Jategaonkar AA, Moubayed S, Moshier E, Urken ML. Epidemiological trends of head and neck Cancer in the United States: a SEER population study. J Oral Maxillofac Surg. 2017. pii:0278-2391(17) 30537-2.
119. Riga M, Chelis L, Danielides V, Vogiatzaki T, Pantazis TL, Pantazis D. Systematic review on T3 laryngeal squamous cell carcinoma; still far from a consensus on the optimal organ preserving treatment. Eur J Surg Oncol. 2017;43:20–31.
120. Hoffman HT, Porter K, Karnell LH, Cooper JS, Weber RS, Langer CJ, Ang KK, Gay G, Stewart A, Robinson RA. Laryngeal cancer in the United States: changes in demographics, patterns of care, and survival. Laryngoscope. 2006;116:1–13.
121. Lassen P, Primdahl H, Johansen J, Kristensen CA, Andersen E, Andersen LJ, Evensen JF, Eriksen JG, Overgaard J, Danish Head and Neck Cancer Group (DAHANCA). Impact of HPV-associated p16-expression on radiotherapy outcome in advanced oropharynx and non-oropharynx cancer. Radiother Oncol. 2014;113(3):310–6.
122. Wittekindt C, Wuerdemann N, Gattenlöhner S, Brobeil A, Wierzbicka M, Wagner S, Klußmann JP. The role of high-risk human papillomavirus infections in laryngeal squamous cell carcinoma. Eur Arch Otorhinolaryngol. 2017;274:3837–42.
123. Xu Y, Liu S, Yi H, Wang J, Dong P, Li X, Yin S. Human papillomavirus infection in 674 Chinese patients with laryngeal squamous cell carcinoma. PLoS One. 2014;9(12):e115914. https://doi.org/10.1371/journal.pone.0115914.
124. Thompson LD. Laryngeal dysplasia, squamous cell carcinoma, and variants. Surg Pathol Clin. 2017;10:15–33.
125. Gale N, Zidar N, Poljak M, Cardesa A. Current views and perspectives on classification of squamous intraepithelial lesions of the head and neck. Head Neck Pathol. 2014;8:16–23.
126. Gale N, Poljak M, Zidar N. Update from the 4th Edition of the World Health Organization Classification of Head and Neck Tumours: What is New in the 2017 WHO Blue Book for Tumours of the Hypopharynx, Larynx, Trachea and Parapharyngeal Space. Head Neck Pathol. 2017;11:23–32.
127. Weller MD, Nankivell PC, McConkey C, et al. The risk and interval to malignancy of patients with laryngeal dysplasia; a systematic review of case series and meta-analysis. Clin Otolaryngol. 2010;35:364–72.
128. Gerry D, Fritsch VA, Lentsch EJ. Spindle cell carcinoma of the upper aerodigestive tract: an analysis of 341 cases with comparison to conventional squamous cell carcinoma. Ann Otol Rhinol Laryngol. 2014;123:576–83.
129. Dubal PM, Marchiano E, Kam D, Dutta R, Kalyoussef E, Baredes S, Eloy JA. Laryngeal spindle cell carcinoma: A population-based analysis of incidence and survival. Laryngoscope. 2015;125:2709–14.
130. Bice TC, Tran V, Merkley MA, Newlands SD, van der Sloot PG, Wu S, Miller MC. Disease-specific survival with spindle cell carcinoma of the head and neck. Otolaryngol Head Neck Surg. 2015;53:973–80.
131. Marioni G, Altavilla G, Marino F, Marchese-Ragona R, Lelli-Mami G, Staffieri A. Squamous cell carcinoma of the larynx with osteosarcoma-like stromal metaplasia. Acta Otolaryngol. 2004;124:870–3.
132. Mosalleum E, Afrogheh A, Stofberg S, Bezuidenhout AF, Schneider J, Hille J. A review of primary osteosarcoma of the larynx and case report. Head Neck Pathol. 2015;9:158–64.

133. Mehrad M, Carpenter DH, Chernock RD, Wang H, Ma XJ, Luo Y, Luo J, Lewis JS Jr, El-Mofty SK. Papillary squamous cell carcinoma of the head and neck: clinicopathologic and molecular features with special reference to human papillomavirus. Am J Surg Pathol. 2013;37:1349–56.
134. Jo VY, Mills SE, Stoler MH, Stelow EB. Papillary squamous cell carcinoma of the head and neck: frequent association with human papillomavirus infection and invasive carcinoma. Am J Surg Pathol. 2009;33:1720–4.
135. Dutta R, Husain Q, Kam D, Dubal PM, Baredes S, Eloy JA. Laryngeal papillary squamous cell carcinoma: a population-based analysis of incidence and survival. Otolaryngol Head Neck Surg. 2015;153:54–9.
136. Dubal PM, Svider PF, Kam D, Dutta R, Baredes S, Eloy JA. Laryngeal verrucous carcinoma: a population-based analysis. Otolaryngol Head Neck Surg. 2015;153:799–805.
137. Huang SH, Lockwood G, Irish J, Ringash J, Cummings B, Waldron J, Kim J, Dawson LA, Bayley A, Hope A, O'Sullivan B. Truths and myths about radiotherapy for verrucous carcinoma of larynx. Int J Radiat Oncol Biol Phys. 2009;73:1110–5.
138. Santoro A, Pannone G, Contaldo M, Sanguedolce F, Esposito V, Serpico R, Lo Muzio L, Papagerakis S, Bufo P. A troubling diagnosis of verrucous squamous cell carcinoma ("the bad kind" of keratosis) and the need of clinical and pathological correlations: a review of the literature with a case report. J Skin Cancer. 2011; 2011:370605. https://doi.org/10.1155/2011/370605.
139. Teymoortash A, Silver CE, Rinaldo A, Cardesa A, Folz BJ, Ferlito A. Verrucous carcinoma: a retrospective diagnosis in three historic patients. Eur Arch Otorhinolaryngol. 2014;271:631–3.
140. Cardesa A, Zidar N, Alos L, Nadal A, Gale N, Klöppel G. The Kaiser's cancer revisited: was Virchow totally wrong? Virchows Arch. 2011;458:649–57.
141. Lewis JS Jr. Not your usual cancer case: variants of laryngeal squamous cell carcinoma. Head Neck Pathol. 2011;5:23–30.
142. Orvidas LJ, Olsen KD, Lewis JE, Suman VJ. Verrucous carcinoma of the larynx: a review of 53 patients. Head Neck. 1998;20:197–203.
143. Ghosh R, Dutta R, Dubal PM, Park RC, Baredes S, Eloy JA. Laryngeal neuroendocrine carcinoma: a population-based analysis of incidence and survival. Otolaryngol Head Neck Surg. 2015;153:966–72.
144. van der Laan TP, Plaat BE, van der Laan BF, Halmos GB. Clinical recommendations on the treatment of neuroendocrine carcinoma of the larynx: a meta-analysis of 436 reported cases. Head Neck. 2015;37:707–15.
145. Perez-Ordonez B, Bishop JA, Gnepp DR, Hunt JL, Thompson LDR: Neuroendocrine tumors. In WHO classifications of head and neck tumours. El-Naggar, AK, Chan JKC, Grandis JR, Takata T, Slootweg PJ, IARC Lyon 2017, pp 95–98.
146. La Rosa S, Sessa F, Uccella S. Mixed neuroendocrine-nonneuroendocrine neoplasms (MiNENs): unifying the concept of a heterogeneous group of neoplasms. Endocr Pathol. 2016;27:284–311.
147. Thompson ED, Stelow EB, Mills SE, Westra WH, Bishop JA. Large cell neuroendocrine carcinoma of the head and neck: a clinicopathologic series of 10 cases with an emphasis on HPV status. Am J Surg Pathol. 2016;40:471–8.
148. Alos L, Hakim S, Larque AB, de la Oliva J, Rodriguez-Carunchio L, Caballero M, Nadal A, Marti C, Guimera N, Fernandez-Figueras MT, Quint W, Ordi J. p16 overexpression in high-grade neuroendocrine carcinomas of the head and neck: potential diagnostic pitfall with HPV-related carcinomas. Virchows Arch. 2016;469:277–84.
149. Dubal PM, Svider PF, Kanumuri VV, Patel AA, Baredes S, Eloy JA. Laryngeal chondrosarcoma: a population-based analysis. Laryngoscope. 2014;124:1877–81.
150. Chin OY, Dubal PM, Sheikh AB, Unsal AA, Park RC, Baredes S, Eloy JA. Laryngeal chondrosarcoma: a systematic review of 592 cases. Laryngoscope. 2017;2017(127):430–9.
151. Choi J, Dharmarajan H, Victores A, Wenaas A, Ongkasuwan J. Chondrosarcoma of the epiglottis: a case report and literature review. J Voice 2017, pii: S0892–1997(17)30244–8. https://doi.org/10.1016/j.jvoice.2017.07.014.
152. Hu R, Xu W, Liu H, Chen X. Laryngeal chondrosarcoma of the arytenoid cartilage presenting as bilateral vocal fold immobility: a case report and literature review. J Voice. 2014; 28(1):129.e13–129.e17.
153. Horta M, Fernandes L, Borges A. Chondrosarcoma of the hyoid bone: an atypical site of a sarcoma of the head and the neck. BMJ Case Rep. 2015;2015:pii:bcr2015212291. https://doi.org/10.1136/bcr-2015-212291.
154. Ciolofan MS, Ioniţă E, Ioniţă I, Mogoantă CA, Anghelina F, Enescu AŞ, Ciobîrcă DM, Osman A, Foarfă MC, Mateescu GO. Chondrosarcoma of the hyoid bone: a case report. Romanian J Morphol Embryol. 2015;56:811–6.
155. Maki D, Mori T, Teshima M, Kobayashi K, Matsumoto F, Sakai A, Okami K, Yoshimoto S. Chondrosarcoma of the hyoid bone - Report of a case and a literature review of the suitable treatment strategy. Auris Nasus Larynx. 2017;44:629–34.
156. Lewis JE, Olsen KD, Inwards CY. Cartilaginous tumors of the larynx: clinicopathologic review of 47 cases. Ann Otol Rhinol Laryngol. 1997;106:94–100.
157. Gökdoğan O, Koybasioglu A, Laryngeal Chondroma IF. An unusual complication endotracheal entubation. J Craniofac Surg. 2016;27:1007–9.
158. Brandwein M, Moore S, Som P, Biller H. Laryngeal chondrosarcomas: a clinicopathologic study of 11 cases, including two "dedifferentiated" chondrosarcomas. Laryngoscope. 1992;102:858–67.
159. Magliocca KR, Edgar MA, Corey A, Villari CR. Dedifferentiated chondrosarcoma of the larynx: radiological, gross, microscopic and clinical features. Ann Diagn Pathol. 2017;30:42–6.
160. Thompson LD, Gannon FH. Chondrosarcoma of the larynx: a clinicopathologic study of 111 cases with a review of the literature. Am J Surg Pathol. 2002;26:836–51.
161. Alexander J, Wakely PE Jr. Primary laryngeal clear cell chondrosarcoma: report of a case and literature review. Head Neck Pathol. 2014;8:307–10.
162. Eble JN, Hull MT, Bojrab D. Laryngeal blastoma. A light and electron microscopic study of a novel entity analogous to pulmonary blastoma. Am J Clin Pathol. 1985;84:378–85.

Supplementary Information

M. S. Brandwein-Weber, *Textbook of Head and Neck Pathology*,
https://doi.org/10.1007/978-3-319-76106-0

Index

A

B

C

D

E

M

N

O

P

R

S

T

V

W

MIX
Papier aus verantwortungsvollen Quellen
Paper from responsible sources
FSC® C105338

If you have any concerns about our products, you can contact us on
ProductSafety@springernature.com

In case Publisher is established outside the EU, the EU authorized representative is:
Springer Nature Customer Service Center GmbH
Europaplatz 3, 69115 Heidelberg, Germany

Printed by Libri Plureos GmbH
in Hamburg, Germany